Immunological Implications and Molecular Diagnostics of Genitourinary Cancer

Graphical abstract

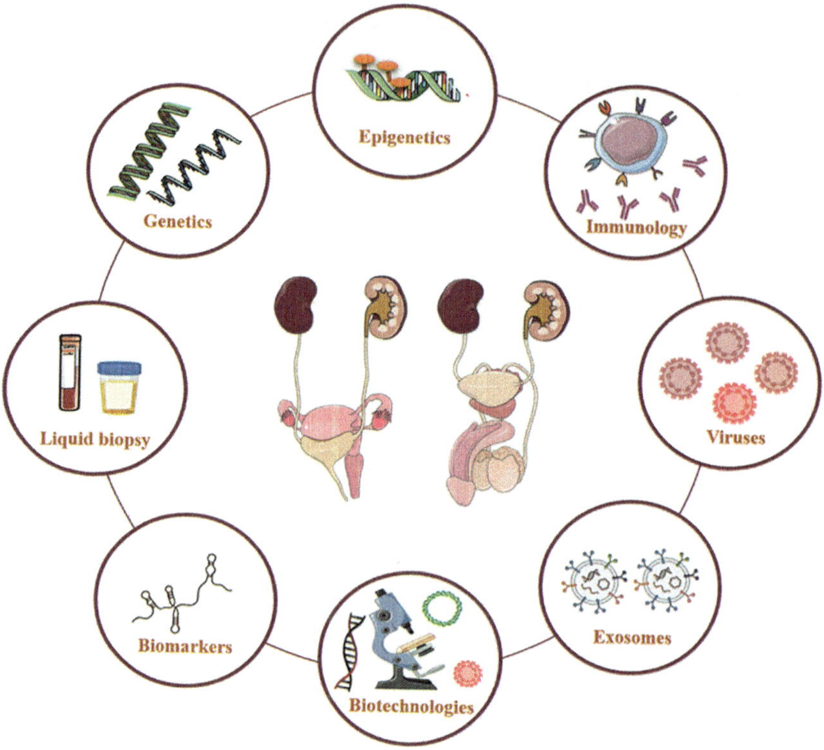

Graphical abstract made by the editor

Immunological Implications and Molecular Diagnostics of Genitourinary Cancer

Edited by

Moulay Mustapha Ennaji

Group Leader Research Team of Virology, Oncology, and Biotechnologies, Head of Laboratory of Virology, Oncology, Biosciences, Environment and New Energies (LVO-BEEN), Faculty of Sciences and Techniques Mohammedia, University Hassan II of Casablanca, Casablanca, Morocco

ELSEVIER

ACADEMIC PRESS

An imprint of Elsevier

Academic Press is an imprint of Elsevier
125 London Wall, London EC2Y 5AS, United Kingdom
525 B Street, Suite 1650, San Diego, CA 92101, United States
50 Hampshire Street, 5th Floor, Cambridge, MA 02139, United States
The Boulevard, Langford Lane, Kidlington, Oxford OX5 1GB, United Kingdom

ISBN: 978-0-323-85496-2

For Information on all Academic Press publications
visit our website at https://www.elsevier.com/books-and-journals

Publisher: Stacy Masucci
Acquisitions Editor: Linda Versteeg-Buschman
Editorial Project Manager: Timothy Bennett
Production Project Manager: Swapna Srinivasan
Cover Designer: Mark Rogers

Typeset by MPS Limited, Chennai, India

Contents

List of contributors

Ferdos Ebrahim Abdul Rahim Faculty of Science, Department of Applied Biology-Biotechnology Program, University of Sharjah, Sharjah, United Arab Emirates

Kawtar Aboulalaa Team of Virology, Oncology, and Biotechnologies, Laboratory of Virology, Oncology, Biosciences, Environment and New Energies (LVO-BEEN), Faculty of Sciences and Techniques Mohammedia, University Hassan II of Casablanca, Casablanca, Morocco

Berjas Abumsimir Team of Virology, Oncology, and Biotechnologies, Laboratory of Virology, Oncology, Biosciences, Environment and New Energies (LVO-BEEN), Faculty of Sciences and Techniques Mohammedia, University Hassan II of Casablanca, Casablanca, Morocco; Pharmacological and Diagnostic Research Centre (PDRC), Department of Medical Laboratory Sciences, Faculty of Allied Medical Sciences, Al-Ahliyya Amman University (AAU), Amman, Jordan

Soukayna Alaoui Sosse Team of Virology, Oncology, and Biotechnologies, Laboratory of Virology, Oncology, Biosciences, Environment and New Energies (LVO-BEEN), Faculty of Sciences and Techniques Mohammedia, University Hassan II of Casablanca, Casablanca, Morocco

Kaoutar Anouar Tadlaoui Team of Virology, Oncology, and Biotechnologies, Laboratory of Virology, Oncology, Biosciences, Environment and New Energies (LVO-BEEN), Faculty of Sciences and Techniques Mohammedia, University Hassan II of Casablanca, Casablanca, Morocco

Hasna Azmi Team of Virology, Oncology, and Biotechnologies, Laboratory of Virology, Oncology, Biosciences, Environment and New Energies (LVO-BEEN), Faculty of Sciences and Techniques Mohammedia, University Hassan II of Casablanca, Casablanca, Morocco

Bouabid Badaoui Biodiversity, Ecology and Genome Laboratory, Faculty of Sciences, Mohammed V University, Rabat, Morocco

Hicham Benaguida Mohammed VI Centre for Treatment of Cancer, University Hospital Ibn Rochd, Casablanca, Morocco

Mohammed Nabil Benchekroun Team of Virology, Oncology, and Biotechnologies, Laboratory of Virology, Oncology, Biosciences, Environment and New Energies (LVO-BEEN), Faculty of Sciences and Techniques Mohammedia, University Hassan II of Casablanca, Casablanca, Morocco

Mustapha Benhessou Team of Virology, Oncology, and Biotechnologies, Laboratory of Virology, Oncology, Biosciences, Environment and New Energies (LVO-BEEN), Faculty of Sciences and Techniques Mohammedia, University Hassan II of Casablanca, Casablanca, Morocco; Mohammed VI Centre for Treatment of Cancer, University Hospital Ibn Rochd, Casablanca, Morocco

Hlima Bessi Team of Virology, Oncology, and Biotechnologies, Laboratory of Virology, Oncology, Biosciences, Environment and New Energies (LVO-BEEN), Faculty of Sciences and Techniques Mohammedia, University Hassan II of Casablanca, Casablanca, Morocco

Thomas Bourlet Laboratory of Infectious Agents and Hygiene (GIMAP), EA3064, University Hospital and University Jean Monnet, Saint-Etienne, France

Rihabe Boussettine Team of Virology, Oncology, and Biotechnologies, Laboratory of Virology, Oncology, Biosciences, Environment and New Energies (LVO-BEEN), Faculty of Sciences and Techniques Mohammedia, University Hassan II of Casablanca, Casablanca, Morocco

Amal Bouziyane Team of Virology, Oncology, and Biotechnologies, Laboratory of Virology, Oncology, Biosciences, Environment and New Energies (LVO-BEEN), Faculty of Sciences and Techniques Mohammedia, University Hassan II of Casablanca, Casablanca, Morocco; University Mohammed VI of Health Science, Casablanca, Morocco

Pierre Cornillon Department of Oncology, North Hospital, CHU Saint Etienne, Saint Etienne, France

Mohamed El Karroumi Mohammed VI Centre for Treatment of Cancer, University Hospital Ibn Rochd, Casablanca, Morocco

Lamyae El Khalki Team of Experimental Oncology and Natural Substances; Cellular & Molecular Immunopharmacology, Faculty of Sciences and Technology, University of Sultan Moulay Slimane, Beni Mellal, Morocco; Department of Microbiology, Immunology, and Inflammation, Temple University, Philadelphia, PA, United States; Center for Inflammation and Lung Research, Temple University, Philadelphia, PA, United States

Mohammed El Mzibri Biology and Medical Research Unit, CNESTEN, Rabat, Morocco; Life Sciences Division CNESTEN, Rabat, Morocco

Oubaida ElBiad Laboratory of Research and Biosafety L3, Military Teaching Hospital Mohammed V, Rabat, Morocco; Sequencing Unit, Laboratory of Virology, Center for Virology, Infectious and Tropical Diseases, Mohammed V Military Teaching Hospital, Faculty of Medicine and Pharmacy, Mohammed V University, Rabat, Morocco; Biodiversity, Ecology and Genome Laboratory, Faculty of Sciences, Mohammed V University, Rabat, Morocco; Laboratory of Biodiversity, Ecology, and Genome, Faculty of Sciences, Mohammed V University, Rabat, Morocco; P3 Research and Biosecurity Laboratory, Mohammed V Military Instruction Hospital, Rabat, Morocco

Mohammed Ennachit Mohammed VI Centre for Treatment of Cancer, University Hospital Ibn Rochd, Casablanca, Morocco

Moulay Mustapha Ennaji Group Leader Research team of Virology, Oncology, and Biotechnologies, Head of Laboratory of Virology, Oncology, Biosciences, Environment and New Energies (LVO-BEEN), Faculty of Sciences and Techniques Mohammedia, University Hassan II of Casablanca, Casablanca, Morocco

Youssef Ennaji Team of Virology, Oncology, and Biotechnologies, Laboratory of Virology, Oncology, Biosciences, Environment and New Energies (LVO-BEEN), Faculty of Sciences and Techniques Mohammedia, University Hassan II of Casablanca, Casablanca, Morocco

Khalid Ennibi Sequencing Unit, Laboratory of Virology, Center for Virology, Infectious and Tropical Diseases, Mohammed V Military Teaching Hospital, Faculty of Medicine and Pharmacy, Mohammed V University, Rabat, Morocco

Pramodkumar Pyarelal Gupta School of Biotechnology and Bioinformatics, D Y Patil Deemed to be University, Navi Mumbai, Maharashtra, India

Najwa Hassou Team of Virology, Oncology, and Biotechnologies, Laboratory of Virology, Oncology, Biosciences, Environment and New Energies (LVO-BEEN), Faculty of Sciences and Techniques Mohammedia, University Hassan II of Casablanca, Casablanca, Morocco

Patrina Joseph Iloukou Mayakia Team of Virology, Oncology, and Biotechnologies, Laboratory of Virology, Oncology, Biosciences, Environment and New Energies (LVO-BEEN), Faculty of Sciences and Techniques Mohammedia, University Hassan II of Casablanca, Casablanca, Morocco; Faculty of Health Sciences, University Marien Ngouabi, Brazzaville, Republic of Congo

Imane Saif Team of Virology, Oncology, and Biotechnologies, Laboratory of Virology, Oncology, Biosciences, Environment and New Energies (LVO-BEEN), Faculty of Sciences and Techniques Mohammedia, University Hassan II of Casablanca, Casablanca, Morocco

Abdeslam Jaafari Team of Experimental Oncology and Natural Substances; Cellular & Molecular Immunopharmacology, Faculty of Sciences and Technology, University of Sultan Moulay Slimane, Beni Mellal, Morocco

Anouar Tadlaoui Kaoutar Team of Virology, Oncology, and Biotechnologies, Laboratory of Virology, Oncology, Biosciences, Environment and New Energies (LVO-BEEN), Faculty of Sciences and Techniques Mohammedia, University Hassan II of Casablanca, Casablanca, Morocco

Yassine Kasmi Team of Virology, Oncology, and Biotechnologies, Laboratory of Virology, Oncology, Biosciences, Environment and New Energies (LVO-BEEN), Faculty of Sciences and Techniques Mohammedia, University Hassan II of Casablanca, Casablanca, Morocco

Moussa Koita Team of Virology, Oncology, and Biotechnologies, Laboratory of Virology, Oncology, Biosciences, Environment and New Energies (LVO-BEEN), Faculty of Sciences and Techniques Mohammedia, University Hassan II of Casablanca, Casablanca, Morocco

Ajay Kumar Department of Zoology, Banaras Hindu University, Varanasi, Uttar Pradesh, India

Maryame Lamsisi Team of Virology, Oncology, and Biotechnologies, Laboratory of Virology, Oncology, Biosciences, Environment and New Energies (LVO-BEEN), Faculty of Sciences and Techniques Mohammedia, University Hassan II of Casablanca, Casablanca, Morocco

Abdelilah Laraqui Laboratory of Human Pathologies Biology, Faculty of Sciences, and Genomic Center of Human Pathologies, Faculty of Medicine and Pharmacy, Mohammed V University, Rabat, Morocco; Bio-Path Laboratory, Faculty of Sciences – Agadl, Mohammed V University, Rabat, Morocco

Guorong Li Laboratory of Infectious Agents and Hygiene (GIMAP), EA3064, University Hospital and University Jean Monnet, Saint-Etienne, France; Department of Urology, North Hospital, CHU Saint Etienne, Saint Etienne, France

Dongdong Liu Department of Laboratory Science, The Second Affiliated Hospital of Guangzhou University of Chinese Medicine, Guangzhou, P.R. China

Sedwige Bernaud Loungouala Sounga Faculty of Health Sciences, University Marien Ngouabi, Brazzaville, Republic of Congo

Ihsane Ali Mahasneh Department of Biotechnology, Faculty of Science, Univeristy of Sharjah, Sharjah, United Arab Emirates; Research and Biosafety Laboratory, Mohammed V Military Teaching Hospital, Laboratory of Human Pathologies Biology, Faculty of Sciences, and Genomic Center of Human Pathologies, Faculty of Medicine and Pharmacy, Mohammed V University, Rabat, Morocco

Nora Mallouk Faculty of Medicine, Center of Electron Microscopy, CMES, Jean Monnet University, Saint Etienne, France

Christophe Mariat Department of Nephrology and Kidney Transplantation, North Hospital, CHU Saint Etienne, Saint Etienne, France

Arundhati Mehta Department of Biotechnology, Guru Ghasidas Vishwavidyalaya, Bilaspur, Chhattisgarh, India

Alami Mohamed Urology Department, Mohammed V Military Hospital, Rabat, Morocco

Donatien Moukassa Faculty of Health Sciences, University Marien Ngouabi, Brazzaville, Republic of Congo

Hassan Ait Mouse Team of Experimental Oncology and Natural Substances; Cellular & Molecular Immunopharmacology. Faculty of Sciences and Technology, University of Sultan Moulay Slimane, Beni Mellal, Morocco

Mohammed Mrabti Research and Biosafety Laboratory, Mohammed V Military Teaching Hospital, Rabat, Morocco; Laboratory of Human Pathologies Biology, Faculty of Sciences, and Genomic Center of Human Pathologies, Faculty of Medicine and Pharmacy, Mohammed V University, Rabat, Morocco; Urology Department, Mohammed V Military Hospital, Rabat, Morocco

Said Abdallah Nabil Group Research leader team of Virology, Oncology, and Biotechnologies, Head of Laboratory of Virology, Oncology, Biosciences, Environment and New Energies (LVO-BEEN), Faculty of Sciences and Techniques Mohammedia, University Hassan II of Casablanca, Casablanca, Morocco

Mouad Najih Group Research leader team of Virology, Oncology, and Biotechnologies, Head of Laboratory of Virology, Oncology, Biosciences, Environment and New Energies (LVO-BEEN), Faculty of Sciences and Techniques Mohammedia, University Hassan II of Casablanca, Casablanca, Casablanca, Morocco

Christy Parfait Nganga Faculty of Health Sciences, University Marien Ngouabi, Brazzaville, Republic of Congo

Dorine Florence Luthera Ngombe Mouabata Group Research leader team of Virology, Oncology, and Biotechnologies, Head of Laboratory of Virology, Oncology, Biosciences, Environment and New Energies (LVO-BEEN), Faculty of Sciences and Techniques Mohammedia, University Hassan II of Casablanca, Casablanca, Morocco; Faculty of Health Sciences, University Marien Ngouabi, Brazzaville, Republic of Congo

Yashwant Ratre (Kumar) Department of Biotechnology, Guru Ghasidas Vishwavidyalaya, Bilaspur, Chhattisgarh, India

Shiv Govind Rawat Department of Zoology, Banaras Hindu University, Varanasi, Uttar Pradesh, India

Dhananjay Shukla Department of Biotechnology, Guru Ghasidas Vishwavidyalaya, Bilaspur, Chhattisgarh, India

Vivek Soni (Kumar) Department of Biotechnology, Guru Ghasidas Vishwavidyalaya, Bilaspur, Chhattisgarh, India; Trivitron Healthcare, Vishakhapatnam, Andhra Pradesh, India

Ikram Tiabi Group Research leader team of Virology, Oncology, and Biotechnologies, Head of Laboratory of Virology, Oncology, Biosciences, Environment and New Energies (LVO-BEEN), Faculty of Sciences and Techniques Mohammedia, University Hassan II of Casablanca, Casablanca, Casablanca, Morocco

Naveen Vishvakarma (Kumar) Department of Biotechnology, Guru Ghasidas Vishwavidyalaya, Bilaspur, Chhattisgarh, India

Jin Wen Department of Urology, Peking Union Medical College Hospital, Beijing, P.R. China

Yang Zhang Guangzhou HopeTech Biological Technology Co, Ltd, Guangzhou, P.R. China

Abdelmajid Zyad Team of Experimental Oncology and Natural Substances; Cellular & Molecular Immunopharmacology, Faculty of Sciences and Technology, University of Sultan Moulay Slimane, Beni Mellal, Morocco

About the editor

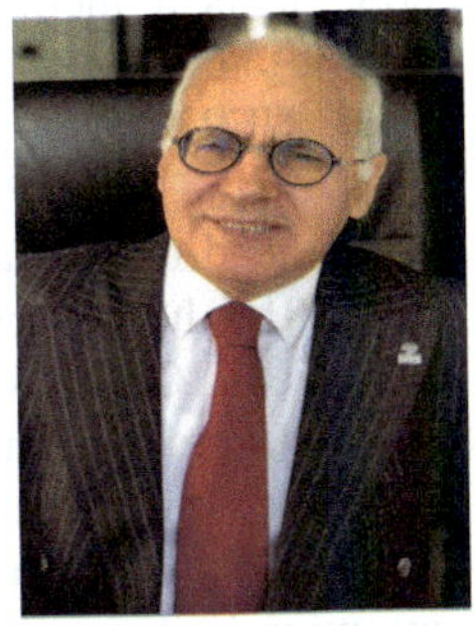

Prof. Dr. Moulay Mustapha Ennaji is a Moroccan and Canadian citizen and a native of Marrakesh, Morocco. He is a scientist specializing in the multiple fields, namely, virology, hygiene, and microbiology. He earned his Master of Science in 1986 and a PhD in virology in 1993 from Armand Frappier Institute, University of Quebec, Canada. Between 1991 and 1993, he completed his postdoctorate at the Canadian Red Cross. He was a research associate (1993–95) and a research officer (1995–96) at the National Council of Research of Canada. He has also worked as a visiting researcher at the University of California, Irvine, United States, and abroad lecturer at the Histochemistry Institutes of Paris, France. He was a guest researcher of the Franklin Foundation in USA NIH Bethesda.

In 1996 he was recruited to the Faculty of Sciences and Techniques, Mohammedia, University Hassan II of Casablanca (UH2C), as a lecturer and enabled professor, where he was the head of the Biology Department from 1997 to 2000. At present, he is professor of higher education in the same faculty. Being a scientist who is deeply concerned with research development, he has given numerous conferences and lectures on virology, cancerology, hygiene, and microbiology since 1986 at various Moroccan, Canadian, and American universities.

Since 2010, he has served as the director of the Laboratory of Virology, Oncology, Biosciences, Environment and New Energies, Faculty of Sciences and Techniques, Mohammedia, University Hassan II of Casablanca, Morocco; leader of Virology Oncology and Biotechnology Team; and deputy director of the Research Centre of Health and Biotechnologies of UH2C. From 2010 to 2016, he was the director of the Laboratory of Virology, Microbiology, Quality, Biotechnologies/Ecotoxicology and Biodiversity, Faculty of Sciences and Techniques, Mohammedia, University Hassan II of Casablanca, Morocco; leader of Virology, Oncology, Total Quality and Medical Biotechnology Team; and deputy director of the Research Centre of Natural Resources and Food (RENSA) of UH2C.

Between 2005 and 2010, he was appointed as the director of Virology, Hygiene, and Microbiology and coordinator of the CONSORTIUM of Biomedical and Environmental Sciences laboratories at UH2C-FSTM. He was also responsible for the master programs in biotechnology and biomedical technologies (2000–03), DESA of microbiology and bioengineering (2005–10), and Master of Science and technology (MST Microbiology, Applied Virology, and Bio-industry Engineering and MST of Livings) (Immuno-Virology and Applied Microbiology) from 2010 to 2015. Since 2008, he is a member of the Council of the Center of Doctoral Studies (CEDoc) at FSTM-UH2C. Between 2005 and 2010, he was the deputy head of the UFR DESA Biomedical Sciences and from 2000 to 2005 deputy leader of the UFR PhD in Health and Environment. Since 2005, he is the deputy head of Life and Environment Sciences Doctoral UFR. Furthermore, since 2010, he is serving as a national expert at CNRST and a member of the National Commission for Scholarships. From 2012 to 2014, he served as a UNESCO expert on governance reform of university systems.

Throughout his career, he has been conferred with 24 awards. He has organized numerous national and international meetings in the fields of virology, microbiology, and hygiene.

At present, he is the vice president of the Moroccan Association of Biosafety, Cancer and Microbiology.

Preface

This book, *Immunological Implications and Molecular Diagnostics of Genitourinary Cancer*, elaborates on the most recent research in the field of genitourinary cancers and the recent advances in the viral therapy in the same field. It elucidates the concepts related to this pathology and highlights the recent tools and techniques in the viral therapy against genitourinary cancers.

This book also describes the numerous studies in the field of molecular diagnostics as the implication of gene suppressor and oncogenes, how growth factor's genes can be associated with genitourinary cancers, and cytokine's gene alterations and genitourinary cancers. The book also discusses the importance of proteomic analysis of genitourinary cancers, genetic diagnostic and prognostic biomarkers of genitourinary cancers, and modern therapeutic targets of genitourinary tumors.

This book is organized into 10 parts, and each part consists of at least one chapter that gives a diversity of subjects and various studies. Each chapter includes relevant definitions and key concepts in addition to a wide description of the subject. An abstract is also provided for each chapter. The contents of each chapter are supported by schematic figures and tables.

This book starts with a general introduction to provide a basic overview of the statistical studies, risk factors, and the state of the art in the field of genitourinary cancers. Subjects of the contents reported are gene suppressor and oncogenes, implications of growth factor's genes in genitourinary cancers, cytokine's gene alterations and genitourinary cancers, proteomic analysis of genitourinary cancers, genetic diagnostic and prognostic biomarkers of genitourinary cancers, exosomes as a tool for genitourinary cancer's diagnostics and prognostics, genitourinary cancer's metabolism defect, clinical genomic relevance of genitourinary cancers, recent advances in viral therapy in genitourinary cancers, and finally, modern therapeutic targets of genitourinary tumors. We hope that we have covered all aspects of molecular and genetic diagnosis as well as the therapeutic targets of genitourinary tumors that will contribute to fighting this disease.

Moulay Mustapha Ennaji
Group Leader Research Team of Virology, Oncology, and Biotechnologies, Head of Laboratory of Virology, Oncology, Biosciences, Environment and New Energies (LVO-BEEN), Faculty of Sciences and Techniques Mohammedia, University Hassan II of Casablanca, Casablanca, Morocco

Acknowledgments

If the only prayer you say in your whole life is thank you, that will be enough.

Maître Eckhart

I am indebted to all the authors who have contributed new chapters describing the novel topics covered in this book, "Immunological Implications and Molecular Diagnostics of Genitourinary Cancer." These researchers have lighted the candles of knowledge so that the entire community can tap into their light and break through knowledge barriers, especially through the participation of a group of eminent/prominent scientists, clinicians, and academicians. I express my special gratitude to the reviewers for offering me help and valuable comments that helped improve the chapter contents and enhance the scientific importance of the contents. This work would not have been possible without the acceptance of the publisher Elsevier and the entire technical team, which has taken diligent care during the different stages of writing, evaluation, and correction, in addition, to the stages of preparation and publication. For this, I would like to express my sincere thanks to both the publishing house and the technical team. I would also like to extend my special thanks to the scientific team, which spared no effort to ensure the success of this work and to all the members of the editorial committee who mobilized all their technical and scientific efforts for the realization of this work.

Editorial advisory board

Editorial management committee

Ennaji Moulay Mustapha, PhD/PES C: His research expertise lies in virology, oncology, molecular biology, and biotechnologies. He is serving as the chief editor of the book. He is currently the head of the Laboratory of Virology, Oncology, Biosciences, Environment and New Energies; he is also the team leader at the Department of Virology, Oncology and Biotechnologies, Faculty of Sciences and Techniques, Mohammedia, University Hassan II of Casablanca, Casablanca, Morocco.

Kasmi Yassine, Bio-Ing.: His research interest lies in virology, oncology, and modelization. He is currently working at the Laboratory of Virology, Oncology, Biosciences, Environment and New Energies, Faculty of Sciences and Techniques, Mohammedia, University Hassan II of Casablanca, Casablanca, Morocco.

Ennaji Youssef, PhD st/M.Sci: His research expertise lies in virology, oncology, molecular biology, and biotechnologies. He is currently working at the Laboratory of Virology, Oncology, Biosciences, Environment and New Energies, Faculty of Sciences and Techniques, Mohammedia, University Hassan II of Casablanca, Casablanca, Morocco.

Abumsimir Berjas, PhD/Professor: Prof. Berjas's research interest lies in virology, oncology, molecular biology, and biotechnologies. He is currently working at the Laboratory of Virology, Oncology, Biosciences, Environment and New Energies, Faculty of Sciences and Techniques, Mohammedia, University Hassan II of Casablanca, Casablanca, Morocco.

Hassou Najwa, PhD: Her research interest lies in virology, environment. She is currently working at the Laboratory of Virology, Oncology, Biosciences, Environment and New Energies, Faculty of Sciences and Techniques, Mohammedia, University Hassan II of Casablanca, Casablanca, Morocco.

Abouchoaib Nabil, MDV: His research interests include virology and molecular biology. He is currently working at ONSSA-Rabat, Morocco.

Ihsan Ali Mahasneh, PhD/Professor: Prof. Mahasneh's research expertise lies in virology, oncology, molecular biology, and biotechnology. He is currently working at the Department of Biotechnology, Faculty of Science, University of Sharjah, Sharjah, UAE.

Amghar Souad, PhD/PES C: Her research interest lies in microbiology. She is a part of the research team Lumbricidae, Improving Soil Productivity and Environment (LAPSE), Centre (Eau, Ressources Naturelles, Environnement et Developpement Durable (CERNE2D)) Mohammed V University in Rabat, Ecole Normale Superieure (ENS), Morocco.

Boussettine Rihabe, PhD: Her research interest lies in virology, environment, and biotechnologies. She is currently working at the Laboratory of Virology, Oncology, Biosciences, Environment and New Energies, Faculty of Sciences and Techniques, Mohammedia, University Hassan II of Casablanca, Casablanca, Morocco.

Max Arella, PhD/Professor: Prof. Arella's research interests include virology, molecular biology, and biotechnologies. He is currently working at the Institut Armand-Frappier, Centre de Recherche en Virologie, Laval, Quebec, Canada H7V 1B7.

Merzouki Abderrahmane, PhD/Professor: Prof. Abderrahmane's research interests include virology, molecular biology, and biotechnologies. He is currently working at the Institut Armand-Frappier, Centre de Recherche en Virologie, Laval, Quebec, Canada H7V 1B7.

Bourlet Thomas, PhD/MD/Professor: Prof. Thomas's research interests include virology, oncology, and immunology. He is currently working at the Laboratory of Infectious Agents and Hygiene GIMAP-EA3064, University Hospital & University Jean Monnet, Saint-Etienne, France.

Gorong Li, PhD/Professor: Prof. Li's research interests include virology, oncology, and immunology. Prof. Li is currently working at the Laboratory of Infectious Agents and Hygiene GIMAP-EA3064, University Hospital & University Jean Monnet, Saint-Etienne, France.

Črtomir Podlipnik, PhD/Professor: Prof. Podlipnik's research interests include chemoinformatics, drug design, and theorical chemistry. He is currently working at the Faculty of Chemistry and Chemical Technology, University of Ljubljana, Večna pot 113, 1000 Ljubljana, Slovenia.

Jalid Sehouli, MD/Professor: Prof. Sehouli's research interests include gynecology and oncology. He is currently working at the Department of

Gynecology. Center for Oncological Surgery, Charité—Universitätsmedizin Berlin, Germany.

Bahraoui Elmostafa, PhD/Professor: Prof. Elmostafa's research interests include virology and immunology. He is currently working at the University of Paul Sabatier Toulouse 3, France.

El Mzibri Mohammed, PhD: His research interests include virology, oncology, molecular biology, and biotechnologies. He is currently working at the Biology and Medical Research Unit, National Center of Energy, Nuclear Sciences and Techniques Rabat, Morocco.

Laraqui Abdelilah, PhD/PES: Prof. Abdelilah's research interests include virology, oncology, molecular biology, and biotechnologies. He is currently working at the Sequencing Unit, Center for Virology, Infectious and Tropical Diseases, Mohammed V Military Hospital, Faculty of Medicine and Pharmacy, Mohammed V University, Rabat, Morocco.

Mohammed Mrabti, MD: His research interests include virology, oncology, molecular biology, and biotechnologies. He is currently working at the Sequencing Unit, Center for Virology, Infectious and Tropical Diseases, Mohammed V Military Hospital, Faculty of Medicine and Pharmacy, Mohammed V University, Rabat, Morocco.

Benchekroun Mohammed Nabil, PhD/PES C: His research interests include oncology and biotechnologies. He is currently working at the Laboratory of Virology, Oncology, Biosciences, Environment and New Energies, Faculty of Sciences and Techniques, Mohammedia, University Hassan II of Casablanca, Casablanca, Morocco.

Bessi Hlima, PhD/PES C: Her research interests include eco-toxicology and environment. She is currently working at the Laboratory of Virology, Oncology, Biosciences, Environment and New Energies, Faculty of Sciences and Techniques, Mohammedia, University Hassan II of Casablanca, Casablanca, Morocco.

Benhessou Mustapha, PhD/MD/PES: Prof. Mustapha's research interests include virology and oncology. He is currently working as permanent member at the Laboratory of Virology, Oncology, Biosciences, Environment and New Energies, Faculty of Sciences and Techniques, Mohammedia, University Hassan II of Casablanca, Casablanca, Morocco. He is acting in parallel in Mohammed VI Centre for Treatment of Cancer, University Hospital Ibn Rochd, Casablanca, Morocco.

Chapter 1

Introduction to the molecular aspects and viral therapy of genitourinary tumors

Moulay Mustapha Ennaji
Group Leader Research team of Virology, Oncology, and Biotechnologies, Head of Laboratory of Virology, Oncology, Biosciences, Environment and New Energies (LVO-BEEN), Faculty of Sciences and Techniques Mohammedia, University Hassan II of Casablanca, Casablanca, Morocco

1.1 Background

According to Dana–Farber Cancer Institute, genitourinary cancer includes (1) adrenal cancer, represented by adrenocortical carcinoma, (2) bladder cancer, including urothelial carcinoma, (3) urachal cancer, (4) kidney cancer, including collecting duct carcinoma, renal cell carcinoma, rhabdoid tumor of the kidney, renal pelvic cancer (ureteral cancer), and Wilms' tumor (nephroblastoma), (5) penile cancer, including urethral cancer, (6) prostate cancer, and finally, (7) testicular cancer (germ cell tumor), which includes seminoma and non-seminoma, wherein the latter includes choriocarcinoma and teratoma.

A wide variety of human tumors are known to infect the reproductive and urinary systems in humans. The urinary system is responsible for removing the body's waste fluid known as urine. This system also ensures that certain chemicals, such as potassium and sodium, stay within our bodies. The male reproductive system is responsible for making and carrying the male reproductive cells (sperm) and its fluid called semen, while female reproductive system is responsible for organizing maturation of sex interior and exterior organs. These systems make sure the male sex cells and hormones are active and balanced.

The identification of driver biomarkers has become the central focus in human tumor research, owing to the necessity of estimating certain variants involved in tumor initiation and progression and to explore potential therapeutic targets in addition to selecting responsive and irresponsive patients against therapy decisions.

Immunological Implications and Molecular Diagnostics of Genitourinary Cancer.
DOI: https://doi.org/10.1016/B978-0-323-85496-2.00006-3

Molecular diagnostic is now extremely important in most human malignancies for accurate diagnosis and prediction of response to targeted biological drugs. Urogenital carcinomas are particularly regarded as part of solid tumors as only a few predictive and molecular prognostic biomarkers have been identified to date in these types of tumors (Maiorano et al., 2021).

Indeed, the prognosis of prostate cancer is still largely dependent on histological features, while therapeutic advances in aggressive prostate cancer still involve primarily hormonal therapy and in a small proportion of drugs targeting genetic changes in the single germ line.

The molecular classification of genitourinary tumors has been a notable achievement in understanding the biological nature of this type of carcinoma. However, the practical application of this molecular classification is still not recognized by most clinicians, and the predictive importance of driver genetic biomarkers in cancer treatment is not well understood. Renal cancer represents the best progress area among solid tumors in terms of change in subtype classification (Al Harthy et al., 2020).

Thus, this classification must also include a large number of other kidney cancers based on molecular distinguishing features. This enhanced understanding of renal carcinomas with different molecular features and common histological features is likely to influence the surgical and diagnostic choices for kidney tumors; however, it is not likely to change the therapeutic decisions for aggressive cases.

Testicular cancer has become prevalent, and a new biological classification associates a similar tissue with a different cancer pathway and the age of onset. Therefore, molecular developments in testicular tumor may fundamentally affect its prognosis as oncology treatment is standardized and correlated with good clinical choices in most aggressive cases (Ding et al., 2021).

Penile cancer has also elevated interests in oncology studies and has been primarily associated with viral infections, especially human papillomavirus. However, studies have focused on nonHPV-related tumors and the relationships between these types of genitourinary tumors and inflammatory microenvironment.

The genetic markers associated with elevated risk of hereditary and sporadic cancer vary significantly between genitourinary tumors. These tumors share many genetic changes, but at different frequencies, which are consistent with their frequent occurrence. These differences likely contribute to the behavior of these types of cancers and mean that their fluctuating frequency and mutation frequency should be treated as related but distinct entities.

Therapeutic cancer vaccines are an important part of the extensive immunotherapy approach to tumor treatment, which aims to boost the immune system to recognize and eliminate cancer cells. Studies in the domain of genitourinary malignancies have demonstrated immense success of therapeutic vaccines against tumors since the implementation of Bacillus Calmette–Guerin for bladder cancer in the 1970s. After the approval from the US Food and Drug Administration for sipuleucel-T for prostate cancer in

2010, several vaccine options have been introduced, such as autologous and allogeneic tumor vaccines, DNA vaccines, use of viral vectors, and peptides as immunostimulating adjuvants. In addition to their mechanism of action, vaccine strategies are of clinical value for having a low adverse effect. Especially in advanced cases, patients who are not candidates for curative therapies, may benefit from treatment with either a vaccine or a combination that keeps tumors in the dormant stage (Guo et al., 2013; Kantoff et al., 2010; Morales et al., 1976; Pal et al., 2013).

The above-mentioned approaches aim to increase antigen production to overcome antigen evasion in the tumor, to generate an intensive immune attack on cold tumors.

References

Al Harthy, M., Redman, J., & Madan, R. A. (2020). Novel immunotherapy combinations for genitourinary cancers. *Expert Opinion on Biological Therapy, 20*(3), 253–262.

Ding, Y., Al-Obaidy, K. I., & Cheng, L. (2021). *Genitourinary neoplasms. Practical Oncologic Molecular Pathology* (pp. 233–244). Cham: Springer.

Guo, C., Manjili, M. H., Subjeck, J. R., Sarkar, D., Fisher, P. B., & Wang, X. Y. (2013). Therapeutic cancer vaccines: Past, present, and future. *Advances in Cancer Research, 119*, 421–475.

Kantoff, P. W., Higano, C. S., Shore, N. D., Berger, E. R., Small, E. J., Penson, D. F., Redfern, C. H., Ferrari, A. C., Dreicer, R., Sims, R. B., et al. (2010). Sipuleucel-T immunotherapy for castration-resistant prostate cancer. *The New England Journal of Medicine, 363*, 411–422.

Maiorano, B. A., et al. (2021). Cancer vaccines for genitourinary tumors: Recent progresses and future possibilities. *Vaccines, 9*(6), 623.

Morales, A., Eidinger, D., & Bruce, A. W. (1976). Intracavitary bacillus calmette-guerin in the treatment of superficial bladder tumors. *The Journal of Urology, 116*, 180–183.

Pal, S. K., Hu, A., & Figlin, R. A. (2013). A new age for vaccine therapy in renal cell carcinoma. *Cancer Journal (Sudbury, Mass.), 19*, 365–370.

Chapter 2

Liquid biopsy of exosome markers for molecular diagnosis of genitourinary cancer

Dongdong Liu[1,*], Guorong Li[2,8,*,†], Jin Wen[3,†], Pierre Cornillon[4], Yang Zhang[5], Nora Mallouk[6] and Christophe Mariat[7]

[1]*Department of Laboratory Science, The Second Affiliated Hospital of Guangzhou University of Chinese Medicine, Guangzhou, P.R. China,* [2]*Department of Urology, North Hospital, CHU Saint Etienne, Saint Etienne, France,* [3]*Department of Urology, Peking Union Medical College Hospital, Beijing, P.R. China,* [4]*Department of Oncology, North Hospital, CHU Saint Etienne, Saint Etienne, France,* [5]*Guangzhou HopeTech Biological Technology Co, Ltd, Guangzhou, P.R. China,* [6]*Faculty of Medicine, Center of Electron Microscopy, CMES, Jean Monnet University, Saint Etienne, France,* [7]*Department of Nephrology and Kidney Transplantation, North Hospital, CHU Saint Etienne, Saint Etienne, France,* [8]*Laboratory of Infectious Agents and Hygiene (GIMAP), EA3064, University Hospital and University Jean Monnet, Saint Etienne, France*

2.1 Introduction

In 1983 exosomal vesicles were first discovered in sheep reticulocytes. The name of exosomes, however, was formally given by Johnstone in 1986 (Harding et al., 2013). Almost all types of cells secret exosomes into the extracellular environment.

There are four steps for the biogenesis of exosomes (Colombo et al., 2014). In the first step, various body cells produce endocytic vesicles through endocytosis. In the second step, the endocytic vesicles fuse to form an early endosome and gradually become a late endosome. In the third step, with the entry of some substances such as nucleic acids and proteins in the cytoplasm, the late endosomes produce many intraluminal vesicles (exosomes) and gradually evolve into multivesicular bodies. In the fourth and final step, the multivesicular bodies fuse with the plasma membrane to release exosomes into

* Dongdong Liu and Guorong Li contributed equally to this work.

† Correspondence: Dr. Jin Wen, Department of Urology, Peking Union Medical College Hospital, Beijing, China. E-mail: wjjxmc@163.com or Dr. Guorong Li, Department of Urology, North Hospital, CHU Saint Etienne, France.

Immunological Implications and Molecular Diagnostics of Genitourinary Cancer.
DOI: https://doi.org/10.1016/B978-0-323-85496-2.00032-4

the extracellular environment. The mechanism of exosomal interaction with recipient cells has not been clarified yet. After the exosomes fuse with the membrane of the recipient cell, they release the "cargoes" into the cytoplasm and re-form multivesicular bodies. Exosomes play an important role in cell-to-cell communications.

At present, there are several methods for the isolation of exosomes such as ultracentrifugation, size exclusion chromatography, magnetic bead immunocapture, precipitation or filtration (Monguió-Tortajada et al., 2019). Each method has its advantages and disadvantages. Different exosome isolation methods are summarized and compared in Table 2.1.

TABLE 2.1 Comparison of different methods for exosome isolation. Each method has its advantages and disadvantages.

	Advantage	Disadvantage
Ultracentrifugation	Easy to use Possible large sample volume High yield Reproducible	Contamination of abundant proteins Possible damage to exosome Expensive equipment Time-consuming
Density gradient centrifugation	High purity Reproducible	Loss of exosome Long processing time Expensive equipment
Size exclusion chromatography	High purity Superior integrity Reproducible	Moderate sample capacity Special equipment needed Costly
Ultrafiltration	Fast Possible high volume Suitable in clinical setting	Moderate purity Possible exosome loss and deterioration Contamination of proteins Possible clogging of membrane
Precipitation	Easy to use Large sample capacity High yield Relatively inexpensive Suitable in clinical setting	Low purity Contaminants Possible long run time
Immunobead method	High purity	Low yield Expensive Possible alteration of exosome markers
Microfluidics	Easy to use Fast Portable	Limited sample capacity Lack of standardization

Minimal information for studies of extracellular vesicles 2018 (MISEV2018) recommends the following test requirements for the characterization of exosomes (Théry et al., 2018):

1. Overall characterization by Western blot or flow cytometry should be performed to analyze at least three positive markers (including at least one transmembrane protein and one cytosolic protein) and one negative protein marker.
2. Individual characterization by nanoparticle tracking analysis (NTA) and transmission electron microscopy (TEM) characterization should be performed. The two methods of NTA and TEM are complementary to each other.

We have developed methods for exosome isolation by using isolation kits. Based on our preliminary works, we provide a typical view of serum and urinary exosomes observed using TEM (Figs. 2.1 and 2.2). Exosomes are cup-shaped. The bilayer lipid membrane is obvious. Their sizes range from 30 to 150 nm.

Most types of living cells can secrete exosomes, which are widely present in various body fluids including blood, saliva, urine, breast milk, and pleural and ascites. Exosomes secreted by different cells can have similar or

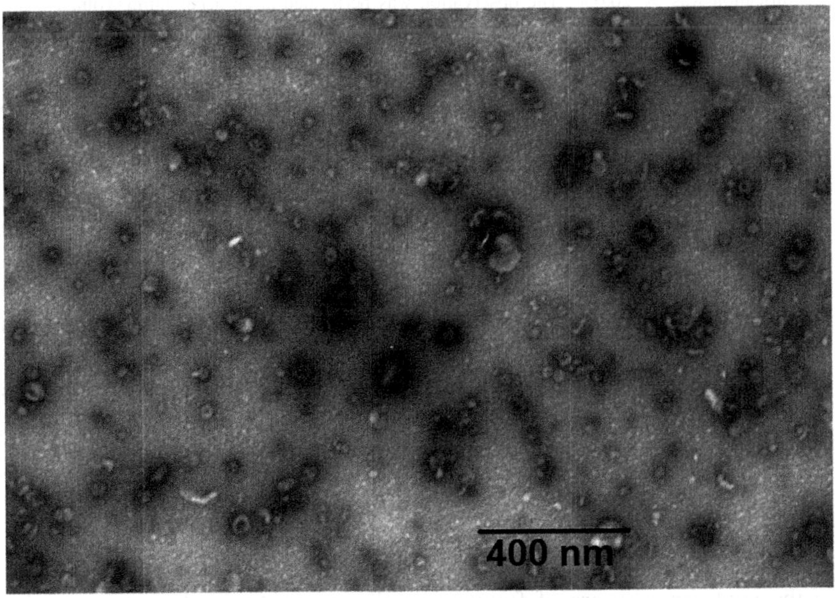

FIGURE 2.1 Transmission electron microscopy view of urinary exosomes. Typical morphology of urinary exosomes was observed. The lipid bilayer membrane was clearly visible. Magnification was × 20,000. The observation was performed at an accelerating voltage value of 100 kV.

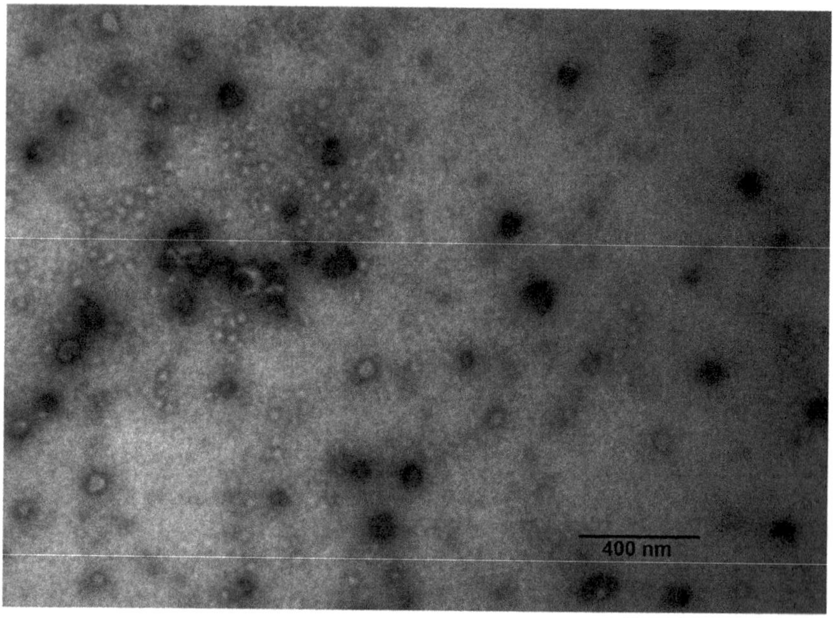

FIGURE 2.2 Transmission electron microscopy view of serum exosomes. Typical morphology of serum exosomes was observed. The lipid bilayer membrane was clearly visible. Magnification was × 20,000. The observation was performed at an accelerating voltage value of 100 kV.

different characteristics and biological functions (Raposo & Stoorvogel, 2013). Exosomes are involved in the regulation of cellular physiological activities, and their roles in immune response, apoptosis, angiogenesis, inflammation, and coagulation have been reported. The phenotype and quantity of exosomes released by different tissue types are different. They can selectively encapsulate intracellular proteins, microRNAs, mRNA, and DNA. Similarly, tumor cells can release tumoral exosomes. The tumor continuously releases exosomes into circulation during its growth process. Exosome is an important source for the interaction between tumor cells and surrounding mesenchymal cells and participates in tumor development and metastasis. Therefore tumor exosomes are promising new tumor biomarkers (Bullock et al., 2015; Melo et al., 2015; LeBleu & Kalluri, 2020).

2.2 Tissue biopsy versus liquid biopsy

In the contemporary era of frequent small tumors, tissue diagnosis remains necessary. There are two routine methods for a tissue biopsy: fine needle aspiration (FNA) biopsy and core biopsy (Yang et al., 2017). Both these routine methods are complementary. FNA is performed by using a negative pressure and mechanical disruption, which may produce more cellular sample than core biopsy. The cellular materials from both FNA and core biopsy can easily be utilized for molecular analysis.

Liquid biopsy has recently garnered massive attention from researchers (Marconi et al., 2016). Liquid biopsy samples include urine, blood (serum/plasma), saliva and other cytoponction liquids such as cerebrospinal and pleural fluid (Fig. 2.3). Liquid biopsy allows the detection of tumor markers in bodily fluids for the diagnosis or monitoring of cancer patients. Compared with tissue biopsy, liquid biopsy is noninvasive. The comparison between tissue biopsy and liquid biopsy is summed up in Table 2.2. Liquid biopsy typically utilizes circulating tumor cells (CTCs), cell-free DNA/RNA, and exosomes. CTCs and cell-free DNA have been studied for a long time, while exosomes are relatively recent but with a rapid development.

Exosomes carry tumor markers such as nucleic acids, proteins, and lipids. Blood is particularly interesting as a source of liquid biopsy as it contains CTC, cell-free DNA/RNA, and exosomes. Currently, most studies are concentrated on blood. Urine is the easiest available bodily fluid. The research on exosomes in the field of liquid biopsy is extensive (Keller et al., 2011; Lodewijk et al., 2018; Palmirotta et al., 2018). Exosomes are involved in multiple processes of tumorigenesis and development, including the promotion of angiogenesis, differentiation and infiltration, regulation of immunity, and response to therapy, etc. Exosomes can not only be used as a source of

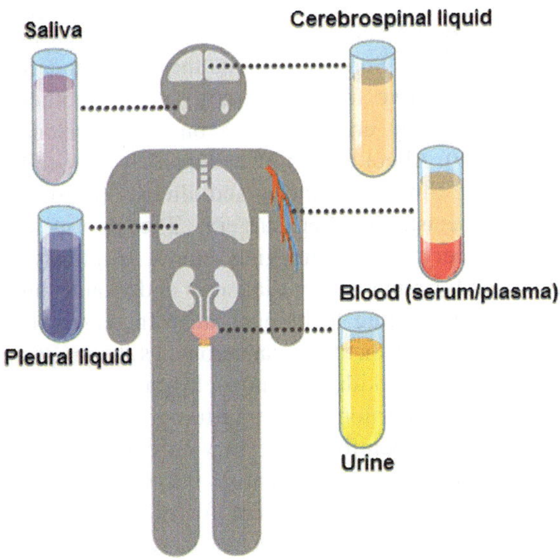

FIGURE 2.3 Analytical samples for liquid biopsy. Liquid biopsy samples include urine, blood (serum/plasma), saliva and other cytoponction liquids such as cerebrospinal and pleural fluid.

TABLE 2.2 Comparison between tissue biopsy and liquid biopsy.

Tissue biopsy	Liquid biopsy
Routine histological diagnosis and staging	Impossible for tumor histology and staging
Painful, invasive, and sometimes difficult	Noninvasive examination
Not representative for the entire tumor owing to tumor heterogeneity	Representative of all malignant clones in the tumor
Difficult in multiple samplings	Easily obtainable and repeatable
Unsuitable for dynamic monitoring	Possible for real-time surveillance of tumor
Gold standard for tumor diagnosis	Most still in laboratory research

liquid biopsy for tumor diagnosis but can also be used as therapeutic means and drug carriers for the treatment of cancers.

2.3 Renal cell cancer

Renal cell cancer originates from renal tubular epithelial cells. About 70%–80% of kidney cancers are clear cell renal cell cancers (ccRCC) (Siegel et al., 2020). Renal cell cancer has almost no conspicuous clinical symptoms at an early stage. Surgery remains the gold standard for the treatment. It is highly insensitive to radiotherapy and chemotherapy. Targeted therapy and immunotherapy are promising but lack personalized markers (Ljungberg et al., 2019). About a third of patients have a locally advanced or metastatic tumor at the time of diagnosis and almost 30% of treated patients develop secondary metastases after surgery. The postoperative followup strategy for renal cancer relies on imaging exams. Clinically, new methods and new technologies for renal cancer diagnosis and monitoring are needed.

Recent advances in imaging techniques have increased the detection of kidney tumors, but not all of them are cancerous, as the proportion of benign tumors is 10%–15% for all kidney tumors. In particular, for renal tumors smaller than 4 cm, the proportion of benign tumors is 20%–30% (Li et al., 2004). A tissue biopsy is therefore necessary to confirm the diagnosis and avoid unnecessary nephrectomy. Currently, the tissue diagnosis of small solid renal mass is a challenging problem for radiologists, urologists, and pathologists. A successful diagnosis depends largely on the tissue obtained from the tumors. For the above reason, many researchers resume the idea of using FNA biopsy for sampling of small solid renal tumors (Yang et al., 2017). The notion of liquid biopsy of renal cancer has been mentioned in recent publications (Dear et al., 2013; Franzen et al., 2016). Liquid biopsies are based on the detection of cancerous biomarkers in body fluid, mostly in the blood, but sometimes also in urine, saliva, or another fluid. Interestingly, the exosomes released by tumoral cells not only have a number of tumor antigens on its surface, but they can also selectively contain small molecules in tumor cytoplasm including proteins and microRNAs (miRNA) during their formation (Lässer, 2013). It is well known that miRNA is a small noncoding RNA with a length of about 22–25 nucleotides. It has been confirmed that many tumor tissues have several specifically expressed miRNAs, which are related to the degree of differentiation and prognosis. Further functional studies have demonstrated that these specifically expressed miRNAs can change the pathological process of tumors by regulating the expression of oncogenes or tumor-suppressor genes (Dear et al., 2013). Although the biological effects of these specific miRNAs after being contained in exosomes and being released outside the cell are still unclear, their applications in tumor diagnosis and treatment monitoring have shown tremendous potential. An example of serum exosome miRNAs in ccRCC is demonstrated (Zhang et al., 2018). In the study under consideration, serum exosomal miR-210 and miR-1233 were investigated. Receiver operating characteristic (ROC) curve analysis was performed for discriminating ccRCC patients from the control individuals. Serum exosomal miR-210 yielded an AUC (the areas under the ROC curve) of 0.69 (95% Cl: 0.61–0.77) with a sensitivity of 70% and a specificity of 62% in discrimination between the ccRCC patients and the controls. Serum exosomal miR-1233 yielded an AUC (Area Under the Curve) of 0.82 (95% Cl: 0.75–0.89) with a sensitivity of 81% and a specificity of 76% in discrimination between the ccRCC patients and the controls.

Previously, we discovered that there was abundant cell-free RNA in the urine of renal cancer patients (Zhao et al., 2015). We believe that these RNAs may come from urinary exosomes. Urine is in close contact with kidney tumor. The search for exosomal markers in urine of renal cancer patients may be interesting. We have launched a study to investigate urinary exosomal mRNAs for the diagnosis of ccRCC (Li et al., 2020).

2.4 Bladder cancer

Bladder cancer is one of the most common malignant tumors worldwide. If it can be detected and treated early, the five-year survival rate is higher than 90% (Ferlay et al., 2015; Kamat et al., 2016; Soukup et al., 2012). Therefore early diagnosis is critical to improve the long-term survival of patients. About 80% of newly diagnosed bladder cancers are nonmuscular invasive tumors (pTa or pT1). These tumors are mainly treated by transurethral resection of bladder tumors and intravesical perfusion. About 20% of bladder cancers are muscular invasive tumors and require radical treatment by cystectomy plus urinary diversion. Furthermore, 70% of nonmuscular invasive bladder tumors will recur after the initial treatment, and a considerable number of patients will progress to muscular invasive tumors. At present, the diagnosis and postoperative followup of bladder cancer rely on the examination of urinary exfoliated cells and cystoscopy. The sensitivity of urinary exfoliated cell examination is very low, especially for low-grade tumors. Although cystoscopy combined with tissue biopsy is very sensitive and accurate, it is traumatic and painful to patients. Therefore looking for markers in urine to detect or diagnose early bladder cancer remains a hot topic in current bladder cancer research in order to reduce or replace cystoscopy.

Urinary tumor markers for bladder cancer have always been a hot subject in the research area. Some tumor markers have been commercialized: UroVyv50 (FISH method), NMP-22 (Elisa method), BTA (Elisa), and ImmunoCyt (Elisa). These diagnostic kits are more or less sensitive. The high false-positive rate or false-negative rate makes them difficult to replace cystoscopy. The current trend is toward DNA or RNA markers. DNA sequencing is under study and has a certain prospect. Theoretically, RNA markers are more sensitive than DNA markers. CxBladder is a new RNA method (Darling et al., 2017). This kit detects five RNA markers in urine exfoliated cells: CDC2, HOXA13, MDK, IGFBP5, and CXCR5. The sensitivity reaches 82%, and the specificity reaches 85%. Therefore it can be used as a supplement to cystoscopy.

Another recent trend is to detect tumor markers in urinary exosomes (Blackwell et al., 2014; Lodewijk et al., 2018). The latest studies have shown that there are a large number of DNA or RNA markers in urine supernatant. The detection of DNA or RNA markers in urine supernatant is expected to provide a new method for the diagnosis of bladder cancer. There are a large number of exosomes secreted from cancer cells into the urine supernatant, and these exosomes are thought to contain a large number of RNA or DNA markers. Recently, it has been found that urinary exosomes contain cell-specific proteins, lipids, and nucleic acids, which can be served as signal molecules to be transmitted to recipient cells. These findings have ignited researcher's interest in urinary exosomes. Recent studies have also found that urinary exosomes play an important role in the physiology and pathology of bladder cancer, such as antigen presentation in immunity, tumor growth and migration, and repair of tissue damage. The exosomes secreted by different cells have different components and functions, which can be served as biomarkers for bladder cancer.

In a pilot study, we combined two techniques: isolation of urinary exosomes and urinary tumoral mRNA markers. We showed the feasibility of detection of tumoral mRNA markers in urinary exosomes of the diagnosis of bladder cancer. By using the gene markers in urinary exosomes, we obtained diagnostic values of an AUC of 0.861 (95% CI: 0.817–0.905) (Fig. 2.4). Preliminary study showed that the sensitivity was 62.03% and the specificity was 96.59% for the diagnosis of bladder cancer. This method can enlarge the

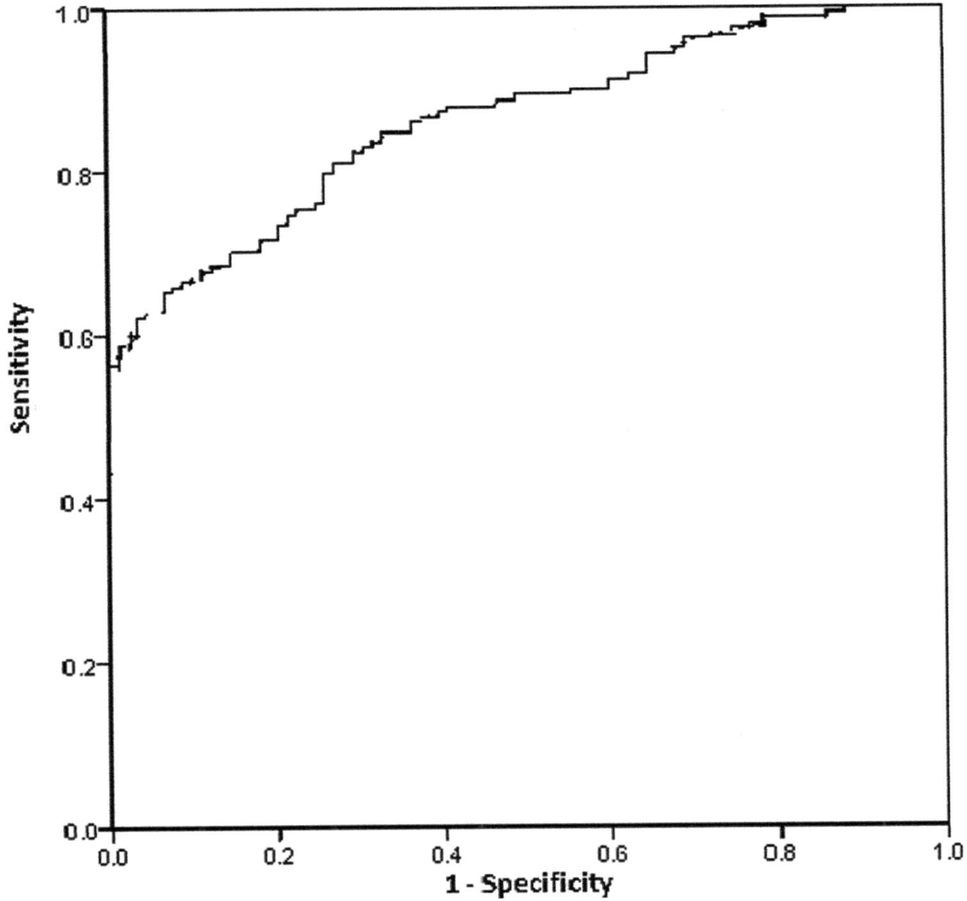

FIGURE 2.4 **Urine exosome markers for the diagnosis of bladder cancer.** Receiver operating characteristic (ROC) curve analysis of urinary exosomal mRNA markers was performed for the diagnosis of bladder cancer. Urinary exosomal mRNA markers yielded an AUC (area under the ROC curve) of 0.861 (95% confidence interval: 0.817–0.905) with a sensitivity of 62.03% and a specificity of 96.59%.

use of urinary mRNA markers in the management of bladder cancer, which depends solely on urinary cells. We agree that urinary exosomes will become a new source of liquid biopsy for bladder cancer. The future work is to study how this technique can improve the urinary cytology as a diagnostic and surveillance method for bladder cancer.

2.5 Prostate cancer

Prostate cancer is one of most common malignant tumors of the male reproductive system, and it is one of the main causes of death from cancer in men in Europe and the United States. The current method of diagnosis of prostate cancer is based on prostate tissue biopsy after blood prostate-specific antigen (PSA) is measured in laboratory. This invasive tissue biopsy is painful to the patient and expensive. PSA is specific to prostate tissue, but it is not a specific marker for prostate cancer. Besides prostate cancer, many other factors can lead to an elevated PSA, including age, prostate infection, benign prostatic hyperplasia, etc. Among prostate tissue biopsies, almost 92% of samples were found to have no cancer or low-to-moderate cancer-graded with Gleason scores between 1 and 6. Therefore a large number of patients find it useless to suffer a prostate biopsy. There is an utmost need to find a method for the accurate diagnosis of clinically significant prostate cancer.

Urine is the easiest liquid to collect that contains abundant exosomes. The prostate is an organ closely related to the urinary tract. At present, researchers try to explore new methods from urine for the diagnosis of prostate cancer. At present, finding markers in urine for an early detection or diagnosis of prostate cancer is an emerging research direction in the world (Pang et al., 2020; Solé et al., 2020). The research on urinary exosomes as prostate cancer markers is still in its infancy. Gen-probe launched PCA3 gene detection reagent (Gen-Probe and Diagnocure company). The kit can assist in the diagnosis of prostate cancer. After digital rectal massage, prostate cancer cells will drop off and enter into the urine. The kit can be used to quantitatively detect PCA3 messenger RNA (mRNA) in these cells (Neveu et al., 2016). PCA3 is not expressed in normal or benign hyperplastic prostate tissue, while the expression in cancerous prostate cells can be significantly increased by 60–100 times. Previous studies have shown that the PCA3 score increased the positive rate of prostate biopsy. The specificity of the urine PCA3 test to diagnose prostate cancer is significantly higher than that of the serum PSA test. However, this test requires a digital rectal massage because the analytical target is prostatic cells. Because the prostate and urine are closely connected, prostatic exosomes can be secreted into the urine. Therefore urinary exosomes may provide a new way for the diagnosis of prostate cancer. Recently, a urine diagnostic kit for prostate cancer (ExoDX Prostate IntelliScore) has just appeared in the United States, which detects three urinary exosomal mRNA (PCA3, ERG, and SPDEF) markers (McKiernan et al., 2016). Digital rectal massage is not needed for this test. This

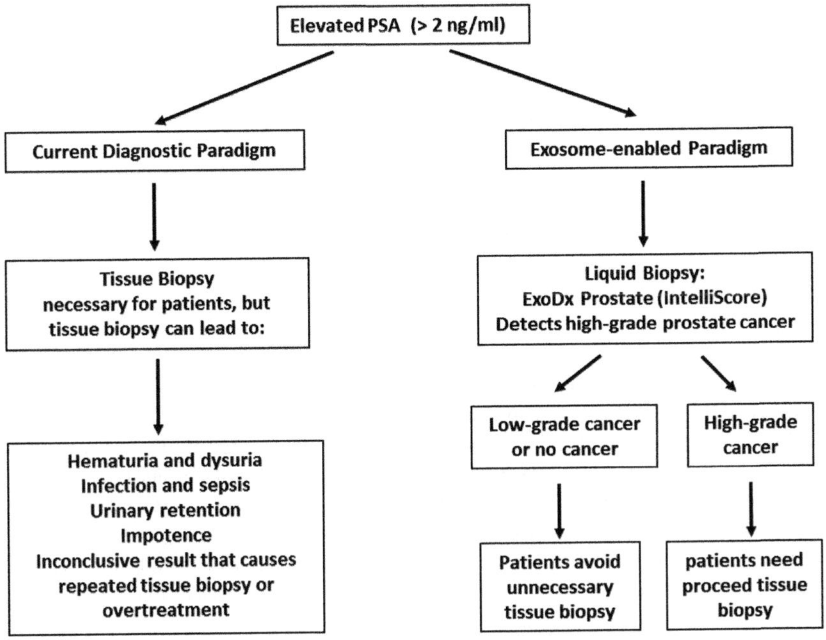

FIGURE 2.5 Urine exosome for the diagnosis of prostate cancer. Urinary exosome test helps the overall decision to defer or proceed with a tissue biopsy and avoids unnecessary prostate tissue biopsy. If the test result indicates a low risk, prostate tissue biopsy may be deferred.

diagnostic kit is especially useful for those who require prostate biopsy among men with an elevated PSA. It is considered to be a major breakthrough in the diagnosis of prostate cancer by avoiding unnecessary tissue biopsy. The diagnostic utility is illustrated in Fig. 2.5.

2.6 Conclusion

In conclusion, genitourinary cancers are diagnosed mainly by tissue biopsy even in the contemporary era. With the rapid development of biologic technology, liquid biopsy will complement or improve the tissue biopsy. Liquid biopsy by means of exosomes will play a potential role to solve the diagnostic problems currently encountered in genitourinary cancers.

References

Blackwell, R. H., Franzen, C. A., Flanigan, R. C., Kuo, P. C., & Gupta, G. N. (2014). The untapped potential of urine shed bladder cancer exosomes: Biomarkers, signaling, and therapeutics. *Bladder*, 7. Available from https://doi.org/10.14440/bladder.2014.38.

Bullock, M. D., Silva, A. M., Kanlikilicer-Unaldi, P., Filant, J., Rashed, M. H., Sood, A. K., Lopez-Berestein, G., & Calin, G. A. (2015). Exosomal non-coding RNAs: Diagnostic, prognostic and therapeutic applications in cancer. *Non-Coding RNA*, *1*(1), 53–68. Available from https://doi.org/10.3390/ncrna1010053.

Colombo, M., Raposo, G., & Théry, C. (2014). Biogenesis, secretion, and intercellular interactions of exosomes and other extracellular vesicles. *Annual Review of Cell and Developmental Biology*, *30*, 255–289. Available from https://doi.org/10.1146/annurev-cellbio-101512-122326.

Darling, D., Luxmanan, C., O'Sullivan, P., Lough, T., & Suttie, J. (2017). Clinical utility of cxbladder for the diagnosis of Urothelial Carcinoma. *Advances in Therapy*, *34*(5), 1087–1096. Available from https://doi.org/10.1007/s12325-017-0518-7.

Dear, J. W., Street, J. M., & Bailey, M. A. (2013). Urinary exosomes: A reservoir for biomarker discovery and potential mediators of intrarenal signalling. *Proteomics*, *13*(10–11), 1572–1580. Available from https://doi.org/10.1002/pmic.201200285.

Ferlay, J., Soerjomataram, I., Dikshit, R., Eser, S., Mathers, C., Rebelo, M., Parkin, D. M., Forman, D., & Bray, F. (2015). Cancer incidence and mortality worldwide: Sources, methods and major patterns in GLOBOCAN 2012. *International Journal of Cancer*, *136*(5), E359–E386. Available from https://doi.org/10.1002/ijc.29210.

Franzen, C. A., Blackwell, R. H., Foreman, K. E., Kuo, P. C., Flanigan, R. C., & Gupta, G. N. (2016). Urinary exosomes: The potential for biomarker utility, intercellular signaling and therapeutics in urological malignancy. *Journal of Urology*, *195*(5), 1331–1339. Available from https://doi.org/10.1016/j.juro.2015.08.115.

Harding, C. V., Heuser, J. E., & Stahl, P. D. (2013). Exosomes: Looking back three decades and into the future. *Journal of Cell Biology*, *200*(4), 367–371. Available from https://doi.org/10.1083/jcb.201212113.

Kamat, A. M., Hahn, N. M., Efstathiou, J. A., Lerner, S. P., Malmström, P. U., Choi, W., Guo, C. C., Lotan, Y., & Kassouf, W. (2016). Bladder cancer. *The Lancet*, *388*(10061), 2796–2810. Available from https://doi.org/10.1016/S0140-6736(16)30512-8.

Keller, S., Ridinger, J., Rupp, A. K., Janssen, J. W. G., & Altevogt, P. (2011). Body fluid derived exosomes as a novel template for clinical diagnostics. *Journal of Translational Medicine*, 9. Available from https://doi.org/10.1186/1479-5876-9-86.

Lässer, C. (2013). Identification and analysis of circulating exosomal microRNA in human body fluids. *Methods in Molecular Biology*, *1024*, 109–128. Available from https://doi.org/10.1007/978-1-62703-453-1_9.

LeBleu, V.S., & Kalluri, R. (2020). Exosomes as a multicomponent biomarker platform in cancer. *Trends Cancer*, *6*(9), 767–774. Available from https://doi.org/10.1016/j.trecan.2020.03.007. Epub 2020 Apr 16. PMID: 32307267.

Li, G., Cuilleron, M., Gentil-Perret, A., & Tostain, J. (2004). Characteristics of image-detected solid renal masses: Implication, for optimal treatment. *International Journal of Urology*, *11*(2), 63–67. Available from https://doi.org/10.1111/j.1442-2042.2004.00750.x.

Li, G., Mallouk, N., Flandrin, P., Garcin, A., Lambert, C., Berremila, S. A., Habchi, H., & Mottet, N. (2020). Evaluation of urinary exosomes' presence for liquid biopsy of clear cell renal cell carcinoma: Protocol for a pilot feasibility study (Preprint). *JMIR Research Protocols*. Available from https://doi.org/10.2196/24423.

Ljungberg, B., Albiges, L., Abu-Ghanem, Y., Bensalah, K., Dabestani, S., Montes, S. F. P., Giles, R. H., Hofmann, F., Hora, M., Kuczyk, M. A., Kuusk, T., Lam, T. B., Marconi, L., Merseburger, A. S., Powles, T., Staehler, M., Tahbaz, R., Volpe, A., & Bex, A. (2019). European association of urology guidelines on renal cell carcinoma: The 2019 update. *European Urology*, *75*(5), 799–810. Available from https://doi.org/10.1016/j.eururo.2019.02.011.

Lodewijk, I., Dueñas, M., Rubio, C., Munera-Maravilla, E., Segovia, C., Bernardini, A., Teijeira, A., Paramio, J. M., & Suárez-Cabrera, C. (2018). Liquid biopsy biomarkers in bladder cancer: A current need for patient diagnosis and monitoring. *International Journal of Molecular Sciences*, *19*(9), 2514. Available from https://doi.org/10.3390/ijms19092514.

Marconi, L., Dabestani, S., Lam, T. B., Hofmann, F., Stewart, F., Norrie, J., Bex, A., Bensalah, K., Canfield, S. E., Hora, M., Kuczyk, M. A., Merseburger, A. S., Mulders, P. F. A., Powles, T., Staehler, M., Ljungberg, B., & Volpe, A. (2016). Systematic review and *meta*-analysis of diagnostic accuracy of percutaneous renal tumour biopsy. *European Urology*, *69* (4), 660–673. Available from https://doi.org/10.1016/j.eururo.2015.07.072.

McKiernan, J., Donovan, M. J., O'Neill, V., Bentink, S., Noerholm, M., Belzer, S., Skog, J., Kattan, M. W., Partin, A., Andriole, G., Brown, G., Wei, J. T., Thompson, I. M., & Carroll, P. (2016). A novel urine exosome gene expression assay to predict high-grade prostate cancer at initial biopsy. *JAMA Oncology*, *2*(7), 882–889. Available from https://doi.org/10.1001/jamaoncol.2016.0097.

Melo, S. A., Luecke, L. B., Kahlert, C., Fernandez, A. F., Gammon, S. T., Kaye, J., LeBleu, V. S., Mittendorf, E. A., Weitz, J., Rahbari, N., Reissfelder, C., Pilarsky, C., Fraga, M. F., Piwnica-Worms, D., & Kalluri, R. (2015). Glypican-1 identifies cancer exosomes and detects early pancreatic cancer. *Nature*, *523*(7559), 177–182. Available from https://doi.org/10.1038/nature14581.

Monguió-Tortajada, M., Gálvez-Montón, C., Bayes-Genis, A., Roura, S., & Borràs, F. E. (2019). Extracellular vesicle isolation methods: Rising impact of size-exclusion chromatography. *Cellular and Molecular Life Sciences*, 2369–2382. Available from https://doi.org/10.1007/s00018-019-03071-y.

Neveu, B., Jain, P., Têtu, B., Wu, L., Fradet, Y., & Pouliot, F. (2016). A PCA3 gene-based transcriptional amplification system targeting primary prostate cancer. *Oncotarget*, *7*(2), 1300–1310. Available from https://doi.org/10.18632/oncotarget.6360.

Palmirotta, R., Lovero, D., Cafforio, P., Felici, C., Mannavola, F., Pellè, E., Quaresmini, D., Tucci, M., & Silvestris, F. (2018). Liquid biopsy of cancer: A multimodal diagnostic tool in clinical oncology. *Therapeutic Advances in Medical Oncology*, 10. Available from https://doi.org/10.1177/1758835918794630.

Pang, B., Zhu, Y., Ni, J., Thompson, J., Malouf, D., Bucci, J., Graham, P., & Li, Y. (2020). Extracellular vesicles: The next generation of biomarkers for liquid biopsy-based prostate cancer diagnosis. *Theranostics*, *10*(5), 2309–2326. Available from https://doi.org/10.7150/thno.39486.

Raposo, G., & Stoorvogel, W. (2013). Extracellular vesicles: Exosomes, microvesicles, and friends. *Journal of Cell Biology*, *200*(4), 373–383. Available from https://doi.org/10.1083/jcb.201211138.

Siegel, R. L., Miller, K. D., & Jemal, A. (2020). Cancer statistics, 2020. *CA Cancer Journal for Clinicians*, *70*(1), 7–30. Available from https://doi.org/10.3322/caac.21590.

Solé, C., Goicoechea, I., Goñi, A., Schramm, M., Armesto, M., Arestin, M., Manterola, L., Tellaetxe, M., Alberdi, A., Nogueira, L., Roumiguie, M., López, J. I., Jaka, J. P. S., Urruticoechea, A., Vergara, I., Loizaga-Iriarte, A., Unda, M., Carracedo, A., Malavaud, B., & Lawrie, C. H. (2020). The urinary transcriptome as a source of biomarkers for prostate cancer. *Cancers*, *12*(2). Available from https://doi.org/10.3390/cancers12020513.

Soukup, V., Babjuk, M., Bellmunt, J., Dalbagni, G., Giannarini, G., Hakenberg, O. W., Herr, H., Lechevallier, E., & Ribal, M. J. (2012). Follow-up after surgical treatment of bladder cancer: A critical analysis of the literature. *European Urology*, *62*(2), 290–302. Available from https://doi.org/10.1016/j.eururo.2012.05.008.

Théry, C., Witwer, K. W., Aikawa, E., Alcaraz, M. J., Anderson, J. D., Andriantsitohaina, R., Antoniou, A., Arab, T., Archer, F., Atkin-Smith, G. K., Ayre, D. C., Bach, J.-M., Bachurski, D., Baharvand, H., Balaj, L., Baldacchino, S., Bauer, N. N., Baxter, A. A., Bebawy, M., & Zuba-Surma, E. K. (2018). Minimal information for studies of extracellular vesicles 2018

(MISEV2018): A position statement of the International Society for Extracellular Vesicles and update of the MISEV2014 guidelines. *Journal of Extracellular Vesicles*, *7*(1), 1535750. Available from https://doi.org/10.1080/20013078.2018.1535750.

Yang, C. S., Choi, E., Idrees, M. T., Chen, S., & Wu, H. H. (2017). Percutaneous biopsy of the renal mass: FNA or core needle biopsy? *Cancer Cytopathology*, *125*(6), 407–415. Available from https://doi.org/10.1002/cncy.21852.

Zhang, W., Ni, M., Su, Y., Wang, H., Zhu, S., Zhao, A., & Li, G. (2018). MicroRNAs in serum exosomes as potential biomarkers in clear-cell renal cell carcinoma. *European Urology Focus*, *4*(3), 412–419. Available from https://doi.org/10.1016/j.euf.2016.09.007.

Zhao, A., Péoc'H, M., Cottier, M., Genin, C., Mottet, N., & Li, G. (2015). Cell-free RNA content in urine as a possible molecular diagnostic tool for clear cell renal cell carcinoma. *International Journal of Cancer*, *136*(11), 2610–2615. Available from https://doi.org/10.1002/ijc.29313.

Chapter 3

The molecular mechanism of novel oncogenes dysregulating signaling pathways associated with cervical carcinoma

Kaoutar Anouar Tadlaoui[1] and Moulay Mustapha Ennaji[2]

[1]*Team of Virology, Oncology, and Biotechnologies, Laboratory of Virology, Oncology, Biosciences, Environment and New Energies (LVO-BEEN), Faculty of Sciences and Techniques Mohammedia, University Hassan II of Casablanca, Casablanca, Morocco,* [2]*Group Leader Research team of Virology, Oncology, and Biotechnologies, Head of Laboratory of Virology, Oncology, Biosciences, Environment and New Energies (LVO-BEEN), Faculty of Sciences and Techniques Mohammedia, University Hassan II of Casablanca, Casablanca, Morocco*

3.1 Introduction

Cervical cancer (CC), that is, the cancer of the cervix, is the second most common cancer in women after breast cancer and its incidence is increasing worldwide (Dasari et al., 2015). In terms of mortality, it ranks fourth among the fatal cancers in women (Liu et al., 2020). According to global statistics, there are approximately 500,000 new cases and 300,000 deaths from CC each year worldwide (Iwata et al., 2016). About 90% of these cases have been reported to occur in developing countries (Zhang & Sun, Zhao, et al., 2019).

Primarily, CC is due to the persistence of *Human papillomavirus* (HPV) infection, which is the most common sexually transmitted infection in the world (Kessler, 2017). HPV comprises more than 200 genotypes (Lizano et al., 2009). Among them, about 50 genotypes cause genitourinary infections (Ljubojevic & Skerlev, 2014), leading to the development of various cancers. Approximately 13 genotypes (HPV 16, 18, 31, 33, 35, 39, 45, 51, 52, 56, 58, 59, and 68) are high-risk oncogenic viruses (HR-HPV), of which the two main ones are HPV-16 and HPV-18, which are involved in 70% of CC incidences (Graham, 2010; Tadlaoui et al., 2020).

Although the most commonly used clinical therapies for CC treatment are surgery, radiotherapy, and chemotherapy, the ineffectiveness and poor

Immunological Implications and Molecular Diagnostics of Genitourinary Cancer.
DOI: https://doi.org/10.1016/B978-0-323-85496-2.00004-X

and severe side effects of these treatments have been observed, and the overall prognosis of patients with CC remains obscure, especially in those with advanced disease(Cáceres-Durán et al., 2020; Luan & Wang, 2018).

However, other factors contribute to the tumor development of CC, including genetic and epigenetic factors of the host, which are mainly involved in the integration of viral DNA into the chromosomal DNA of the host (Liu et al., 2020). This involves a variety of cell signaling pathways and a series of genetic and epigenetic alterations where certain oncogenes are activated and other tumor suppressor genes are deactivated (S. Yang et al., 2020). Therefore it increases the progression of cell proliferation and reduces apoptosis, thereby promoting CC pathogenesis and metastasis.

Nevertheless, the exploration of novel oncogenic factors and signaling pathways associated with invasiveness and metastases has provided a potential target for the development of an antitumor therapeutic strategy against advanced CC.

Recent studies have identified new oncogenes discussed in this chapter such as calponin 3 (CNN3), antisilencing function 1B (ASF1B), colorectal neoplasia differentially expressed (CRNDE), proline-rich protein 11 (PRR11), which play important biological roles in the development and progression of CC by inducing various molecular changes in CC tissues and aberrant dysregulation of cell signaling pathways involved in CC.

3.2 Cervical cancer overview

3.2.1 Epidemiology of cervical cancer

Globally, CC is the fourth most common cancer among women. In 2018 the World Health Organization (WHO) estimated the number of new cases at 570,000 (Ferlay et al., 2018), while in terms of mortality, the WHO estimated the number of deaths as 311,000. Almost 90% of this death rate has occurred in developing countries (Ferlay et al., 2018).

On November 17, 2020, the WHO released a global strategy to accelerate the elimination of CC as a public health problem and described it as a disease that can be prevented in the future. This global strategy is based on vaccination, screening, and treatment of CC (Zhang et al., 2020).

If these are successfully implemented, WHO estimates by means of new measures, the annual incidence rate of CC is expected to increase from 570,000 to 700,000 new cases between 2018 and 2030, and the annual number of deaths is expected to increase from 311,000 to 400,000 deaths (2020).

3.2.2 Anatomopathology of the cervix

The uterus (Fig. 3.1) is a smooth, hollow female muscular organ, approximately 10 cm in length, pear-shaped, and thick-walled. It is composed of a body and a cervix; the former is made up of the myometrium, lined with serosa (connective tissue), enveloping the uterine cavity, which is lined by

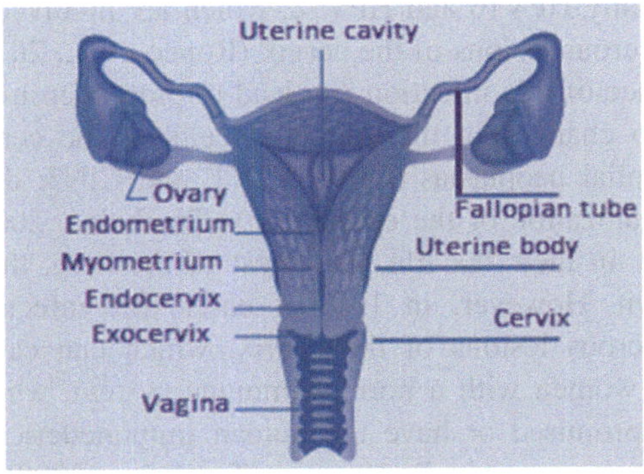

FIGURE 3.1 **The structure of the uterus (longitudinal section). The anatomy of the female reproductive system shows the uterine cavity, the ovary, the fallopian tubes, the cervix, the vagina, and three distinct tissue layers making up the wall of the uterus body.**

the endometrium. Thus on both sides of the upper part of the body of the uterus, the fallopian tubes open up. These lead the egg to the uterus. Below the body is the cervix, made up of dense fibromuscular tissue. The cervical canal crossing the middle of the cervix contains a viscous mucus secreted by the mucous membrane. The cervix opens into the vagina via an intravaginal part known as the "tench muzzle" (Balaya et al., 2016).

CC or cervical carcinoma is a tumor of epithelial origin. Most often (around 80%), it is a squamous cell carcinoma following the involvement of "slice snout" cells, while at times (between 10% and 20%) it is an adenocarcinoma when the cells of the cervical canal are affected. However, nonepithelial cervical tumors such as sarcomas, melanomas, and lymphomas, are not included (Balaya et al., 2016).

3.2.3 The different cancers of the cervix

CC develops precisely in the lower, narrow part of the uterus. The most common form of these cancers (around 80% of cases) develops from cells of the Malpighian epithelium: these are squamous cell carcinomas, whereas cancers that develop from the glandular epithelium are called adenocarcinomas (Pointreau et al., 2010). These types of CC usually develop from precancerous lesions inside the cervix, called cervical dysplasias, linked in particular to an HR-HPV infection. Upon being treated early according to a specific protocol, these tumors provide a good prognosis.

3.2.4 Risk factors of cervical cancer

The main cause of the development of CC is the persistence of a genital infection, sexually transmitted and generated by certain types of the

HR-HPV, especially HPV16 and HPV18, which are involved in 82% of cancers and precancerous lesions of the cervix (Ronco et al., 2010).

The persistence of this infection can lead to precancerous cervical lesions corresponding to changes in the epithelial cells of the cervix, particularly called intraepithelial neoplasias (CIN1, CIN2, and CIN3: depending on the degree of disorganization of the epithelium) (Tranbaloc, 2008). Women can be infected early in their sex life, and most of the time, the infection goes away on its own. However, in 10% of cases, the infection persists and induces precancerous lesions of the cervix, which can cause cancer after 15–20 years in women with a normal immune system, while in those who are immunocompromised or have the human immunodeficiency virus, that is, HIV, cancer may appear in 5–10 years (Tranbaloc, 2008).

However, under the influence of other factors such as early sexual intercourse, multiple sexual partners, multiparity, precocious puberty, late menopause, certain infections (Chlamydia or herpes virus), alcohol consumption or smoking, the risk of developing CC is higher (Tranbaloc, 2008).

There is also another important risk factor involved in the development of CC, which is the prolonged use of hormonal contraceptives (pill, implant, and patch or hormonal intrauterine device). The longer the duration of administration of oral contraceptives, the greater the risk of developing CC. However, this risk decreases when treatment is stopped until it becomes almost zero for 10 years (IARC, 2012).

3.3 The leading oncogenes related to cervical cancer development

3.3.1 Calponin 3

CNN3 is one of the three isoforms of calponin, actin filament binding proteins with broad tissue distributions. CNN3 is involved in the rearrangement of the cytoskeleton (Junghans & Herzog, 2018) and the development of the central nervous system (Flemming et al., 2015). Subsequent studies provided evidence for other functions of CNN3, such as downregulation of trophoblast cell fusion, inhibition of myoblast cell fusion during differentiation (Shibukawa et al., 2010), as well as alteration of the formation of primary skin fibroblasts stress fibers and consequently decrease in cell motility and contractile capacity of fibroblasts (Daimon et al., 2013). CNN3 plays a role in cell differentiation, cell migration, and cell proliferation through remodeling of cytoskeleton and stress fiber formation (Daimon et al., 2013; Shibukawa et al., 2013).

However, CNN3 was related to lymph node and peritoneal metastases in colorectal cancer (Nakarai et al., 2015), and it regulates cell invasion and doxorubicin resistance in gastric cancer (Hong et al., 2019).

According to recent studies, CNN3 mRNA expression has been elevated in CC tissue. CNN3 has been implicated in the proliferation, migration, and invasion of CC cells and in the acceleration of the growth and metastasis of xenografted tumors in immunodeficient mice (Xia et al., 2020). In addition, CNN3 controls the genetic transcription of the ribosomal protein P1 lateral stem subunit (RPLP1) and mediates the regulation of the viability and motility of CC cells (Xia et al., 2020).

In brief, CNN 3 acts as an oncogene to promote the viability and motility of CC cells, as well as accelerate cell proliferation and metastasis, by affecting the expression of RPLP1 (Xia et al., 2020).

3.3.2 Antisilencing function 1B

ASF1B is one of the two paralogy proteins (ASF1A and ASF1B) of antisilencing function 1 (ASF1). The latter is a major histone H3-H4 chaperone protein that plays a role in chromatin-based cell progression of DNA replication, repair of DNA damage, and regulation of transcription (Messiaen et al., 2016; Peng et al., 2010). The role of ASF1A is to participate in DNA repair and cell senescence, while ASF1B is involved in cell proliferation (Messiaen et al., 2016; Paul et al., 2016).

Different studies have shown that ASF1B acts as an oncogene to promote the development of various cancers and progression, including prostate cancer, renal cell carcinoma, breast cancer, and CC (Corpet et al., 2011; Han et al., 2018; Jiangqiao et al., 2019; Liu et al., 2020).

Corpet and her research team showed that ASF1B mRNA overexpression correlates with tumor progression in breast cancer. Therefore they proposed that ASF1B may be a novel proliferation biomarker and serve for the early diagnosis and good prognosis of breast cancer (Corpet et al., 2011).

However, another research group revealed that ASF1B was overexpressed in cancerous tissues of CC as well as in CC cell lines: CaSki and HeLa cells. They also reported for the first time that ASF1B and cyclin-dependent kinase 9 (CDK9) could bind and function as factors in a nuclear complex to promote cancerous progression of CC via coimmunoprecipitation technique and the colocalization of ASF1B and CDK9 in the nucleus (Liu et al., 2020). CDK9 is a cyclin-dependent kinase associated with positive transcription elongation factor b (P-TEFb) and is a transcriptional activator to upgrade RNA polymerase II (RNAPII) promoter-proximal break release (Zhang, Pandey, et al., 2018). CDK9 is involved in many cancers such as CC (Xu et al., 2019), breast cancer (Schlafstein et al., 2018), ovarian cancer (Wang, Dean, et al., 2019), acute myeloid leukemia (Zhang & Tao, 2019), prostate cancer (Rahaman et al., 2016), and osteosarcoma (Ma et al., 2019).

A study showed that CDK9 was a protein ubiquitinated and degraded by the proteasome, and its ubiquitination was modulated by cyclin T1 and $p45^{SKP2}$ (Kiernan et al., 2001). Liu's team proposed a new mechanism in their research on CC, where they investigated the link between CDK9 stabilization and the ASF1B-CDK9 cofactor relationship (Liu et al., 2020). Thus they indicated that CDK9 was unstable with a half-life of 12 h and proposed a new molecular mechanism by which ASF1B could promote CC progression through stabilization of CDK9 protein while inhibiting its ubiquitination and proteasome-mediated degradation (Liu et al., 2020).

Furthermore, Liu's team found in their research that ASF1B is an oncogene involved in the tumor cell proliferation, migration, and antiapoptosis of CC cells (Liu et al., 2020). Therefore ASF1B can be regarded as a novel potential marker and therapeutic target for the diagnosis and prognosis of CC.

3.3.3 Long noncoding RNA colorectal neoplasia differentially expressed

CRNDE is an RNA gene, located at human chromosome 16q12.2 and affiliated with the long noncoding RNA (lncRNA) class (Zhang, Yin, et al., 2018).

Different studies have reported that CRNDE is upregulated in different malignant tumors such as colorectal cancer, gastrointestinal cancers, bladder, hepatocellular carcinoma, and other cancers (Cheng et al., 2018; Han et al., 2017; He et al., 2019; Ji et al., 2019; Liang et al., 2018). CRNDE has been found to be highly upregulated in CC tissues and cell lines. Its overexpression was positively correlated with advanced stage of FIGO, lymph node metastases, and low rate of overall survival. In addition, CRNDE has been shown to influence proliferation and apoptosis in CC cells by targeting the PI3K/AKT pathway (Yang et al., 2018).

Furthermore, CRNDE acts as an oncogene in CC by mop up miR-183 while modulating expression of CCNB1 (cyclin B1) proteins (Bai et al., 2020). CCNB1 is a regulatory protein linked to mitosis by competitively binding to miR-183 (Bai et al., 2020).

lncRNAs play a major role in the progression of CC by absorbing tumor suppressor miRNAs and by involving certain proteins and cell signaling pathways, thus inducing several alterations at the cell cycle level. (m) lncRNA CRNDE acts as an oncogene in CC by blotting miR-183.

The function of the CRNDE/miR-183/CCNB1 axis in regulating the proliferation, migration, invasion, and apoptosis of cancer cells presents a promising diagnostic strategy for the treatment of CC (Zhang, Yin, et al., 2018). Thus the oncogenic effect of CRNDE inhibits the expression of the upregulated apoptosis modulator p53 (PUMA) and reduces the PUMA signaling pathway, suggesting that CRNDE can act as not only a diagnostic biomarker with high sensitivity and specificity in tissues and plasma but also an effective prognostic and therapeutic potential target to prevent the progression of CC (Yang et al., 2018).

3.3.4 Proline-rich Protein 11

PRR11 is a relatively new molecular gene, located on human chromosome 17q22 region, which plays a key role in the carcinogenesis (Chen et al., 2015). In 2013 PRR11 was first identified and functionally characterized by Ji et al., who discovered its main role in cell cycle progression and pathogenesis of cancer (Ji et al., 2013).

Several studies show that this gene is conserved throughout evolution and is upregulated in various tumors, including cancerous tumors of the brain, breast, cervix, ovaries, lungs, esophagus, stomach, pancreas, colorectal, hilar cholangiocarcinoma, and tongue squamous cell carcinoma (Chen et al., 2015; Chen et al., 2020; Ji et al., 2013; Song et al., 2015; Tan et al., 2017; Wang Zhang et al., 2019; Zhang et al., 2015; Zhou et al., 2014; Zhu et al., 2018).

However, previous studies have shown that the recurrence of PRR11 and its aggressiveness in several types of cell lines and cancerous tissues is due to its overexpression, which induces the transcriptional regulation of related genes, subsequently promoting cell cycle progression and apoptosis (Larance et al., 2013; Zhu et al., 2018).

According to a study on the effect of PRR11 on cell migration through the epithelial–mesenchymal transition (EMT), and among biological processes, genes associated with cell adhesion and cell migration were mainly altered in PRR11 cells -KO. Since the vimentin protein (VIM) is a marker for EMT, knockdown of PRR11 resulted in decreased expression of VIM and increased expression of E-cadherin. Therefore PRR11 is well involved in cell migration/invasion (Tan et al., 2017; Zhou et al., 2014).

PRR11, a candidate oncogene, regulates key genes associated with the development of tumors (Song et al., 2015; Wang et al., 2015; Zhu et al., 2018). It has been implicated in cell cycle progression, apoptosis, and tumorigenesis of CC and other tumors. The high expression of PRR11 was correlated with CC tumor size, histological grade, and poor prognosis, thus playing a biological role in CC proliferation (Xu & Li, 2020).

Studies have reported that PRR11 may participate in cell cycle regulation by altering the expression of cell cyclin A1, RRM1, MAP4K4, and DHRS2, and alterations in cyclin expression affect cell cycle progression (Ji et al., 2013).

However, silencing of PRR11 blocks cells in phase G1 downregulates expression of the cyclin D1 protein (Xu & Li, 2020). The latter is a key protein for cells to switch from S phase to G1 phase and promotes upregulation of cells entering the proliferative phase (Yi et al., 2017). As a result, the CC cell viability and tumorigenic potential are inhibited.

Furthermore, Xu and li have showed that PRR11 can regulate apoptosis in CC cells by influencing the expression of the caspase-3 protein (Xu & Li, 2020).

Therefore PRR11 may serve as a potential new target for the diagnosis and the treatment of CC, by regulating the main genes involved in cell cycles and tumorigenesis.

3.4 Conclusion

Accumulating evidence has confirmed the aberrant overexpression of several oncogenes in various human cancers including CC, which correlated with advanced clinic-pathological features and poor prognosis.

Besides the oncogenes mentioned in this chapter, many other novel oncogenes have been reported to be dysregulated in CC and playing multiple roles in its tumor progression and pathogenesis. Each oncogene, according to its own mechanism of action, promotes the proliferation, differentiation, migration, or invasion of cancer cells and in particular metastases, and suppresses apoptosis.

Nevertheless, the detailed regulatory mechanisms of those oncogenes remain to be elucidated, and further experimental and clinical studies are necessary to offer new alternative approaches for developing an antitumor CC therapeutic strategy for early prognosis, and better diagnosis in the near future.

Acknowledgment

I would like to extend my deep thanks and gratitude for support, encouragement, and contribution adopted by Faculty of Sciences and Techniques of Mohammedia, University Hassan II of Casablanca, Morocco, my Professor My Mustapha ENNAJI and my team research of Virology, Oncology, Total Quality and Medical Biotechnology.

References

Bai, X., Wang, W., Zhao, P., Wen, J., Guo, X., Shen, T., Shen, J., & Yang, X. (2020). LncRNA CRNDE acts as an oncogene in cervical cancer through sponging miR-183 to regulate CCNB1 expression. *Carcinogenesis*, *41*(1), 111–121. Available from https://doi.org/10.1093/carcin/bgz166.

Balaya, V., Uhl, J. F., Lanore, A., Salachas, C., Samoyeau, T., Ngo, C., Bensaid, C., Cornou, C., Rossi, L., Douard, R., Bats, A. S., Lecuru, F., & Delmas, V. (2016). Modélisation anatomique 3D du pelvis féminin par dissection anatomique assistée par ordinateur: Applications et perspectives. *Journal de Gynecologie Obstetrique et Biologie de La Reproduction*, *45*(5), 467–477. Available from https://doi.org/10.1016/j.jgyn.2016.01.006.

Cáceres-Durán, M. Á., Ribeiro-Dos-santos, Â., & Vidal, A. F. (2020). Roles and mechanisms of the long noncoding RNAs in cervical cancer. *International Journal of Molecular Sciences*, *21*(24), 1–20. Available from https://doi.org/10.3390/ijms21249742.

Chen, J., Yang, H. M., Zhou, H. C., Peng, R. R., Niu, Z. X., & Kang, C. Y. (2020). PRR11 and SKA2 promote the proliferation, migration and invasion of esophageal carcinoma cells. *Oncology Letters*, *20*(1), 639–646. Available from https://doi.org/10.3892/ol.2020.11615.

Chen, Y., Cha, Z., Fang, W., Qian, B., Yu, W., Li, W., Yu, G., & Gao, Y. (2015). The prognostic potential and oncogenic effects of PRR11 expression in hilar cholangiocarcinoma. *Oncotarget*, *6*(24), 20419–20433. Available from https://doi.org/10.18632/oncotarget.3983.

Cheng, J., Chen, J., Zhang, X., Mei, H., Wang, F., & Cai, Z. (2018). Overexpression of CRNDE promotes the progression of bladder cancer. *Biomedicine and Pharmacotherapy*, *99*, 638–644. Available from https://doi.org/10.1016/j.biopha.2017.12.055.

Corpet, A., De Koning, L., Toedling, J., Savignoni, A., Berger, F., Lemaître, C., O'Sullivan, R. J., Karlseder, J., Barillot, E., Asselain, B., Sastre-Garau, X., & Almouzni, G. (2011). Asf1b, the necessary Asf1 isoform for proliferation, is predictive of outcome in breast cancer. *The EMBO Journal, 30*(3), 480–493. Available from https://doi.org/10.1038/emboj.2010.335.

Daimon, E., Shibukawa, Y., & Wada, Y. (2013). Calponin 3 regulates stress fiber formation in dermal fibroblasts during wound healing. *Archives of Dermatological Research, 305*(7), 571–584. Available from https://doi.org/10.1007/s00403-013-1343-8.

Dasari, S., Wudayagiri, R., & Valluru, L. (2015). Cervical cancer: Biomarkers for diagnosis and treatment. *Clinica Chimica Acta, 445*, 7–11. Available from https://doi.org/10.1016/j.cca.2015.03.005.

Ferlay, J., Ervik, M., Lam, Colombet, M., Mery, Piñeros, M., Znaor, Soerjomataram, Bray (2018). Global Cancer Observatory: Cancer Today.

Flemming, A., Huang, Q. Q., Jin, J. P., Jumaa, H., & Herzog, S. (2015). A conditional knockout mouse model reveals that Calponin-3 is dispensable for early B cell development. *PLoS One, 10*(6). Available from https://doi.org/10.1371/journal.pone.0128385.

Graham, S. V. (2010). Human papillomavirus: Gene expression, regulation and prospects for novel diagnostic methods and antiviral therapies. *Future Microbiology, 5*(10), 1493–1506. Available from https://doi.org/10.2217/fmb.10.107.

Han, G., Zhang, X., Liu, P., Yu, Q., Li, Z., Yu, Q., & Wei, X. (2018). Knockdown of anti-silencing function 1B histone chaperone induces cell apoptosis via repressing PI3K/Akt pathway in prostate cancer. *International Journal of Oncology, 53*(5), 2056–2066. Available from https://doi.org/10.3892/ijo.2018.4526.

Han, P., Li, J. w, Zhang, B. m, Lv, J. c, Li, Y. m, Gu, X. y, Yu, Z. w, Jia, Y. h, Bai, X. f, Li, L., Liu, Y. L., & Cui, B. B. (2017). The lncRNA CRNDE promotes colorectal cancer cell proliferation and chemoresistance via miR-181a-5p-mediated regulation of Wnt/β-catenin signaling. *Molecular Cancer, 16*(1). Available from https://doi.org/10.1186/s12943-017-0583-1.

He, T. Y., Li, S. H., Huang, J., Gong, M., & Li, G. (2019). Prognostic value of long non-coding RNA crnde in gastrointestinal cancers: A *meta*-analysis. *Cancer Management and Research, 11*, 5629–5642. Available from https://doi.org/10.2147/CMAR.S201646.

Hong, K. S., Kim, H., Kim, S. H., Kim, M., & Yoo, J. (2019). Calponin 3 regulates cell invasion and doxorubicin resistance in gastric cancer. *Gastroenterology Research and Practice, 2019*. Available from https://doi.org/10.1155/2019/3024970.

IARC. (2012). GLOBOCAN: Estimated cancer incidence, mortality and prevalence worldwide in 2012. Available from <http://globocan.iarc.fr/Pages/online.aspx>.

Iwata, T., Miyauchi, A., Suga, Y., Nishio, H., Nakamura, M., Ohno, A., Hirao, N., Morisada, T., Tanaka, K., Ueyama, H., Watari, H., & Aoki, D. (2016). Neoadjuvant chemotherapy for locally advanced cervical cancer. *Chinese Journal of Cancer Research, 28*(2), 235–240. Available from https://doi.org/10.21147/j.issn.1000-9604.2016.02.13.

Ji, D., Jiang, C., Zhang, L., Liang, N., Jiang, T., Yang, B., & Liang, H. (2019). LncRNA CRNDE promotes hepatocellular carcinoma cell proliferation, invasion, and migration through regulating miR-203/ BCAT1 axis. *Journal of Cellular Physiology, 234*(5), 6548–6560. Available from https://doi.org/10.1002/jcp.27396.

Ji, Y., Xie, M., Lan, H., Zhang, Y., Long, Y., Weng, H., Li, D., Cai, W., Zhu, H., Niu, Y., Yang, Z., Zhang, C., Song, F., & Bu, Y. (2013). PRR11 is a novel gene implicated in cell cycle progression and lung cancer. *International Journal of Biochemistry and Cell Biology, 45*(3), 645–656. Available from https://doi.org/10.1016/j.biocel.2012.12.002.

Jiangqiao, Z., Tao, Q., Zhongbao, C., Xiaoxiong, M., Long, Z., Jilin, Z., & Tianyu, W. (2019). Anti-silencing function 1B histone chaperone promotes cell proliferation and migration via activation of the AKT pathway in clear cell renal cell carcinoma. *Biochemical and Biophysical Research Communications*, *511*(1), 165–172. Available from https://doi.org/10.1016/j.bbrc.2019.02.060.

Junghans, D., & Herzog, S. (2018). Cnn3 regulates neural tube morphogenesis and neuronal stem cell properties. *The FEBS Journal*, *285*(2), 325–338. Available from https://doi.org/10.1111/febs.14338.

Kessler, T. A. (2017). Cervical cancer: Prevention and early detection. *Seminars in Oncology Nursing*, *33*(2), 172–183. Available from https://doi.org/10.1016/j.soncn.2017.02.005.

Kiernan, R. E., Emiliani, S., Nakayama, K., Castro, A., Labbé, J. C., Lorca, T., Nakayama, K. I., & Benkirane, M. (2001). Interaction between cyclin T1 and SCFSKP2 targets CDK9 for ubiquitination and degradation by the proteasome. *Molecular and Cellular Biology*, *21*(23), 7956–7970. Available from https://doi.org/10.1128/MCB.21.23.7956-7970.2001.

Larance, M., Ahmad, Y., Kirkwood, K. J., Ly, T., & Lamond, A. I. (2013). Global subcellular characterization of protein degradation using quantitative proteomics. Molecular and Cellular. *Proteomics*, *12*(3), 638–650. Available from https://doi.org/10.1074/mcp.M112.024547.

Liang, C., Zhang, B., Ge, H., Xu, Y., Li, G., & Wu, J. (2018). Long non-coding RNA CRNDE as a potential prognostic biomarker in solid tumors: A *meta*-analysis. *Clinica Chimica Acta*, *481*, 99–107. Available from https://doi.org/10.1016/j.cca.2018.02.039.

Liu, X., Song, J., Zhang, Y., Wang, H., Sun, H., Feng, X., Hou, M., Chen, G., Tang, Q., & Ji, M. (2020). ASF1B promotes cervical cancer progression through stabilization of CDK9. *Cell Death & Disease*, *11*(8). Available from https://doi.org/10.1038/s41419-020-02872-5.

Lizano, M., Berumen, J., & García-Carrancá, A. (2009). HPV-related carcinogenesis: Basic concepts, viral types and variants. *Archives of Medical Research*, *40*(6), 428–434. Available from https://doi.org/10.1016/j.arcmed.2009.06.001.

Ljubojevic, S., & Skerlev, M. (2014). HPV-associated diseases. *Clinics in Dermatology*, *32*(2), 227–234. Available from https://doi.org/10.1016/j.clindermatol.2013.08.007.

Luan, X., & Wang, Y. (2018). LncRNA XLOC_006390 facilitates cervical cancer tumorigenesis and metastasis as a ceRNA against miR-331-3p and miR-338-3p. *Journal of Gynecologic Oncology*, *29*(6). Available from https://doi.org/10.3802/jgo.2018.29.e95.

Ma, H., Seebacher, N. A., Hornicek, F. J., & Duan, Z. (2019). Cyclin-dependent kinase 9 (CDK9) is a novel prognostic marker and therapeutic target in osteosarcoma. *EBioMedicine*, *39*, 182–193. Available from https://doi.org/10.1016/j.ebiom.2018.12.022.

Messiaen, S., Guiard, J., Aigueperse, C., Fliniaux, I., Tourpin, S., Barroca, V., Allemand, I., Fouchet, P., Livera, G., & Vernet, M. (2016). Loss of the histone chaperone ASF1B reduces female reproductive capacity in mice. *Reproduction*, *151*(5), 477–489. Available from https://doi.org/10.1530/REP-15-0327.

Nakarai, C., Osawa, K., Akiyama, M., Matsubara, N., Ikeuchi, H., Yamano, T., Hirota, S., Tomita, N., Usami, M., & Kido, Y. (2015). Expression of AKR1C3 and CNN3 as markers for detection of lymph node metastases in colorectal cancer. *Clinical and Experimental Medicine*, *15*(3), 333–341. Available from https://doi.org/10.1007/s10238-014-0298-1.

Paul, P. K., Rabaglia, M. E., Wang, C. Y., Stapleton, D. S., Leng, N., Kendziorski, C., Lewis, P. W., Keller, M. P., & Attie, A. D. (2016). Histone chaperone ASF1B promotes human β-cell proliferation via recruitment of histone H3.3. *Cell Cycle*, *15*(23), 3191–3202. Available from https://doi.org/10.1080/15384101.2016.1241914.

Peng, H., Nogueira, M. L., Vogel, J. L., & Kristie, T. M. (2010). Transcriptional coactivator HCF-1 couples the histone chaperone Asf1b to HSV-1 DNA replication components. *Proceedings of the National Academy of Sciences*, *107*(6), 2461–2466. Available from https://doi.org/10.1073/pnas.0911128107.

Pointreau, Y., Denis, F., & Barillot, I. (2010). Cervix cancer. *Cancer Radiotherapie: Journal de la Societe francaise de Radiotherapie Oncologique*, *14*, 147–153.

Rahaman, M. H., Kumarasiri, M., Mekonnen, L. B., Yu, M., Diab, S., Albrecht, H., Milne, R. W., & Wang, S. (2016). Targeting CDK9: A promising therapeutic opportunity in prostate cancer. *Endocrine-Related Cancer*, T211–T226. Available from https://doi.org/10.1530/erc-16-0299.

Ronco, G., Giorgi-Rossi, P., Carozzi, F., Confortini, M., Palma, P. D., Del Mistro, A., Ghiringhello, B., Girlando, S., Gillio-Tos, A., De Marco, L., Naldoni, C., Pierotti, P., Rizzolo, R., Schincaglia, P., Zorzi, M., Zappa, M., Segnan, N., & Cuzick, J. (2010). Efficacy of human papillomavirus testing for the detection of invasive cervical cancers and cervical intraepithelial neoplasia: A randomised controlled trial. *The Lancet Oncology*, *11* (3), 249–257. Available from https://doi.org/10.1016/S1470-2045(09)70360-2.

Schlafstein, A. J., Withers, A. E., Rudra, S., Danelia, D., Switchenko, J. M., Mister, D., Harari, S., Zhang, H., Daddacha, W., Ehdaivand, S., Li, X., Torres, M. A., & Yu, D. S. (2018). CDK9 expression shows role as a potential prognostic biomarker in breast cancer patients who fail to achieve pathologic complete response after neoadjuvant chemotherapy. *International Journal of Breast Cancer*, *2018*. Available from https://doi.org/10.1155/2018/6945129.

Shibukawa, Y., Yamazaki, N., Daimon, E., & Wada, Y. (2013). Rock-dependent calponin 3 phosphorylation regulates myoblast fusion. *Experimental Cell Research*, *319*(5), 633–648. Available from https://doi.org/10.1016/j.yexcr.2012.12.022.

Shibukawa, Y., Yamazaki, N., Kumasawa, K., Daimon, E., Tajiri, M., Okada, Y., Ikawa, M., & Wada, Y. (2010). Calponin 3 regulates actin cytoskeleton rearrangement in trophoblastic cell fusion. *Molecular Biology of the Cell*, *21*(22), 3973–3984. Available from https://doi.org/10.1091/mbc.E10-03-0261.

Song, Z., Liu, W., Xiao, Y., Zhang, M., Luo, Y., Yuan, W., Xu, Y., Yu, G., Hu, Y., & Xie, K. (2015). PRR11 is a prognostic marker and potential oncogene in patients with gastric cancer. *PLoS One*, *10*(8), e0128943. Available from https://doi.org/10.1371/journal.pone.0128943.

Tadlaoui, K. A., Hassou, N., Bennani, B., & Ennaji, M. M. (2020). Emergence of oncogenic high-risk human papillomavirus types and cervical cancer. In *Emerging and Reemerging Viral Pathogens*, (pp. 539–570). Academic Press. Available from https://doi.org/10.1016/B978-0-12-819400-3.00024-7.

Tan, S., Jiang, Z., Hou, A., Wang, J., Zhang, J., & Dai, L. (2017). Expression of PRR11 protein and its correlation with pancreatic cancer and effect on survival. *Oncology Letters*, *13*(6), 4117–4122. Available from https://doi.org/10.3892/ol.2017.5974.

Tranbaloc, P. (2008). Histoire naturelle des lésions précurseurs du cancer du col utérin. *Gynecologie Obstetrique et Fertilite*, *36*(6), 650–655. Available from https://doi.org/10.1016/j.gyobfe.2008.03.016.

Wang, J., Dean, D. C., Hornicek, F. J., Shi, H., & Duan, Z. (2019). Cyclin-dependent kinase 9 (CDK9) is a novel prognostic marker and therapeutic target in ovarian cancer. *FASEB Journal*, *33*(5), 5990–6000. Available from https://doi.org/10.1096/fj.201801789RR.

Wang, Y., Zhang, C., Mai, L., Niu, Y., Wang, Y., & Bu, Y. (2019). PRR11 and SKA2 gene pair is overexpressed and regulated by p53 in breast cancer. *BMB Reports*, *52*(2), 157–162. Available from https://doi.org/10.5483/BMBRep.2019.52.2.207.

Wang, Y., Zhang, Y., Zhang, C., Weng, H., Li, Y., Cai, W., Xie, M., Long, Y., Ai, Q., Liu, Z., Du, G., Wang, S., Niu, Y., Song, F., Ozaki, T., & Bu, Y. (2015). The gene pair PRR11 and SKA2 shares a NF-Y-regulated bidirectional promoter and contributes to lung cancer development. *Biochimica et Biophysica Acta – Gene Regulatory Mechanisms*, *1849*(9), 1133–1144. Available from https://doi.org/10.1016/j.bbagrm.2015.07.002.

WHO (2020). A cervical cancer-free future: first-ever global commitment to eliminate a cancer. Available from <https://www.who.int/news/item/17-11-2020-a-cervical-cancer-free-future-first-ever-global-commitment-to-eliminate-a-cancer>.

Xia, L., Yue, Y., Li, M., Zhang, Y. N., Zhao, L., Lu, W., Wang, X., & Xie, X. (2020). CNN3 acts as a potential oncogene in cervical cancer by affecting RPLP1 mRNA expression. *Scientific Reports*, *10*(1). Available from https://doi.org/10.1038/s41598-020-58947-y.

Xu, J., Xu, S., Fang, Y., Chen, T., Xie, X., & Lu, W. (2019). Cyclin-dependent kinase 9 promotes cervical cancer development via AKT2/p53 pathway. *IUBMB Life*, *71*(3), 347–356. Available from https://doi.org/10.1002/iub.1983.

Xu, M., & Li, C. (2020). The expression significance of PRR11 in cervical cancer and its effect on the proliferation and apoptosis of cervical cancer cells. *Marker Immunoassay and Clinic*, *27*(2), 349–355.

Yang, H. Y., Huang, C. P., Cao, M. M., Wang, Y. F., & Liu, Y. (2018). Long non-coding RNA CRNDE may be associated with poor prognosis by promoting proliferation and inhibiting apoptosis of cervical cancer cells through targeting PI3K/AKT. *Neoplasma*, *65*(6), 872–880. Available from https://doi.org/10.4149/neo_2018_171225N841.

Yang, S., Liu, L., Xu, D., & Li, X. (2020). The relationship of the TLR9 and TLR2 genetic polymorphisms with cervical cancer risk: A *Meta*-analysis of case-control studies. *Pathology and Oncology Research*, *26*(1), 307–315. Available from https://doi.org/10.1007/s12253-018-0465-x.

Yi, Q., Liang, L., & Rongmiao, Z. (2017). Study on the cell cycle arrest effect of artesunate-induced gastric adenocarcinoma SGC-7901. Chinese. *Journal of Coal Industry Medicine*, *20*(6).

Zhang, C., Zhang, Y., Li, Y., Zhu, H., Wang, Y., Cai, W., Zhu, J., Ozaki, T., & Bu, Y. (2015). PRR11 regulates late-S to G2/M phase progression and induces premature chromatin condensation (PCC). *Biochemical and Biophysical Research Communications*, *458*(3), 501–508. Available from https://doi.org/10.1016/j.bbrc.2015.01.139.

Zhang, H., Pandey, S., Travers, M., Sun, H., Morton, G., Madzo, J., Chung, W., Khowsathit, J., Perez-Leal, O., Barrero, C. A., Merali, C., Okamoto, Y., Sato, T., Pan, J., Garriga, J., Bhanu, N. V., Simithy, J., Patel, B., Huang, J., & Issa, J. P. J. (2018). Targeting CDK9 reactivates epigenetically silenced genes in cancer. *Cell*, *175*(5), 1244–1258. Available from https://doi.org/10.1016/j.cell.2018.09.051, e26.

Zhang, J., Yin, M., Peng, G., & Zhao, Y. (2018). CRNDE: An important oncogenic long non-coding RNA in human cancers. *Cell Proliferation*, *51*(3), e12440. Available from https://doi.org/10.1111/cpr.12440.

Zhang, S., Xu, H., Zhang, L., & Qiao, Y. (2020). Cervical cancer: Epidemiology, risk factors and screening. *Chinese Journal of Cancer Research*, *32*(6), 720–728. Available from https://doi.org/10.21147/j.issn.1000-9604.2020.06.05.

Zhang, X., & Tao, W. (2019). Long noncoding RNA LINC00152 facilitates the leukemogenesis of acute myeloid leukemia by promoting CDK9 through miR-193a. *DNA and Cell Biology*, *38*(3), 236–242. Available from https://doi.org/10.1089/dna.2018.4482.

Zhang, Y., Sun, B., Zhao, L., Liu, Z., Xu, Z., Tian, Y., & Hao, C. (2019). Up-regulation of miRNA-148a inhibits proliferation, invasion, and migration while promoting apoptosis of cervical cancer cells by down-regulating RRS1. *Bioscience Reports*, *39*(5). Available from https://doi.org/10.1042/BSR20181815.

Zhou, F., Liu, H., Zhang, X., Shen, Y., Zheng, D., Zhang, A., Lai, Y., & Li, H. (2014). Proline-rich protein 11 regulates epithelial-to-mesenchymal transition to promote breast cancer cell invasion. *International Journal of Clinical and Experimental Pathology*, *7*(12), 8692–8699. Available from http://www.ijcep.com/files/ijcep0003244.pdf.

Zhu, J., Hu, H., Wang, J., Yang, Y., & Yi, P. (2018). PRR11 overexpression facilitates ovarian carcinoma cell proliferation, migration, and invasion through activation of the PI3K/AKT/β-catenin pathway. *Cellular Physiology and Biochemistry*, *49*(2), 696–705. Available from https://doi.org/10.1159/000493034.

Chapter 4

Role of epigenetic factors in cancer progression induced by inactivation of tumor suppressors genes

Imane Saif[4], Youssef Ennaji[4], Mohammed El Mzibri[2,3] and Moulay Mustapha Ennaji[1]

[1]Group Leader Research team of Virology, Oncology, and Biotechnologies, Head of Laboratory of Virology, Oncology, Biosciences, Environment and New Energies (LVO-BEEN), Faculty of Sciences and Techniques Mohammedia, University Hassan II of Casablanca, Casablanca, Morocco, [2]Life Sciences Division CNESTEN, Rabat, Morocco, [3]Biology and Medical Research Unit, CNESTEN, Rabat, Morocco, [4]Team of Virology, Oncology, and Biotechnologies, Laboratory of Virology, Oncology, Biosciences, Environment and New Energies (LVO-BEEN), Faculty of Sciences and Techniques Mohammedia, University Hassan II of Casablanca, Casablanca, Morocco

4.1 Introduction

Breast cancer's incidents is 36% worldwide, while ovary cancer is 5% (Siegel et al., 2016). The reports state that approximately 5%–10% of the cases of cancers (breast, colon, and ovary) are due to epigenetic modifications among other causes.

The frequency of cancers could still increase by 50%, and a study anticipated 15 million new cases per year in 2020. The same study estimated 1,685,210 new cancer cases diagnosed in 2016. Lung cancer is by far the leading cause of cancer death among female (26%), followed by breast (14%) and colorectal (8%) cancers (Siegel et al., 2016).

Recent studies have identified important mechanisms of gene expression regulation, investigating how they are active and repressed according to cell type. These codes to lock in gene expression, DNA methylation, and certain posttranslational changes in histones (acetylation and methylation), these factors are studied by molecular biology techniques. Not to mention microRNAs, which are an actor of epigenetics. This modification is called epigenetic

Immunological Implications and Molecular Diagnostics of Genitourinary Cancer.
DOI: https://doi.org/10.1016/B978-0-323-85496-2.00014-2

because it modulates the activity of the genome without affecting its sequence. However, methylation is a major phenomenon in several biological processes. As a gene mutation-induced tumorigenesis process, methylation can lead to cancer by inactivation of tumor suppressor genes. The latter is identified by methyltransferases, which are enzymes that catalyze the transfer reaction of methyl residues on cytosines and are often expressed in cancer (Fang et al., 2007). Other studies have shown that inhibition of transcription results in addition to DNA methylation, posttranslational modification, which affects chromatin, and methylation of histones (Nicolas et al., 2001). Though the correlation between these mechanisms has been investigated, no such correlation has been revealed until now except for a few cases or microRNAs. The development of molecular biology research has shown that changes in DNA sequences cannot explain the entire transmission of phenotypic traits. The concept of epigenetic intervention is thus regarded as a complement of classical genetics, which is concerned with the transmission of acquired features associated with modifications that do not relate to the sequence of the DNA but with the chemical structure of the DNA, the histones which surround it or certain noncoding RNA (Joffin, 2015). Each cell of the human body initially contains the same number of genes; however, only a small number is expressed in a cell, according to the stage of development of the organization or the cellular type considered. To understand how the genes are expressed in a particular cellular type, it is essential to understand at the same time how these genes are activated and repressed (Jones & Takai, 2001).

4.2 Methylation of DNA

Genes that play a crucial role in the malignant transformation process are classified as oncogenes and tumor suppressor genes. The latter ones are genes that contribute to the elimination of tumors as they act on the repression of the cell cycle and are involved in the induction of apoptosis.

Studies have classified genes implied with the release of gynecologic–mammary cancers (breast and ovary) according to their degree of penetrance, as described in Table 4.1. The genes associated with high penetrance have relative risk (rr) of cancer higher than 5 of 10, while the genes with intermediate penetrance have a rr of cancer from 1.5 to 5, as shown in Table 4.1.

There exists a large body of evidence that normal chromosome structure may be affected by methylation, and these human diseases, including cancer, are caused and impacted by abnormal methylation. The clusters of CpGs, called CpG islands, are often found in association with genes, most often in the promoters and first exons but also in regions more toward the 3'end region (Larsen et al., 1992).

There are field mammal genomes, called CpG islets, where these dinucleotides are more strongly concentrated. Small CpG blocks are 0.5–3 KB sequences with G + C contents greater than 50% and an observed/expected CpG ratio equal to or greater than 0.6 (Aerts et al., 2004). These small islets are frequently found upstream, in the promoter and the first exon.

TABLE 4.1 List of tumor suppressor genes most often inactivated by the hypermethylation of CpG located in their promoter region at the time of the tumorogenesis.

Tumor type	Biological role	Gene	Locus	Possibility of long-term risk (%)	References
Genes with strong penetrance					
Breast/ovarian cancer	DNA repair	BRCA1	17q12–21	40–80	Flower et al. (2015)
	DNA repair	BRCA2	13q12–13	20–85	Dhillon et al. (2004)
	Cellular cycle	STK11	19p13.3	32–54	Trojan et al. (2000)
Breast cancer	Cellular cycle	P53	17p13.1	56–90	Suh et al. (2011)
	Response to the growth factors and the hormones	PTEN	10q23.3	25–50	Siddiqui et al. (2016)
Genes with intermediate penetrance					
Breast/ovarian cancer	DNA repair	PALB2	16p12.1	20–40	Potapova et al. (2008)
	Cellular cycle	CHEK2	22q12.1	25–37	Zhang et al. (2010)
	DNA repair	ATM	11q22.3	15–20	Rigi-Ladiz et al. (2011)
	DNA repair	MLH1	3p	At the moderate risk	Koutsimpelas et al. (2012)
	DNA repair	MGMT	10q26.3		Koutsimpelas et al. (2012)
	DNA repair	RASSF1A	3p21.3		Koutsimpelas et al. (2012)

BRCA1, breast cancer 1; *BRCA2*, breast cancer 2; *STK11*, Serine/threonine kinase 11; *TP53*, tumor protein 53; *PTEN*, phosphatase and tensin homolog; *PALB2*, Partner and localizer of BRCA2; *ATM*, ataxia telangiectasia mutated; *CHEK2*, Checkpoint kinase 2; *MLH1*, human mutant L homolog; *MGMT*, O6-methyl guanine DNA methyl transferase; *RASSF1A*, Ras-effector homolog.

Bioinformatic analyses of human genome sequencing have detected 29,000 small islets of CpG throughout the genome (Lander et al., 2001).

The precise mechanisms by which small CpG islets are protected from methylation are unclear, but this lack of methylation appears to be a prerequisite for active transcription. However, the nature of the affected sequences and the absence of associations between these two aberrations strongly support an independent role of hypo- and hypermethylation in tumor initiation and progression (Ehrlich et al., 2003).

The methylation of the DNA is catalyzed by specific enzymes called DNA methyltransferases or DNMT (DNA methyltransferases). The DNMT family is divided into three classes: DNMT1, DNMT2, and DNMT3. All these enzymes use a common catalytic mechanism allowing the transfer of a methyl group (CH3) on carbon 5 of a residue cytosine and employ the cofactor S-Adenosyl L-Methionine (AdoMet) like main source of methyl group (Eden et al., 2003).

For the catalysis to occur, enzyme DNMT must bind at the same time to its target, a cytosine of the DNA, and with donor AdoMet the methyl. The reaction begins when target cytosine is extracted from the double helix of DNA by a phenomenon of inversion and is inserted in the catalytic field of the DNMT (Cheng & Roberts, 2001).

An intermediate covalent complex between the enzyme and the DNA is thus formed. This attack is facilitated by the transitory protonation of the N3 nitrogen of cytosine. A reactive cytosine is created, which then tackles the group in its turn methyl brought by the cofactor AdoMet. Following the loss of its methyl, AdoMet becomes S-adenosyl-L-homocysteine (AdoHcy). The transfer of the methyl group in C5 position is carried out, and the proton present is released and then collected by a basic group of the enzyme. Thus a double connection between carbons 5 and 6 is reformed. Finally, the enzyme is released by E-elimination (Bestor & Ingram, 1983). This reaction leads to the formation of 5-methylcytosine (Jang & Shin, 2013) (Fig. 4.1).

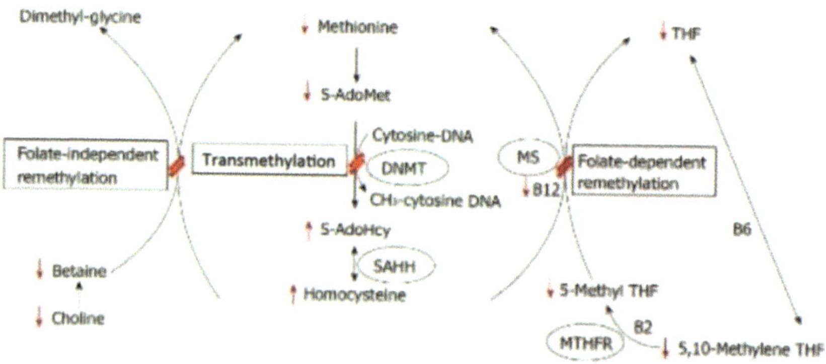

FIGURE 4.1 Effect of methyl-deficiency on biological methylation pathway (Jang and Shin, 2013). S-AdoMet, S-adenosylmethionine; S-AdoHcy, S-adensylhomocysteine; *DNMT*, DNA methyltransferases; *SAHH*, S-adensylhomocysteine hydrolase; *Ms*, Methionine synthase; *THF*, Tetrahydrofolate; *MTHFR*, Methylenetetrahydrofolate reductase.

Subsequently, the association of methylation/transcriptional repression was verified for many genes. The mechanisms by which DNA methylation can occur in gene transcription are based on the modulation of DNA–protein interactions. Changes in methylation patterns can transform a cell from one cell type to another. These changes have variable effects on chromatin structure by modulating histone–DNA interactions (Bird, 2002).

Bird (2002) revealed a mechanistic correlation between DNA methylation and a posttranslational modification of chromatin. An MBD domain repressor (methyl-CpG-binding domain) binds specifically to methylated DNA and recruits histone deacetylases (HDAC). The fusion of DNMTs to a DNA-binding domain leads to maintaining the chromatin in the condensed form and consequently repress the transcription.

4.3 Histone code

Histones are small basic proteins (11–22 kDa) containing a hydrophobic globular field called histone field. This field, formed of three helices, is involved in histone dimerization. Nucleosomes are an alternation between a fully coiled state and several more or less partial states of coiling. In these states, nucleoside DNA is no longer transiently in contact with surface histones. Nucleosome particles are connected to each other by short segments of binding DNA of 15–80 base pairs in length, and the whole forms a chain of nucleosomes (Fig. 4.2) (Fuks et al., 2000).

Chromatin compaction is a dynamic phenomenon stabilized by multiple proteins associated with chromatin (Morillon et al., 2005). Posttranslational changes in histones are covalent. They deteriorate the electrostatic loads of histones and change their structural properties and/or modify the interactions of their extremities. Several types of changes exist: acetylation, methylation, phosphorylation, sumoylation, ADP-ribosylation, ubiquitination, and biotinylation. Changes such as acetylation and methylation have been known and

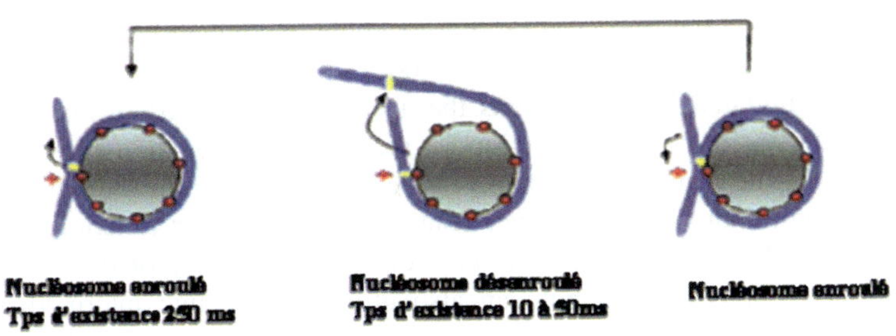

FIGURE 4.2 The dynamic nucleosome: The points of contacts between the DNA (*blue*) and the heart histone (gray) are symbolized by small *red* circles. The *red* arrow shows the entrance points and the exit of the nucleosomal DNA. For more simplicity, only one bit of DNA is represented in the diagram (Morillon et al., 2005).

identified for over 30 years. They were particularly studied on the NH2-final ends of histones H3 and H4 (Morillon et al., 2005).

All the histones are likely to be acetylated on specific lysins in their amino-terminal field. The neutralization of the positive load of NH^{3+} group of lysin can lead to the reduction in the contacts with the nucleosomic DNA since it has a negative charge because of PO_4^{3-} group, with close nucleosomes and certain regulating proteins stabilizing chromatin. These modifications produce a more flexible chromatin, where the DNA is more accessible (Zhang & Reinberg, 2001).

Two families of enzymes influence the levels of acetylation of histones: the histones acetyltransferases (HATs), which add acetyls groups to lysins, and the histones deacetylases (HDACs), which play a role contrary to HATs, which remove the acetyls groups of histones. This phenomenon finally gives place with a hypoacetylation, which leads to the repression of the transcription of genes (Morillon et al., 2005).

One currently distinguishes 18 HDACs human dividing itself into three distinct big classes: HDACs of class I: HDACs 1, 2, 3, and 8; HDACs of class II: HDACs 4, 5, 6, 7, 9, and 10; and HDACs class III: they do not show any similarity with HDACs of class I and II, one finds SIRT 1, 2, 3, 4, 5, 6, and 7 (Morillon et al., 2005). This class of HDACs is the least characterized. Histones can also undergo other modifications such as the methylation of lysins or the arginines located on the amino-final ends of the histones H3 and H4.

The methylation of histones occurs at various levels on the residues lysin and arginine. The methylation of the histones H3 and H4 is best described. The histones methyl-transferases (HMT) catalyze the transfer of methyl groups starting from S-adenosyl methionine toward an amino-terminal groups of residues lysin or arginine. Lysins can be mono, di-, or trimethyl, whereas the arginines exist only in the mono and dimethyl forms (Humphrey et al., 2001).

The specific lysin methylation often plays a part in the formation of heterochromatin. On its side, the methylation of the arginines seems to have a positive effect on the transcription. For example, methylase can modify lysin 9 of the H3 histone (Drummond et al., 2005).

This methylated lysine prevents the acetylation of lysins in histones H3 and H4 and has an inhibitory action on the expression of the genes. During transduction, the histone code involves the transformation of the data by the histone modifications in an answer controlling the cellular functions related to the DNA. This transduction can be a direct consequence of the change in the structure of chromatin but can also utilize a proteinic intermediary, a transducer, which interacts specifically with the modified histone (Drummond et al., 2005).

The H3 histone is recognized by proteins with chromodomaine, such as heterochromatin protein 1 (HP1), when its lysin 9 is methylated. The acetylated histones interact as for them specifically with proteins with chromodomaine. The methylation of lysin 9 on the H3 histone constitutes a brand—or signature—associated with the inactive regions of the genome transcription, while the hyperacetylate state of histones generally corresponds to the active regions (Drummond et al., 2005).

The existence of several modifications on the same histone brings an additional dimension to the code histone. Indeed, a modification on a site can influence the capacity of another site to being modified in a synergistic way or on the contrary antagonistic (Drummond et al., 2005). Besides the methylation of the DNA and the code histone, a small sequence has a broad mechanism that interferes with proteins in order to control the form of genes: microRNAs. The discovery of these small regulating RNA revolutionized the study of the biological mechanisms related on the development of the organizations and the diseases, in particular, cancer (Morillon et al., 2005).

It was recently shown that in mammals, the methylation of DNA is dependent on the methylation of histones, conversely. The locking of transcription by DNA methylation is intimately connected to chromatin remodeling by histone-modifying enzymes: DNMTs interfere with HDAC and HMT in order to modify chromatin and make it permissive for transcription.

Tumor suppressor genes repressed by hypermethylation in a cancer process are necessarily associated with hypoacetylation of histones (Humphrey et al., 2001). miRNAs may play a role in regulating histone acetylation.

Another form of posttranslational modification is microRNAs. MicroRNAs are involved in translational regulation by binding to messenger RNAs and blocking their translation (Drummond et al., 2005).

4.4 The microRNAs

The miRNAs (miRNAs or miRs) are one of the three classes of small RNAs simple not-coding bit, composed of 21–23 nucleotides, which join proteins to control the form of genes (Liu et al., 2009) (Fig. 4.3).

They are small RNAs noncoding ensuring the posttranscriptional regulation of the genic expression. Their expression is fabric-specific. miRNAs react in the tumoral processes by two mechanisms: amplification or deletion of chromosomal areas containing the gene cluster coding of the miRNAs (quantitative effect) or modification the effects of the miRNAs on their target genes by change in the site of interaction with RNAms (qualitative effect). A number of studies have revealed that in the human one, there are more than 500 miRNA, which can target potentially nearly 30% of human RNAm (Jones & Laird, 1999).

On the other hand, if the complementarity is imperfect, a repression of the translation of target RNAm is generally observed. There exist however, several cases for which an imperfect complementarity causes a degradation of target RNAm, showing that this rule is not always respected

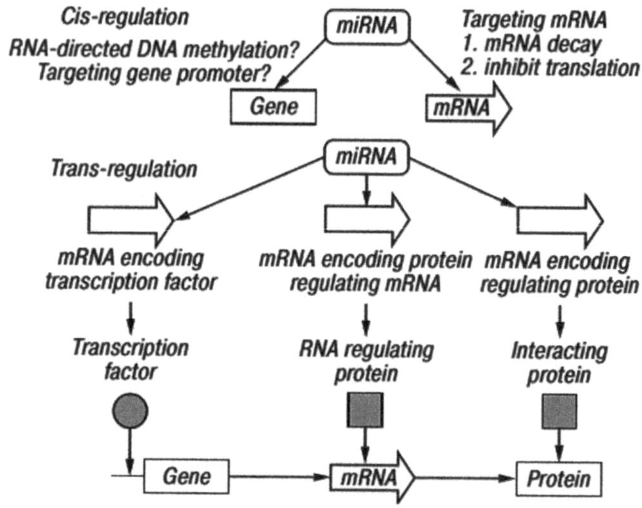

FIGURE 4.3 Potential microRNA regulation mechanisms (Liu et al., 2009).

(MacFarlane & Murphy, 2010). The cartography of genes coding for these miRNA confirmed these observations by revealing that they are present in chromosomal areas amplified or deleted in the tumoral cells (Wiemer, 2007). The relationship between different miRNA and cancer was first revealed by Professor G. Calin in 2002 (Calin et al., 2004).

Their existence also made it possible to understand why some of these areas were associated neither with suppressors' tumors nor with known oncogenes. It has been hypothesized that deregulated synthesis of microRNAs is one of the most important factors contributing to cancer development (Liu et al., 2009).

Nevertheless, two examples (in the table below), namely, miR-17–92 and let-7, are among best characterized in the research conducted heretofore, and they illustrate the way in which the small RNA can act like oncogenes or tumor suppressors (Wiemer, 2007) (Table 4.2).

In the case as of miRNA, it seems that a reduction of their expression reaching a threshold is sufficient to generate an increase in targeted oncogene and thus a phenotype of cancer. Moreover, the artificial expression of this miRNA in this kind of tumor involves a reduction in the proliferation of the cells (Wiemer, 2007). Cellular differentiation is the result of a balance extinction/activation of groups of genes. This balance is controlled not only by factors of transcription that bind to the DNA according to the cellular needs but also by epigenetic information, which includes mainly modifications of the methylation of the DNA and the histone code (Fig. 4.4).

Deteriorations of the profiles of methylation of the DNA were associated a long time with the abnormal expression of the DNMT in various types of

TABLE 4.2 miRNA tumor suppressor in the breast cancer (Wiemer, 2007).

Micro-ARN	Functions	Types of cancer	ARNm targets	References
mir-17–92	Tumor suppressors	Breast cancer	AIB1	Calin et al. (2004)
Let-7	Tumor suppressor	Breast cancer	RAS, CDK6, CDC25A, HMGA2, c-MYC	Hossain et al. (2006)

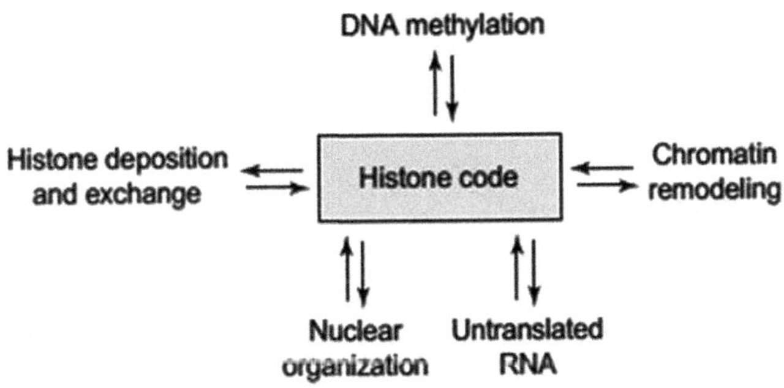

FIGURE 4.4 Schematic representation of the factors that interact with modified histones to establish the epigenetic regulation of transcription through the histone code (Wiemer, 2007).

cancers and tumors. However, clear or somewhat clear correlation between the level of expression of the DNMT and the degree of tumorigenicity still could be established. Reversibility of the histone modifications, just like that of the modification by methylation of CpG of the DNA, the plasticity of epigenetic information highlights, contrary to stable genetic code apart from the events of mutagenesis. In cancers, while being protected (CpG small islands) from methylation, the factors of transcription can bind to the target DNA sequence to initiate the transcription process. On the other hand, when there is an abnormal level of methyl group in the promoter region, there is a nonrecognition of the site, and the transcription factors cannot bind to the promoter region. Thus there is no expression of the gene. The inhibition of the transcription of tumor suppressor genes confers an advantage on the tumoral cells. Any protein histone modification could repress transcription (Calin et al., 2004). The nucleosomal DNA is not accessible (Hossain et al., 2006); in addition, the factors of transcription would be unable to bind to a nucleosome; moreover, the histonic field could act like a signal for the recruitment and the assembly of specific complexes, which would involve the creation of areas transcriptional inactive (Yu et al., 2007). However, the operation of a histonic protein depends on the work of mRNA, whose repression is under the intervention of the miRNAs. The study of the function of a miRNA is a complex task, in so far as the same miRNA can target several RNAm, and a variation in the level of a miRNA can have broad repercussions on the expression of several genes. Future studies will investigate whether only a few miRNA target mRNAs are responsible for the observed physiological effect or whether it is the set of target mRNAs.

4.5 Conclusion

The extinction of gene expression in an oncology process is the result of a correlation between epigenetic factors and chromatin. Any cell type expresses a precise number of genes for its functioning. An anomaly is observed during various biological process, which until now demands to define how this correlation is maintained stochastically in epigenetic terms.

Acknowledgment

Authors would like to thank University Hassan II of Casablanca, Faculty of Sciences and Techniques Mohammedia, Team of Virology, Oncology, and Medical Biotechnologies and Laboratory of Virology, Microbiology, Quality and Biotechnologies/Ecotoxicology and Biodiversity for all their efforts for their kind support in completing this work.

References

Aerts, S., Thijs, G., Dabrowski, M., Moreau, Y., & De Moor, B. (2004). Comprehensive analysis of the base composition around the transcription start site in Metazoa. *BMC Genomics*, *5*(1). Available from https://doi.org/10.1186/1471-2164-5-34.

Bestor, T. H., & Ingram, V. M. (1983). Two DNA methyltransferases from murine erythroleukemia cells: Purification, sequence specificity, and mode of interaction with DNA. *Proceedings of the National Academy of Sciences of the United States of America*, *80*(181), 5559–5563. Available from https://doi.org/10.1073/pnas.80.18.5559.

Bird, A. (2002). DNA methylation patterns and epigenetic memory. *Genes and Development*, *16* (1), 6–21. Available from https://doi.org/10.1101/gad.947102.

Calin, G. A., Sevignani, C., Dumitru, C. D., Hyslop, T., Noch, E., Yendamuri, S., Shimizu, M., Rattan, S., Bullrich, F., Negrini, M., & Croce, C. M. (2004). Human microRNA genes are frequently located at fragile sites and genomic regions involved in cancers. *Proceedings of the National Academy of Sciences of the United States of America*, *101*(9), 2999–3004. Available from https://doi.org/10.1073/pnas.0307323101.

Cheng, X., & Roberts, R. J. (2001). AdoMet-dependent methylation, DNA methyltransferases and base flipping. *Nucleic Acids Research*, *29*(18), 3784–3795. Available from https://doi.org/10.1093/nar/29.18.3784.

Dhillon, V. S., Shahid, M., & Husain, S. A. (2004). CpG methylation of the FHIT, FANCF, cyclin-D2, BRCA2 and RUNX3 genes in granulosa cell tumors (GCTs) of ovarian origin. *Molecular Cancer*, *3*. Available from https://doi.org/10.1186/1476-4598-3-33.

Drummond, D. C., Noble, C. O., Kirpotin, D. B., Guo, Z., Scott, G. K., & Benz, C. C. (2005). Clinical development of histone deacetylase inhibitors as anticancer agents. *Annual Review of Pharmacology and Toxicology*, *45*, 495–528. Available from https://doi.org/10.1146/annurev.pharmtox.45.120403.095825.

Eden, A., Gaudet, F., Waghmare, A., & Jaenisch, R. (2003). Chromosomal instability and tumors promoted by DNA hypomethylation. *Science (New York, N.Y.)*, *300*(5618), 455. Available from https://doi.org/10.1126/science.1083557.

Ehrlich, M., Hopkins, N. E., Jiang, G., Dome, J. S., Yu, M. C., Woods, C. B., Tomlinson, G. E., Chintagumpala, M., Champagne, M., Dillerg, L., Parham, D. M., & Sawyer, J. (2003). Satellite DNA hypomethylation in karyotyped wilms tumors. *Cancer Genetics and Cytogenetics*, *141*(2), 97–105. Available from https://doi.org/10.1016/S0165-4608(02)00668-4.

Fang, M., Chen, D., & Yang, C. S. (2007). Dietary polyphenols may affect DNA methylation. *The Journal of Nutrition*, *137*(1), 223S–228S. Available from https://doi.org/10.1093/jn/137.1.223S.

Flower, K. J., Shenker, N. S., El-Bahrawy, M., Goldgar, D. E., Parsons, M. T., Spurdle, A. B., Morris, J. R., Brown, R., & Flanagan, J. M. (2015). DNA methylation profiling to assess pathogenicity of BRCA1 unclassified variants in breast cancer. *Epigenetics: Official Journal of the DNA Methylation Society*, *10*(12), 1121–1132. Available from https://doi.org/10.1080/15592294.2015.1111504.

Fuks, F., Burgers, W. A., Brehm, A., Hughes-Davies, L., & Kouzarides, T. (2000). DNA methyltransferase Dnmt1 associates with histone deacetylase activity. *Nature Genetics*, *24*(1), 88–91. Available from https://doi.org/10.1038/71750.

Hossain, A., Kuo, M. T., & Saunders, G. F. (2006). Mir-17-5p regulates breast cancer cell proliferation by inhibiting translation of AIB1 mRNA. *Molecular and Cellular Biology*, *26*(21), 8191–8201. Available from https://doi.org/10.1128/MCB.00242-06.

Humphrey, G. W., Wang, Y., Russanova, V. R., Hirai, T., Qin, J., Nakatani, Y., & Howard, B. H. (2001). Stable histone deacetylase complexes distinguished by the presence of SANT domain proteins CoREST/kiaa0071 and Mta-L1. *Journal of Biological Chemistry*, *276*(9), 6817–6824. Available from https://doi.org/10.1074/jbc.M007372200.

Jang, H., & Shin, H. (2013). Current trends in the development and application of molecular technologies for cancer epigenetics. *World Journal of Gastroenterology*, *19*(7), 1030–1039. Available from https://doi.org/10.3748/wjg.v19.i7.1030.

Joffin, N. (2015). Impact de la citrulline sur le métabolisme du tissu adipeux, (Doctoral dissertation), vol. 5.

Jones, P. A., & Laird, P. W. (1999). Cancer epigenetics comes of age. *Nature Genetics*, *21*(2), 163–167. Available from https://doi.org/10.1038/5947.

Jones, P. A., & Takai, D. (2001). The role of DNA methylation in mammalian epigenetics. *Science (New York, N.Y.)*, *293*(5532), 1068–1070. Available from https://doi.org/10.1126/science.1063852.

Koutsimpelas, D., Pongsapich, W., Heinrich, U., Mann, S., Mann, W. J., & Brieger, J. (2012). Promoter methylation of MGMT, MLH1 and RASSF1A tumor suppressor genes in head and neck squamous cell carcinoma: Pharmacological genome demethylation reduces proliferation of head and neck squamous carcinoma cells. *Oncology Reports*, *27*(4), 1135–1141. Available from https://doi.org/10.3892/or.2012.1624.

Lander, E. S., Linton, L. M., Birren, B., Nusbaum, C., Zody, M. C., Baldwin, J., Devon, K., Dewar, K., Doyle, M., Fitzhugh, W., Funke, R., Gage, D., Harris, K., Heaford, A., Howland, J., Kann, L., Lehoczky, J., Levine, R., McEwan, P., & Morgan, M. J. (2001). Initial sequencing and analysis of the human genome. *Nature*, *409*(6822), 860–921. Available from https://doi.org/10.1038/35057062.

Larsen, F., Gundersen, G., Lopez, R., & Prydz, H. (1992). CpG islands as gene markers in the human genome. *Genomics*, *13*(4), 1095–1107. Available from https://doi.org/10.1016/0888-7543(92)90024-M.

Liu, X., Chen, Z., Yu, J., Xia, J., & Zhou, X. (2009). MicroRNA profiling and head and neck cancer. *Comparative and Functional Genomics*, *15*(7), 1–11. Available from https://doi.org/10.1155/2009/837514.

MacFarlane, L. A., & Murphy, P. R. (2010). MicroRNA: Biogenesis, function and role in cancer. *Current Genomics*, *11*(7), 537–561. Available from https://doi.org/10.2174/138920210793175895.

Morillon, A., Karabetsou, N., Nair, A., & Mellor, J. (2005). Dynamic lysine methylation on histone H3 defines the regulatory phase of gene transcription. *Molecular Cell*, *18*(6), 723–734. Available from https://doi.org/10.1016/j.molcel.2005.05.009.

Nicolas, E., Vandel, L., Trouche, D. (2001). Quand la méthylation des histones entre en scène.

Potapova, A., Hoffman, A. M., Godwin, A. K., Al-Saleem, T., & Cairns, P. (2008). Promoter hypermethylation of the PALB2 susceptibility gene in inherited and sporadic breast and ovarian cancer. *Cancer Research*, *68*(4), 998–1002. Available from https://doi.org/10.1158/0008-5472.CAN-07-2418.

Rigi-Ladiz, M. A., Kordi-Tamandani, D. M., & Torkamanzehi, A. (2011). Analysis of hypermethylation and expression profiles of APC and ATM genes in patients with oral squamous cell carcinoma. *Clinical Epigenetics*, *3*(3). Available from https://doi.org/10.1186/1868-7083-3-6.

Siddiqui, S., Akhter, N., Deo, S. V. S., Shukla, N. K., & Husain, S. A. (2016). A study on promoter methylation of PTEN in sporadic breast cancer patients from North India. *Breast Cancer (Tokyo, Japan)*, *23*(6), 922–931. Available from https://doi.org/10.1007/s12282-015-0665-0.

Siegel, R. L., Miller, K. D., & Jemal, A. (2016). Cancer statistics, 2016. *CA Cancer Journal for Clinicians*, *66*(1), 7–30. Available from https://doi.org/10.3322/caac.21332.

Suh, S. O., Chen, Y., Zaman, M. S., Hirata, H., Yamamura, S., Shahryari, V., Liu, J., Tabatabai, Z. L., Kakar, S., Deng, G., Tanaka, Y., & Dahiya, R. (2011). MicroRNA-145 is regulated by DNA methylation and p53 gene mutation in prostate cancer. *Carcinogenesis*, *32*(5), 772–778. Available from https://doi.org/10.1093/carcin/bgr036.

Trojan, J., Brieger, A., Raedle, J., Esteller, M., & Zeuzem, S. (2000). 5'-CpG island methylation of the LKB1/STK11 promoter and allelic loss at chromosome 19p13.3 in sporadic colorectal cancer. *Gut*, *47*(2), 272–276. Available from https://doi.org/10.1136/gut.47.2.272.

Wiemer, E. A. C. (2007). The role of microRNAs in cancer: No small matter. *European Journal of Cancer*, *43*(10), 1529–1544. Available from https://doi.org/10.1016/j.ejca.2007.04.002.

Yu, F., Yao, H., Zhu, P., Zhang, X., Pan, Q., Gong, C., Huang, Y., Hu, X., Su, F., Lieberman, J., & Song, E. (2007). let-7 regulates self renewal and tumorigenicity of breast cancer cells. *Cell*, *131*(6), 1109–1123. Available from https://doi.org/10.1016/j.cell.2007.10.054.

Zhang, S., Lu, J., Zhao, X., Wu, W., Wang, H., Lu, J., Wu, Q., Chen, X., Fan, W., Chen, H., Wang, F., Hu, Z., Jin, L., Wei, Q., Shen, H., Huang, W., & Lu, D. (2010). A variant in the CHEK2 promoter at a methylation site relieves transcriptional repression and confers reduced risk of lung cancer. *Carcinogenesis*, *31*(7), 1251–1258. Available from https://doi.org/10.1093/carcin/bgq089.

Zhang, Y., & Reinberg, D. (2001). Transcription regulation by histone methylation: Interplay between different covalent modifications of the core histone tails. *Genes and Development*, *15*(18), 2343–2360. Available from https://doi.org/10.1101/gad.927301.

Chapter 5

Exosomes as diagnostic and prognostic tools in prostate cancer

Youssef Ennaji[4], Maryame Lamsisi[4], Ikram Tiabi[4], Soukayna Alaoui Sosse[4], Imane Saif[4], Berjas Abumsimir[3,4], Abdelilah Laraqui[2], Kawtar Aboulalaa[4] and Moulay Mustapha Ennaji[1]

[1]Group Leader Research team of Virology, Oncology, and Biotechnologies, Head of Laboratory of Virology, Oncology, Biosciences, Environment and New Energies (LVO-BEEN), Faculty of Sciences and Techniques Mohammedia, University Hassan II of Casablanca, Casablanca, Morocco, [2]Laboratory of Human Pathologies Biology, Faculty of Sciences, and Genomic Center of Human Pathologies, Faculty of Medicine and Pharmacy, Bio-Path Laboratory, Faculty of sciences-Agdal, Mohammed V University, Rabat, Morocco, [3]Pharmacological and Diagnostic Research Centre (PDRC), Department of Medical Laboratory Sciences, Faculty of Allied Medical Sciences, Al-Ahliyya Amman University (AAU), Amman, Jordan, [4]Team of Virology, Oncology, and Biotechnologies, Laboratory of Virology, Oncology, Biosciences, Environment and New Energies (LVO-BEEN), Faculty of Sciences and Techniques Mohammedia, University Hassan II of Casablanca, Casablanca, Morocco

5.1 Introduction

Prostate cancer (PCa) is the most common solid malignancy with a high mortality in men (Ingrosso et al., 2018), and it is the only one of the four solid tumor types, namely, breast, lung, and colorectal cancer, which has a clinical useful protein biomarker for diagnostics and follow-up after treatment. Prostate-specific antigen (PSA) has shown reasonable sensitivity for the screening and detection of incipient cancer and can also predict response to treatment (Freedland et al., 2005). However, it is recognized that PSA lacks specificity and sensitivity to discriminating benign prostate diseases (e.g., benign prostatic hyperplasia and infection), indolent PCa, and aggressive PCa. Thus, additional PCa biomarkers are required, especially the ones that furnish information about the severity of the disease and can predict high or low risk for future metastases. Searching for novel biomarkers has been the focus of a number of research groups, and the studies have become more extensive and sophisticated. Liquid biopsies, circulating tumor cells,

Immunological Implications and Molecular Diagnostics of Genitourinary Cancer.
DOI: https://doi.org/10.1016/B978-0-323-85496-2.00017-8

exosomes, and circulating nucleic acids have been developed as minimally invasive assays for monitoring PCa patients (Lu et al., 2019).

Urine is a promising source of new biomarkers of PCa, and several urinary markers have been reported, such as PCA3 and the TMPRSS2-fusion gene (Fujita et al., 2016). Recently, urine collected after prostate massage was reported to contain extracellular vesicles (EVs) that are secreted from PCa cells (Zijlstra & Stoorvogel, 2016). Two types of microvesicles are present in prostate secretions: (1) prostasomes (150–500 nm), produced by prostatic ductal epithelial cells that are a normal component of seminal fluid and play a role in male fertility (Burden et al., 2006); and (2) exosomes, specialized nanovesicles (30–100 nm) with a cup-shaped morphology, actively secreted by a variety of normal and tumor cells. EVs, such as exosomes and microvesicles contain microRNAs, proteins, and mRNAs and play a role in intercellular communications via the mechanisms of exocytosis and endocytosis (Liu et al., 2016).

5.2 Structure, biogenesis, and function of exosomes

5.2.1 Structure and biogenesis of exosomes

Although observed for several decades, the release of membrane-enclosed vesicles by cells into their surrounding environment has been the subject of increasing interest in the few past years, which led to the creation of a scientific society dedicated to this subject in 2012: The International Society for EVs. Convincing evidence that vesicles enable exchange of complex information has further stimulated this interest. However, it has also become clear that different types of secreted vesicles coexist, with different intracellular origins and modes of formation and thus probably different compositions and functions (Kowal et al., 2014).

Exosomes are small (from 30 to 120 nm in diameter) EVs. Their lipid bilayer membrane, with a size of 5 nm, protects them from the negative action of RNases and proteases (Fig. 5.1). Exosomes have double-membrane structures containing various cargo proteins, such as miRNAs, proteins (e.g., tetraspanin CD63, CD81, CD82, CD53, and CD37, as well as cytosolic proteins), lipids (e.g., sphingomyelin, cholesterol, and generally saturated fats), and viral particles (Qin & Xu, 2014). Initial proteomic studies revealed that exosomes contain a specific subset of proteins from endosomes, the plasma membrane (PM), and the cytosol (Théry et al., 2001).

The exact mechanisms involved in exosome biogenesis are not fully elucidated; however, certain factors have been reported to play a role. First, specific lipids and transmembrane proteins are grouped in the cellular membrane (De Gassart et al., 2003). The biogenesis of these vesicles starts from the internalization of cellular membrane that forms an early endosome. During the formation of this endosome, cytoplasmic content is taken up by inward budding of endosomal membranes, resulting in exosome formation. Exosomes are formed as intraluminal vesicles (ILVs) by budding into early

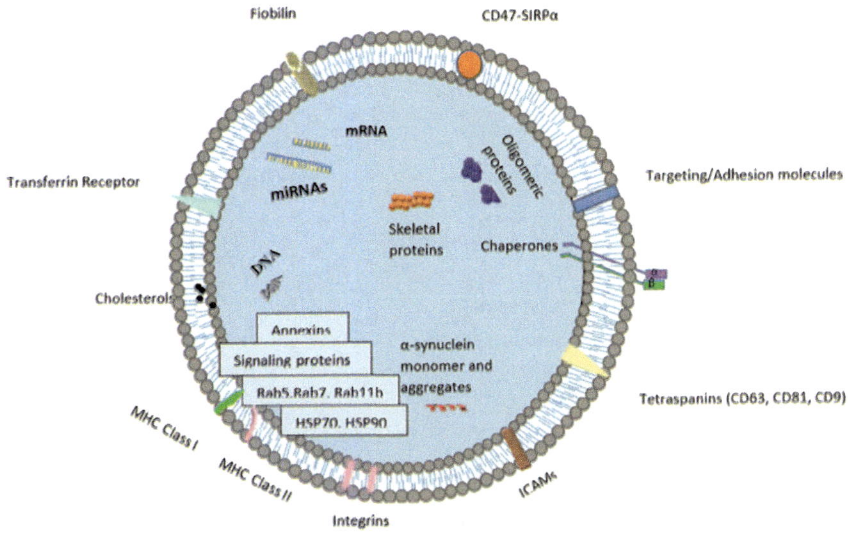

FIGURE 5.1 Schematic diagram of an exosome (Lorenc et al., 2020).

endosomes and multivesicular body (MVB). Several molecules are involved in the biogenesis of ILVs, such as the endosomal sorting complex required for transport machinery, lipids (such as ceramide), and the tetraspanins. It is still unknown whether these mechanisms act simultaneously on the same MVB or on different MVBs. The fate of MVBs can be either fusion with lysosomes or fusion with the PM, which allows the release of their content to the extracellular environment. Several RAB proteins (RAB11, RAB27, and RAB35) have been shown to be involved in the transport of MVBs to the PM and in exosome secretion. Herein, we propose that these proteins can act on different MVBs. In addition, soluble NSF-attachment protein receptors are probably involved in fusion of these MVBs with the PM (Fig. 5.2).

When the MVB fuses with the cellular membrane, the vesicles are secreted (Duijvesz et al., 2011). MVBs, which appear along the endocytic pathway, are characterized by the presence of vesicles in their lumen ILVs formed by inward budding from the limiting membrane (Klumperman & Raposo, 2014).

5.2.2 Functions of exosomes

Exosomes are released by the exocytosis of MVBs, developed from early and then late endosomes (Panigrahi & Deep, 2017), and serve to exchange genetic material through RNA between cells, intercellular communication, propagation of pathogens, contribution to the immune system, and antigen presentation (Beach et al., 2014; Valadi et al., 2007). Exosomes are widely involved in material transport and signal transmission between cells through

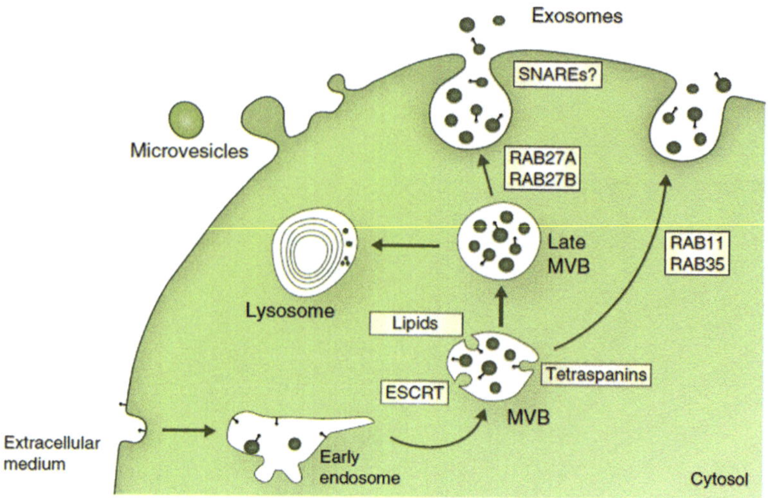

FIGURE 5.2 Schematic representation of the origin and release of exosomes by eukaryotic cells (Kowal et al., 2014).

the release of the specific components they carry into the recipient cells (Kalluri & LeBleu, 2020). With these discoveries, scientists developed a better understanding of the composition and function of exosomes and began to see how they might be used in disease diagnosis and treatment. Those naturally occurring membrane particles mediate intercellular communication by delivering molecular information between cancer and stromal cells, especially cancer-associated fibroblasts (Pullan et al., 2019). Cancer cell-derived EVs cause very diverse effects and may depend on their target cells, which appear to take them up in several ways, such as receptor/lipid raft endocytosis, phagocytosis, micropinocytosis, or fusion with the PM (Guo et al., 2017). Some exosomes can reduce the anticancer immune response, interact with specific membrane receptors, and promote a suitable microenvironment, while others may cause drug resistance and the failure of antibody therapy involving RNA species and protein delivery (Filella & Foj, 2016; Saari et al., 2015). Studies have revealed that exosomes are enriched with specific antigens, compared to whole-cell lysates (Clayton & Mason, 2009). Moreover, exosomes can provide candidate biomarkers for PCa, contribute to tumor progression, and promote tumor metastasis (Liu et al., 2016).

5.3 The functional roles and tumor-derived exosomes in prostate cancer progression

Tumor metastasis usually indicates a poor prognosis and is the leading cause of cancer-related deaths (Hanahan & Weinberg, 2011). Exosomes derived from PCa cells, which have become the common object of scientists' interest, are implicated in creating a premetastatic niche (Pan et al., 2017). Normal human cells can express prostate-specific genes after culturing with exosomes derived from PCa tissues (Renzulli et al., 2010). It is a microenvironment that is especially favorable to cancer cells composed of different cell types, like fibroblasts, lymphocytes, epithelial cells, matrix molecules, growth factors, and cytokines (Egeblad et al., 2010).

Chronic inflammation is a driving force for tumor development and metastasis. Thus, the local inflammatory microenvironment is one of the basic factors for the formation of a premetastatic niche. Exosomes influence the immune system in a premetastatic niche through various mechanisms. The local inflammatory microenvironment can induce tumor cells to produce tumor-derived secreted factors (TDSFs), such as vascular endothelial growth factor (VEGF), tumor necrosis factor alpha (TNF-α), transforming growth factor-β (TGF-β), and interleukin (IL). The expression of inflammatory factors is upregulated by stromal cells under the influence of TDSFs. Furthermore, tumor-derived exosome content enhances the premetastatic niche (Guo et al., 2019). Immune cells are recruited to the premetastatic niche and accelerate the secretion of inflammatory factors. In addition, tumor-derived exosomes carry inflammatory factors into the bloodstream, which in turn reach the premetastatic niche. Through the above possible ways, an inflammatory microenvironment favorable for tumors is finally formed in the premetastatic niche (Guo et al., 2019). Tumor exosomes possess the capacity to support the migration of immune cells, like neutrophils, macrophages, and regulatory T to secondary sites, thereby reducing immune response against tumors and inhibiting antigen-presenting cells, such as dendritic cells. These nanoparticles could impair the function of T cells and NK cells via the blocking, proliferation, activation, and provision of apoptosis (Liu et al., 2010) (Fig. 5.3).

5.3.1 The diagnosis potential of exosomes in prostate cancer

Present diagnostic markers such as PSA and carbohydrate antigens have substantial drawbacks such as false negatives, false positives, and lack of tumor-type specificity (Perkins et al., 2003). Tumor biopsy is the only definitive method of diagnosis, but it is invasive. Novel PCa biomarkers are required for clinical application. Exosomes can be isolated from human body fluids such as the blood, urine, and saliva (Keller et al., 2011). Exosomes may be the key biomarkers in the early diagnosis of PCa and in a personalized approach to treatment and to future patients' prognosis (Vlaeminck-Guillem., 2018). Exosomes present many different proteins on their surface. These proteins can act as epitopes, which are recognized using different mono- or polyclonal antibodies. In Nilsson et al. (2009) reported that PCa-derived exosomes, which contain PCa-specific markers of PCA3 and TMPRSS-ERG, were detected in urine after prostate massage of PCa patients.

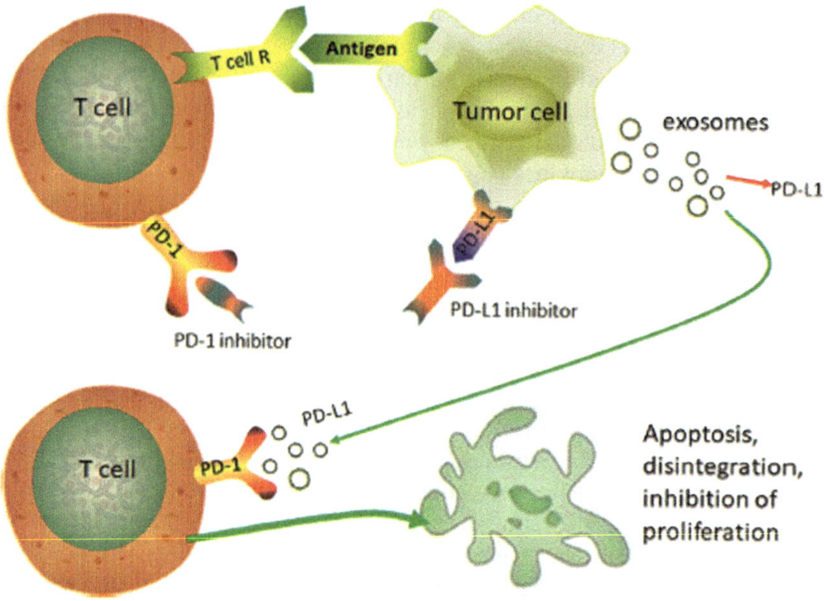

FIGURE 5.3 Exosome PD-L1 has a similar function to tumor PD-L1. The former can also bind to PD-1 on T cells, induce T cell apoptosis, and inhibit T cell activation and proliferation (Guo et al., 2019).

The ExoDx prostate test is a commercially available urinary test for the detection of PCa. This urinary exosome gene expression assay measures the three genes prostate cancer antigen 3 (PCA3), ERG (including the TMPRSS2-ERG fusion gene), and SPDEF (sterile alpha motif-pointed domain containing Ets transcription factor) by reverse transcriptase polymerase chain reaction (Fig. 5.4). Nilsson et al. reported in 2009 that The TMPRSS2-ERG fusion transcripts were detected in urinary exosomes from two patients with high Gleason scores but not in those from two patients with low Gleason scores. Other nucleic acids, such as mRNA, miRNA, have all been found in exosomes. In PCa, plasma vesicles were isolated using the precipitation-based ExoQuick method. Several studies identified miR-1290 and miR-375 as potential prognostic biomarkers in castration-resistant prostate cancer (CRPC), since their level correlates with a poorer overall survival ($P < .004$) (Huang et al., 2013, 2015). Exosomal miR-34a could induce docetaxel sensitivity in docetaxel-resistant PCa cells by inhibiting Bcl-2 (Carmeliet & Jain, 2000), and exosomal miR-34a can be used as a predictive biomarker for the response to docetaxel (Corcoran et al., 2014).

Noninvasive and simple diagnostic methods are required for PCa diagnosis. A novel noninvasive urine exosome gene expression assay has been applied to reduce the number of unnecessary biopsies (McKiernan et al., 2016). Additionally, a polymerase chain reaction-free efficient diagnostic

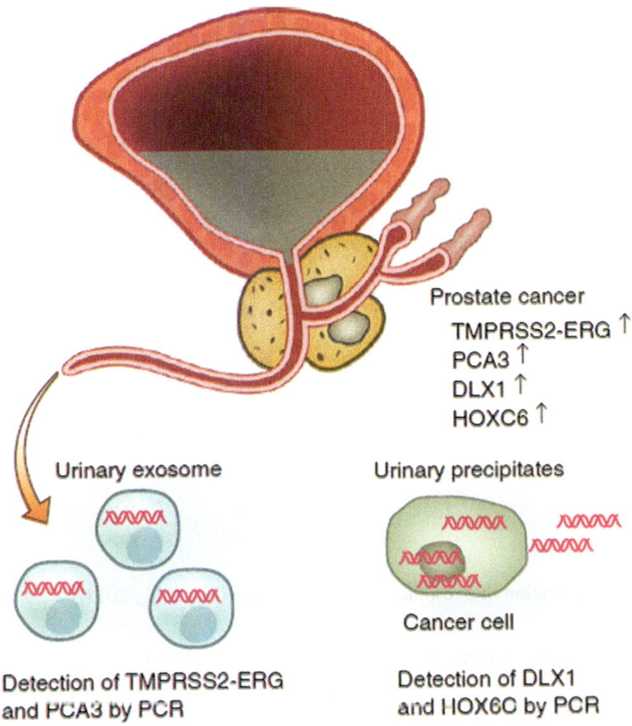

FIGURE 5.4 ExoDx prostate measures exosomal PCA3 and ERG in first-catch urine without prostatic manipulations. SelectMDx measures HOXC6 and DLX1 in urine after prostatic massage (Fujita & Nonomura, 2018).

method was developed for simultaneous and multiplexed detection of exosomal miRNAs (Lee et al., 2016). These improvements of detection technology aid and facilitate the application of exosomes for PCa diagnosis.

5.3.2 Future directions and applications of exosomes in prostate cancer

Studies have been increasingly confirming the potential therapeutic role of exosomes in cancer treatment. Exosomes have a high potential for both as diagnostic and therapeutic agents in immune therapy, vaccination trials, and regenerative medicine. The native structure and unique cellular functions of exosomes give them a great potential as natural drug/gene delivery vehicles, but developing efficient and reliable isolation methods is necessary to fully use their potential (Li et al., 2019). Exosomes can be used as a delivery vector to target cancer cells, and the contents can escape the attack by immune system (Yim et al., 2016). Several studies used exosomes as the carriers to deliver paclitaxel to autologous PCa cells and showed increased cytotoxic

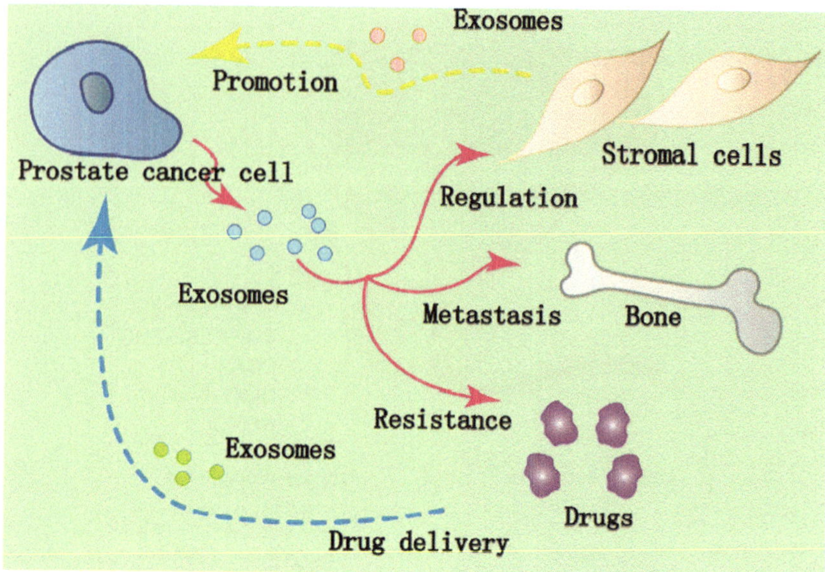

FIGURE 5.5 Implication of exosomes in prostate cancer (Pan et al., 2017).

effect (Saari et al., 2015). Exosomes are also applied in tumor vaccination. Tumor-derived exosomes often contain tumor-specific antigens to activate dendritic cells, which induce antitumor response of T lymphocytes, and dendritic cell-derived exosomes activate NK cells (Andre et al., 2002; Viaud et al., 2010). As a conclusion, exosomes are very promising tools for the future therapeutic and diagnostics of PCa (Fig. 5.5), but their use first requires solutions for the many challenging issues remaining.

Acknowledgments

Authors would like to thank the Ministry of National Education, Professional Training, Higher Education and Scientific Research and express gratitude to members of Virology, Oncology and Medical Biotechnology team at FSTM-Hassan II University of Casablanca, for their support during all work stages on this research.

References

Andre, F., Schartz, N. E. C., Movassagh, M., Flament, C., Pautier, P., Morice, P., Pomel, C., Lhomme, C., Escudier, B., Le Chevalier, T., Tursz, T., Amigorena, S., Raposo, G., Angevin, E., & Zitvogel, L. (2002). Malignant effusions and immunogenic tumour-derived exosomes. *Lancet*, *360*(9329), 295–305. Available from https://doi.org/10.1016/S0140-6736(02)09552-1.

Beach, A., Zhang, H. G., Ratajczak, M. Z., & Kakar, S. S. (2014). Exosomes: An overview of biogenesis, composition and role in ovarian cancer. *Journal of Ovarian Research*, *7*(1). Available from https://doi.org/10.1186/1757-2215-7-14.

Burden, H. P., Holmes, C. H., Persad, R., & Whittington, K. (2006). Prostasomes – Their effects on human male reproduction and fertility. *Human Reproduction Update*, *12*(3), 283–292. Available from https://doi.org/10.1093/humupd/dmi052.

Carmeliet, P., & Jain, R. K. (2000). Angiogenesis in cancer and other diseases. *Nature*, *407* (6801), 249–257. Available from https://doi.org/10.1038/35025220.

Clayton, A., & Mason, M. D. (2009). Exosomes in tumour immunity. *Current Oncology*, *16*(3), 46–49. Available from https://doi.org/10.3747/co.v16i3.367.

Corcoran, C., Rani, S., & O'Driscoll, L. (2014). miR-34a is an intracellular and exosomal predictive biomarker for response to docetaxel with clinical relevance to prostate cancer progression. *The Prostate*, *74*(13), 1320–1334. Available from https://doi.org/10.1002/pros.22848.

De Gassart, A., Géminard, C., Février, B., Raposo, G., & Vidal, M. (2003). Lipid raft-associated protein sorting in exosomes. *Blood*, *102*(13), 4336–4344. Available from https://doi.org/10.1182/blood-2003-03-0871.

Duijvesz, D., Luider, T., Bangma, C. H., & Jenster, G. (2011). Exosomes as biomarker treasure chests for prostate cancer. *European Urology*, *59*(5), 823–831. Available from https://doi.org/10.1016/j.eururo.2010.12.031.

Egeblad, M., Nakasone, E. S., & Werb, Z. (2010). Tumors as organs: Complex tissues that interface with the entire organism. *Developmental Cell*, *18*(6), 884–901. Available from https://doi.org/10.1016/j.devcel.2010.05.012.

Filella, X., & Foj, L. (2016). Prostate cancer detection and prognosis: From prostate specific antigen (PSA) to exosomal biomarkers. *International Journal of Molecular Sciences*, *17*(11). Available from https://doi.org/10.3390/ijms17111784.

Freedland, S. J., Mangold, L. A., Walsh, P. C., & Partin, A. W. (2005). The prostatic specific antigen era is alive and well: Prostatic specific-antigen and biochemical progression following radical prostatectomy. *Journal of Urology*, *174*(4 I), 1276–1281. Available from https://doi.org/10.1097/01.ju.0000173907.84852.ec.

Fujita, K., Hayashi, T., Matsuzaki, K., Nakata, W., Masuda, M., Kawashima, A., & Nonomura, N. (2016). Decreased fucosylated PSA as a urinary marker for high Gleason score prostate cancer. *Oncotarget*, *7*(35), 56643.

Fujita, K., & Nonomura, N. (2018). Urinary biomarkers of prostate cancer. *International Journal of Urology*, *25*(9), 770–779. Available from https://doi.org/10.1111/iju.13734.

Guo, W., Gao, Y., Li, N., Shao, F., Wang, C., Wang, P., Yang, Z., Li, R., & He, J. (2017). Exosomes: New players in cancer. *Oncology Reports*, *38*(2), 665–675. Available from https://doi.org/10.3892/or.2017.5714.

Guo, Y., Ji, X., Liu, J., Fan, D., Zhou, Q., Chen, C., Wang, W., Wang, G., Wang, H., Yuan, W., Ji, Z., & Sun, Z. (2019). Effects of exosomes on pre-metastatic niche formation in tumors. *Molecular Cancer*. Available from https://doi.org/10.1186/s12943-019-0995-1.

Hanahan, D., & Weinberg, R. A. (2011). Hallmarks of cancer: The next generation. *Cell*, *144*(5), 646–674. Available from https://doi.org/10.1016/j.cell.2011.02.013.

Huang, X., Yuan, T., Liang, M., Du, M., Xia, S., Dittmar, R., Wang, D., See, W., Costello, B. A., Quevedo, F., Tan, W., Nandy, D., Bevan, G. H., Longenbach, S., Sun, Z., Lu, Y., Wang, T., Thibodeau, S. N., Boardman, L., … Wang, L. (2015). Exosomal miR-1290 and miR-375 as prognostic markers in castration-resistant prostate cancer. *European Urology*, *67* (1), 33–41. Available from https://doi.org/10.1016/j.eururo.2014.07.035.

Huang, X., Yuan, T., Tschannen, M., Sun, Z., Jacob, H., Du, M., Liang, M., Dittmar, R. L., Liu, Y., Liang, M., Kohli, M., Thibodeau, S. N., Boardman, L., & Wang, L. (2013).

Characterization of human plasma-derived exosomal RNAs by deep sequencing. *BMC Genomics*, *14*(1). Available from https://doi.org/10.1186/1471-2164-14-319.

Ingrosso, G., Detti, B., Scartoni, D., Lancia, A., Giacomelli, I., Baki, M., Carta, G., Livi, L., & Santoni, R. (2018). Current therapeutic options in metastatic castration-resistant prostate cancer. *Seminars in Oncology*, *45*(5–6), 303–315. Available from https://doi.org/10.1053/j.seminoncol.2018.10.001.

Kalluri, R., & LeBleu, V. S. (2020). The biology, function, and biomedical applications of exosomes. *Science (New York, N.Y.)*, *6478*.

Keller, S., Ridinger, J., Rupp, A. K., Janssen, J. W. G., & Altevogt, P. (2011). Body fluid derived exosomes as a novel template for clinical diagnostics. *Journal of Translational Medicine*, *9*. Available from https://doi.org/10.1186/1479-5876-9-86.

Klumperman, J., & Raposo, G. (2014). The complex ultrastructure of the endolysosomal system. *Cold Spring Harbor Perspectives in Biology*, *6*(10). Available from https://doi.org/10.1101/cshperspect.a016857.

Kowal, J., Tkach, M., & Théry, C. (2014). Biogenesis and secretion of exosomes. *Current Opinion in Cell Biology*, *29*(1), 116–125. Available from https://doi.org/10.1016/j.ceb.2014.05.004.

Lee, J. H., Kim, J. A., Jeong, S., & Rhee, W. J. (2016). Simultaneous and multiplexed detection of exosome microRNAs using molecular beacons. *Biosensors and Bioelectronics*, *86*, 202–210. Available from https://doi.org/10.1016/j.bios.2016.06.058.

Li, X., Corbett, A. L., Taatizadeh, E., Tasnim, N., Little, J. P., Garnis, C., Daugaard, M., Guns, E., Hoorfar, M., & Li, I. T. S. (2019). Challenges and opportunities in exosome research-Perspectives from biology, engineering, and cancer therapy. *APL Bioengineering*, *3*(1). Available from https://doi.org/10.1063/1.5087122.

Liu, C. M., Hsieh, C. L., Shen, C. N., Lin, C. C., Shigemura, K., & Sung, S. Y. (2016). Exosomes from the tumor microenvironment as reciprocal regulators that enhance prostate cancer progression. *International Journal of Urology*, *23*(9), 734–744. Available from https://doi.org/10.1111/iju.13145.

Liu, Y., Xiang, X., Zhuang, X., Zhang, S., Liu, C., Cheng, Z., Michalek, S., Grizzle, W., & Zhang, H. G. (2010). Contribution of MyD88 to the tumor exosome-mediated induction of myeloid derived suppressor cells. *American Journal of Pathology*, *176*(5), 2490–2499. Available from https://doi.org/10.2353/ajpath.2010.090777.

Lorenc, T., Klimczyk, K., Michalczewska, I., Słomka, M., Kubiak-Tomaszewska, G., & Olejarz, W. (2020). Exosomes in prostate cancer diagnosis, prognosis and therapy. *International Journal of Molecular Sciences*, *21*(6), 1–14. Available from https://doi.org/10.3390/ijms21062118.

Lu, Y. T., Delijani, K., Mecum, A., & Goldkorn, A. (2019). Current status of liquid biopsies for the detection and management of prostate cancer. *Cancer Management and Research*, *11*.

McKiernan, J., Donovan, M. J., O'Neill, V., Bentink, S., Noerholm, M., Belzer, S., Skog, J., Kattan, M. W., Partin, A., Andriole, G., Brown, G., Wei, J. T., Thompson, I. M., & Carroll, P. (2016). A novel urine exosome gene expression assay to predict high-grade prostate cancer at initial biopsy. *JAMA Oncology*, *2*(7), 882–889. Available from https://doi.org/10.1001/jamaoncol.2016.0097.

Nilsson, J., Skog, J., Nordstrand, A., Baranov, V., Mincheva-Nilsson, L., Breakefield, X. O., & Widmark, A. (2009). Prostate cancer-derived urine exosomes: A novel approach to biomarkers for prostate cancer. *British Journal of Cancer*, *100*(10), 1603–1607. Available from https://doi.org/10.1038/sj.bjc.6605058.

Pan, J., Ding, M., Xu, K., Yang, C., & Mao, L. J. (2017). Exosomes in diagnosis and therapy of prostate cancer. *Oncotarget*, *8*(57), 97693–97700. Available from https://doi.org/10.18632/oncotarget.18532.

Panigrahi, G. K., & Deep, G. (2017). Exosomes-based biomarker discovery for diagnosis and prognosis of prostate cancer. *Frontiers in Bioscience - Landmark*, *22*(10), 1682–1696. Available from https://doi.org/10.2741/4565.

Perkins, G. L., Slater, E. D., Sanders, G. K., & Prichard, J. G. (2003). Serum tumor markers. *American Family Physician*, *68*(6), 1075–1082.

Pullan, J. E., Confeld, M. I., Osborn, J. K., Kim, J., Sarkar, K., & Mallik, S. (2019). Exosomes as Drug Carriers for Cancer Therapy. *Molecular Pharmaceutics*, *16*(5), 1789–1798. Available from https://doi.org/10.1021/acs.molpharmaceut.9b00104.

Qin, J., & Xu, Q. (2014). Functions and applications of exosomes. *Acta Poloniae Pharmaceutica - Drug Research*, *71*(4), 537–543. Available from http://www.ptfarm.pl/pub/File/Acta_Poloniae/1998/acta4-2014.pdf.

Renzulli, J. F., Del Tatto, M., Dooner, G., Aliotta, J., Goldstein, L., Dooner, M., Colvin, G., Chatterjee, D., & Quesenberry, P. (2010). Microvesicle Induction of Prostate Specific Gene Expression in Normal Human Bone Marrow Cells. *Journal of Urology*, *184*(5), 2165–2171. Available from https://doi.org/10.1016/j.juro.2010.06.119.

Saari, H., Lázaro-Ibáñez, E., Viitala, T., Vuorimaa-Laukkanen, E., Siljander, P., & Yliperttula, M. (2015). Microvesicle- and exosome-mediated drug delivery enhances the cytotoxicity of Paclitaxel in autologous prostate cancer cells. *Journal of Controlled Release*, *220*, 727–737. Available from https://doi.org/10.1016/j.jconrel.2015.09.031.

Théry, C., Boussac, M., Véron, P., Ricciardi-Castagnoli, P., Raposo, G., Garin, J., & Amigorena, S. (2001). Proteomic analysis of dendritic cell-derived exosomes: A secreted subcellular compartment distinct from apoptotic vesicles. *Journal of Immunology*, *166*(12), 7309–7318. Available from https://doi.org/10.4049/jimmunol.166.12.7309.

Valadi, H., Ekström, K., Bossios, A., Sjöstrand, M., Lee, J. J., & Lötvall, J. O. (2007). Exosome-mediated transfer of mRNAs and microRNAs is a novel mechanism of genetic exchange between cells. *Nature Cell Biology*, *9*(6), 654–659. Available from https://doi.org/10.1038/ncb1596.

Viaud, S., Théry, C., Ploix, S., Tursz, T., Lapierre, V., Lantz, O., Zitvogel, L., & Chaput, N. (2010). Dendritic cell-derived exosomes for cancer immunotherapy: What's next? *Cancer Research*, *70*(4), 1281–1285. Available from https://doi.org/10.1158/0008-5472.CAN-09-3276.

Vlaeminck-Guillem, V. (2018). Extracellular vesicles in prostate cancer carcinogenesis, diagnosis, and management. *Frontiers in Oncology*, *8*. Available from https://doi.org/10.3389/fonc.2018.00222.

Yim, N., Ryu, S. W., Choi, K., Lee, K. R., Lee, S., Choi, H., Kim, J., Shaker, M. R., Sun, W., Park, J. H., Kim, D., Do Heo, W., & Choi, C. (2016). Exosome engineering for efficient intracellular delivery of soluble proteins using optically reversible protein-protein interaction module. *Nature Communications*, *7*. Available from https://doi.org/10.1038/ncomms12277.

Zijlstra, C., & Stoorvogel, W. (2016). Prostasomes as a source of diagnostic biomarkers for prostate cancer. *Journal of Clinical Investigation*, *126*(4), 1144–1151. Available from https://doi.org/10.1172/JCI81128.

Chapter 6

Adenovirus vectors for vaccination and cancer gene therapy

Rihabe Boussettine[1], Najwa Hassou[2], Hlima Bessi[1] and Moulay Mustapha Ennaji[1]

[1]Team of Virology, Oncology, and Biotechnologies, Laboratory of Virology, Oncology, Biosciences, Environment and New Energies (LVO-BEEN), Faculty of Sciences and Techniques Mohammedia, University Hassan II of Casablanca, Casablanca, Morocco, [2]Group Leader Research team of Virology, Oncology, and Biotechnologies, Head of Laboratory of Virology, Oncology, Biosciences, Environment and New Energies (LVO-BEEN), Faculty of Sciences and Techniques Mohammedia, University Hassan II of Casablanca, Casablanca, Morocco

6.1 Introduction

Cancer is one of the leading causes of death worldwide, with 7.6 million deaths, or about 13% of all deaths, reported in 2008 (WHO, 2011). Despite its treatment with conventional treatments such as surgery, chemotherapy, and radiotherapy, the total number of deaths continues to increase. In addition to treatment modalities, gene therapy is expected to play a key role in next-generation cancer. Since 1990, the total number of gene therapy clinical trials has increased, after this technique was first used to treat a patient with adenosine deaminase defect (Hunt & Anderson, 1990). Currently, the total number of clinical protocols involving gene therapy has exceeded 1700, that is, almost two-third of the therapy protocols.

The vectors most frequently used in gene therapy for cancer are adenoviruses (Adv) because of their many useful characteristics (Higuchi et al., 2004). Adv can be produced in very high titles with ease, have a relatively high capacity for the transgene insertion, and effectively transduce both division and not divide the cells without incorporating viral DNA into the host genome (Higuchi et al., 2004). Adv are the most used vectors against various cancers in which they therapeutically transduce genes, including tumor suppressor genes, cytokine genes, and suicide genes. However, despite preclinical encouragement and early clinical results (Li et al., 2009), successful clinical utility of the gene therapy has been

Immunological Implications and Molecular Diagnostics of Genitourinary Cancer.
DOI: https://doi.org/10.1016/B978-0-323-85496-2.00029-4

achieved heretofore. The application of gene therapy in the treatment of cancer is confronted with several barriers to widespread acceptance and use of Adv. The first obstacle is ineffective Adv-mediating gene transfer in tumor cells missing from the primary Adv receptor, coxsackievirus, and adenovirus receptor (CAR). It is well known that the expression CAR is highly variable (and often low) in many malignant tumors (Korn et al., 2009). The second obstacle is the rapid accumulation of the injected Adv in the liver and its induction of serious side effects due to undesirable transgenic expression (Yao et al., 2007). Because the transfer of primary and metastatic lesions is essential for successful gene therapy of cancer, Adv targeted against cancer with high levels of accumulation in tumor tissue and negligible distribution to normal tissue after systemic injection should be developed (Yao et al., 2007; Okada et al., 2005). In addition, most people have Adv-neutralizing antibodies, which hinder the effectiveness of gene expression (Zheng et al., 2010). Adequate transgenic expression, currently available Adv should be given at a sufficiently high dose, which has caused negative side effects (Lehrman, 1999). These problems have complicated the clinical application of Adv. Therefore, more effective and safer Adv require stricter in vivo regulation of Adv to obtain selective expression of its therapeutic effect.

In this chapter, we will present several approaches to overcome the problems associated with targeting Adv. First, a genetic modification method, the host range for adenoviral transfection, is reviewed.

Subsequently, a transcriptional regulatory approach for effective gene therapy using Adv is described. The chemical conjugation of Adv surface proteins with targeting ligands or polymers to control in vivo kinetics and alter the distribution of these viruses is summarized. Finally, an active targeting strategy by adding ligands such as antibodies, peptides, and sugars to the end of polymers, which are conjugated with Adv, is discussed.

6.2 Several approaches to overcome problems associated with the targeting of adenoviruses

The hydrophilic nature and size of nucleic acids imposes constraints that distinguish them from conventional drugs. Their inclusion in liposomes or their formulation with cationic lipids protects them from degradation in vivo and increases their affinity for lipid bilayers. If these formulations increase the effectiveness of membrane transit, the complexes end inexorably in the endosome and lysosome, where they are mostly degraded. An astronomical number of complexes is in fact necessary to allow the expression of nucleic acids in a limited number of cells (Felgner et al., 1987). Although the emergence of viruses is a real enigma for geneticists, they are nevertheless nature's solution to the formidable challenge of gene transfer. The viral genome is protected within a nucleoprotein complex (the viral "core"), specially adapted for transit and through all biological barriers that separate it from cell compartments in which it can be expressed: cytoplasm (RNA) or cell nucleus. It is therefore not surprising if researchers and practitioners are trying to understand various viral strategies to better reproduce them. Two major strategies allow viruses to release their genetic information into the cell cytoplasm. Nonenveloped viruses penetrate through endocytosis and encode functions, allowing them to escape from endosmosis trapping. Enveloped viruses encode proteins that can fuse two membranes lipids and release a nucleo-protein complex directly into the cytoplasm (Latta et al., 1995). Table 6.1 presents the different approaches to overcome problems associated with the targeting of Adv.

6.3 General properties of adenovirus and adenovirus vector

Adv belong to the family of Adenoviridae. Those affecting mammals belong to the genus mastadenovirus (Ishibashi & Yasue, 1984); Among the 100 different serotypes, 51 are pathogenic for humans (Ray et al., 2004). Seven subgroups or species named A to G and 52 serotypes are identified for human Adv (Ghebremedhin, 2014).

Adenovirus is a nonenveloped, 80–110 nm diameter virus presenting icosahedral symmetry (Fig. 6.1) Fig. 6.1. Adv contain a linear, double-stranded DNA genome, with a terminal protein (TP) attached covalently to the 5' termini (van Regenmortel et al., 2000). The protein capsid encloses the nucleoid (core or heart) containing the viral DNA. Two major components, or capsomeres, make up the bulk of the viral capsid hexon, which forms the faces (12 hexon per side, 240 per particle) and the penton located at 12 vertices. These two capsomers use 3 of the 12 major polypeptides constituting the viral particle. Hexon is a trimer of polypeptide II; the penton, encased between five contiguous hexons, is formed by the noncovalent assembly of a pentameric polypeptide III, the base of the penton (or penton-base), associated with the fiber. The fiber is a spicular projection emanating from the base of the penton; it consists of a polypeptide trimer IV. The heart contains 4 proteins in close contact with the viral DNA. The other constituent polypeptides participate in this structure by stabilizing the capsomeres with each other or with the heart (Molinier-Frenkel et al., 2003; Hassou et al., 2020).

The hexon, penton base, and knobbed fiber, are the most important capsid proteins for gene delivery. Hexon is the major protein forming the 20 triangular faces of the viral capsid. The 240 hexon capsomers in the capsid are trimers, each interacting with six other trimers. The 12 vertices are formed by the penton capsomere, a complex of five copies of the penton base, and three copies of fiber. Each penton capsomere interacts with five hexon capsomeres, one from each of the five faces that converge at the vertex. The knobbed fiber protrudes from the fiber base (Fig. 6.2).

The genome of the Adv consists of a linear and double-stranded DNA molecule and corresponds to 30–40 open reading frames, circularized during replication by a TP and carrying at each of its ends an inverted terminal repeat (ITR) sequence of 43–369 nucleotides.

TABLE 6.1 Several approaches to overcome problems associated with the targeting of adenoviruses.

Strategies	Description	Advantages	Disadvantages	Reference
Genetic modification	Genetic modification of adenovirus capsid proteins to alter transfection range	Enhanced transduction efficiency in car-negative cells	Unknown biological risk	Barnett et al. (2002)
				Mizuguchi et al. (2001)
Transcriptional regulation	Driven transgene expression of Adv By transcriptional level	Tumor-specific expression	Should not alter the distribution of Adv	Qiu et al. (1998)
				Mizuguchi and Hayakawa (2002a,b)
				Okada et al. (2005)
Physical coating and chemical conjugation	1. Physical coating of Adv with liposomes or é with nanoparticles	Mask surface epitopes, prevent antibody neutralization, control in vivo kinetics and alter distribution of Adv	Steric hindrance to transduction of Adv	Lee et al. (2007)
	2. Chemical conjugation of surface protein of Adv with (1) ligands (2) polymers			Weaver and Barry (2008)

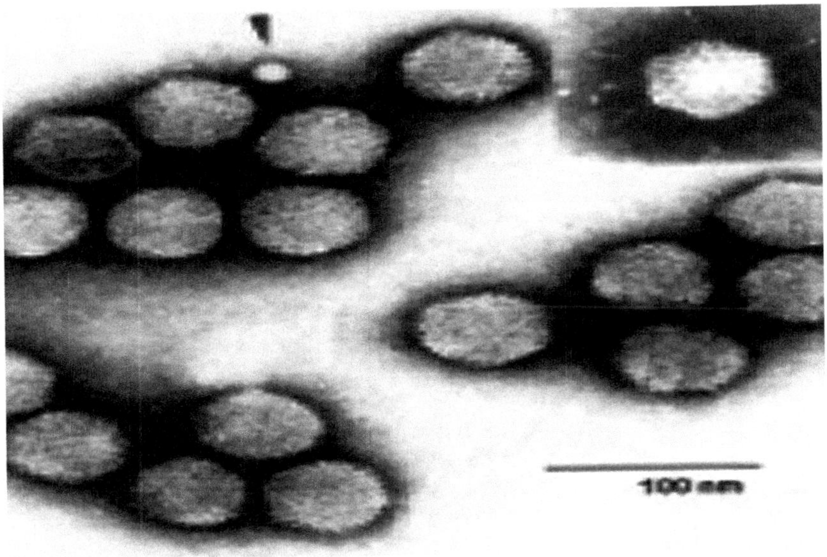

FIGURE 6.1 A virus image from the International Committee on Taxonomy of Viruses, from "The Big Picture Book of Viruses," available at http://www.virology.net/Big_Virology/BVDNAadeno.html.

The genome size varies from 26 to 45 kbp (it is about 36 kbp for human Adv 2 and 5) and is subdivided into early (E for early), intermediate (protein IX and IVa2) and late (L for late), organized into blocks of genes operating in transcription units.

Protein TP, 55 kDa is covalently bound to the 5 'ends of the DNA. The binding between the TP and the viral DNA is via a phosphodiester bridge between the beta-hydroxyl group of a serine residue (position 562) of the TP protein and the 5'-hydroxyl terminal of a deoxycytosine. The TP allows replication to begin. The transcript of the genome is made on both strands (Enligne Vénard et al., 2001).

The capsid is composed of 240 hexon capsomeres and 12 penton capsomeres with spike-shaped protrusions or fibers (Rux & Burnett, 2004). The N-terminus of fiber, the tail domain, binds to a penton base, which acts as an anchor. The C-terminus of fiber, the knob domain, binds to CAR on target cells during infection (Rux & Burnett, 2004). The binding between the fiber on Ad and CAR on target cells is the first step of adenoviral infection (Rux & Burnett, 2004). After this binding, interaction between an RGD motif on the surface of the penton base protein and a cell-surface integrin molecule promotes the uptake of the virus by endocytosis which is induced by clathrin receptors (Meier et al., 2002) Shortly after viral capsid in the endosome, the fibers fall. The release of the penton bases of the capsid is caused by the decrease of the pH of the endosome, and their release causes the lysis of the

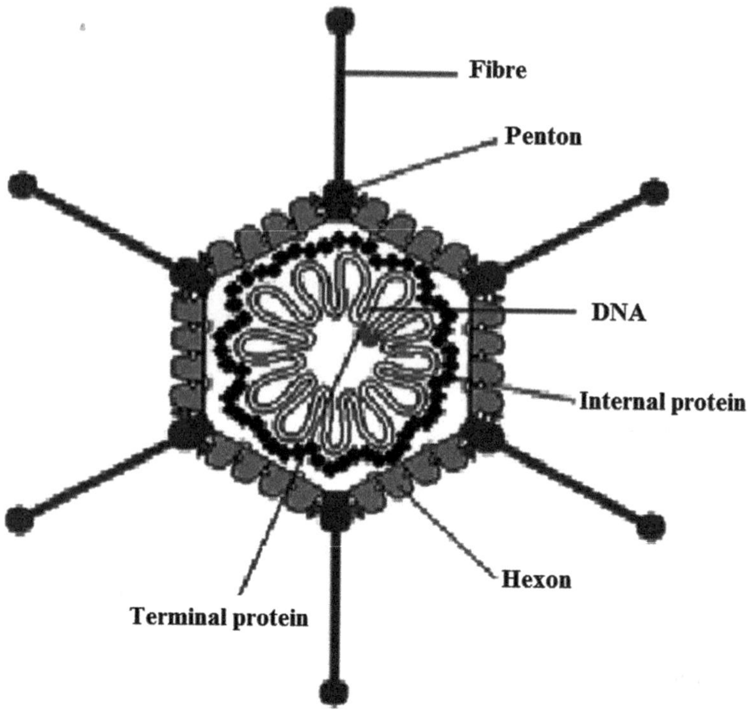

FIGURE 6.2 Viral particles of adenovirus (http://www.micro.msb.le.acv.uk/335/Adenoviruses).

endosome. After entry into cell cytoplasm, Ad virions dock with nuclear pore complex (Meier & Greber, 2003). Adenoviral DNA is then extruded into the nucleus.

Currently, more than 50 human Ad serotypes have been identified. Ad serotype 2 and 5 (Ad2 and Ad5, respectively) have the desired characteristics for gene transfer vectors for gene therapy, in particular, the ability to generate high-quality, low pathogenicity virus solutions and high efficiency of nuclear transfer. To use Ad as a gene transfer vector, the suppression of the E1 gene, which contributes to reproduction, is necessary. Deficient conventional replication, known as first generation. First-generation vectors contain deletions in the E1 region, often lacking E1A and E1B, while second-generation vectors lack even more nonessential regions, such as E2 and E4 transcription units, to increase the capacity for exogenous DNA. Helper-dependent adenovirus vectors, also referred to as gutted vectors, contain only viral sequences that are essential for DNA replication, including the inverted terminal repeats that serve as DNA replication origins and viral packaging sequences. These vectors have an even greater cloning capacity than the first- and second-generation adenovirus vectors. Because they lack early and late genes that are essential for the production of virus particles, helper-dependent adenovirus vectors must be grown in the presence of a complementing helper adenovirus that provides these missing elements. Various techniques have been developed to ensure that only the vector DNA is packaged and to separate the helper-dependent adenovirus vector from the helper adenovirus (Shiravi et al., 2021). The advanced values are based on the substitution of the E1 region by the therapeutic gene. First-generation Adv usually have an additional deletion in the E3 region, which is not necessary for replication approximately 8 kb (Bett et al., 1994). Deletion of both E1 and E3 negate adenoviral pathogenicity while maintaining high transduction efficiency (Fig. 6.3).

6.4 Adenovirus tumor-selective replication

The study and design of Adv, which replicate selectively in tumor cells, is the most intensive area of research in adenovirus cancer virotherapy before analyzing what has been achieved in selective replication, it is useful to comment on the assays that were used.

Selective replication of a CRAd has generally been studied by comparison of different human cell lines in vitro. While different cell lines can show varying levels of susceptibility to adenovirus infection and virus production, these variables have not always been taken into account. This deficiency can be corrected by including a comparison with a nonselective adenovirus such

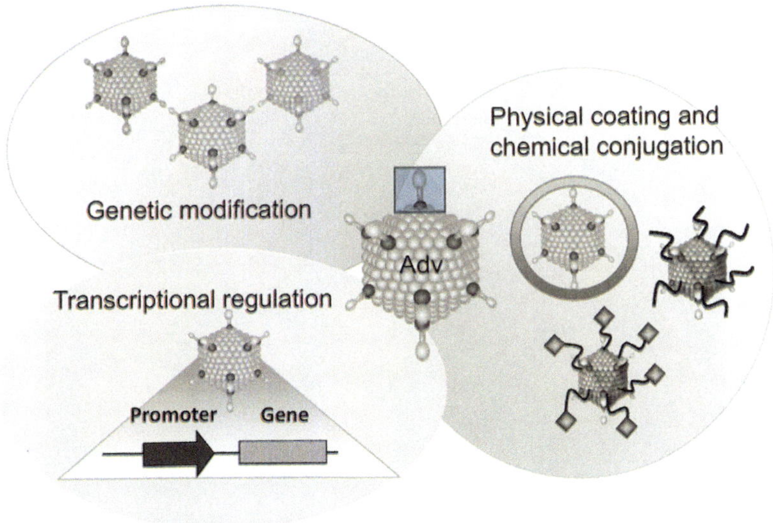

FIGURE 6.3 Targeting strategies of adenoviruses.

as wild type (Adwt), although not all studies incorporate this control. The effect of a CRAd in vitro was measured at the level of viral DNA replication, late gene expression, cell death, and production of offspring. These parameters are not always correlated. Replication of viral DNA, hexon expression, and cell death can occur without the production of offspring. Conversely, in some types of cells, such as fibroblasts and keratinocytes, virus production may occur without obvious cytopathic effect.

Therefore although crystal violet staining, exclusion of trypan blue, and other living dead tests provide information on the effects of CRAd in each cell type, from the standpoint of oncolysis, the offspring production is the most relevant. In addition, the progeny released into the supernatant is likely to have more oncolytic predictive value than if we measure it after releasing virus from cells by freeze/thaw cycles. For a given cell type, burst size or number of infectious particles produced per cell is a quantitative measure of progeny production (Ramón et al., 2001) (Fig. 6.4).

Perhaps the best and easiest way to numerically express selectivity of a CRAd between a tumor and normal cell line is as follows:

(CRAd burst size in tumor cell / CRAd burst size in normal cell) × (Adwt burst size in normal cell / Adwt burst size in tumor cell)

Using this formula, if a CRAd produces 1000 plaque units (m.p.u.)/cell in a tumor cell and 1 m.p.u./cell in a normal cell, and Adwt produces 10,000 and 100, respectively, then this CRAd is 10 times more selective than Adwt.

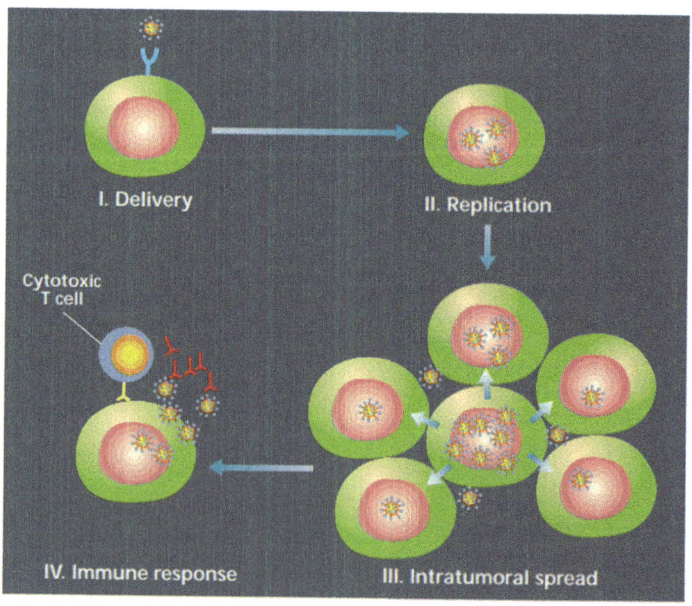

FIGURE 6.4 Oncolysis steps that provide opportunities for intervention.

The presence of Adwt in this formula corrects the difference in infectivity and virus production between different types of cells. In contrast, the choice of normal cells is critical. Primary human embryonic kidney cells are the most susceptible adenovirus types 2 and 5 (Lucher et al., 1995) Human fibroblast cell lines and endothelial cell lines employed in different studies (Hay et al., 1999; Heise et al., 1997; Yu et al., 1999) show poor infectivity and delayed cytopathic effect. Mammary and bronchial epithelial cells used in other reports (Rothmann et al., 1998) are more permissive to adenovirus infection and production.

Biodistribution of adenovirus is not based solely on CAR. In fact, the results of intravascular adenovirus administration have been reported mainly for the liver, spleen, heart, lungs, and kidneys of mice, although these tissues are not necessarily the most in the CAR expression. Instead, the degree of vascularization structure in each organ probably contributes to biodistribution. Tissue macrophages, such as Kupffer cells of the liver, play a major role in the suppression of adenovirus from the blood (Alemany et al., 2001). This is a nonCAR-mediated process and results in rapid blood clearance and virus degradation. However, Kupffer cells can be saturated with around 1–2 10^{10} viral particles in mice, and thereafter, virus delivery to other organs is increased (Tao et al., 2001). Alternatively, Kupffer cells can be depleted (Alemany et al., 2001). It is currently unknown if these aspects are similar in humans (Fig. 6.5).

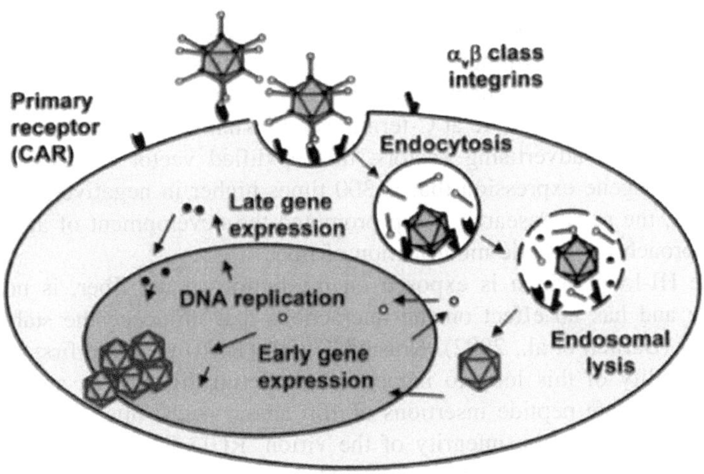

FIGURE 6.5 The adenovirus infection pathway. Cell entry is initiated by high-affinity binding of the fiber knob domain to its primary receptor, CAR. CAR binding is followed by endocytosis mediated by penton-base RGD interaction with cellular v integrins. After endosomal lysis, viral DNA is transported to the nucleus through a microtubule-mediated process, and viral genes or transgenes are expressed.

6.5 Genetic modification to alter transfection range of adenoviruses

The first stage of Adv infection involves an interaction between the Adv fiber protein and CAR. Although Adv could infect many types of cells, several cell populations remain difficult to infect, especially dendritic cells (DCs), hematopoietic cells, and malignant tumor cells with very low expression (or not) RAC (Murakami et al., 2007). Reduction of RAC expression in advanced tumor stages is one of the main barriers to the use of Adv for cancer gene therapy. Fortunately, the attachment itself is not essential for Adv infection and serves only as a means of viral particle in intimate contact with the cell surface.

6.5.1 1-Insertion of foreign ligand into fiber protein

The button domain of the fiber protein Ad is the main site for binding with the native primary receptor, CAR. Many research groups have therefore focused on fiber modification to optimize viral transfection.

The successful modification of the fiber must follow some basic guidelines to not structure the protein. In particular, the inserted ligand must be displayed on the surface of the fiber to access its ligand and receptor should not inhibit trimeration of the natural fiber structure.

Michael et al. (1995) made the first modifications of the Ad5 fiber before the crystalline structure of the fiber protein was confirmed. These researchers inserted the peptide-releasing gastrin gene in the C-terminus of the fibrous protein using a flexible bond. This vector has retained the ability to bind both GRP and CAR without interruption of fiber trimerization. These studies were continued by Wickham et al. (1993) who inserted polylysine residues that bind to heparan sulfate at C-terminus (Wickham et al., 1997). Compared to conventional advertising vectors, this modified vector induces approximately transgene expression that is 300 times higher in negative CAR cells. However, the same research group promoted the development of an alternative approach for genetic modification of fiber.

The HI-loop, which is exposed on the button of the fiber, is normally flexible and has no effect on the interactions that influence the stability of the fiber (Barnett et al., 2002). Krasnykh et al. (1998) were the first to report the suitability of this loop to incorporate targeting ligands. In addition, HI loop can tolerate peptide insertions of 100 amino acids, often with minimal negative effects on the integrity of the virion. RGD-4C (CDCRGDCFC) is the best known peptide in the HI loop. This peptide was selected for its ability to bind with a number of integral cells and for its small size (Wickham et al., 1997; Hidaka et al., 2006; Krasnykh et al., 2000) without disrupting the three-dimensional structure of the fibrous protein or its ability to trimerize (Krasnykh et al., 1998). Because the Adv-encoded RGD-4C peptide in the HI loop retained the ability to recognize CAR but was able to transduce target cells via a v integrin-mediated, CAR-independent pathway, it showed better transfection ability for various cancer cells, such as primary cells and established ovarian cancer cells (Kanerva et al., 2002), squamous cell carcinoma (Kasono et al.,1999), and myelocytic leukemia (García-Castro et al., 2001). By integrin binding, this vector enabled efficient transgene expression in CAR-deficient cells, which are difficult to transduce with conventional Adv (Okada et al., 2005). A simple method was developed by Mizuguchi and Hayakawa (2004) based on in vitro ligation to construct Adv containing heterologous foreign peptides both in the HI loop and at the C end of the fiber button (Koizumi et al., 2003). They demonstrated that advertising vectors containing RGD, poly-lysine (KKKKKKK; K7) or Tat peptides from the HI loop or from the C-terminus showed high transgene expression with wider tropism (Kurachi et al., 2007). This simple method promoted the further development of Mutated Adv.

Many research groups have adapted fiber-mutant Adv to various applications, such as suicide gene therapy and cytokine gene therapy, for CAR-negative tumor cells (Mizuguchi & Hayakawa, 2002a,b; Kurachi et al., 2007). This type of vector containing an RGD motif in the HI loop has been shown to be effective in immunizing DCs for cancer immunotherapy (Okada et al., 2001). DCs, the most effective antigen present in cells, are being investigated as antigen delivery vehicles for eliciting T cell-mediated antitumor immunity. Recent studies have demonstrated genetic utility of immunotherapy based on Adv-modified DC, but the gene transduction efficiency of conventional Adv is insufficient for clinical use owing to lack of expression of CAR on the DC surface (Okada et al., 2001). Therefore Adv was constructed with RGD peptides in the HI loop (Adv-RGD), which encoded a cytokine or chemokine gene to activate DC function or cancer antigenic gene for cancer vaccination (Okada et al., 2003). Compared to that of DC transduced with conventional Adv, Adv-RGD transduit DC function or a cancer antigen gene for cancer vaccination demonstrated an increased antitumor effect or effective vaccination against cancer (Okada et al., 2005). These results suggest that Adv fiber-targeted mutant v-integrin is a potent tool for DC-based immunotherapy.

6.5.2 2-Fiber mutation for generating targeted adenoviruses

Even though the main determinant of adenoviral transfection range is the level of expression of CAR at the surface cell level, it should be noted that removal of the binding between Adv and CAR does not completely prevent Adv from binding nontarget cells (Okada et al., 2005). It has recently been shown that it is essential to inhibit Adv binding of v integrins, which are secondary receptors and heparan sulfate glycosaminoglycans (HSGs), which are subsidiary receptors, to untarget Adv (Nakamura et al., 2003). In this light, Koizumi et al. reported Adv with ablation of CAR, v integrin and HSG binding due to mutation of the AB loop in the fiber button, removal of the RGD motif in the penton base, and substitution of the domain of the fiber tree for it derived from the Adv type 35 (Koizumi et al., 2003; Koizumi et al., 2006). Compared to conventional Adv, intravenous injection of these Adv triple mutants induces significantly lower transgene expression in murine liver (approximately 30,000 fold) and other organs. Insertion of targeting ligands into these vectors could achieve cell-specific gene transfer. From these results, triple mutant Adv appear to be fundamental prototype vectors for targeted Adv.

Successful cancer targeting therapy requires an effective targeting ligand that produces high affinity and specificity against a target receptor expressed on the surface of the tumor cell. The phage display system, in which libraries of random peptides expressed on phages can be screened either in vitro (Nicklin et al., 2000) or in vivo (Lee et al., 2007), is a promising approach to identify a desirable ligand from a large number of candidates. Candidate peptides can be inserted into Adv capsid proteins. If the incorporated peptides retain their native binding capacity, Adv can also target the same molecule (Nicklin et al., 2001). Xia et al. (1994) used phage display to identify 10 candidate peptides that targeted the human transferrin receptor and were highly expressed in tumor tissue (Xia et al., 2000). Although one half of the candidates showed specific binding, the other half were difficult to bind to Adv. These results show that the inserted peptides can disrupt the structure of the fiber, thus abrogating the natural tropism of the CAR binding capacity of the button domain. Conformational changes in the fiber button domain that disrupt the binding capacity of the inserted peptides is another potential problem of Adv. Therefore, it is essential to develop a screening system to identify targeting ligands that retain their binding capacity upon insertion into advertisements.

6.5.3 3-Fiber exchange

Because Adv based on serotypes 2 and 5 recognizes CAR as a primary receptor, retargeting of Adv may be possible by replacing the entire fiber protein with that of another serotype (Denby et al., 2004; Rea et al., 2001; Takayama et al., 2003). Although the fibrous protein has serotypic characteristics, the similarity in the basic structure of the protein (especially between the fiber tail domain and penton base) among the serotypes allows the exchange of fibers. Gall et al. were the first to report the successful use of this approach, when they replaced the native fiber of Ad5 with that of Ad7 (Gall et al., 1996). The fiber-exchanged Adv showed an altered viral transfection behavior compared to conventional Ad5.

Subsequently, several research groups demonstrated the serotypic characteristics of fiber infectivity for constructing a novel fiber-exchanged Adv, which can be used to transfect CAR-negative cells. Mizuguchi and

Hayakawa (2004) used an Ad5F35 vector: a fiber-substituted Ad5 vector containing the protein fiber of Ad35 (an Ad subgroup B) to efficiently transduce not only human CAR-positive cells but also CAR-negative cells, such as CD34 cells + human bone marrow (Mizuguchi & Hayakawa, 2002a,b). In addition, these researchers used homozygotes and hemizygous human CD46 transgenic mice to clarify that Ad5F35 vectors recognize human CD46 as a CAR (Gall et al., 1996). These vectors are likely to have wide utility against CAR-negative cells, including several malignant tumors.

6.5.4 4-Modification of other capsid proteins

Although modification of fiber is currently the most advanced genetic approach for altering the adenoviral transfection range, several research groups have sought to mutate other capsid proteins, such as hexon, the penton base, and capsid protein IX. Hexon is a particularly attractive target for genetic modification because it is the most abundant capsid protein of Adv and because it has a hypervariable region that is displayed on the Adv surface.

For a successful approach to retargeting cancer, all of these characteristics must be taken into account. Adv with an RGD motif in the hypervariable region of the hexone protein could transduce vascular smooth muscle by a fiber-independent mechanism (Vigne et al., 1999). Wickham et al. (1993) constructed mutated Ad vectors with a penton base, wherein they replaced the RGD motif of the penton base with LDV, an integrin-specific binding motif (Wickham et al., 1995); this Adv obtained increased expression of the transgene against B lymphocytes and T lymphocytes expressing integrin. These results suggest that the base proteins hexon and penton are candidates for modification to modify adenoviral transfection behavior. Targeting ligands can also be inserted into the C-terminus of capsid protein IX, which stabilizes the conformation of the adenoviral capsid and plays a critical role in viral DNA packaging (Rosa-Calatrava et al., 2001; Douglas et al., 1999). The C-terminus of capsid protein IX faces the outer surface of the viral capsid, making it a reasonable site for insertion of a targeting ligand.

Dmitriev et al. (1998) inserted polylysine, a motif that binds heparan sulfate, into the C-terminus of capsid protein IX to enhance transfection of CAR-deficient human breast cancer cell lines and human umbilical vein endothelial cells (Dmitriev et al., 2002; Kurachi, Tashiro, et al., 2007). Another research group constructed Adv containing the FLAG tag or an RGD peptide in protein IX by a simple in vitro ligation-based method (Kurachi et al., 2007). Although expression of the foreign peptides on the virus surface was detected, the transduction efficiency of these Adv was very low. These results suggest that protein IX has the potential to be used in capsid modification strategies for Adv targeting, despite the existence of some unknown factor that compromises the gene transduction ability of protein

IX-mutated Adv. Combination of any of the described technologies for broadening the transfection range of Adv will enable the simultaneous display of multiple, functionally different molecules on the Adv surface. This kind of Adv would not only have the targeting ability of one molecule but also the additional benefit afforded by another molecule (e.g., a tag peptide to facilitate virus purification). Limitations of these vectors include the stability of their binding with adapter molecules in vivo, extra immune response induced by genetic modification of adenoviral capsid protein. These drawbacks must be carefully addressed before these vectors gain clinical utility.

6.6 Conclusion

At the beginning of the use of gene therapy, monogenic diseases were mainly taken into consideration. Currently, clinical trials are mostly focused on cancer diseases. Gene therapy could indeed stimulate the immune system of patients in order to fight tumor cells more effectively. Many trials also concern cardiovascular diseases: gene therapy could allow the regeneration of heart tissue. Hematological or neurological diseases (such as multiple sclerosis or Alzheimer's disease) may also benefit from treatment with gene therapy. Finally, gene therapy may be effective in the treatment of some infectious diseases, and Adv offer a great advantage in this regard.

Acknowledgment

The authors would like to express gratitude for the support from the Ministry of High Education of Morocco, the University Hassan II of Casablanca and Faculty of Sciences and Techniques Mohammedia. They would also like to thank the entire staff of Laboratory of Virology, Microbiology, Quality and Biotechnologies/Ecotoxicology and Biodiversity, and the team of Virology for their technical assistance.

References

Alemany, R., & Curiel, D. T. (2001). CAR-binding ablation does not change biodistribution and toxicity of adenoviral vectors. *Gene Therapy*, *8*(17), 1347–1353.

Barnett, B. G., Crews, C. J., & Douglas, J. T. (2002). Targeted adenoviral vectors. *Biochimica et Biophysica Acta – Gene Structure and Expression*, *1575*(1–3), 1–14. Available from https://doi.org/10.1016/S0167-4781(02)00249-X.

Bett, A. J., Haddara, W., Prevec, L., & Graham, F. L. (1994). An efficient and flexible system for construction of adenovirus vectors with insertions or deletions in early regions 1 and 3. *Proceedings of the National Academy of Sciences of the United States of America*, *91*(19), 8802–8806. Available from https://doi.org/10.1073/pnas.91.19.8802.

Denby, L., Work, L. M., Graham, D., Hsu, C., Von Seggern, D. J., Nicklin, S. A., & Baker, A. H. (2004). Adenoviral serotype 5 vectors pseudotyped with fibers from subgroup D show modified tropism in vitro and in vivo. *Human Gene Therapy*, *15*(11), 1054–1064. Available from https://doi.org/10.1089/1043034042431083.

Dmitriev, I., Krasnykh, V., Miller, C. R., Wang, M., Kashentseva, E., Mikheeva, G., Belousova, N., & Curiel, D. T. (1998). An adenovirus vector with genetically modified fibers demonstrates expanded tropism via utilization of a coxsackievirus and adenovirus receptor- independent cell entry mechanism. *Journal of Virology, 72*(12), 9706–9713. Available from https://doi.org/10.1128/jvi.72.12.9706-9713.1998.

Dmitriev, I. P., Kashentseva, E. A., & Curiel, D. T. (2002). Engineering of adenovirus vectors containing heterologous peptide sequences in the C terminus of capsid protein IX. *Journal of Virology, 76*(14), 6893–6899. Available from https://doi.org/10.1128/JVI.76.14.6893-6899.2002.

Douglas, J. T., Miller, C. R., Kim, M., Dmitriev, I., Mikheeva, G., Krasnykh, V., & Curiel, D. T. (1999). A system for the propagation of adenoviral vectors with genetically modified receptor specificities. *Nature Biotechnology, 17*(5), 470–475. Available from https://doi.org/10.1038/8647.

Enligne Vénard, V., Bordigoni, P., & Le Faou, A. (2001). Adenovirus infections in the hospital setting. *Virology, 5*(4), 245–253.

Felgner, P. L., Gadek, T. R., Holm, M., Roman, R., Chan, H. W., Wenz, M., & Danielsen, M. (1987). Lipofection: a highly efficient, lipid-mediated DNA-transfection procedure. *Proceedings of the National Academy of Sciences, 84*(21), 7413–7417.

Gall, J., Kass-Eisler, A., Leinwand, L., & Falck-Pedersen, E. (1996). Adenovirus type 5 and 7 capsid chimera: Fiber replacement alters receptor tropism without affecting primary immune neutralization epitopes. *Journal of Virology, 70*(4), 2116–2123. Available from https://doi.org/10.1128/jvi.70.4.2116-2123.1996.

García-Castro, J., Segovia, J. C., García-Sánchez, F., Lillo, R., Gómez-Navarro, J., Curiel, D. T., & Bueren, J. A. (2001). Selective transduction of murine myelomonocytic leukemia cells (WEHI-3B) with regular and RGD-adenoviral vectors. *Molecular Therapy, 3*(1), 70–77. Available from https://doi.org/10.1006/mthe.2000.0221.

Ghebremedhin, B. (2014). Human adenovirus: Viral pathogen with increasing importance. *European Journal of Microbiology and Immunology, 4*(1), 26–33.

Hassou, N., Bouseettine, R., Abouchoaib, N., et, E. 2020. Adénovirus entériques: Émergence d'une menace pour la santé publique. In Emerging and Reemerging Viral Pathogens (pp. 879–905).

Hay, C. M., Ruhl, D. J., Basgoz, N. O., Wilson, C. C., Billingsley, J. M., DePasquale, M. P., & Walker, B. D. (1999). Lack of viral escape and defective in vivo activation of human immunodeficiency virus type 1-specific cytotoxic T lymphocytes in rapidly progressive infection. *Journal of Virology, 73*(7), 5509–5519.

Heise, C., Sampson-Johannes, A., Williams, A., Mccormick, F., Von Hoff., & Kirn, D. H. (1997). ONYX-015, an E1B gene-attenuated adenovirus, causes tumor-specific cytolysis and antitumoral efficacy that can be augmented by standard chemotherapeutic agents. *Nature Medicine, 3*(6), 639–645.

Hidaka, C., Milano, E., Leopold, P. L., Bergelson, J. M., Hackett, N. R., Finberg, R. W., Wickham, T. J., Kovesdi, I., Roelvink, P., & Crystal, R. G. (2006). CAR-dependent and CAR-independent pathways of adenovirus vector-mediated gene transfer and expression in human. *Human Gene Therapy, 17*, 264–279.

Higuchi, M., Pischke, M. S., Mähönen, A. P., Miyawaki, K., Hashimoto, Y., Seki, M., Kobayashi, M., Shinozaki, K., Kato, T., Tabata, S., Helariutta, Y., Sussman, M. R., & Kakimoto, T. (2004). In planta functions of the *Arabidopsis cytokinin* receptor family. *Proceedings of the National Academy of Sciences of the United States of America, 101*(23), 8821–8826. Available from https://doi.org/10.1073/pnas.0402887101.

Hunt, S. J., & Anderson, W. D. (1990). Malignant rhabdoid tumor of the liver. A distinct clinicopathologic entity. *American Journal of Clinical Pathology*, *94*(5), 645–648. Available from https://doi.org/10.1093/ajcp/94.5.645.

Ishibashi, M., & Yasue, H. (1984). Adenoviruses of animals. In The adenoviruses, (pp. 497–562). Boston, MA: Springer.

Kanerva, A., Wang, M., Bauerschmitz, G. J., Lam, J. T., Desmond, R. A., Bhoola, S. M., Barnes, M. N., Alvarez, R. D., Siegal, G. P., Curiel, D. T., & Hemminki, A. (2002). Gene transfer to ovarian cancer vs normal tissues with fiber-modified adenoviruses. *Molecular Therapy*, *5*(6), 695–704. Available from https://doi.org/10.1006/mthe.2002.0599.

Kasono, K., Blackwell, J. L., Douglas, J. T., Dmitriev, I., Strong, T. V., Reynolds, P., Kropf, D. A., Carroll, W. R., Peters, G. E., Bucy, R. P., Curiel, D. T., & Krasnykh, V. (1999). Selective gene delivery to head and neck cancer cells via an integrin targeted adenoviral vector. *Clinical Cancer Research*, *5*(9), 2571–2579.

Koizumi, N., Kawabata, K., Sakurai, F., Watanabe, Y., Hayakawa, T., & Mizuguchi, H. (2006). Modified adenoviral vectors ablated for coxsackievirus-adenovirus receptor, αv integrin, and heparan sulfate binding reduce in vivo tissue transduction and toxicity. *Human Gene Therapy*, *17*(3), 264–279. Available from https://doi.org/10.1089/hum.2006.17.264.

Koizumi, N., Mizuguchi, H., Sakurai, F., Yamaguchi, T., Watanabe, Y., & Hayakawa, T. (2003). Reduction of natural adenovirus tropism to mouse liver by fiber-shaft exchange in combination with both CAR- and αv integrin-binding ablation. *Journal of Virology*, *77*(24), 13062–13072. Available from https://doi.org/10.1128/JVI.77.24.13062-13072.2003.

Koizumi, N., Mizuguchi, H., Utoguchi, N., Watanabe, Y., & Hayakawa, T. (2003). Generation of fiber-modified adenovirus vectors containing heterologous peptides in both the HI loop and C terminus of the fiber knob. *Journal of Gene Medicine*, *5*(4), 267–276. Available from https://doi.org/10.1002/jgm.348.

Korn, T., Bettelli, E., Oukka, M., & Kuchroo, V. K. (2009). IL-17 and Th17 cells. *Annual Review of Immunology*, *27*, 485–517. Available from https://doi.org/10.1146/annurev.immunol.021908.132710.

Krasnykh, V., Dmitriev, I., Mikheeva, G., Miller, C. R., Belousova, N., & Curiel, D. T. (1998). Characterization of an adenovirus vector containing a heterologous peptide epitope in the HI loop of the fiber knob. *Journal of Virology*, *72*(3), 1844–1852. Available from https://doi.org/10.1128/jvi.72.3.1844-1852.1998.

Krasnykh, V., Dmitriev, I., Navarro, J. G., Belousova, N., Kashentseva, E., Xiang, J., Douglas, J. T., & Curiel, D. T. (2000). Advanced generation adenoviral vectors possess augmented gene transfer efficiency based upon coxsackie adenovirus receptor-independent cellular entry capacity. *Cancer Research*, *60*(24), 6784–6787.

Kurachi, S., Koizumi, N., Sakurai, F., Kawabata, K., Sakurai, H., Nakagawa, S., Hayakawa, T., & Mizuguchi, H. (2007). Characterization of capsid-modified adenovirus vectors containing heterologous peptides in the fiber knob, protein IX, or hexon. *Gene Therapy*, 266–274. Available from https://doi.org/10.1038/sj.gt.3302859.

Kurachi, S., Tashiro, K., Sakurai, F., Sakurai, H., Kawabata, K., Yayama, K., Okamoto, H., Nakagawa, S., & Mizuguchi, H. (2007). Fiber-modified adenovirus vectors containing the TAT peptide derived from HIV-1 in the fiber knob have efficient gene transfer activity. *Gene Therapy*, *14*(15), 1160–1165. Available from https://doi.org/10.1038/sj.gt.3302969.

Latta, K., Jamieson, N. V., Scheinman, J. I., Schärer, K., Bensman, A., Cochat, P., & Mansell, M. A. (1995). Selection of transplantation procedures and perioperative management in primary hyperoxaluria type 1. *Nephrology Dialysis Transplantation*, *10*(supp 8), 53–57.

Lee, T. Y., Lin, C. T., Kuo, S. Y., Chang, D. K., & Wu, H. C. (2007). Peptide-mediated targeting to tumor blood vessels of lung cancer for drug delivery. *Cancer Research*, *67*(22), 10959–10965. Available from https://doi.org/10.1158/0008-5472.CAN-07-2233.

Lehrman, S. (1999). Virus treatment questioned after gene therapy death. *Nature*, *401*(6753), 517–518. Available from https://doi.org/10.1038/43977.

Li, H., Handsaker, B., Wysoker, A., Fennell, T., Ruan, J., Homer, N., Marth, G., Abecasis, G., & Durbin, R. (2009). The sequence alignment/map format and SAM tools. *Bioinformatics (Oxford, England)*, *25*(16), 2078–2079. Available from https://doi.org/10.1093/bioinformatics/btp352.

Lucher, L. A. (1995). Abortive adenovirus infection and host range determinants. *The Molecular Repertoire of Adenoviruses I*, 119–152.

Meier, O., Boucke, K., Hammer, S. V., Keller, S., Stidwill, R. P., Hemmi, S., & Greber, U. F. (2002). Adenovirus triggers macropinocytosis and endosomal leakage together with its clathrin-mediated uptake. *Journal of Cell Biology*, *158*(6), 1119–1131. Available from https://doi.org/10.1083/jcb.200112067.

Meier, O., & Greber, U. F. (2003). Adenovirus endocytosis. *The Journal of Gene Medicine*, *6*, 1891–1902.

Michael, S. I., Hong, J. S., Curiel, D. T., & Engler, J. A. (1995). Addition of a short peptide ligand to the adenovirus fiber protein. *Gene Therapy*, *2*(9), 660–668.

Mizuguchi, H., & Hayakawa, T. (2002a). Adenovirus vectors containing chimeric type 5 and type 35 fiber proteins exhibit altered and expanded tropism and increase the size limit of foreign genes. *Gene*, *285*(1–2), 69–77. Available from https://doi.org/10.1016/S0378-1119(02)00410-9.

Mizuguchi, H., & Hayakawa, T. (2002b). Enhanced antitumor effect and reduced vector dissemination with fiber-modified adenovirus vectors expressing herpes simplex virus thymidine kinase. *Cancer Gene Therapy*, *9*(3), 236–242. Available from https://doi.org/10.1038/sj.cgt.7700440.

Mizuguchi, H., & Hayakawa, T. (2004). Targeted adenovirus vectors. *Human Gene Therapy*, *15*(11), 1034–1044. Available from https://doi.org/10.1089/hum.2004.15.1034.

Mizuguchi, H., Koizumi, N., Hosono, T., Utoguchi, N., Watanabe, Y., Kay, M. A., & Hayakawa, T. (2001). A simplified system for constructing recombinant adenoviral vectors containing heterologous peptides in the HI loop of their fiber knob. *Gene Therapy*, *8*(9), 730–735. Available from https://doi.org/10.1038/sj.gt.3301453.

Molinier-Frenkel, V., Prévost-Blondel, A., Hong, S. S., Lengagne, R., Boudaly, S., Magnusson, M. K., & Guillet, J. G. (2003). The maturation of murine dendritic cells induced by human adenovirus is mediated by the fiber knob domain. *Journal of Biological Chemistry*, *278*(39), 37175–37182.

Murakami, S., Sakurai, F., Kawabata, K., Okada, N., Fujita, T., Yamamoto, A., Hayakawa, T., & Mizuguchi, H. (2007). Interaction of penton base Arg-Gly-Asp motifs with integrins is crucial for adenovirus serotype 35 vector transduction in human hematopoietic cells. *Gene Therapy*, *14*(21), 1525–1533. Available from https://doi.org/10.1038/sj.gt.3303019.

Nakamura, T., Sato, K., & Hamada, H. (2003). Reduction of natural adenovirus tropism to the liver by both ablation of fiber-coxsackievirus and adenovirus receptor interaction and use of replaceable short fiber. *Journal of Virology*, *77*(4), 2512–2521. Available from https://doi.org/10.1128/JVI.77.4.2512-2521.2003.

Nicklin, S. A., Von Seggern, D. J., Work, L. M., Pek, D. C. K., Dominiczak, A. F., Nemerow, G. R., & Baker, A. H. (2001). Ablating adenovirus type 5 fiber-CAR binding and HI loop insertion of the SIGYPLP peptide generate an endothelial cell-selective adenovirus. *Molecular Therapy*, *4*(6), 534–542. Available from https://doi.org/10.1006/mthe.2001.0489.

Nicklin, S. A., White, S. J., Watkins, S. J., Hawkins, R. E., & Baker, A. H. (2000). Selective targeting of gene transfer to vascular endothelial cells by use of peptides isolated by phage display. *Circulation*, *102*(2), 231–237. Available from https://doi.org/10.1161/01.CIR.102.2.231.

Okada, N., Iiyama, S., Okada, Y., Mizuguchi, H., Hayakawa, T., Nakagawa, S., Mayumi, T., Fujita, T., & Yamamoto, A. (2005). Immunological properties and vaccine efficacy of murine dendritic cells simultaneously expressing melanoma-associated antigen and interleukin-12. *Cancer Gene Therapy*, *12*(1), 72–83. Available from https://doi.org/10.1038/sj.cgt.7700772.

Okada, N., Masunaga, Y., Okada, Y., Mizuguchi, H., Iiyama, S., Mori, N., Sasaki, A., Nakagawa, S., Mayumi, T., Hayakawa, T., Fujita, T., & Yamamoto, A. (2003). Dendritic cells transduced with gp100 gene by RGD fiber-mutant adenovirus vectors are highly efficacious in generating anti-B16BL6 melanoma immunity in mice. *Gene Therapy*, *10*(22), 1891–1902. Available from https://doi.org/10.1038/sj.gt.3302090.

Okada, N., Mori, K., Saito, T., Fujita, T., Yamamoto, A., Tsukada, Y., Nakagawa, S., Mayumi, T., Mizuguchi, H., & Hayakawa, T. (2001). Efficient gene delivery into dendritic cells by fiber-mutant adenovirus vectors. *Biochemical and Biophysical Research Communications*, *282*(1), 173–179. Available from https://doi.org/10.1006/bbrc.2001.4527.

Okada, N., Mori, N., Koretomo, R., Okada, Y., Nakayama, T., Yoshie, O., Mizuguchi, H., Hayakawa, T., Nakagawa, S., Mayumi, T., Fujita, T., & Yamamoto, A. (2005). Augmentation of the migratory ability of DC-based vaccine into regional lymph nodes by efficient CCR7 gene transduction. *Gene Therapy*, *12*(2), 129–139. Available from https://doi.org/10.1038/sj.gt.3302358.

Okada, N., Saito, T., Masunaga, Y., Mori, K., Fujita, T., Yamamoto, A., Tsukada, Y., Nakagawa, S., Mayumi, T., Mizuguchi, H., Hayakawa, T., & Okada, Y. (2001). Efficient antigen gene transduction using Arg-Gly-Asp fiber-mutant adenovirus vectors can potentiate antitumor vaccine efficacy and maturation of murine dendritic cells. *Cancer Research*, *61*(21), 7913–7919.

Okada, Y., Feng, Q., Lin, Y., Jiang, Q., Li, Y., Coffield, V. M., Su, L., Xu, G., & Zhang, Y. (2005). hDOT1L links histone methylation to leukemogenesis. *Cell*, *121*(2), 167–178. Available from https://doi.org/10.1016/j.cell.2005.02.020.

Qiu, Y., Sharma, A., & Stein, R. (1998). p300 mediates transcriptional stimulation by the basic helix-loop-helix activators of the insulin gene. *Molecular and Cellular Biology*, *18*(5), 2957–2964.

Ramón, S., Moreno, A., de Felipe, J., Sola, R. G., & Navarro, A. (2001). Neuronal and mixed neuronal glial tumors associated to epilepsy. A heterogeneous and related group of tumours. *Histology and Histopathology*, *16*(2), 613–622.

Ray, P., De, A., Min, J. J., Tsien, R. Y., & Gambhir, S. S. (2004). Imaging tri-fusion multimodality reporter gene expression in living subjects. *Cancer Research*, *64*(4), 1323–1330.

Rea, D., Havenga, M. J. E., VandenAssem, M., Sutmuller, R. P. M., Lemckert, A., Hoeben, R. C., Bout, A., Melief, C. J. M., & Offringa, R. (2001). Highly efficient transduction of human monocyte-derived dendritic cells with subgroup B fiber-modified adenovirus vectors enhances transgene-encoded antigen presentation to cytotoxic T cells. *Journal of Immunology*, *166*(8), 5236–5244. Available from https://doi.org/10.4049/jimmunol.166.8.5236.

Rosa-Calatrava, M., Grave, L., Puvion-Dutilleul, F., Chatton, B., & Kedinger, C. (2001). Functional analysis of adenovirus protein IX identifies domains involved in capsid stability, transcriptional activity, and nuclear reorganization. *Journal of Virology*, *75*(15), 7131–7141. Available from https://doi.org/10.1128/JVI.75.15.7131-7141.2001.

Rothmann, K., Schnölzer, M., Radziwill, G., Hildt, E., Moelling, K., & Schaller, H. (1998). Host cell-virus cross talk: phosphorylation of a hepatitis B virus envelope protein mediates intracellular signaling. *Journal of Virology*, *72*(12), 10138–10147.

Rux, J. J., & Burnett, R. M. (2004). Adenovirus structure. *Human Gene Therapy*, *15*(12), 1167–1176. Available from https://doi.org/10.1089/hum.2004.15.1167.

Shiravi, A. A., Ardekani, A., Sheikhbahaei, E., & Heshmat-Ghahdarijani, K. (2021). Complications cardiovasculaires des vaccins contre le SRAS-CoV-2 : un aperçu. *Cardiologie et Thérapie*, 1–9.

Takayama, K., Reynolds, P. N., Short, J. J., Kawakami, Y., Adachi, Y., Glasgow, J. N., Rots, M. G., Krasnykh, V., Douglas, J. T., & Curiel, D. T. (2003). A mosaic adenovirus possessing serotype Ad5 and serotype Ad3 knobs exhibits expanded tropism. *Virology*, *309*(2), 282–293. Available from https://doi.org/10.1016/S0042-6822(03)00067-9.

Tao, K., Li, J., Warner, J., MacLeod, K., Miller, F. R., & Sahagian, G. G. (2001). Multiple lysosomal trafficking phenotypes in metastatic mouse mammary tumor cell lines. *International Journal of Oncology*, *19*(6), 1333–1339.

van Regenmortel., Fauquet, C. M., Bishop, D. H., Carstens, E. B., Estes, M. K., Lemon, S. M., & Wickner, R. B. (2000). Virus taxonomy: classification and nomenclature of viruses. In *Seventh report of the International Committee on Taxonomy of Viruses*, Academic Press.

Vigne, E., Mahfouz, I., Dedieu, J. F., Brie, A., Perricaudet, M., & Yeh, P. (1999). RGD inclusion in the hexon monomer provides adenovirus type 5-based vectors with a fiber knob-independent pathway for infection. *Journal of Virology*, *73*(6), 5156–5161. Available from https://doi.org/10.1128/jvi.73.6.5156-5161.1999.

Weaver, E. A., & Barry, M. A. (2008). Effects of shielding adenoviral vectors with polyethylene glycol on vector-specific and vaccine-mediated immune responses. *Human Gene Therapy*, *19*(12), 1369–1382.

Wickham, T. J., Carrion, M. E., & Kovesdi, I. (1995). Targeting of adenovirus penton base to new receptors through replacement of its RGD motif with other receptor-specific peptide motifs. *Gene Therapy*, *2*(10), 750–756.

Wickham, T. J., Mathias, P., Cheresh, D. A., & Nemerow, G. R. (1993). Integrins $\alpha v\beta 3$ and $\alpha v\beta 5$ promote adenovirus internalization but not virus attachment. *Cell*, *73*(2), 309–319. Available from https://doi.org/10.1016/0092-8674(93)90231-E.

Wickham, T. J., Tzeng, E., Shears, L. L., Roelvink, P. W., Li, Y., Lee, G. M., Brough, D. E., Lizonova, A., & Kovesdi, I. (1997). Increased in vitro and in vivo gene transfer by adenovirus vectors containing chimeric fiber proteins. *Journal of Virology*, *71*(11), 8221–8229. Available from https://doi.org/10.1128/jvi.71.11.8221-8229.1997.

Xia, D., Henry, L. J., Gerard, R. D., & Deisenhofer, J. (1994). Crystal structure of the receptor-binding domain of adenovirus type 5 fiberprotein at 1.7 Å resolution. *Structure (London, England: 1993)*, *2*(12), 1259–1270. Available from https://doi.org/10.1016/S0969-2126(94)00126-X.

Xia, H., Anderson, B., Mao, Q., & Davidson, B. L. (2000). Recombinant human adenovirus: Targeting to the human transferrin receptor improves gene transfer to brain microcapillary endothelium. *Journal of Virology*, *74*(23), 11359–11366. Available from https://doi.org/10.1128/JVI.74.23.11359-11366.2000.

Yao, X., Panichpisal, K., Kurtzman, N., & Nugent, K. (2007). Cisplatin nephrotoxicity: A review. *American Journal of the Medical Sciences*, *334*(2), 115–124. Available from https://doi.org/10.1097/MAJ.0b013e31812dfe1e.

Yao, X., Yoshioka, Y., Eto, Y., Morishige, T., Okada, Y., Mizuguchi, H., Mukai, Y., Okada, N., & Nakagawa, S. (2007). TERT promoter-driven adenovirus vector for cancer gene therapy via systemic injection. *Biochemical and Biophysical Research Communications*, *362*(2), 419–424. Available from https://doi.org/10.1016/j.bbrc.2007.08.001.

Yu, M. W., Horng, I. S., Hsu, K. H., Chiang, Y. C., Liaw, Y. F., & Chen, C. J. (1999). Plasma selenium levels and risk of hepatocellular carcinoma among men with chronic hepatitis virus infection. *American Journal of Epidemiology*, *150*(4), 367–374.

Zheng, C., Nikolov, N. P., Alevizos, I., Cotrim, A. P., Liu, S., McCullagh, L., Chiorini, J. A., Illei, G. G., & Baum, B. J. (2010). Transient detection of E1-containing adenovirus in saliva after the delivery of a first-generation adenoviral vector to human parotid gland. *Journal of Gene Medicine*, *12*(1), 3–10. Available from https://doi.org/10.1002/jgm.1416.

Chapter 7

Molecular diagnosis of human oncogenic viruses associated with prostate cancer: Human Papillomavirus and Epstein–Barr virus

Dorine Florence Luthera Ngombe Mouabata[2,3], Christy Parfait Nganga[2], Sedwige Bernaud Loungouala Sounga[2], Donatien Moukassa[2] and Moulay Mustapha Ennaji[1]

[1]Group Leader Research team of Virology, Oncology, and Biotechnologies, Head of Laboratory of Virology, Oncology, Biosciences, Environment and New Energies (LVO-BEEN), Faculty of Sciences and Techniques Mohammedia, University Hassan II of Casablanca, Casablanca, Morocco, [2]Faculty of Health Sciences, University Marien Ngouabi, Brazzaville, Republic of Congo, [3]Team of Virology, Oncology, and Biotechnologies, Laboratory of Virology, Oncology, Biosciences, Environment and New Energies (LVO-BEEN), Faculty of Sciences and Techniques Mohammedia, University Hassan II of Casablanca, Casablanca, Morocco

7.1 Introduction

Prostate cancer (PCa) is one of the major causes of morbidity and mortality in men around the world and constitutes a line of research for pathologists, urologists, and uro-oncologists. It is the second most common cancer and the eighth leading cause of cancer death in men. Although the lifetime risk of developing a PCa is about ~16% (David Crawford et al., 2014; Howlader et al., 2012), the risk of dying from the disease is only about 2%. The discrepancy between the incidence and lethality of PCa has led to an in-depth review of the management of patients with PCa. The main known risk factors in PCa include increased age, ethnicity, and family history of the disease. PCa is both a biologically and clinically heterogeneous disease that develops amid various genetic and epigenetic changes (Barbieri et al., 2013; Berger et al., 2011). It develops in a minority of people who are persistently infected and only after many years of chronic infection (Schiller & Lowy, 2014). Viral involvement

Immunological Implications and Molecular Diagnostics of Genitourinary Cancer.
DOI: https://doi.org/10.1016/B978-0-323-85496-2.00025-7

as essential factors or cofactors in the carcinogenesis of PCa worldwide has aroused scientific interest for decades. Oncoviruses generally maintain chronic infections in which there is little or no production of viral particles by mechanisms of viral persistence and/or latency. These mechanisms are biologically compatible with the carcinogenic process, as they prevent cell death while keeping the infectious agent hidden from the immune system. Oncogenic viruses are necessary but not sufficient for the development of all types of malignant tumors.

Currently, around 15% of cancer cases worldwide and around 20% of cases in developing countries are associated with infectious agents (zur Hausen, 2009), and 12% of all cancers can be caused by oncoviruses (Bouvard et al., 2009), the vast majority of which (>85%) are likely occur in developing countries and regions (Grinstein et al., 2002; Lin et al., 2011). Human oncogenic viruses are made up of both RNA and DNA viruses and include several different taxonomic groups. Human oncogenic RNA viruses include HCV and HTLV-1, and human oncogenic DNA viruses include HBV, HPV, EBV, and KSHV. A number of viruses associated with PCa have been identified and can interact with host proteins, causing genetic, immunological, and inflammatory changes, which in turn lead to the initiation or progression of PCa. PCa has been reported to have several indications based on the analysis of prostatic secretions of men with and without PCa among which we have the human papillomavirus (HPV) and herpesviruses including cytomegalovirus (Cohen et al., 2007; Hagensee et al., 2011; Khalili et al., 2003; Liu et al., 2005).

The oncogenic potential of high-risk HPV and Epstein–Barr virus (EBV) is well established. In addition, there is recent experimental evidence that has demonstrated that HPV and EBV may increase the oncogenicity of HPV-positive cervical cancer cell cultures (Hagensee et al., 2011), suggesting that the same is true for the epithelial cells of the prostate. HPV and EBV gene sequences have been identified in a very high proportion of samples in benign and malignant prostate tissues. These sequences were localized in the nuclei of epithelial cells of the prostate. These observations confirm the frequent identification in many studies of high-risk HPV in PCa and the identification in three studies of EBV in PCa (Bergh et al., 2007; Grinstein et al., 2002; Sfanos et al., 2008).

7.2 Molecular epidemiology of human papillomavirus and Epstein–Barr virus associated with prostate cancer worldwide

The number and percentage of human cancers linked to persistent unidentified viral infections is increasing (zur Hausen, 2009). This may hold true in the case of PCa. Although the prostate is an opening for several viral infections, some of which have oncogenic potential, only a few studies have focused on the relationship between PCa and viral infection. More concrete data are required to clarify the role of HPV and EBV in PCa carcinogenesis as well as their coinfection (Fatemipour et al., 2021).

7.2.1 Prostate cancer

PCa is the second most common cancer in men, with 1,414,259 (14.1%) new cases diagnosed in the world in 2020 (Fig. 7.1) (https://gco.iarc.fr/today/data/factsheets/populations/900-world-fact-sheets). In terms incidence, it is placed in 3rd position for both sexes combined after lung and breast cancer according to statistics from the International Agency for Research on Cancer in 2020 worldwide (Fig. 7.2) (https://gco.iarc.fr/today/data/factsheets/populations/900-world-fact-sheets). However, in terms of mortality, PCa ranks eighth, with an estimate of 375,304 deaths in 2020. Lung cancer is the cancer with the highest death rate than any other cancer in the world, with 1,796,144 deaths in 2020. According to the World Health Organization (WHO), recent data show a higher incidence of PCa in Europe and America in men estimated respectively at 500,827 and 454,096 new cases and lower in Africa, while in Asia, the highest death rate has been recorded with 120,593 deaths (Fig. 7.3) (https://gco.iarc.fr/today/data/factsheets/cancers/27-Prostate-fact-sheet). In Africa, the incidence of PCa is heterogeneous and varies considerably between regions. PCa ranks first in terms of incidence in males (Fig. 7.4) (https://gco.iarc.fr/today/data/factsheets/populations/903-africa-fact-sheets). It is one of the leading causes of death in men in many African countries, representing 93,173 (29.7%) new cases. It is placed in the second position after breast cancer for both sexes combined. In terms of incidence, it is among the top 10 cancers (Fig. 7.5) (https://gco.iarc.fr/today/data/factsheets/populations/903-africa-fact-sheets). A more refined analysis of the distribution of PCa by region in 2021 shows that the highest incidence is in East and West Africa with an estimate of 26,392 and 23,622 new cases.

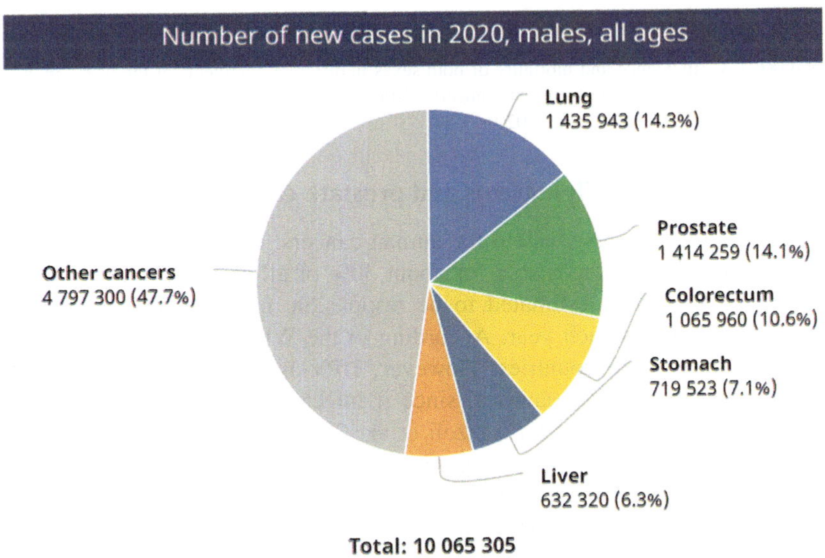

FIGURE 7.1 Estimated incidence of all male cancers in 2020 https://gco.iarc.fr/today/data/factsheets/populations/900-world-fact-sheets Number of new cases in 2020, males, all ages (Globocan, 2020).

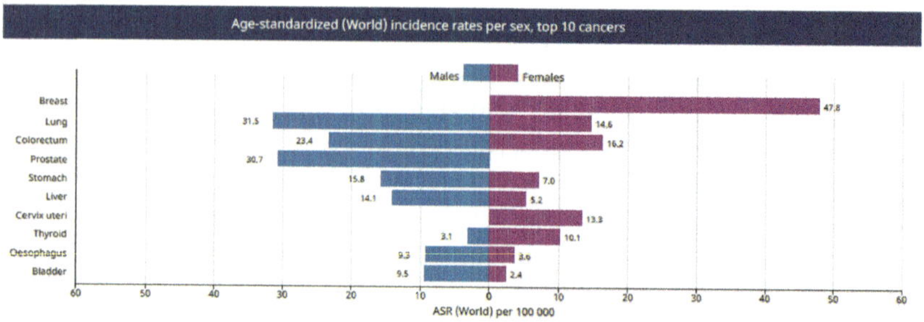

FIGURE 7.2 Estimated incidence of prostate cancer (third rank) among both sexes in the world in 2020 https://gco.iarc.fr/today/data/factsheets/populations/900-world-fact-sheets. Age-standardized (world) incidence rates per sex, top 10 cancers; per 100,000 (Globocan, 2020).

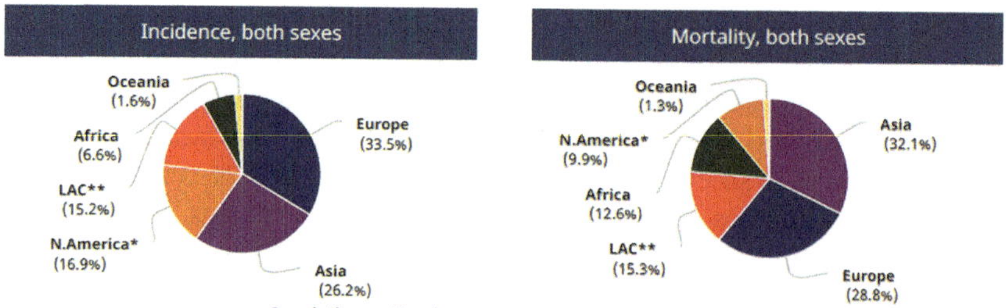

Population	Number
Europe	473 344
Asia	371 225
*Northern America	239 574
**Latin America and the Caribbean	214 522
Africa	93 173
Oceania	22 421
Total	1 414 259

Population	Number
Asia	120 593
Europe	108 088
**Latin America and the Caribbean	57 415
Africa	47 249
*Northern America	37 192
Oceania	4 767
Total	375 304

FIGURE 7.3 Incidence and mortality of both sexes in different continents of the world in 2020 https://gco.iarc.fr/today/data/factsheets/cancers/27-Prostate-fact-sheet. Incidence and mortality both sexes worldwide (Globocan, 2020).

7.2.2 Human papillomavirus and prostate cancer

Among the viruses responsible for human cancers, HPV occupies a preponderant place, being responsible for about 30% of all cancers linked to infectious agents. HPV is estimated to be responsible for 610,000 cancer cases and 250,000 deaths each year. According to the WHO, 85% of these deaths occur in developing countries. However, HPV is not just a public health problem in developing countries, since it infects approximately 6.2 million people in the United States (Mazzoli et al., 2008). HR-HPV infection is the most common infection in young sexually active individuals. Indeed, it is estimated that around 75%–80% of sexually active people will be infected during their lifetime. HPV is the established etiological factor in cancers: of the cervix, vulva, vagina, penis, and anus (de Sanjosé et al., 2014). Given its

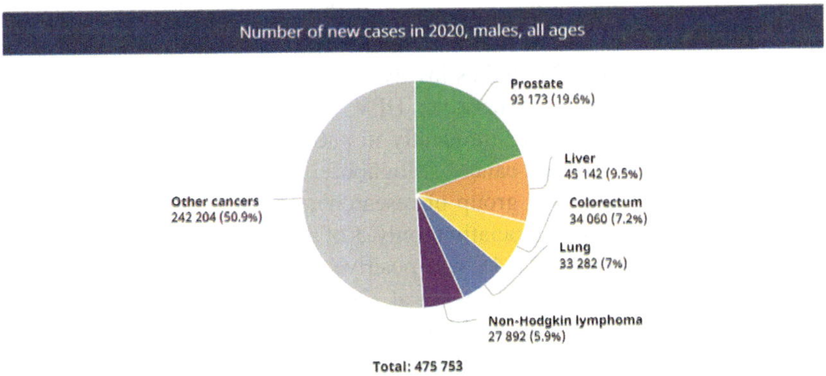

FIGURE 7.4 Estimated incidence of PCa among males in Africa in 2020 https://gco.iarc.fr/today/data/factsheets/populations/903-africa-fact-sheets. Number of new cases in 2020 among males (all ages) in Africa (Globocan, 2020).

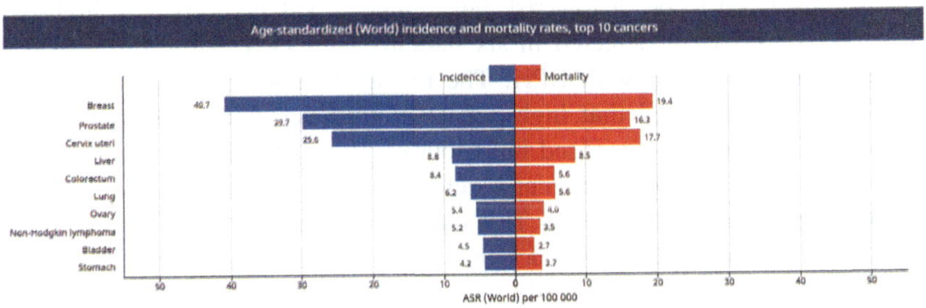

FIGURE 7.5 Estimated rate of incidence (second rank) and mortality of PCa among both sexes in Africa in 2020 https://gco.iarc.fr/today/data/factsheets/populations/903-africa-fact-sheets Age-standardized (world) incidence rates per sex, top 10 cancers; per 100,000 (Globocan, 2020).

anatomical proximity to the anogenital and urinary sites, the prostate has been extensively studied for HPV infection. Although the link between HPV and cervical cancer is clearly established, the link between HPV to PCa is still questionable and hotly debated by researchers.

Studies in Mediterranean and Asian populations have suggested a link between HPV, particularly high-risk subtypes 16 and 18, and PCa (Atashafrooz & Rokhbakhsh-Zamin, 2016; Michopoulou et al., 2014; Singh et al., 2015; Whitaker et al., n.d.). The strength of the association varies according to geographic distribution. In addition, studies have found positive associations of PCa with sexual activity and sexually transmitted diseases (Chung et al., 2013; Huang et al., 2008; Spence et al., 2014), including HPV, suggesting that an infectious etiology may be involved in prostate carcinogenesis. HPV justifies a more rigorous investigation, in particular, to reconcile the diversity of the results reported within the same populations. Several recent metaanalysis studies have shown that HPV infection is associated with an increasing risk in the occurrence of PCa, which indicates a potential link between HPV and PCa. Another metaanalysis with an overall systematic review, using data from 24 studies involving 5546 cases of PCa, found a significant positive association between HPV infection and the risk of PCa. Genotype 16 was found more frequently in patients with PCa, which significantly increased the risk of cancer (Moghoofei et al., 2019). The discovery of another study made by a group of researchers, aiming to explore the role of HPV in PCa found no association, only 3 of 133 samples analyzed in total were positive; high-risk HPV-18 was positive in 2 (3.4%) of 58 cases and 1 (1.3%) of 75 controls (Abdolmaleki et al., 2018).

In 2018, Martha I Dávila Rodriguez detected the high-risk HPV in PCa. This was a case-control study using normal and benign prostate tissue as a control, which showed the presence of HPV in 13 of 87 samples (62 with primary PCa and 25 with benign prostatic hyperplasia, i.e., BPH), with a statistically significant high frequency in prostatic adenocarcinoma (19.4%) than patients with BPH (4%). The HPV genotype detected was HPV-11, and it was considered to be of low risk but higher prevalence (46.1%); high-risk HPV 51, 52, 66 were detected in six patients with PCa, while HPV-18 was detected in one patient with BPH. The result of another study on Mexican population also showed that high-risk HPV was detected in 37 out of 189 (19.6%) PCa samples compared to 16 out of 167 of the BPH samples. HPV 52 and 58 were the most frequently detected genotypes in the study population (Medel-Flores et al., 2018). This causal inference for HPV in male cancer is corroborated by (1) evidence that HPV infection can be quite common in the male population, up to 20% in a recent study of young Italian men by Mazzoli et al. (Mazzoli et al., 2008); (2) epidemiological studies demonstrating a clear protective effect of circumcision in men and women; and (3) a series of epidemiological studies demonstrating an association between infection by HPV and PCa (Al-Maghrabi, 2007).

7.2.3 Epstein–Barr virus

EBV is an ubiquitous human herpesvirus infecting over 90% of the world's adult population with oncogenic activity (Tsao et al., 2015). It has been reported to be a contributing factor in 1%–2% of all cancers (Fitzsimmons & Kelly, 2017). It is involved in the development of a large number of lymphoid and epithelial cancers, including Hodgkin's and non-Hodgkin's lymphomas, Burkitt's lymphoma, carcinoma of the nasopharynx, and posttransplant lymphoproliferative disorder (Shah & Young, 2009) (Malekshahi et al., 2020). It has been proposed that various epithelial carcinomas such as those of breast, kidney, colon, lung, stomach, and prostate could also be included in the list of EBV-related neoplasms (Tsao et al., 2015). Few attempts have been made to investigate the possible association of EBV with PCa (Bergh et al., 2007; Grinstein et al., 2002; Sfanos et al.,

2008; Smelov et al., 2016; Whitaker et al., n.d.). Although EBV has a high distribution in the global population with known oncogenic potential, only a few studies have explored the possible association of EBV with PCa. Grinstein et al. confirmed the presence of EBV in 7 (37%) of the 18 adenocarcinomas of the prostate in American patients. Another study also identified EBV in 8% of malignant prostate tissue in American men (Sfanos et al., 2008). A result concerning the development of PCa by EBV was obtained by Bergh et al. They demonstrated the presence of EBV infection in 31 (9.4%) benign, malignant, and normal 352 prostate tissues in Sweden. In 2019, Malekshahi et al. conducted a case-control study to identify the presence of the BK virus and EBV genome in BPH and PCa prostate samples in Iran. EBV was only detected in one PCa tissue sample among the 121 prostate tissues examined. These results provide further evidence against a causal role of EBV in the development of PCa (Malekshahi et al., 2020). Whitaker et al. identified EBV in equal proportion (40%, 4/10 cases) in malignant and normal prostate tissue in Australia. Sfanos and et al. also identified EBV in 16 of 200 (8%) normal, benign, and malignant prostate tissue in American men.

7.2.4 Human papillomavirus and Epstein–Barr virus coinfection

HPV and EBV are human DNA oncogenic viruses. The International Agency for Research on Cancer has included both EBV and HPV as viruses causing neoplastic disease (Perera et al., 2010). Viral infections are estimated to contribute to 15%–20% of all human cancers such as PCa, breast cancer, and brain cancer (Alibek et al., 2013). EBV and HPV are believed to be linked to 38% of all cancers associated with viruses (Mesri et al., 2014). Numerous studies have shown that HPV infection is linked to NPC as an etiological factor (Giannoudis et al., 1995; Punwaney et al., 1999; Rassekh et al., 1998; Singhi et al., 2012) and that EBV is also present in cervical cancer uterus (Prayitno, 2006) and PCa (Whitaker et al., n.d.). In addition, experimental evidence also shows that HPV and EBV work together to promote the proliferation of cultured cervical cells, suggesting that the same holds true for prostate epithelial cells (Ammatuna et al., 2000).

These observations are consistent with those of studies on high-risk HPV and studies on EBV in PCa (Sfanos et al., 2008). The HPV type 18 and EBV gene (EBNA1) sequences have been identified in a high and approximately equal proportion of malignant, benign, and normal prostate samples. The sequences were localized in the nuclei of prostate epithelial cells. EBV alone was identified in 4/10 (40%) of malignant samples, 2/10 (20%) of benign, and 4/10 (40%) of normal fixed archival prostates. HPV alone has been identified in 7/10 (70%) smart samples, 7/10 (70%) benign, and 1/10 (10%) of normal samples, and these differences were statistically significant. The frequency of EBV and HPV coinfection was significantly higher in PCa 22/40 (55%) than in benign 6/40 (15%) and normal samples from the prostate

12/40 (30%). The study of Whitaker et al. helped to understand the association of HPV with EBV and the potential oncogenic influences of each other (Whitaker et al., n.d.). The identification of EBV and HPV in the fresh samples was confirmed by sequencing the PCR product of selected samples of DNA extracts from the fresh frozen samples. Variations were observed in the sequences, indicating that there was probably no contamination. Only HPV type 18 has been identified. The frequency of infections with these viruses can vary by geographic region.

7.3 Molecular diagnosis and prognostic biomarkers of prostate cancer

After nearly two decades of PSA-based PCa screening, methods currently used in the diagnosis of PCa include digital rectal examination (DRE), prostate-specific antigen (PSA) test, and followup from transrectal ultrasound (TRUS)-guided biopsies (Briganti et al., 2002; Gardiner, 2006), these data allow us to support the hypothesis that screening for PCa may reduce PCa mortality. Despite its good performance and apparently favorable impact on PCa mortality, the measurement of serum PSA concentration as a screening tool for the early diagnosis of PCa is far from perfect. As PSA and DRE are abnormal in 20% to 30% of most populations to be screened, screening for PCa results in a large number of unnecessary prostate biopsies (Catalona et al., 1994). In addition, the complex relationship between PSA, PCa, BPH, and an enlarged prostate, which is the most common cause of elevated PSA, results in difficulty in interpretation of highly problematic PSA results (Canto et al., n.d.). Many molecular biomarkers of PCa have been identified; however, only a few are approved by the Food and Drug Administration (FDA) – PSA in 1994, Prostate Health Index (phi) in 2012, and PCA3 in 2012. To improve the detection of aggressive PCa and reduce unnecessary biopsies, additional protein-based assays such as the phi and the four-kallikrein panel (4K) have been developed and incorporate various combinations of isoforms of PSA and human kallikrein. The phi and 4K assays have been shown to improve cancer detection compared to total PSA alone (Nordström et al., 2015). DNA- and RNA-based sequencing efforts have identified several new biomarkers for the early detection of PCa.

7.3.1 Blood biomarkers

7.3.1.1 Prostate-specific antigen

PSA is a 33 kDa serine protease encoded by the kallikrein 3 (KLK3) gene on chromosome 19q 13.3–13.4. It is produced and secreted by the ductal and acinar epithelium of the prostate. PSA was initially identified and characterized as a marker of human sperm (Lilja et al., 1991; Ornstein et al., 2000).

However, there are inherent limitations in using the PSA test for PCa screening. First, the test can give false positive or false negative results.

Most men with high PSA levels (greater than 4.0 ng/mL) do not have PCa; only about 25% of men who have a prostate biopsy for high PSA actually have a PCa. Conversely, a negative result can give false assurances that PCa is not detected, when in fact cancer may exist. Also, early detection of PCa may not reduce a man's risk of succumbing to the disease (PSA Test – National Cancer Institute). To improve the sensitivity and specificity of the serum PSA test, several derivatives and isoforms of PSA can be used. PSA density can be useful in determining the presence of PCa. Shortly after molecular cloning of the complementary DNA for PSA, it was discovered that the PSA isolated from serum existed in a bound form (i.e., to α-1 antichymotrypsin) or in an unbound form enzymatically inactive. The former was nicknamed complex PSA (cPSA), and the latter as fPSA. Initial studies have shown that serum cPSA concentrations are correlated with the presence of PCa and that serum fPSA levels are elevated in patients with BPH (Rannikko et al., 1991). Mostly, PSA screening has significantly contributed to early detection and treatment, leading to a decline in PCa mortality over the past three decades (Etzioni et al., 2008; Polascik et al., 1999). It is interesting to note that at the start of the PSA tests, the African American (AA) men with newly diagnosed PCa had higher serum PSA levels at the time of initial diagnosis than Caucasian American (CA) men, which corresponded to a larger tumor volume observed in AA men treated in an equal-access healthcare system (Moul et al., 1995).

7.3.1.2 Prostate health index

The Prostate Health Index (phi; Beckman Coulter, Brea, CA, USA) is a blood test that analyzes the levels of fPSA, tPSA, and [−2] proPSA (p2PSA) to predict the risk of Gleason ≥7 disease in a biopsy sample (Loeb et al., 2015). It was developed as an additional diagnostic biomarker in men with a serum PSA level of 2−10 ng/mL. Previous studies have shown that high proPSA/fPSA ratios are associated with PCa. In a recent prospective cohort of men enrolled in active surveillance for PCA, higher serum and tissue levels of proPSA at diagnosis were associated with the need for further treatment (Stephan et al., 2013).

7.3.1.3 4Kscore

The 4Kscore is a score that represents a combination of the four kallikrein proteins: tPSA, fPSA, intact PSA, and hK2. The 4Kscore test has been included in the National Comprehensive Cancer Network (NCCN) PCa early detection guidelines since 2015 (Carroll et al., 2016). The 4Kscore, along with clinical information (age and previous negative biopsy history) provides an estimate of the likelihood of biopsy-positive PCa. Vickers et al. reported that 4Kscore improved the predictive accuracy of clinically diagnosed PCa, relative to total PSA and age. In 50- and 60-year-old men with elevated PSA, a low-risk 4Kscore predicts a low risk of metastasis (Stattin et al., 2015; Vickers et al., 2011). Sixty-year-old men with a PSA ≥ 3 ng/mL and a 4Kscore $<7.5\%$ had a $<1\%$ chance of developing metastatic PCa at age 15 (Ravipaty et al., 2017). The 4Kscore has not yet been approved by the FDA so far (Kohaar et al., 2019).

7.3.1.4 Serum protein panel

A recent study evaluating 500 serum samples reported the development of a new panel of serum proteins from three PCa biomarkers, filamin A, filamin B, and keratin-19 (FLNA, FLNB, and KRT19) at using multivariate models for disease detection and prognosis (Ravipaty et al., 2017). The combination of these prostate biomarkers with the PSA test was better than PSA alone in identifying PCa and improved the prediction of high-risk and low-risk disease and cancer compared to BPH.

7.3.2 Urinary biomarker

7.3.2.1 PCa antigen

PCa antigen 3 (PCA3) is a noncoding messenger RNA that was found to be elevated in $>90\%$ of men with PCa but not significantly elevated in normal prostate glands or in BPH. PCA3 is unique as it can be measured in urine and adds to diagnostic information obtained from the PSA test, with higher area under the curve (AUC) values from 0.66 to 0.72, compared to 0.54–0.63 for serum PSA alone (De La Taille et al., 2011). PCA3, also known as DD3, remains the only biomarker that has been extensively evaluated and studied for its diagnostic potential. A test measuring the expression of PCA3 in urine has generated significant interest and has been introduced clinically are released from the prostate in urine. PCA3 RNA can be measured not only in prostate tissue samples but also in urine and sediment urinary after DRE. To assess the probability of detection of PCa in the prostate biopsy sample, the quantitative PCA3 score was developed. The score is defined as the PCA3 ratio PSA 1000 mRNA/mRNA, which means that PCA3 expression is normalized with the expression of PSA serving as the prostate housekeeping gene (Salagierski & Schalken, 2012).

7.3.2.2 Fusion TMPRSS2-ERG

The most common genomic rearrangement that occurs in PCa is the fusion of the androgen-regulated gene TMPRSS2 with a member of the ETS family of transcription factors (ERG, ETV1, ETV4, ETV5, FLI1) (Petrovics et al., 2007; Sanguedolce et al., 2016; Sreenath et al., 2011). TMPRSS2-ERG is a fusion between the transmembrane protease serine 2 (TMPRSS2) gene and the homolog of the E26 oncogene of the erythroblastosis virus v-ets (avian; ERG) gene. This gene fusion is the predominant variant in about 40% to 80% of PCa. The quantitative levels of urinary TMPRSS2-ERG appear to be associated with a clinically significant PCa based on the Epstein criteria, which stratifies the aggressiveness of the disease using the density of PSA and the characteristics of the patient's biopsy (Gleason score), the percentage of tumor relative to normal prostate tissue observed, and the number of nuclei with tumor (Park et al., 2010). A multicenter study of TMPRSS2: ERG (T2-ERG) and PCA3 in the post-DRE urine of 1312 men showed significant improvement over serum PSA for the detection of clinically relevant cancer in biopsy sample (Rice et al., 2010). Recently, three studies demonstrated the diagnostic utility of TMPRSS2: ERG and PCA3 in urine (Leyten et al., 2014; Sanda et al., 2017; Tomlins et al., 2016). Taken together, the data from these studies suggest that a combination of urine PCA3 and T2-ERG as well as serum PSA can significantly improve the detection of aggressive disease (Gleason score $\geq$ 7) through the initial biopsy sample and a reduction of 42% of unnecessary biopsies (Miettinen et al., 2011; Park et al., 2010).

7.3.3 Tissue biomarker

7.3.3.1 PTEN gene

PTEN is a tumor suppressor gene involved in cell cycle regulation. Among the common molecular alterations seen in primary PCa, loss of PTEN has emerged as one of the most robust prognostic biomarkers and is consistently associated with a poor prognosis in PCa. The PTEN protein functions primarily as a lipid phosphatase, in contrast with the oncogenic PI3K/AKT signaling cascade. The PTEN test is a prognostic fluorescence in situ hybridization (FISH) test typically ordered in conjunction with prostate biopsy tests to indicate partial (hemizygous) or complete (homozygous) deletions in the gene. In primary PCa, PTEN is most often lost by genomic deletion, although genomic rearrangements and more rarely truncation mutations leading to inactivation of PTEN have been described (Chaux et al., 2012). As with many prognostic biomarkers, including Ki-67, the frequency of PTEN loss is associated with a higher Gleason grade as well as pathological stage (Lotan et al., 2011) and risk of progression and recurrence after treatment. In addition, it is associated with localized or advanced metastatic disease and death.

7.3.3.2 ConfirmMDx

ConfirmMDx (MDxHealth, Inc, Irvine, CA, USA) is a DNA methylation test based on prostate tissue biopsy. This multiplexed epigenetic test evaluates glutathione S-transferase Pi 1 (GSTP1), adenomatous polyposis coli (APC), and the associated Ras (RalGDS/AF-6) member of the domain 2 family (RASSF2). These genes are also commonly found in PCa. The test is included in the NCCN guidelines for men with at least one previous negative biopsy. It has been validated by two studies: the methylation assay to localize occult cancer assay (MATLOC), where the test was significantly associated with patient outcome with an odds ratio of 3.17 (Stewart et al., 2013).

7.3.3.3 Oncotype DX Genomic Prostate Score

The Oncotype DX Genomic Prostate Score (GPS) Test (Genomic Health, Redwood City, CA, USA) is a biopsy-based genomic test that measures the mRNA expression of 17 genes responsible for tumor cell growth and survival. Improved prognostic tests enable better stratification of patients based on their risk of disease-specific mortality and likelihood of progression. The Oncotype DX GPS test has been validated independently from a biopsy cohort of 431 men of various races (with very low, low, or intermediate risk PCa) treated in medical centers of the Ministry of Defense (Cullen et al., 2015). These results confirmed that GPS was strongly correlated with BCR, metastasis, and unwanted pathology in samples of RP. It should be noted that this study highlighted the observation that the GPS test worked similarly in AA and CA patients. Together, these studies continue to demonstrate the prognostic value of the Oncotype DX GPS test in the management of low- and intermediate-risk patients.

7.3.3.4 ProMark

Promark (Metamark, Cambridge, MA, USA) is a protein-based prognostic biopsy test that can predict cancer aggressiveness in patients with biopsy Gleason scores of $3+3$ and $3+4$. It uses immunofluorescence imaging analysis to quantify biomarker expression and classify patient tumors. The assay evaluates eight protein markers using an automated, quantitative, multiplex immunofluorescence assay on FFPE fabrics (Shipitsin et al., 2014). A clinical validation study demonstrated that ProMark can differentiate between indolent and aggressive diseases using data from standard formalin fixed and paraffin embedded tissues.

7.3.4 Exosomes as a diagnostic and prognostic tool for prostate

7.3.4.1 Exosomal biomarkers

Exosomes are small extracellular vesicles bound to the double lipid membrane (30–150 nm) containing proteins, lipids, and nucleic acid and are secreted by most cell types. They are released from cells during the fusion between an intermediate endocytic compartment, the multivesicular body, and the plasma membrane. This leads to the release of intraluminal vesicles into the extracellular medium. These liberated vesicles are called exosomes.

It is suggested that exosomes play an essential role in intercellular communication and the transmission of macromolecules between cells. These vesicles also allow the propagation of proteins, lipids, mRNA, microRNAs, and DNA, and contribute to the development of several pathologies. There is significant interest in the discovery of biomarkers using exosomes as they can be detected and are remarkably stable in bodily fluids, including blood, urine, semen, saliva, and the environment cell culture (Duijvesz et al., 2011; Filella & Foj, 2016). Prostate-derived exosomes are a rich source of molecular markers (proteins, RNA, miRNA) for the diagnosis and prognosis of PCa. Prostate-derived exosomes are higher in patients with PCa and correlate with high Gleason scores (Tavoosidana et al., 2011). Urinary exosome-derived PCA3 and TMPRSS2-ERG have been shown to be associated with PCa diagnosis [Nilsson] and PCa risk stratification (McKiernan et al., 2016; Urabe et al., 2019). Changes in miR concentration can be detected in plasma and serum samples, which may be useful to aid in the diagnosis of PCa (Bryant et al., 2012; Mitchell et al., 2008; Valentino et al., 2017). miR-141 and miR-375 from serum-derived exosomes have been shown to be associated with metastatic PCa. miR 34a has also been shown to be a predictive marker of response to docetaxel (Corcoran et al., 2014). Like mRNA or miRNA, exosomal proteins are also found to be useful biomarkers for PCa. Exosomal survivin and plasma-derived claudin 3 have also been shown to be elevated in patients with PCa, suggesting its role in the diagnosis of PCa (Intasqui et al., 2018; Khan et al., 2012; Worst et al., 2017).

7.3.4.2 Cellular factors promoting the emergence and development of tumors via exosomes in cells infected with Epstein–Barr virus

Nanbo et al. studied the mode of internalization of exosomes derived from EBV-negative epithelial cells, or infected in EBV latency I or III program. As a result, exosomes derived from all three cell types are internalized in the same way in target epithelial cells (Nanbo et al., 2013). The exosomes from EBV latency III cells induce an increase in the proliferation and expression of the intercellular adhesion molecule-1 (ICAM-1) of the recipient cells, and this is in a more significant way than for the exosomes produced by uninfected or latently infected cell lines of type I. Ahmed and his collaborators have shown that the two noncoding RNA subtypes of EBV, EBER-1 and -2, are present in the exosomal purified fractions of all EBV-infected cell lines of the study, compared to lines not transformed by the virus. In addition, they discovered that the fractions of the purified exosomes also contain the La protein, having the function of binding to EBERs. These results show that EBERs are probably released from cells infected with EBV in the form of EBER–La complexes in exosomal particles. These results suggest that this may be one of the mechanisms of EBV to hijack the host's immune system whose function is to link to the EBERs. (Ahmed et al., 2014). Gallo and his collaborators studied the global profile of viral and cellular noncoding RNAs in lymphoblastoid lines induced by EBV. The authors identified that all the viral microRNAs expressed in the lymphoblastoid cell lines (LCLs) are packaged in the exosomes. More specifically, the authors observed that two microRNAs, ebv-miR-BART3 and ebv-miR-BHRF1, are more abundant in exosomal particles, which suggests a transfer of viral microRNAs by microvesicles (Gallo et al., 2017). These data reveal new mechanisms on how EBV can manipulate the cellular microenvironment through the exosomal transfer of viral and cellular factors (Meckes, 2015). Important signaling functions of exosomes are altered by LMP1 in infected B cells. In EBV-associated cancers, these virus-modified exosomes can influence tumor growth in neighboring cells, inhibit immune function, or stimulate angiogenesis.

7.4 Conclusion

PCa is the most frequently diagnosed cancer among men. The prostate gland in men represents a complex niche where multiple virus infections occur at DNA oncogenics like HPV and EBV, implying the potential role of these viruses in the progression of PCa. Recent advances in genomic and molecular assays have identified an increasing number of molecular biomarkers of PCa, which play an important role in improving diagnosis, prognosis, and targeted therapy. The challenges of the development of PCa biomarkers require in-depth and cross-validation, direct comparisons of potential biomarkers, and the development of panels of markers applicable to multiple clinical contexts and therapies. Potential biomarkers should provide additional information from already established clinical and pathological variables, in order to improve the predictive accuracy of diagnosis.

References

Abdolmaleki, K., Ramezanzadeh., & Roshani, D. (2018). No association between human papillomavirus and prostate cancer. *International Journal of Cancer Management, 30.*

Ahmed, W., Philip, P. S., Tariq, S., & Khan, G. (2014). Epstein-Barr virus-encoded small RNAs (EBERs) are present in fractions related to exosomes released by EBV-transformed cells. *PLoS One*, *9*(6). Available from https://doi.org/10.1371/journal.pone.0099163.

Alibek, K., Kakpenova, A., & Baiken, Y. (2013). Role of infectious agents in the carcinogenesis of brain and head and neck cancers. *Infectious Agents and Cancer*, *8*(1). Available from https://doi.org/10.1186/1750-9378-8-7.

Al-Maghrabi, J. A. (2007). The role of human papillomavirus infection in prostate cancer. *Saudi Medical Journal*, *28*(3).

Ammatuna, P., Giovannelli, L., Giambelluca, D., Mancuso, S., Rubino, E., Colletti, P., Mazzola, G., Belfiore, P., & Lima, R. (2000). Presence of human papillomavirus and Epstein-Barr virus in the cervix of women infected with the human immunodeficiency virus. *Journal of*

Medical Virology, *62*(4), 410–415. Available from https://doi.org/10.1002/1096-9071(200012)62: 4<410::aid-jmv3>3.0.co;2-j.

Atashafrooz, F., & Rokhbakhsh-Zamin, F. (2016). Frequency and type distribution of human papilloma virus in patients with prostate cancer, Kerman, southeast of Iran. *Asian Pacific Journal of Cancer Prevention*, *17*(8), 3951–3956. Available from http://www.apocpcontrol.org/paper_file/issue_abs/Volume17_No8/3951-3956%205.28%20Fatemeh%20Atashafrooz.pdf.

Barbieri, C. E., Bangma, C. H., Bjartell, A., Catto, J. W. F., Culig, Z., Grönberg, H., Luo, J., Visakorpi, T., & Rubin, M. A. (2013). The mutational landscape of prostate cancer. *European Urology*, *64*(4), 567–576. Available from https://doi.org/10.1016/j.eururo.2013.05.029.

Berger, M. F., Lawrence, M. S., Demichelis, F., Drier, Y., Cibulskis, K., Sivachenko, A. Y., Sboner, A., Esgueva, R., Pflueger, D., Sougnez, C., Onofrio, R., Carter, S. L., Park, K., Habegger, L., Ambrogio, L., Fennell, T., Parkin, M., Saksena, G., Voet, D., & Garraway, L. A. (2011). The genomic complexity of primary human prostate cancer. *Nature*, *470*(7333), 214–220. Available from https://doi.org/10.1038/nature09744.

Bergh, J., Marklund, I., Gustavsson, C., Wiklund, F., Grönberg, H., Allard, A., Alexeyev, O., & Elgh, F. (2007). No link between viral findings in the prostate and subsequent cancer development. *British Journal of Cancer*, *96*(1), 137–139. Available from https://doi.org/10.1038/sj.bjc.6603480.

Bouvard, V., Baan, R., Straif, K., Grosse, Y., Secretan, B., El Ghissassi, F., Benbrahim-Tallaa, L., Guha, N., Freeman, C., Galichet, L., & Cogliano, V. (2009). A review of human carcinogens—part B: Biological agents. *The Lancet Oncology*, *10*(4), 321–322. Available from https://doi.org/10.1016/s1470-2045(09)70096-8.

Briganti, E. M., Russ, G. R., McNeil, J. J., Atkins, R. C., & Chadban, S. J. (2002). Risk of renal allograft loss from recurrent glomerulonephritis. *New England Journal of Medicine*, *347*(2), 103–109. Available from https://doi.org/10.1056/NEJMoa013036.

Bryant, R. J., Pawlowski, T., Catto, J. W. F., Marsden, G., Vessella, R. L., Rhees, B., Kuslich, C., Visakorpi, T., & Hamdy, F. C. (2012). Changes in circulating microRNA levels associated with prostate cancer. *British Journal of Cancer*, *106*(4), 768–774. Available from https://doi.org/10.1038/bjc.2011.595.

Canto, E., Shariat, S., & Slawin, K.M. (n.d.). *Molecular diagnosis of prostate cancer*.

Carroll, P. R., Parsons, J. K., Andriole, G., Bahnson, R. R., Castle, E. P., Catalona, W. J., Dahl, D. M., Davis, J. W., Epstein, J. I., Etzioni, R. B., Farrington, T., Hemstreet, G. P., Kawachi, M. H., Kim, S., Lange, P. H., Loughlin, K. R., Lowrance, W., Maroni, P., Mohler, J., & Freedman-Cass, D. A. (2016). NCCN guidelines insights: Prostate cancer early detection, Version 2.2016. *Journal of the National Comprehensive Cancer Network*, 509–519. Available from https://doi.org/10.6004/jnccn.2016.0060.

Catalona, W. J., Richie, J. P., Ahmann, F. R., Hudson, M. A., Scardino, P. T., Flanigan, R. C., DeKernion, J. B., Ratliff, T. L., Kavoussi, L. R., Dalkin, B. L., Waters, W. B., MacFarlane, M. T., & Southwick, P. C. (1994). Comparison of digital rectal examination and serum prostate specific antigen in the early detection of prostate cancer: Results of a multicenter clinical trial of 6,630 men. *Journal of Urology*, *151*(5), 1283–1290. Available from https://doi.org/10.1016/S0022-5347(17)35233-3.

Chaux, A., Peskoe, S. B., Gonzalez-Roibon, N., Schultz, L., Albadine, R., Hicks, J., De Marzo, A. M., Platz, E. A., & Netto, G. J. (2012). Loss of PTEN expression is associated with increased risk of recurrence after prostatectomy for clinically localized prostate cancer. *Modern Pathology*, *25*(11), 1543–1549. Available from https://doi.org/10.1038/modpathol.2012.104.

Chung, S. D., Lin, Y. K., Huang, C. C., & Lin, H. C. (2013). Increased risk of prostate cancer following sexually transmitted infection in an Asian population. *Epidemiology and Infection, 141*(12), 2663–2670. Available from https://doi.org/10.1017/S0950268813000459.

Cohen, S. B., Graham, M. E., Lovrecz, G. O., Bache, N., Robinson, P. J., & Reddel, R. R. (2007). Protein composition of catalytically active human telomerase from immortal cells. *Science, 315*(5820), 1850–1853. Available from https://doi.org/10.1126/science.1138596.

Corcoran, C., Rani, S., & O'Driscoll, L. (2014). MiR-34a is an intracellular and exosomal predictive biomarker for response to docetaxel with clinical relevance to prostate cancer progression. *Prostate, 74*(13), 1320–1334. Available from https://doi.org/10.1002/pros.22848.

Crawford, E. D., Ventii, K., & Shore, N. D. (2014). New biomarkers in prostate cancer. *Oncology (Williston Park), 28*(2), 135–142.

Cullen, J., Rosner, I. L., Brand, T. C., Zhang, N., Tsiatis, A. C., Moncur, J., Ali, A., Chen, Y., Knezevic, D., Maddala, T., Lawrence, H. J., Febbo, P. G., Srivastava, S., Sesterhenn, I. A., & McLeod, D. G. (2015). A biopsy-based 17-gene genomic prostate score predicts recurrence after radical prostatectomy and adverse surgical pathology in a racially diverse population of men with clinically low- and intermediate-risk prostate cancer. *European Urology, 68*(1), 123–131. Available from https://doi.org/10.1016/j.eururo.2014.11.030.

David Crawford, E., Ventii, K., & Shore, N. D. (2014). New biomarkers in prostate cancer. *Oncology (United States), 28*(2). Available from http://www.cancernetwork.com/printpdf/196735.

De La Taille, A., Irani, J., Graefen, M., Chun, F., De Reijke, T., Kil, P., Gontero, P., Mottaz, A., & Haese, A. (2011). Clinical evaluation of the PCA3 assay in guiding initial biopsy decisions. *Journal of Urology, 185*(6), 2119–2125. Available from https://doi.org/10.1016/j.juro.2011.01.075.

de Sanjosé, S., Bruni, L., & Alemany, L. (2014). HPV in genital cancers (at the exception of cervical cancer) and anal cancers. *La Presse Médicale*, e423–e428. Available from https://doi.org/10.1016/j.lpm.2014.10.001.

Duijvesz, D., Luider, T., Bangma, C. H., & Jenster, G. (2011). Exosomes as biomarker treasure chests for prostate cancer. *European Urology, 59*(5), 823–831. Available from https://doi.org/10.1016/j.eururo.2010.12.031.

Etzioni, R., Tsodikov, A., Mariotto, A., Szabo, A., Falcon, S., Wegelin, J., diTommaso, D., Karnofski, K., Gulati, R., Penson, D. F., & Feuer, E. (2008). Quantifying the role of PSA screening in the US prostate cancer mortality decline. *Cancer Causes & Control, 19*(2), 175–181. Available from https://doi.org/10.1007/s10552-007-9083-8.

Fatemipour, M., Nahand, J. S., Fard Azar, M. E., Baghi, H. B., Taghizadieh, M., Sorayyayi, S., Hussen, B. M., Mirzaei, H., Moghoofei, M., & Bokharaei-Salim, F. (2021). Human papillomavirus and prostate cancer: The role of viral expressed proteins in the inhibition of anoikis and induction of metastasis. *Microbial Pathogenesis*, 152. Available from https://doi.org/10.1016/j.micpath.2020.104576.

Filella, X., & Foj, L. (2016). Prostate cancer detection and prognosis: From prostate specific antigen (PSA) to exosomal biomarkers. *International Journal of Molecular Sciences, 17*(11). Available from https://doi.org/10.3390/ijms17111784.

Fitzsimmons, L., & Kelly, G. L. (2017). EBV and apoptosis: The viral master regulator of cell fate? *Viruses, 9*(11). Available from https://doi.org/10.3390/v9110339.

Gallo, A., Vella, S., Miele, M., Timoneri, F., Di Bella, M., Bosi, S., Sciveres, M., & Conaldi, P. G. (2017). Global profiling of viral and cellular non-coding RNAs in Epstein–Barr virus-induced lymphoblastoid cell lines and released exosome cargos. *Cancer Letters, 388*, 334–343. Available from https://doi.org/10.1016/j.canlet.2016.12.003.

Gardiner, R. A. (2006). *Development of a Novel, Non-Invasive Diagnostic Test for Prostate Cancer*. QUEENSLAND: UNIV BRISBANE AUSTRALIA.

Giannoudis, A., Ergazaki, M., Segas, J., Giotakis, J., Adamopoulos, G., Gorgoulis, V., & Spandidos, D. A. (1995). Detection of Epstein-Barr virus and human papillomavirus in nasopharyngeal carcinoma by the polymerase chain reaction technique. *Cancer Letters*, *89*(2), 177–181. Available from https://doi.org/10.1016/0304-3835(94)03667-8.

Grinstein, S., Preciado, M. V., Gattuso, P., Chabay, P. A., Warren, W. H., de Matteo, E., & Gould, V. E. (2002). Demonstration of Epstein-Barr virus in carcinomas of various sites. *Cancer Research*, *62*(17), 4876–4878.

Hagensee, M., Clark, R., Cameron, J., & Angelo, D. (2011). Epstein Barr virus interacts with human papilloma virus to decrease apoptosis in vitro and increase cervical dysplasia in vivo. *International Centre Genetic Engineering Biotechnology DNA Tumour Virus Meeting Proceedings Trieste*.

Huang, W. Y., Hayes, R., Pfeiffer, R., Viscidi, R. P., Lee, F. K., Wang, Y. F., Reding, D., Whitby, D., Papp, J. R., & Rabkin, C. S. (2008). Sexually transmissible infections and prostate cancer risk. *Cancer Epidemiology Biomarkers and Prevention*, *17*(9), 2374–2381. Available from https://doi.org/10.1158/1055-9965.EPI-08-0173.

Intasqui, P., Bertolla, R. P., & Sadi, M. V. (2018). Prostate cancer proteomics: Clinically useful protein biomarkers and future perspectives. *Expert Review of Proteomics*, *15*(1), 65–79. Available from https://doi.org/10.1080/14789450.2018.1417846.

Khalili, K., Del Valle, L., Wang, J. Y., Darbinian, N., Lassak, A., Safak, M., & Reiss, K. (2003). T-antigen of human polyomavirus JC cooperates with IGF-IR signaling system in cerebellar tumors of the childhood-medulloblastomas, In *Anticancer Research*, *23* (3A), 2035–2041.

Khan, S., Jutzy, J. M. S., Valenzuela, M. M. A., Turay, D., Aspe, J. R., Ashok, A., Mirshahidi, S., Mercola, D., Lilly, M. B., & Wall, N. R. (2012). Plasma-derived exosomal survivin, a plausible biomarker for early detection of prostate cancer. *PLoS One*, *7*(10). Available from https://doi.org/10.1371/journal.pone.0046737.

Kohaar, I., Petrovics, G., & Srivastava, S. (2019). A rich array of prostate cancer molecular biomarkers: Opportunities and challenges. *International Journal of Molecular Sciences*, *20*(8). Available from https://doi.org/10.3390/ijms20081813.

Leyten, G. H. J. M., Hessels, D., Jannink, S. A., Smit, F. P., De Jong, H., Cornel, E. B., De Reijke, T. M., Vergunst, H., Kil, P., Knipscheer, B. C., Van Oort, I. M., Mulders, P. F. A., Hulsbergen-Van De Kaa, C. A., & Schalken, J. A. (2014). Prospective multicentre evaluation of PCA3 and TMPRSS2-ERG gene fusions as diagnostic and prognostic urinary biomarkers for prostate cancer. *European Urology*, *65*(3), 534–542. Available from https://doi.org/10.1016/j.eururo.2012.11.014.

Lilja, H., Christensson, A., Dahlén, U., Matikainen, M. T., Nilsson, O., Pettersson, K., & Lövgren, T. (1991). Prostate-specific antigen in serum occurs predominantly in complex with alpha 1-antichymotrypsin. *Clinical Chemistry*, *37*(9), 1618–1625. Available from https://doi.org/10.1093/clinchem/37.9.1618.

Lin, Y., Mao, Q., Zheng, X., Yang, K., Chen, H., Zhou, C., & Xie, L. (2011). Human papillomavirus 16 or 18 infection and prostate cancer risk: A *meta*-analysis. *Irish Journal of Medical Science*, *180*(2), 497–503. Available from https://doi.org/10.1007/s11845-011-0692-6.

Liu, B., Hong, S., Tang, Z., Yu, H., & Giam, C.-Z. (2005). HTLV-I Tax directly binds the Cdc20-associated anaphase-promoting complex and activates it ahead of schedule. *Proceedings of the National Academy of Sciences*, *102*(1), 63–68. Available from https://doi.org/10.1073/pnas.0406424101.

Loeb, S., Sanda, M. G., Broyles, D. L., Shin, S. S., Bangma, C. H., Wei, J. T., Partin, A. W., Klee, G. G., Slawin, K. M., Marks, L. S., Van Schaik, R. H. N., Chan, D. W., Sokoll, L. J., Cruz, A. B., Mizrahi, I. A., & Catalona, W. J. (2015). The prostate health index selectively identifies clinically significant prostate cancer. *Journal of Urology*, *193*(4), 1163–1169. Available from https://doi.org/10.1016/j.juro.2014.10.121.

Lotan, T. L., Gurel, B., Sutcliffe, S., Esopi, D., Liu, W., Xu, J., Hicks, J. L., Park, B. H., Humphreys, E., Partin, A. W., Han, M., Netto, G. J., Isaacs, W. B., & De Marzo, A. M. (2011). PTEN protein loss by immunostaining: Analytic validation and prognostic indicator for a high risk surgical cohort of prostate cancer patients. *Clinical Cancer Research*, *17*(20), 6563–6573. Available from https://doi.org/10.1158/1078-0432.CCR-11-1244.

Malekshahi, S. S., Yavarian, J., Salehi, R., Babaei, F., Ahmadi, S. A., Ghavami, N., Naseri, M., Hosseini, M., Mokhtari-Azad, T., & Shafiei-Jandaghi, N. Z. (2020). Epstein-Barr and BK virus in cancerous and noncancerous prostate tissue. *Future Virology*, *15*(1), 13–17. Available from https://doi.org/10.2217/fvl-2019-0140.

Mazzoli, S., Cai, T., Mondaini, N., & Bartoletti, R. (2008). HPV vaccination program: Women's health under male protection. *European Urology Supplements*, 156. Available from https://doi.org/10.1016/s1569-9056(08)60338-3.

McKiernan, J., Donovan, M. J., O'Neill, V., Bentink, S., Noerholm, M., Belzer, S., Skog, J., Kattan, M. W., Partin, A., Andriole, G., Brown, G., Wei, J. T., Thompson, I. M., & Carroll, P. (2016). A novel urine exosome gene expression assay to predict high-grade prostate cancer at initial biopsy. *JAMA Oncology*, *2*(7), 882–889. Available from https://doi.org/10.1001/jamaoncol.2016.0097.

Meckes, D. G. (2015). Exosomal communication goes viral. *Journal of Virology*, *89*(10), 5200–5203. Available from https://doi.org/10.1128/JVI.02470-14.

Medel-Flores, O., Valenzuela-Rodríguez, V. A., Ocadiz-Delgado, R., Castro-Muñoz, L. J., Hernández-Leyva, S., Lara-Hernández, G., Silva-Escobedo, J. G., Vidal, P. G., & Sánchez-Monroy, V. (2018). Association between HPV infection and prostate cancer in a Mexican population. *Genetics and Molecular Biology*, *41*(4), 781–789. Available from https://doi.org/10.1590/1678-4685-gmb-2017-0331.

Mesri, E. A., Feitelson, M. A., & Munger, K. (2014). Human viral oncogenesis: A cancer hallmarks analysis. *Cell Host and Microbe*, *15*(3), 266–282. Available from https://doi.org/10.1016/j.chom.2014.02.011.

Michopoulou, V., Derdas, S. P., Symvoulakis, E., Mourmouras, N., Nomikos, A., Delakas, D., Sourvinos, G., & Spandidos, D. A. (2014). Detection of human papillomavirus (HPV) DNA prevalence and p53 codon 72 (Arg72Pro) polymorphism in prostate cancer in a Greek group of patients. *Tumor Biology*, *35*(12), 12765–12773. Available from https://doi.org/10.1007/s13277-014-2604-7.

Miettinen, M., Wang, Z. F., Paetau, A., Tan, S. H., Dobi, A., Srivastava, S., & Sesterhenn, I. (2011). ERG transcription factor as an immunohistochemical marker for vascular endothelial tumors and prostatic carcinoma. *American Journal of Surgical Pathology*, *35*(3), 432–441. Available from https://doi.org/10.1097/PAS.0b013e318206b67b.

Mitchell, P. S., Parkin, R. K., Kroh, E. M., Fritz, B. R., Wyman, S. K., Pogosova-Agadjanyan, E. L., Peterson, A., Noteboom, J., O'Briant, K. C., Allen, A., Lin, D. W., Urban, N., Drescher, C. W., Knudsen, B. S., Stirewalt, D. L., Gentleman, R., Vessella, R. L., Nelson, P. S., Martin, D. B., & Tewari, M. (2008). Circulating microRNAs as stable blood-based markers for cancer detection. *Proceedings of the National Academy of Sciences of the United States of America*, *105*(30), 10513–10518. Available from https://doi.org/10.1073/pnas.0804549105.

Moghoofei, M., Keshavarz, M., Ghorbani, S., Babaei, F., Nahand, J. S., Tavakoli, A., Mortazavi, H. S., Marjani, A., Mostafaei, S., & Monavari, S. H. (2019). Association between human papillomavirus infection and prostate cancer: A global systematic review and *meta*-analysis. *Asia-Pacific Journal of Clinical Oncology*, *15*(5), e59–e67. Available from https://doi.org/10.1111/ajco.13124.

Moul, J. W., Douglas, T., Mcleod, D. G., Sesterhenn, I. A., Mostofi, F. K., Connelly, R. R., & Srivastava, S. (1995). Prostate-specific antigen values at the time of prostate cancer diagnosis in African-American men. *JAMA: The Journal of the American Medical Association*, *274*(16), 1277–1281. Available from https://doi.org/10.1001/jama.1995.03530160029029.

Nanbo, A., Kawanishi, E., Yoshida, R., & Yoshiyama, H. (2013). Exosomes derived from Epstein-Barr virus-infected cells are internalized via caveola-dependent endocytosis and promote phenotypic modulation in target cells. *Journal of Virology*, *87*(18), 10334–10347. Available from https://doi.org/10.1128/JVI.01310-13.

Nordström, T., Vickers, A., Assel, M., Lilja, H., Grönberg, H., & Eklund, M. (2015). Comparison between the four-kallikrein panel and prostate health index for predicting prostate cancer. *European Urology*, *68*(1), 139–146. Available from https://doi.org/10.1016/j.eururo.2014.08.010.

Ornstein, D. K., Englert, C., Gillespie, J. W., Paweletz, C. P., Linehan, W. M., Emmert-Buck, M. R., & Petricoin, E. F. (2000). Characterization of intracellular prostate-specific antigen from laser capture microdissected benign and malignant prostatic epithelium. *Clinical Cancer Research*, *6*(2), 353–356.

Park, K., Tomlins, S. A., Mudaliar, K. M., Chiu, Y. L., Esgueva, R., Mehra, R., Suleman, K., Varambally, S., Brenner, J. C., MacDonald, T., Srivastava, A., Tewari, A. K., Sathyanarayana, U., Nagy, D., Pestano, G., Kunju, L. P., Demichelis, F., Chinnaiyan, A. M., & Rubin, M. A. (2010). Antibody-based detection of ERG rearrangement-positive prostate cancer. *Neoplasia*, *12*(7), 590–598. Available from https://doi.org/10.1593/neo.10726.

Perera, R. A. P. M., Samaranayake, L. P., & Tsang, C. S. P. (2010). Shedding dynamics of Epstein-Barr virus: A type 1 carcinogen. *Archives of Oral Biology*, *55*(9), 639–647. Available from https://doi.org/10.1016/j.archoralbio.2010.06.009.

Petrovics, G., Liu, A., Shaheduzzaman, S., Furusato, B., Sun, C., Chen, Y., et al. (2007). Frequent overexpression of ETS-related gene-1 (ERG1) in prostate cancer transcriptome. *Oncogene-Basingstoke*, *26*(46).

Polascik, T. J., Oesterling, J. E., & Partin, A. W. (1999). Prostate specific antigen: A decade of discovery – what we have learned and where we are going. *Journal of Urology*, *162*(2), 293–306. Available from https://doi.org/10.1016/S0022-5347(05)68543-6.

Prayitno, A. (2006). Cervical cancer with human papilloma virus and Epstein Barr virus positive. *Journal of Carcinogenesis*, 5. Available from https://doi.org/10.1186/1477-3163-5-13.

Punwaney, R., Brandwein, M. S., Zhang, D. Y., Urken, M. L., Cheng, R., Park, C. S., Li, H. B., & Li, X. (1999). Human papillomavirus may be common within nasopharyngeal carcinoma of Caucasian Americans: Investigation of Epstein-Barr virus and human papillomavirus in eastern and western nasopharyngeal carcinoma using ligation-dependent polymerase chain reaction. *Head and Neck*, *21*(1), 21–29. Available from https://doi.org/10.1002/(SICI)1097-0347(199901)21: 1 <21::AID-HED3>3.0.CO;2-Z

Rannikko, S., Tuhkanen, K., & Alfthan, O. (1991). A complex between prostate-specific antigen and α1-antichymotrypsin is the major form of prostate-specific antigen in serum of patients with prostatic cancer: Assay of the complex improves clinical sensitivity for cancer. *Cancer Research*, *51*(1), 222–226.

Rassekh, C. H., Rady, P. L., Arany, I., Tyring, S. K., Knudsen, S., Calhoun, K. H., Seikaly, H., & Bailey, B. J. (1998). Combined Epstein-Barr virus and human papillomavirus infection in nasopharyngeal carcinoma. *Laryngoscope*, *108*(3), 362–367. Available from https://doi.org/10.1097/00005537-199803000-00010.

Ravipaty, S., Wu, W., Dalvi, A., Tanna, N., Andreazi, J., Friss, T., Klotz, A., Liao, C., Garren, J., Schofield, S., Diamandis, E. P., Klein, E. A., Dobi, A., Srivastava, S., Tekumalla, P., Kiebish, M. A., Vishnudas, V., Sarangarajan, R. P., Narain, N. R., & Akmaev, V. R. (2017). Clinical validation of a serum protein panel (FLNA, FLNB and KRT19) for diagnosis of prostate cancer. *Journal of Molecular Biomarkers & Diagnosis*. Available from https://doi.org/10.4172/2155-9929.1000323.

Rice, K. R., Chen, Y., Ali, A., Whitman, E. J., Blase, A., Ibrahim, M., Elsamanoudi, S., Brassell, S., Furusato, B., Stingle, N., Sesterhenn, I. A., Petrovics, G., Miick, S., Rittenhouse, H., Groskopf, J., McLeod, D. G., & Srivastava, S. (2010). Evaluation of the ETS-related gene mRNA in urine for the detection of prostate cancer. *Clinical Cancer Research*, *16*(5), 1572–1576. Available from https://doi.org/10.1158/1078-0432.CCR-09-2191.

Salagierski, M., & Schalken, J. A. (2012). Molecular diagnosis of prostate cancer: PCA3 and TMPRSS2:ERG gene fusion. *Journal of Urology*, *187*(3), 795–801. Available from https://doi.org/10.1016/j.juro.2011.10.133.

Sanda, M. G., Feng, Z., Howard, D. H., Tomlins, S. A., Sokoll, L. J., Chan, D. W., Regan, M. M., Groskopf, J., Chipman, J., Patil, D. H., Salami, S. S., Scherr, D. S., Kagan, J., Srivastava, S., Thompson, I. M., Siddiqui, J., Fan, J., Joon, A. Y., Bantis, L. E., & Taneja, S. (2017). Association between combined TMPRSS2:ERG and PCA3 RNA urinary testing and detection of aggressive prostate cancer. *JAMA Oncology*, *3*(8), 1085–1093. Available from https://doi.org/10.1001/jamaoncol.2017.0177.

Sanguedolce, F., Cormio, A., Brunelli, M., D'Amuri, A., Carrieri, G., Bufo, P., & Cormio, L. (2016). Urine TMPRSS2: ERG fusion transcript as a biomarker for prostate cancer: Literature review. *Clinical Genitourinary Cancer*, *14*(2), 117–121. Available from https://doi.org/10.1016/j.clgc.2015.12.001.

Schiller, J. T., & Lowy, D. R. (2014). Virus infection and human cancer: An overview. *Recent Results in Cancer Research*, *193*, 1–10. Available from https://doi.org/10.1007/978-3-642-38965-8_1.

Sfanos, K. S., Sauvageot, J., Fedor, H. L., Dick, J. D., De Marzo, A. M., & Isaacs, W. B. (2008). A molecular analysis of prokaryotic and viral DNA sequences in prostate tissue from patients with prostate cancer indicates the presence of multiple and diverse microorganisms. *Prostate*, *68*(3), 306–320. Available from https://doi.org/10.1002/pros.20680.

Shah, K. M., & Young, L. S. (2009). Epstein-Barr virus and carcinogenesis: Beyond Burkitt's lymphoma. *Clinical Microbiology and Infection*, *15*(11), 982–988. Available from https://doi.org/10.1111/j.1469-0691.2009.03033.x.

Shipitsin, M., Small, C., Choudhury, S., Giladi, E., Friedlander, S., Nardone, J., Hussain, S., Hurley, A. D., Ernst, C., Huang, Y. E., Chang, H., Nifong, T. P., Rimm, D. L., Dunyak, J., Loda, M., Berman, D. M., & Blume-Jensen, P. (2014). Identification of proteomic biomarkers predicting prostate cancer aggressiveness and lethality despite biopsy-sampling error. *British Journal of Cancer*, *111*(6), 1201–1212. Available from https://doi.org/10.1038/bjc.2014.396.

Singh, N., Hussain, S., Kakkar, N., Singh, S. K., Sobti, R. C., & Bharadwaj, M. (2015). Implication of high risk Human papillomavirus HR-HPV infection in prostate cancer in Indian population – a pioneering case-control analysis. *Scientific Reports*. Available from https://doi.org/10.1038/srep07822.

Singhi, A. D., Califano, J., & Westra, W. H. (2012). High-risk human papillomavirus in nasopharyngeal carcinoma. *Head and Neck*, *34*(2), 213–218. Available from https://doi.org/10.1002/hed.21714.

Smelov, B., Mühr, A., Eklund., Komyakov, G., et al. (2016). Detection of DNA viruses in prostate cancer. *Scientific Reports*, *28*.

Spence, A. R., Rousseau, M. C., & Parent, M. É. (2014). Sexual partners, sexually transmitted infections, and prostate cancer risk. *Cancer Epidemiology*, *38*(6), 700–707. Available from https://doi.org/10.1016/j.canep.2014.09.005.

Sreenath, T., Dobi, A., Petrovics, G., & Srivastava, S. (2011). Oncogenic activation of ERG: A predominant mechanism in prostate cancer. *Journal of Carcinogenesis*, *10*, 10–21. Available from https://doi.org/10.4103/1477-3163.91122.

Stattin, P., Vickers, A. J., Sjoberg, D. D., Johansson, R., Granfors, T., Johansson, M., Pettersson, K., Scardino, P. T., Hallmans, G., & Lilja, H. (2015). Improving the specificity of screening for lethal prostate cancer using prostate-specific antigen and a panel of kallikrein markers: A nested case-control study. *European Urology*, *68*(2), 207–213. Available from https://doi.org/10.1016/j.eururo.2015.01.009.

Stephan, C., Vincendeau, S., Houlgatte, A., Cammann, H., Jung, K., & Semjonow, A. (2013). Multicenter evaluation of [-2]proprostate-specific antigen and the prostate health index for detecting prostate cancer. *Clinical Chemistry*, *59*(1), 306–314. Available from https://doi.org/10.1373/clinchem.2012.195784.

Stewart, G. D., Van Neste, L., Delvenne, P., Delrée, P., Delga, A., McNeill, S. A., O'Donnell, M., Clark, J., Van Criekinge, W., Bigley, J., & Harrison, D. J. (2013). Clinical utility of an epigenetic assay to detect occult prostate cancer in histopathologically negative biopsies: Results of the MATLOC study. *Journal of Urology*, *189*(3), 1110–1116. Available from https://doi.org/10.1016/j.juro.2012.08.219.

Tavoosidana, G., Ronquist, G., Darmanis, S., Yan, J., Carlsson, L., Wu, D., Conze, T., Ek, P., Semjonow, A., Eltze, E., Larsson, A., Landegren, U. D., & Kamali-Moghaddam, M. (2011). Multiple recognition assay reveals prostasomes as promising plasma biomarkers for prostate cancer. *Proceedings of the National Academy of Sciences of the United States of America*, *108*(21), 8809–8814. Available from https://doi.org/10.1073/pnas.1019330108.

Tomlins, S. A., Day, J. R., Lonigro, R. J., Hovelson, D. H., Siddiqui, J., Kunju, L. P., Dunn, R. L., Meyer, S., Hodge, P., Groskopf, J., Wei, J. T., & Chinnaiyan, A. M. (2016). Urine TMPRSS2:ERG Plus PCA3 for individualized prostate cancer risk assessment. *European Urology*, *70*(1), 45–53. Available from https://doi.org/10.1016/j.eururo.2015.04.039.

Tsao, S. W., Tsang, C. M., To, K. F., & Lo, K. W. (2015). The role of Epstein-Barr virus in epithelial malignancies. *Journal of Pathology*, *235*(2), 323–333. Available from https://doi.org/10.1002/path.4448.

Urabe, F., Ochiya, T., & Egawa, S. (2019). Re: A prospective adaptive utility trial to validate performance of a novel urine exosome gene expression assay to predict high-grade prostate cancer in patients with prostate-specific antigen 2–10 ng/mL at initial biopsy. *European Urology*, *76*(2), 254–255. Available from https://doi.org/10.1016/j.eururo.2019.02.036.

Valentino, A., Reclusa, P., Sirera, R., Giallombardo, M., Camps, C., Pauwels, P., Crispi, S., & Rolfo, C. (2017). Exosomal microRNAs in liquid biopsies: Future biomarkers for prostate cancer. *Clinical and Translational Oncology*, *19*(6), 651–657. Available from https://doi.org/10.1007/s12094-016-1599-5.

Vickers, A. J., Gupta, A., Savage, C. J., Pettersson, K., Dahlin, A., Bjartell, A., Manjer, J., Scardino, P. T., Ulmert, D., & Lilja, H. (2011). A panel of kallikrein marker predicts prostate cancer in a large, population-based cohort followed for 15 years without screening.

Cancer Epidemiology Biomarkers and Prevention, *20*(2), 255–261. Available from https://doi.org/10.1158/1055-9965.EPI-10-1003.

Howlader N., Noone A. M, Krapcho M., Garshell J., Neyman N., Altekruse S. F, Kosary C. L, Yu M., Ruhl J., Tatalovich Z., Cho H., Mariotto A., Lewis D. R, Chen H. S, Feuer E. J, Cronin K. A, editors. SEER Cancer Statistics Review, 1975–2010. National Cancer Institute; Bethesda, MD: http://seer.cancer.gov/csr/1975_2010/, based on November 2012 SEER data submission, posted to the SEER web site, April 2013.

Whitaker, Glenn, W., Sahrudin, A., Orde, M., Delprado, W., & Lawson, J.S. (n.d.). Human papillomavirus and Epstein Barr virus in prostate cancer: Koilocytes indicate potential oncogenic influences of human papillomavirus in prostate cancer. *The Prostate*.

Worst, T. S., Von Hardenberg, J., Gross, J. C., Erben, P., Schnölzer, M., Hausser, I., Bugert, P., Michel, M. S., & Boutros, M. (2017). Database-augmented mass spectrometry analysis of exosomes identifies claudin 3 as a putative prostate cancer biomarker. *Molecular and Cellular Proteomics*, *16*(6), 998–1008. Available from https://doi.org/10.1074/mcp.M117.068577.

zur Hausen, H. (2009). Papillomaviruses in the causation of human cancers – A brief historical account. *Virology*, *384*(2), 260–265. Available from https://doi.org/10.1016/j.virol.2008.11.046.

Chapter 8

Molecular characterization of oncogenic biomarkers associated with genitourinary cancers: the case of prostate cancer

Ikram Tiabi[2], Youssef Ennaji[2], Soukayna Alaoui Sosse[2], Berjas Abumsimir[2,3], Abdelilah Laraqui[4], Mohammed Mrabti[4], Mohammed Nabil Benchekroun[2] and Moulay Mustapha Ennaji[1]

[1]Group Leader Research team of Virology, Oncology, and Biotechnologies, Head of Laboratory of Virology, Oncology, Biosciences, Environment and New Energies (LVO-BEEN), Faculty of Sciences and Techniques Mohammedia, University Hassan II of Casablanca, Casablanca, Morocco, [2]Team of Virology, Oncology, and Biotechnologies, Laboratory of Virology, Oncology, Biosciences, Environment and New Energies (LVO-BEEN), Faculty of Sciences and Techniques Mohammedia, University Hassan II of Casablanca, Casablanca, Morocco, [3]Pharmacological and Diagnostic Research Centre (PDRC), Department of Medical Laboratory Sciences, Faculty of Allied Medical Sciences, Al-Ahliyya Amman University (AAU), Amman, Jordan, [4]Laboratory of Human Pathologies Biology, Faculty of Sciences, and Genomic Center of Human Pathologies, Faculty of Medicine and Pharmacy, Bio-Path Laboratory, Faculty of sciences-Agdal, Mohammed V University, Rabat, Morocco

8.1 Introduction

All types of cancer are the product of changes in the DNA sequence of the cancer cell's genome. Over the past quarter-century, we have learned a great deal about these mutations and the abnormal genes involved in cancer.

Genitourinary cancers are the second leading cause of death among men after lung cancer. Prostate cancer, bladder cancer, and testicular cancer are becoming increasingly prevalent. Bladder cancer is currently the second most common urological cancer in France (Ferlay et al., 2014).

Bladder cancer is the second most frequent cancer in the urogenital cancer group in the world, after prostate cancer. In 2008 386,300 new cases of bladder cancer and 150,200 associated deaths were reported worldwide. The highest incidences are reported in Europe, North America, and North Africa. In France, bladder cancer is the seventh most prevalent cancer (WHO).

Immunological Implications and Molecular Diagnostics of Genitourinary Cancer.
DOI: https://doi.org/10.1016/B978-0-323-85496-2.00022-1

The world is currently at a stage where it is possible to read the complete genetic sequence of many cancer genomes. These studies open up a new perspective on the study of the evolution of individual cancers. Prostate cancer has become the most common cancer and the second leading cause of death among men (WHO). This public health phenomenon is becoming more and more important owing to the increase in life expectancy. Currently, one man in eight is likely to develop prostate cancer during his lifetime. Prostate cancer is the second most common cancer in men and the fourth most common cancer overall. There were 1.3 million new cases reported in 2018 and 20 countries had the highest rates of prostate cancer in 2018 (Khazaei et al., 2019). In sub-Saharan Africa, the average age of prostate cancer diagnosis ranges from 68 years in Senegal to 70 years in South Africa. These values are comparable to those observed in North Africa, with a mean age of 72.8 years in Tunisia and 71.4 years in Egypt (Ferlay et al., 2014). In Morocco, and according to the Greater Casablanca registry, the mean age is 70.4 years with a maximum incidence rate above 75 years (Greater Casablanca registry).

Until now, little work has been done to identify the genetic mutations that cause prostate cancer in human tissues. However, more rapid and sensitive molecular biology techniques such as real-time polymerase chain reaction (PCR) tests are now available.

8.2 General information about prostate cancer

8.2.1 Definition

The term "cancer" refers to all malignant tumors. A tumor is a pathological multiplication of cells. A distinction can be made between benign and malignant tumors (Gérin et al., 2003).

Benign tumors are formed in situ. In principle, the nomenclature of benign cancers uses the suffix (*ome*) added to the name of the tissue from which the tumor originates; thus, the benign tumor of the gland (*adeno* in Greek) will be called adenoma (Gérin et al., 2003).

8.2.2 Carcinogenesis

The pathophysiology of prostate cancer is primarily related to the discovery of abnormalities in gene function or structure as a result of several parameters. These result in mutations, deletions, or methylations of DNA (Lonergan & Tindall, 2011). The most well known factor with a definite role in prostate cancer is the presence of androgens (specifically testosterone). These are cholesterol-synthesizing hormones, which originate from the testes (95%) or the adrenal glands (5%).

The androgen receptor is an essential component of normal prostate proliferation and development, as well as cancer. It is expressed in most primary prostate cancers (Fig. 8.1).

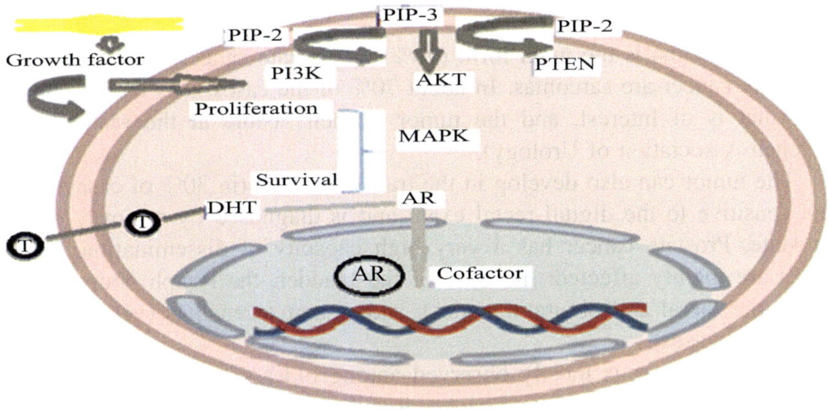

FIGURE 8.1 Mechanism of carcinogenesis in prostate cancer.

Circulating testosterone is bound to a particular transport protein called SHBG (steroid hormone-binding globulin). When it reaches the cytoplasm of prostate cells, it is transformed by an enzyme, namely, 5-alpha reductase. The metabolite produced is dihydro-testosterone (DHT) (Lonergan et al., 2013).

The binding of the ligand (DHT) to the androgen receptor causes a change in the configuration of the androgen receptor and its entry into the nucleus. Once in the nucleus, the receptor will bind to specific recognition sequences called ARES at the promoter and enhancer regions of target genes encoding proteins that increase cell survival and proliferation.

Indeed, in the absence of androgens, it is also possible that other factors can stimulate the androgen receptor. This is referred to as "alternative stimulation" (Lonergan & Tindall, 2011).

These molecules are:

Growth factors such as epidermal growth factor or insulin growth factor that activate the androgen receptor through the MAP kinase pathway.

- Phosphatidylinositol 3 kinase (PI3K): Its activation leads to the generation of PIP3, which allows the recruitment of Akt. This kinase is involved in the process of cell maintenance and multiplication (Akamatsu et al., 2012).
- Interleukins (IL-6 and IL-8 in particular) are likely to phosphorylate a Janus kinase, which stimulates the androgen receptor through a transcriptional activator (STAT-3).
- A mutation in the tumor suppressor gene PTEN (phosphatase and tensin homolog deleted on chromosome 10): This is thought to be a tensin and phosphatase homolog whose mutations lead to an increase in PIP3 and activation of a chain response resulting in increased survival, growth, and cell invasion (Lonergan et al., 2013).

8.2.3 Tumor development

Adenocarcinoma is the main form (90%) of prostate cancer, while the other forms of cancer are sarcomas. In about 70% of the cases, it is the peripheral part that is of interest, and the tumor is then visible at the rectal touch (French Association of Urology).

The tumor can also develop in the transition zone (in 30% of cases). It is not sensitive to the digital rectal exam and is diagnosed by a biopsy of the prostate. Prostate cancer has a very high capacity of dissemination. Three areas are mainly affected: the base of the bladder, the lymph nodes (especially the sacral and obturator nodes), and distant extensions (very frequent bone metastases).

Prostate cancer is mostly observed among older men, and the high frequency of histological prostate cancer found after autopsy shows that a high proportion of men have prostate cancer that remains subclinical (French Association of Urology).

Approximately 75% of prostate cancers develop in the peripheral zone of the prostate, causing urological manifestations only at a very late stage, 20% in the transition zone and 5% in the central zone, causing imminent urinary pathologies.

Prostatic carcinoma starts from the epithelial cells of the prostate; its development is slow and includes several stages (Fig. 8.2).

Prostate cancer can multiply beyond the prostate capsule by directly invading tissues and organs near the prostate. It can also colonize more

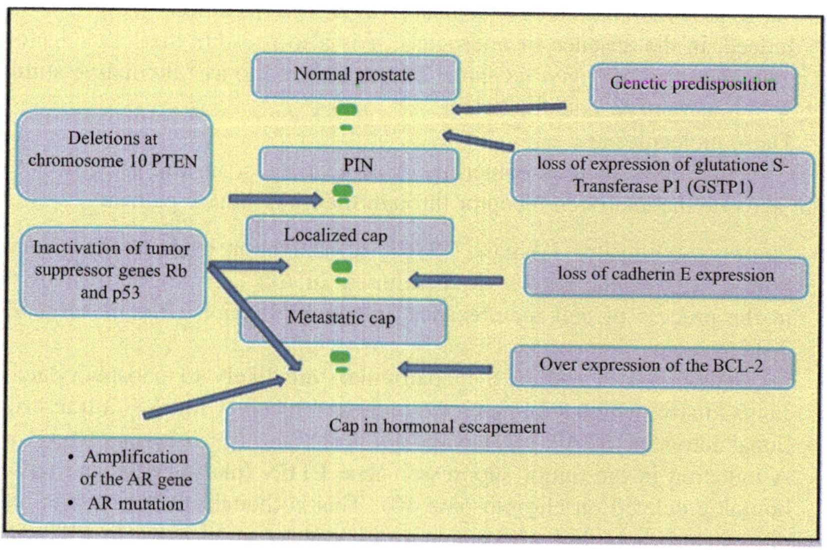

FIGURE 8.2 Prostatic carcinogenesis consisting of a succession of steps that can be linked to molecular events (Akamats et al., 2012).

distant organs when the cancer cells have acquired the ability to enter lymphatic and blood vessels.

Its diffusion in the bloodstream leads to distant metastasis, mainly in the bones (spine, ribs, pelvis, and sternum) and much less frequently in other organs such as the lungs, liver, skin, or brain. Lymphatic diffusion leads to lymph node metastasis, most often pelvic and more rarely lumbo-aortic (Akamats et al., 2012).

Prostate carcinogenesis consists of a sequence of steps that may be related to molecular events. "Genetic factors" are likely to be associated with the development of intraepithelial neoplasia (PIN), the high-grade form of which may be linked to prostate cancer. PIN can progress to so-called "histological" prostate cancer, which is often asymptomatic and discovered incidentally at autopsy.

Blood androgens promote RA in stromal and limbal cells. Stromal cells have a paracrine influence on epithelial cells by releasing growth and survival factors. Stimulated luminal cells secrete PSA in an androgen-dependent manner.

CaP is therefore considered a hormone-dependent cancer, which means that there is a relationship between the progression of prostate cancer cells and the presence of male sex hormones such as testosterone and DHT.

Treatment that inhibits or significantly reduces the secretion of these hormones is very effective in reducing the severity of the disease (French Association of Urology).

Thus, patients with locally advanced CaP, local recurrence after prostatectomy, or metastatic CaP undergo first-approach hormonal therapy or medical sterilization, the goal of which is to significantly decrease plasma levels of testosterone and its equivalent, DHT.

8.2.4 Epidemiology of prostate cancer

8.2.4.1 Epidemiology of prostate cancer on a global scale

Prostate cancer has thus become a real human health concern, which leads us to define the main indicators and epidemiological parameters of this cancer. Age-adjusted prevalence indices for prostate cancer have increased significantly, primarily because of the increased availability of the prostate-specific antigen (PSA) test in men with no symptoms of the disease. This test can identify many small and/or unidentified prostate cancers that may or may not progress to advanced disease (Fig. 8.3).

8.2.4.2 Epidemiology of prostate cancer in Africa

A closer look at the context of the African continent shows that, among men and against the global trend, prostate cancer has the highest incidence in the world, with about 80,971 new cases in 2018 (Fig. 8.4), which represents 18.1% of all cancers. Liver cancer is the second most common cancer and

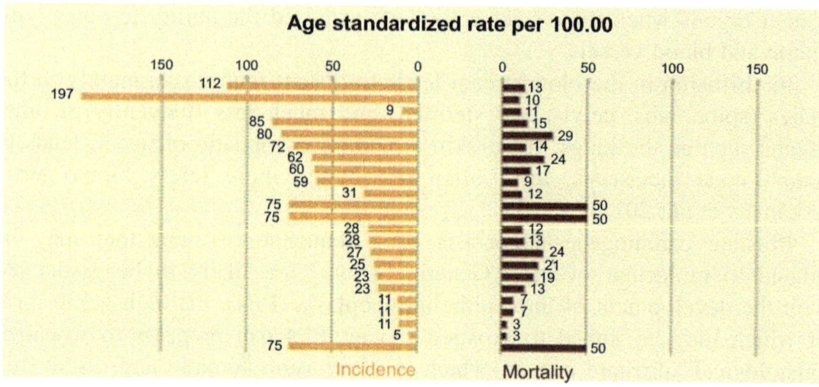

FIGURE 8.3 World age-standardized prostate cancer incidence by country (rate per 100,000 men) (Antoni et al., 2016).

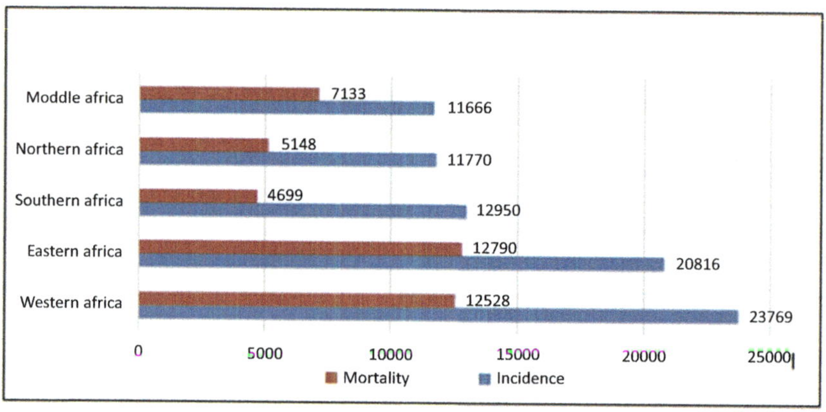

FIGURE 8.4 Estimated number of prostate incidents and deaths, men, all ages (Abumsimir et al., 2019).

also makes up a significant proportion of the incidence with 43,530 (9.7%) new cases in 2018. This cancer also has the highest number of deaths in the African continent, with 42,786 deaths in 2018 and prostate cancer with 42,298 deaths assessed in 2018 (Abumsimir et al., 2020).

8.2.4.3 Epidemiology of prostate cancer in Morocco

In Morocco, and according to the Registry of Greater Casablanca, the average duration is 70.4 years for an optimal incidence above 75 years. Prostate cancer has evolved between 2004 and 2012. The number of new cases increased from 124 to 296. The crude incidence rate increased from 7 to 296 cases (Abumsimir et al., 2019) per 100,000 in 2004 to 14.4 per 100,000 in 2012 (Fig. 8.5).

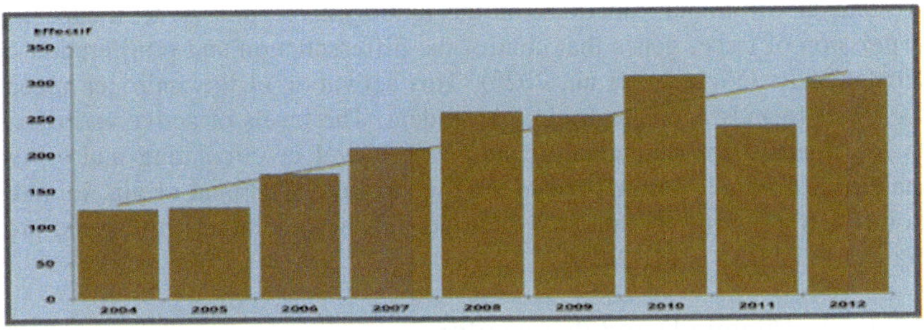

FIGURE 8.5 Evolution of the number of new cases of prostate cancer between 2004 and 2012 in Morocco (Greater Casablanca Cancer Registry).

8.3 Tumor development

8.3.1 Risk factors for prostate cancer

The major risk factors determined with some certainty are age, family history of prostate or breast cancer, and ethnicity (populations of African descent such as African Americans or Caribbean populations) (Fournier et al., 2004).

Other risk factors have also been reported, mainly related to the environment. It is a combination of genetic and environmental factors that would explain the ethnic and geographic variations in the incidence of the disease. The ethnic factor seems to be linked to the genetic determinism of certain hormonal factors and to the permissive factors of the carcinogenic environment and sociocultural behaviors, particularly dietary (Fournier et al., 2004).

8.3.1.1 Family history

There are three different types of prostate cancer as a result of family history, namely, hereditary form, familial form, and sporadic form (Fournier et al., 2004).

8.3.1.2 Hormonal and other growth factors

Hormonal factors were logically considered because of the very strong interactions between the androgens on the one hand and the normal prostate or prostate cancer on the other hand.

8.3.1.2.1 Androgens

The role of androgens in the course of the normal prostate and in the progression (promotion) of prostate cancer has been very generally established since the work of Huggins in the 1940s. It is at the origin of the hormonal treatment of prostate cancer. Finally, a metaanalysis concluded that high testosterone levels induce a higher than normal risk (Fournier et al., 2004).

One of the major functions of the androgen receptor is to induce the expression of target genes that control the differentiation and proliferation of prostate cells (Vickman et al., 2020). This activation of the androgen receptor by its ligands is concentration-dependent. The levels of active androgens in the prostate are thus conditioned by the level of circulating androgens, mainly of testicular origin, and to a lesser degree of adrenal origin, in addition to intraprostatic mutation of androgens from circulating androgenic precursors (Vickman et al., 2020).

8.3.1.2.2 Vitamin D and its receptor

In contrast to androgens, vitamin D has some inhibitory effect on prostate tumor multiplication. Epidemiological studies have shown that high levels of vitamin D are associated with a lower risk of prostate cancer, which is consistent with the higher incidence of this condition in countries with low sunlight. Thus, one would expect UV radiation to have a protective effect through vitamin D metabolism (Khammissa et al., 2018).

8.3.1.2.3 Insulin growth factor 1

The androgen receptor and the vitamin D receptor produce their effects in part through insulin growth factor 1 (IGF-1). In the prostate, IGF-1's function is regulated by binding proteins such as IGF-binding protein-3 (BP-3), which determine its bioavailability, the latter being negatively regulated by androgens and positively regulated by vitamin D analogs. The circulating blood level of IGF-1 is related to the risk of prostate cancer and certain polymorphisms in the gene regulating IGF-1 transcription that correlates with the circulating level (Fournier et al., 2004).

8.3.1.3 Environmental factors: diet and other factors

Although the subclinical incidence is broadly similar, evidence of variability in clinical cancer proliferation suggests that environmental factors may influence cancer progression. The peculiarity of progression to clinical cancer raises the possibility that environmental factors are involved in the progression of this neoplasia. The influence of these factors is also confirmed by the fact that Japanese and Chinese immigrants present in one generation an incidence of prostate cancer four to nine times higher than in their country of origin, which goes against the implication of genetic factors to justify the differences in incidence. In this context, nutrition could be an essential factor, inhibiting or stimulating, depending on the type of nutrient, the proliferation of microscopic prostate cancer (Boyle et al., 2003).

8.3.1.3.1 Foods at risk

Red meat has been implicated, especially if prepared at high temperatures (Norrish et al., 1999).

A diet very rich in fats would promote the risk mainly by polyunsaturated fatty acids (alpha linolenic acid) according to several mechanisms: increase in the level of sex hormones, immune response, constitution of cell membranes in phospholipids, formation of free radicals, decrease in vitamin D, elevation of IGF-1, or action on 5-alpha-reductase type 2 (Boyle et al., 2003). Similarly, calcium intake and consumption of dairy products are associated with an increased risk of cancer (Chan et al., 1998; Grönberg, 2003).

8.3.1.3.2 Protective foods

Indeed, some foods have been presented as preventive factors or even as real drugs for the prevention of prostate cancer (Giovannucci et al., 2002). The have been reported for prostate cancer prevention, insofar as their consumption is correlated with a reduced risk of prostate cancer (Miller et al., 2002).

8.3.1.4 Other factors

Exposure to UV rays have been shown to have a protective effect through vitamin D. It has not been established that people who smoke have a higher incidence of prostate cancer (Giovannucci et al., 1999; Gleason and Mellinger, 1974), but as far as prostate cancer mortality is concerned, alcohol is not a risk factor, nor are the various toxic products used in the workplace, such as pesticides (Boyle et al., 2003).

8.3.2 Genetic mutations responsible for prostate cancer

8.3.2.1 HOXB13 variants

A large number of authors have confirmed the correlation between the G84E variant and the risk of prostate cancer (Breyer et al., 2012). Although the reported probability depends on the population analyzed (Karlsson et al., 2014; Xu et al., 2013), the frequency of gene carriage appears to be generally higher in patients with early-onset disease or a family history of prostate cancer and higher in the group with both family history and early-onset disease (Laitinen et al., 2013, Witte et al., 2013). According to several studies, the G84E variant is not represented in men without European ancestry (Alanee et al., 2013), whereas other HOXB13 mutations have been reported in patients of African and Asian ancestry (Ewing et al., 2012; Kote-Jarai et al., 2015). A systematic study of HOXB13 mutations in prostate cancer patients from southern Europe is lacking; in fact, the only study available for populations from this same region is the absence of the G84E gene in 183 men who were part of the REDUCE chemo-prevention trial, 165 of whom were from Portugal, with no indication of how many of them developed prostate cancer during followup (Chen et al., 2013; Alanee et al., 2013).

8.3.2.2 Mutations in the BRAF gene

The most common mutation found in codon 600 of the BRAF gene was a GTG–GCG mutation, which causes an amino acid change from valine to alanine. The second most common mutation was a GTG–ATG (valine to methionine) mutation. The remaining two mutations were GTG–GAG (valine to glutamic acid).

8.4 Methods for studying genetic polymorphisms

8.4.1 Classical genotyping methods

8.4.1.1 High-throughput genotyping

8.4.1.1.1 Spoligotyping

Spoligotyping is the technique of "typing by means of oligonucleotides of the spacers of the Dr locus." Spoligotyping was carried out at the University Hospital of Angers on cells prepared at the Pasteur Institute of Guadeloupe according to a published protocol (Kamerbeek et al., 1997).

8.4.1.2 VNTR typing

VNTR (variable number of DNA tandem repeats) typing technique is based on the amplification of five polymorphic loci (exact tandem repeats or ETR) ETR-A to ETR-E, whose copy number is easily determined by PCR from the size of the products thus obtained. The resulting product is a five-digit code based on the number of copies of each ETR (e.g., 32,333). This technique has been shown to have excellent interlaboratory replication, although it is less discriminating than spoligotage (Kremer et al., 1999).

8.4.1.3 Double-repetitive-element-polymerase chain reaction

The DRE-PCR (double-repetitive-element-PCR) technique is based on the amplification between PGRS (polymorphic GC-rich sequence) and IS6110 insertions with four specific and previously described primers. The amplification products are then analyzed on agarose gel and placed side by side with the results of spoligotyping and VNTR to identify identical profiles. Although highly discriminating, this method is only moderately reproducible (Montoro et al., 1998).

8.4.1.4 Biochips, multiparametric biosensors

8.4.1.4.1 Biosensors

The mode of operation of a biosensor, is based on an association between a bioreceptor, which allows the specific molecular taking into account of an analyte, with a transducer, which transforms the physicochemical signal generated during the phenomenon of recognition into a physical signal interpretable and quantifiable. The term "biosensor" appeared in the 1950s with the development by Leland Clark of a device to measure glucose in blood (Clark and Lyons, 1962). For this purpose, he had glucose oxidase immobilized in a membrane next to a platinum electrode and used it as a bioelement for the precise detection of glucose in a sample, in combination with an electrochemical electrode. sample, in combination with electrochemical transduction.

8.4.1.5 DNA chips and oligonucleotide chips

The first chips developed were the so-called "DNA" chips. They quickly became an essential analytical tool. The market for DNA chips thus grew from 48 million dollars in 1997 to 670 million in 2008 (Biophoenix 2009). It was valued at $2.25 billion in 2014. The recognition agents are DNA strands or oligonucleotides (a few tens of bases) (MacBeath and Schreiber, 2000). These are able to hybridize, by a very particular base coupling, with complementary target sequences in solution in the sample. Determination of the double strands formed enables identification of the targets present. The wide range of accessible spot densities gives access to a wide range of applications (Table 8.1).

TABLE 8.1 Microarray applications by probe density.

Degree of complexity	Number of hybridization spots	Target application
Low complexity	10–1000	Diagnostic
Average complexity	1000–10,000	Mutation study, genotyping
High complexity	10,000–100,000	Gene sequencing, study of gene expression
Very high complexity	>100,000	Gene sequencing, study of gene expression

8.4.1.6 *Protein chips*

The development of nucleic acid microarray technology has led to a desire to transfer these results to the development of miniaturized multiparametric immunoassays, this time using immobilized proteins, peptides or antibodies. Using this equipment and the slide scanners developed for DNA chips, MacBeath and Schreiber in 2000 developed a protein chip on a glass slide and demonstrated their applicability to a high-throughput study of protein/protein, enzyme/substrate, and protein/small molecule interactions (MacBeath and Schreiber, 2000). After disrupting genomics, microarrays are opening up new avenues in functional proteomics (study or discovery of new functions) (Phizicky et al., 2003; Pandey and Mann, 2000).

8.5 Conclusion

Quantitative and structural genetic alterations lead to the development and progression of prostate cancer. A number of genes have been associated with prostate cancer through genetic alterations and the functional consequences of these genetic alterations.

Acknowledgments

The authors would like to thank the Minister of National Education, Professional Training, Higher Education and Scientific Research and express gratitude to members of Virology, Oncology and Medical Biotechnology team at FSTM-Hassan II University of Casablanca, for all their efforts in supporting us during all work stages on this research.

References

Abumsimir, B., & Ennaji, M. M. (2019). Suggested parameters to setup Y chromosome microsatellites markers as a prostate cancer genetic risk indicator. *Future Oncology*, *15*(30), 3423–3426.

Abumsimir, B., Abualala, K., Jroundi, C., Tiabi, I., Kasmi, Y., Bessi, H., & Ennaji, M. M. (2020). Gynecomammary and Prostate Tumors: Epidemiology and Viral Etiology. In Emerging and Reemerging Viral Pathogens, (pp. 1063–1084). Academic Press.

Akamatsu, G., Ishikawa, K., Mitsumoto, K., Taniguchi, T., Ohya, N., Baba, S., & Sasaki, M. (2012). Improvement in PET/CT image quality with a combination of point-spread function and time-of-flight in relation to reconstruction parameters. *Journal of Nuclear Medicine*, *53* (11), 1716–1722.

Alanee, S., Shah, S., Vijai, J., Schrader, K., Hamilton, R., Rau-Murthy, R., Sarrel, K., Manschreck, C., Eastham, J., & Offit, K. (2013). Prevalence of HOXB13 mutation in a population of Ashkenazi Jewish men treated for prostate cancer. *Familial Cancer*, *12*(4), 597–600. Available from https://doi.org/10.1007/s10689-013-9618-y.

Antoni, S., Soerjomataram, I., Møller, B., Bray, F., & Ferlay, J. (2016). An assessment of GLOBOCAN methods for deriving national estimates of cancer incidence. *Bulletin of the World Health Organization*, *94*(3), 174.

Boyle, P., Severi, G., & Giles, G. G. (2003). The epidemiology of prostate cancer. *Urologic Clinics of North America*, *30*(2), 209–217. Available from https://doi.org/10.1016/S0094-0143(02)00181-7.

Breyer, J. P., Avritt, T. G., McReynolds, K. M., Dupont, W. D., & Smith, J. R. (2012). Confirmation of the HOXB13 G84E germline mutation in familial prostate cancer. *Cancer Epidemiology Biomarkers and Prevention*, *21*(8), 1348–1353. Available from https://doi.org/10.1158/1055-9965.EPI-12-0495.

Chan, J. M., Giovannucci, E., Andersson, S. O., Yuen, J., Adami, H. O., & Wolk, A. (1998). Dairy products, calcium, phosphorous, vitamin D, and risk of prostate cancer (Sweden). *Cancer Causes and Control*, *9*(6), 559–566. Available from https://doi.org/10.1023/A:1008823601897.

Chen, Z., Greenwood, C., Isaacs, W. B., Foulkes, W. D., Sun, J., Zheng, S. L., Condreay, L. D., & Xu, J. (2013). The G84E mutation of HOXB13 is associated with increased risk for prostate cancer: Results from the REDUCE trial. *Carcinogenesis*, *34*(6), 1260–1264. Available from https://doi.org/10.1093/carcin/bgt055.

Clark, L. C., & Lyons, C. (1962). Electrode systems for continuous monitoring in cardiovascular surgery. *Annals of the New York Academy of Sciences*, *102*(1), 29–45. Available from https://doi.org/10.1111/j.1749-6632.1962.tb13623.x.

Ewing, C. M., Ray, A. M., Lange, E. M., Zuhlke, K. A., Robbins, C. M., Tembe, W. D., Wiley, K. E., Isaacs, S. D., Johng, D., Wang, Y., Bizon, C., Yan, G., Gielzak, M., Partin, A. W., Shanmugam, V., Izatt, T., Sinari, S., Craig, D. W., Zheng, S. L., & Cooney, K. A. (2012). Germline mutations in HOXB13 and prostate-cancer risk. *New England Journal of Medicine*, *366*(2), 141–149. Available from https://doi.org/10.1056/NEJMoa1110000.

Ferlay, J., Soerjomataram, I., Ervik, M., Dikshit, R., Eser, S., Mathers, C., … & Bray, F. (2014). GLOBOCAN 2012 v1. 0, Cancer incidence and mortality worldwide: IARC CancerBase No. 11. 2013.

Fournier, G., Valeri, A., Mangin, P., & Cussenot, O. (2004). Cancer de la prostate. Épidémiologie. Facteurs de risques. Anatomopathologie. *Annales d'Urologie*, 187–206. Available from https://doi.org/10.1016/j.anuro.2004.07.001.

Gérin, M., Gosselin, P., Cordier, S., Viau, C., Quénel, P., & Dewailly, É. (2003). *Environnement et santé publique: Fondements et pratiques. Édisem/Tec & Doc.*

Giovannucci, E., Rimm, E. B., Ascherio, A., Colditz, G. A., Spiegelman, D., Stampfer, M. J., & Willett, W. C. (1999). Smoking and risk of total and fatal prostate cancer in United States health professionals. *Cancer Epidemiology Biomarkers and Prevention*, *8*(4), 277–282.

Giovannucci, E., Rimm, E. B., Liu, Y., Stampfer, M. J., & Willett, W. C. (2002). A prospective study of tomato products, lycopene, and prostate cancer risk. *Journal of the National Cancer Institute*, *94*(5), 391–398. Available from https://doi.org/10.1093/jnci/94.5.391.

Gleason, D. F., & Mellinger, G. T. (1974). Prediction of prognosis for prostatic adenocarcinoma by combined histological grading and clinical staging. *Journal of Urology*, 58–64. Available from https://doi.org/10.1016/s0022-5347(17)59889-4.

Grönberg, H. (2003). Prostate cancer epidemiology. *Lancet*, *361*(9360), 859–864. Available from https://doi.org/10.1016/S0140-6736(03)12713-4.

Kamerbeek, J., Schouls, L., Kolk, A., Van Agterveld, M., Van Soolingen, D., Kuijper, S., Bunschoten, A., Molhuizen, H., Shaw, R., Goyal, M., & Van Embden, J. (1997). Simultaneous detection and strain differentiation of *Mycobacterium tuberculosis* for diagnosis and epidemiology. *Journal of Clinical Microbiology*, *35*(4), 907–914. Available from https://doi.org/10.1128/jcm.35.4.907-914.1997.

Karlsson, R., Aly, M., Clements, M., Zheng, L., Adolfsson, J., Xu, J., Grönberg, H., & Wiklund, F. (2014). A population-based assessment of germline HOXB13 G84E mutation and prostate cancer risk. *European Urology*, *65*(1), 169–176. Available from https://doi.org/10.1016/j.eururo.2012.07.027.

Khammissa, R. A. G., Fourie, J., Motswaledi, M. H., Ballyram, R., Lemmer, J., & Feller, L. (2018). The biological activities of vitamin D and its receptor in relation to calcium and bone homeostasis, cancer, immune and cardiovascular systems, skin biology, and oral health. *BioMed research international*, *2018*.

Khazaei, Z., Sohrabivafa, M., Momenabadi, V., Moayed, L., & Goodarzi, E. (2019). Global cancer statistics 2018: Globocan estimates of incidence and mortality worldwide prostate cancers and their relationship with the human development index. *Advances in Human Biology*, *9*(3), 245.

Kote-Jarai, Z., Mikropoulos, C., Leongamornlert, D. A., Dadaev, T., Tymrakiewicz, M., Saunders, E. J., Jones, M., Jugurnauth-Little, S., Govindasami, K., Guy, M., Hamdy, F. C., Donovan, J. L., Neal, D. E., Lane, J. A., Dearnaley, D., Wilkinson, R. A., Sawyer, E. J., Morgan, A., Antoniou, A. C., & Nordestgaard, B. G. (2015). Prevalence of theHOXB13 G84E germline mutation in British men and correlation with prostate cancer risk, tumour characteristics and clinical outcomes. *Annals of Oncology*, *26*(4), 756–761. Available from https://doi.org/10.1093/annonc/mdv004.

Kremer, K., Van Soolingen, D., Frothingham, R., Haas, W. H., Hermans, P. W. M., Martín, C., Palittapongarnpim, P., Plikaytis, B. B., Riley, L. W., Yakrus, M. A., Musser, J. M., & Van Embden, J. D. A. (1999). Comparison of methods based on different molecular epidemiological markers for typing of *Mycobacterium tuberculosis* complex strains: Interlaboratory study of discriminatory power and reproducibility. *Journal of Clinical Microbiology*, *37*(8), 2607–2618. Available from https://doi.org/10.1128/jcm.37.8.2607-2618.1999.

Laitinen, V. H., Wahlfors, T., Saaristo, L., Rantapero, T., Pelttari, L. M., Kilpivaara, O., Laasanen, S. L., Kallioniemi, A., Nevanlinna, H., Aaltonen, L., Vessella, R. L., Auvinen, A., Visakorpi, T., Tammela, T. L. J., & Schleutker, J. (2013). HOXB13 G84E mutation in Finland: Population-based analysis of prostate, breast, and colorectal cancer risk. *Cancer Epidemiology Biomarkers and Prevention*, *22*(3), 452–460. Available from https://doi.org/10.1158/1055-9965.EPI-12-1000-T.

Lonergan, P. E., & Tindall, D. J. (2011). Androgen receptor signaling in prostate cancer development and progression. *Journal of carcinogenesis*, *10*.

Lonergan, M. H., Olivera-Figueroa, L. A., Pitman, R. K., & Brunet, A. (2013). Propranolol's effects on the consolidation and reconsolidation of long-term emotional memory in healthy participants: a meta-analysis. *Journal of Psychiatry and Neuroscience*, *38*(4), 222–231.

MacBeath, G., & Schreiber, S. L. (2000). Printing proteins as microarrays for high-throughput function determination. *Science*, *289*(5485), 1760–1763.

Miller, E. C., Giovannucci, E., Erdman, J. W., Bahnson, R., Schwartz, S. J., & Clinton, S. K. (2002). Tomato products, lycopene, and prostate cancer risk. *Urologic Clinics of North America*, *29*(1), 83–93. Available from https://doi.org/10.1016/S0094-0143(02)00020-4.

Montoro, E., Valdivia, J., & Leão, S. C. (1998). Molecular fingerprinting of *Mycobacterium tuberculosis* isolates obtained in Havana, Cuba, by IS6110 restriction fragment length polymorphism analysis and by the double-repetitive-element PCR method. *Journal of Clinical Microbiology*, *36*(10), 3099–3102. Available from https://doi.org/10.1128/jcm.36.10.3099-3102.1998.

Norrish, A. E., Ferguson, L. R., Knize, M. G., Felton, J. S., Sharpe, S. J., & Jackson, R. T. (1999). Heterocyclic amine content of cooked meat and risk of prostate cancer. *Journal of the National Cancer Institute*, *91*(23), 2038–2044. Available from https://doi.org/10.1093/jnci/91.23.2038.

Pandey, A., & Mann, M. (2000). Proteomics to study genes and genomes. *Nature*, *405*(6788), 837–846. Available from https://doi.org/10.1038/35015709.

Phizicky, E., Bastiaens, P. I. H., Zhu, H., Snyder, M., & Fields, S. (2003). Protein analysis on a proteomic scale. *Nature*, *422*(6928), 208–215. Available from https://doi.org/10.1038/nature01512.

Vickman, R. E., Franco, O. E., Moline, D. C., Vander Griend., Thumbikat, P., & Hayward, S. W. (2020). The role of the androgen receptor in prostate development and benign prostatic hyperplasia: A review. *Asian Journal of Urology*, *7*(3), 191–202.

Witte, J. S., Mefford, J., Plummer, S. J., Liu, J., Cheng, I., Klein, E. A., Rybicki, B. A., & Casey, G. (2013). HOXB13 mutation and prostate cancer: Studies of siblings and aggressive disease. *Cancer Epidemiology Biomarkers and Prevention*, *22*(4), 675–680. Available from https://doi.org/10.1158/1055-9965.EPI-12-1154.

Xu, J., Lange, E. M., Lu, L., Zheng, S. L., Wang, Z., Thibodeau, S. N., Cannon-Albright, L. A., Teerlink, C. C., Camp, N. J., Johnson, A. M., Zuhlke, K. A., Stanford, J. L., Ostrander, E. A., Wiley, K. E., Isaacs, S. D., Walsh, P. C., Maier, C., Luedeke, M., Vogel, W., & Isaacs, W. B. (2013). HOXB13 is a susceptibility gene for prostate cancer: Results from the international consortium for prostate cancer genetics (ICPCG). *Human Genetics*, *132*(1), 5–14. Available from https://doi.org/10.1007/s00439-012-1229-4.

Chapter 9

Diagnostic screening of the microdeleation mutations in the azoospermia factor-gene cluster of the Y chromosome and; prostate cancer among Arabs: toward establishment of gene therapy platform in the region ☆

Ihsane Ali Mahasneh[1], Ferdos Ebrahim Abdul Rahim[1], Moulay Mustapha Ennaji[2], Berjas Abumsimir[3,4] and Yassine Kasmi[3]

[1]*Faculty of Science, Department of Applied Biology-Biotechnology Program, University of Sharjah, Sharjah, United Arab Emirates,* [2]*Group Leader Research team of Virology, Oncology, and Biotechnologies, Head of Laboratory of Virology, Oncology, Biosciences, Environment and New Energies (LVO-BEEN), Faculty of Sciences and Techniques Mohammedia, University Hassan II of Casablanca, Casablanca, Morocco,* [3]*Team of Virology, Oncology, and Biotechnologies, Laboratory of Virology, Oncology, Biosciences, Environment and New Energies (LVO-BEEN), Faculty of Sciences and Techniques Mohammedia, University Hassan II of Casablanca, Casablanca, Morocco,* [4]*Pharmacological and Diagnostic Research Centre (PDRC), Department of Medical Laboratory Sciences, Faculty of Allied Medical Sciences, Al-Ahliyya Amman University (AAU), Amman, Jordan*

9.1 Background for our hypothesis on the azoospermia factor gene cluster among Arabs for future gene therapy of infertility

The evolution of DNA technology during the last several years has become evident, and thus this therapy is used to analyze various aspects of human DNA.

☆In the Book: Genitourinary cancer: Molecular diagnostic immunological implications: genetic aspect and viral therapy.

Immunological Implications and Molecular Diagnostics of Genitourinary Cancer.
DOI: https://doi.org/10.1016/B978-0-323-85496-2.00008-7

Our research outcomes, using the latest technology such as next-generation sequencing, microsatellite analysis, and biochip microarray have shown conclusively that the epidemiology of cancers is correlated to the genealogy and ethnicity of the population's clusters around the world (Mahasneh, 2016, 2018). More recently, we have reported the genealogical-genetic map of the Y chromosome and determined the genography of Arabian population (Mahasneh & Zuriegat, 2020; Mahasneh et al., 2021). Currently and since the last decade, there has been a worldwide growing interest on the diagnostic screening of the microdeletion mutations on the azoospermia factor (AZF) region of Y-chromosome as a driving force for male infertility (Alkhalaf & Al-Shoumer, 2010; Hellani et al., 2006; Liu et al., 2016; Arafa et al., 2017; Khabour et al., 2014; Shafae et al., 2018; Ghorbel et al., 2012; Naasse et al., 2010). Heretofore, there is a lack of information among gynecologists with respect to the genetic complexity of the AZF microdeletions and their correlations with the ancestor genealogical lineages of males as reflected by the microsatellite analysis for the short tandem repeats of Y chromosome (Y-STRs).

The human Y chromosome uniquely and strictly harbors all genes responsible for male fertility including testis development, initiation and maintenance of spermatogenesis in adulthood. More precisely, it is the long arm of Y chromosome (Yq), the nonrecombined region specific for and therefore exposed to self-recombination during spermatogenesis, making it more venerable to the inter-chromosomal deletion, thus resulting in male infertility. The most common Yq deletions causing infertile males are termed as AZF microdeletions and abbreviated as AZFa, AZFb, AZFc, AZFd, and AZFe. Therefore the Yq deletions and/or mutations are considered to be the driving genetic force causing male infertility due to its direct effect on the expression level of spermatogenesis.

In different nations and populations around the world, the AZFa, AZFb, AZFc, AZFd, and AZFe microdeletion has been extensively studied to detect the frequency of male infertility; a few studies were performed on AZF microdeletions among Arab males including Saudi Arabia, Kuwait, Qatar, Jordan, Egypt, Tunisia, and Morocco (Alkhalaf & Al-Shoumer, 2010; Arafa et al., 2017; Ghorbel et al., 2012; Hellani et al., 2006; Khabour et al., 2014; Naasse et al., 2010; Shafae et al., 2018). This chapter is the first attempt to address the urgency for diagnostic infertility AZF diagnosis and gene therapy comprehensive point of view from which that we can conclude the most common pattern of these mutations of microdeletions among Arab genealogical lineages.

As both AZF region and the nonrecombined region of YSTRs (Y-short tandem repeats forming the YDNA haplogroups) are strictly inherited by future generations as Y-linked pattern, we hypothesize that it is highly plausible that the familial-wize progression of the Yq mutations/microdeletions on the AZF region is associated with the step-wize mutation patterns of the YSTRs, which determine the familial genealogical lineage on family level. Therefore a comparative diagnostic screening is urgently needed to determine the male infertility pattern among Arab males in particular as compared to other worldwide nations in a wider spectrum.

Due to the fact that Y chromosome infertility is strictly inherited by future generations as Y chromosome-linked pattern, the clinical importance of the diagnostic screening in the gynecologist and the in-vitro fertilization (IVF) clinics is tremendous and so are its implications on populations. Therefore diagnostic screening of Y chromosome deletions in different ethnic groups and families will help tremendously to understand the deletion patterns and its negative effect on infertility rates among different lineages of populations, which will help the clinicians to promote a rational management strategy for their patients and thus the global infertility prevalence. Furthermore, as these deletions are inherited by male offspring born through assisted reproduction by IVF clinics and hospitals, testing for the infertility deletion is investable and must be conducted prior to couple marriage to allow couples to make their own informed choice regarding the familial concerns on the male infertility perpetuation in the future generation.

9.2 Landscape of the azoospermia factor gene cluster and chromosome Y chromosome structure

The structure diagram of the Y chromosome and the landscape of the AZF (a,b,c,d,e) gene cluster is presented in Fig. 9.1. The genome size of Y chromosome is the smallest in terms of the functional genes and is composed of 59 Mbp, which larger in size than the smallest chromosome 21 (spanning 48 Mbp).

The Y chromosome contains the maleness development SRY gene, which triggers male development and is passed only from father to son. It carries an estimated 100–200 genes, out of which between 45 and 73 are protein-coding genes. During male meiosis, recombination only takes place in the pseudoautosomal regions at the tips of both arms of Y and X chromosomes (PAR1, with 2.6 Mb, and PAR 2, with 0.32 Mb). Along ~95% of its length, the Y chromosome is male-specific and effectively haploid, since it is exempt from meiotic recombination. Therefore this Y chromosome segment where X-Y crossing over is absent has been designated as the nonrecombining region of the Y chromosome or NRY. Because of the high nonhomologous recombination occurring within this Y chromosome specific region, a more appropriate name of male-specific region or MSY is nowadays used to designate it.

The historical terminology of the male-specific region of the Y chromosome, the MSY, goes back to 1976 when a conserved, terminal deletion within MSY located at the long arm (11q) was identified in a group of infertility patients diagnosed in azoospermic men based on the terminal deletions in this series and their corresponding phenotypes. It was hypothesized that the 11q region of the Y chromosome performed vital functions in spermatogenesis and was termed the "azoospermia factor." Several years after the identification of AZF, "microdeletions" at 76 discrete DNA loci were mapped into three subregions of Yq11 based on their presentation in azoospermic men as well as their putative action in different phases of male germ

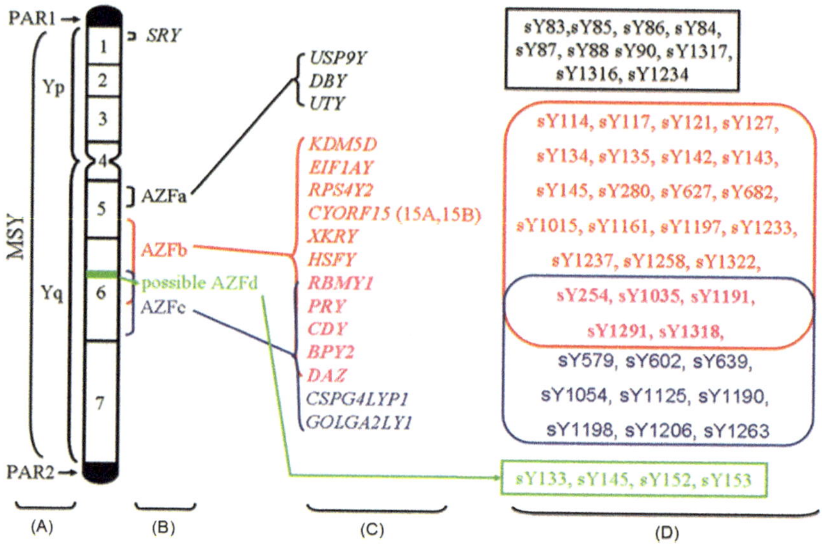

FIGURE 9.1 Diagram of the human Y chromosome showing the azoospermia factor (AZF) loci, associated genes, and sequence-tagged sites (STSs) markers. (A) Schematic representation of the structure of the human Y chromosome showing the pseudo autosomal regions (PAR1, PAR2), Yp (short arm), Yq (long arm), and MSY (male-specific region). (B) Schematic locations of the four AZF loci. (C) Corresponding candidate genes in the AZFa, AZFb, and AZFc regions. The black, red, blue, and pink colors represent the genes in the AZFa, AZFb, AZFc, and overlapping AZFb/AZFc regions, respectively. (D) Conventional STS markers associated with the AZFa, AZFb, AZFc, and AZFd regions. The black, red, blue, pink, and green colors represent the STS markers for the genes in the AZFa, AZFb, AZFc, overlapping AZFb/AZFc, and AZFd regions, respectively (Yu et al., 2015). *After Yu, X. W., Wei, Z. T., Jiang, Y. T., Zhang, S. L. 2015. Y chromosome azoospermia factor region microdeletions and transmission characteristics in azoospermic and severe oligozoospermic patients. International Journal of Clinical and Experimental Medicine, 8(9), 14634–14646.*

cell development; they were termed AZFa (the most proximal segment), AZFb (middle), and AZFc (most distal; Fig. 9.1). Several years later, partial deletions in regions of AZFc, such as gr/gr and b2/b3, have been frequently identified in men and added to the AZF standard testing by the multiplex polymerase chain reaction (PCR) technology as provided in the commercial kit of Promega Company for the last 20 years in the market.

MSY is a mosaic of heterochromatic and euchromatic regions; besides the centromeric heterocromatin, a large heterochromatic region is located on the distal long arm of the Y chromosome (Yq) and constitutes more than half of the chromosome in some normal males, but is virtually undetectable in others. A third heterochromatic region interrupts the euchromatic sequences of proximal Yq. These regions are composed of highly repeated sequences of nonfunctional DNA: DYZ1, DYZ2, DYZ3, DYZ17, DYZ18, and DYZ19. In contrast, the euchromatin is a constant size region and includes sequences homologous to the X chromosome, Y-specific repetitive sequences, and all the genes identified in the Y chromosome, which include the now identified 27 distinct protein-coding genes or gene families.

The PAR regions exchange genetic material with the PAR region on the X PAR region during meiosis. PAR1 and PAR2, located on the telomeres of Y_p and Y_q, respectively, represent 5% of the chromosome, whereas the majority of the Y chromosome is made up of the NRY, region which includes the SRY gene (also known as the MSY chromosome), as this portion does not recombine with the X chromosome and composes 95% of the Y chromosome (Jégou & Skinner, 2018). Because of the fact that the Y chromosome has only one copy of its critical genetic material, any deletion or mutation of this material may have a severe impact on a man's spermatogenesis potential. Microdeletions may occur when two palindromic sequences of the Y chromosome recombine inadvertently, deleting the intervening genetic material (Hotaling & Carrell, 2014) (Fig. 9.1).

The human Y chromosome, with the size of ~60 Mb, is the smallest chromosome in terms of the number of functional genes representing around 2%–3% of the total haploid genome (Quintana-Murci & Fellous, 2001). Cytogenetically, it is an acrocentric chromosome composed of a short arm (Yp) and long arm (Yq) clearly joined by a centromere (Lahn et al., 2001; Navarro-Costa et al., 2010). Cytogenic banding studies allowed for the identification of the three sites of the Y chromosome known as pseudoautosomal region (PAR1 and PAR2), euchromatic, and heterochromatic regions.

The Y chromosome, particularly AZF region, is composed of highly repetitive sequences, amplicons, and massive palindromes allowing for intrachromosomal recombination to occur more commonly (Kuroda-Kawaguchi et al., 2001; Vogt, 2005). The intrachromosomal recombination in this region thus provokes partial or complete microdeletions in the AZF region in the Y chromosome (Rozen et al., 2003; Sun et al., 2000; Vogt, 2005). As a result, the deletion of candidate genes from AZF subdivision is associated with different degree of clinical consequences. AZFc deletion is most commonly detected among infertile males, which may probably be due to the presence of high repetitive sequences compared to other intervals (Kuroda-Kawaguchi et al., 2001).

9.3 Global heterogeneity and ethnicity of familial infertility clustering of azoospermia factor microdeletion variants among different genealogical lineages of populations

In our previous publications, we have underlined the importance of ethnicity and the genealogical lineages of chromosome Y haplogroups as driving force in allelic heterogeneity not only for the AZF gene cluster but also for prostate cancer (Mahasneh, 2016, 2018; Mahasneh et al., 2018, 2021; Mahasneh & Zuriegat, 2020). About a decade ago, it was also suggested by Cocuzza et al. (2013) that an accurate diagnosis of azoospermia and systematic evaluation of the patient to establish the disease etiology are required to guide appropriate management options and to determine the associated cost benefits, risks, and prognosis for treatment success. The global prevalence among infertile men displays a wide range of heterogeneity—from 2% to 24% based on region and ethnicity with the fact that AZFc is the most commonly identified microdeletion, and fortunately, its medical condition provides the highest chance for fertility through artificial reproductive protocols applied worldwide. In contrast with AZFc, the deletions in the subregions of either AZFa and AZFb or any combination are associated with low probabilities of achieving pregnancy. This situation underlines the importance of gene therapy to overcome the problem of infertility globally. The latest review published by a research group (Rabinowitz et al., 2021) reported that the frequency of Y chromosome microdeletions in MSY is within the range of 5% and 10% of severe oligospermic and azoospermic men, respectively.

The global frequency of azoospermia affects about 1% of male population and accounts for 20% of male infertility cases, and at least four semen samples should be examined before diagnosing a male with azoospermia (Rabinowitz et al., 2021). The latest international criteria available nowadays for definition for the infertility classification and stratification is the one that has been set in the manual of the World Health Organization (WHO) and several authors more than a decade ago. Initially, infertility was defined as the inability to conceive after 12 months of unprotected intercourse or 6 months of unprotected sex in the setting of advanced maternal age (Cooper, Noonan, von Eckardstein, Auger, et al., 2010; Cooper, Noonan, von Eckardstein, 2010; Kumar & Singh, 2015; Rabinowitz et al., 2021; Rutstein & Shah, 2004). It is estimated that infertility will affect one of every 12 men in their lifetimes, and of men presenting with infertility, 90% will have an underlying oligospermia or azoospermia.

The medical condition azoospermia is divided into obstructive azoospermia (a posttesticular obstruction of the ductal system impeding the movement of sperm at any location in the reproductive tract—sperm is classically seen on testicular biopsy) and nonobstructive azoospermia (NOA; absence of sperm in the ejaculate due to primary testicular failure and is commonly diagnosed by testicular biopsy suggestive of spermatogenic failure). Thus azoospermia is defined as the absence of sperm in the ejaculate, and it is identified in approximately 1% of all men and in 10%–15% of infertile males (Cooper, Noonan, von Eckardstein, Auger, et al., 2010; Cooper, Noonan, von Eckardstein, 2010; Kumar & Singh, 2015; Rabinowitz et al., 2021). In contrast, oligospermia is defined as a sperm concentration of less than 15 million sperms per milliliter of ejaculate, below the fifth percentile of fertile men, and therefore this category can be further stratified into mild, moderate, and severe categories defined as 10–15 million sperm/mL, 5–10 million sperms/mL, and any sperm to 5 million sperm/mL, respectively.

The practical results in the IVF clinics around the world suggest that the must cut-off criterion must be revised and that a new criterion must bet set to replace that proposed by Cooper, Noonan, von Eckardstein (2010). The new criterion should recommend a lower cut-off value for diagnosis the azoospermia stratification, which would be more accurate on the basis of ethnicity and genealogical requirements, for example, to set a threshold from 5 million sperm/mL of ejaculate to 1 million/mL as the frequency of Y chromosome microdeletions in men with sperm concentrations between 1 and 5 million sperm/mL is very low (~0.8%). The prevalence of AZF microdeletion in azoospermic or severe oligospermic males (sperm count $<5 \times 10^6$/mL) is evaluated to be 10%–15%, whereas it is very rarely detected in males with normal fertility rate or those with sperm density greater than 5 million/mL. The AZF genes contribute to differences in their genomic arrangement and functional role. Studies have reported the DDX3Y in AZFa, KDM5D and RBMY1A1 in AZFb, and DAZ and CDY in AZFb/c as biomarkers in determining the genetic health of spermatogenesis. The remaining genes in AZF region need more studies to be associated with male infertility. Although the exact genotype–phenotype relationship is not fully understood, microdeletions in intervals of AZF result in variable degrees of spermatogenic failure reflecting different clinical manifestations. Accordingly, advances in genomic approach of male reproductive system are clearly significant to determine the clinical management of males diagnosed with infertility.

The global frequency of the infertility problem is affecting 15% of couples of reproductive age, and 50% of the infertility is attributed to men. This problem shows higher prevalence among Arabs than any other nation worldwide due to the consanguineous marriages (40%–60%), which represent males as the driving force of population's reproduction according to the cultural structure of the Arabian societies on a global level. Despite the availability of the advanced diagnostic gene testing of the mutations/microdeletions on the AZF a,b,c,d region of the Yq region, male diagnosis and medical conditions in the reproductive health sector in Arabian countries is still being evaluated and thus determined using the classical diagnostic methodology as descriptive parameters (sperm count, sperm morphology, sperm motility, including total and progressive motility), which do not determine the genetic pathogenesis of the infertility reproductive issues.

The global prevalence of the Yq microdeletions is 7.5% in infertile males, and the European infertile men are less susceptible, whereas the highest prevalence is among Americans and East Asian infertile men. In addition, partial deletions of the AZFc locus seems to be dependent on the ethnicity as gr/gr deletions are significantly associated with male infertility among Caucasians in Europe, Western Pacific regions and Mongolian men, while the b2/b3 deletion is associated with males of African and Dravidian genealogical origin.

9.4 Familial infertility clustering and consanguinity among Arabian populations

Ethnic and tribal factors greatly influence consanguineous marriages, which are socially supported practice in several global communities as Middle East and North Africa region (MENA), particularly in Arab population. The rate of consanguinity in UAE has been detected to be 50% with the coefficient of inbreeding of 0.0222 based on study performed Al Ain and Dubai cities between October 1994 and March 1995 (AlGazali et al., 1997).

The most recent statistics (Ben-Halim et al., 2013) reveal that the consanguinity frequency among Arabian populations is much higher than previously reported: Egypt (68%), Jordan (51%–58%), Qatar (52%), UAE (50%), Kuwait (54%), Saudi Arabia (58%), Yemen (40%–47%), and Oman (50%). These findings reflect the fact that the first cousins and double first (F is greater than or equal to 0.0625) are the predominant marriages among Arabian populations. Increased rates of consanguinity marriages among Arabs increase the prevalence of chromosomal alterations associated with disorders in reproductive and developmental health factors, thus resulting in infertility in males. Although the genetics of the Arab literature exhibits several gaps, especially in fields of infertility, several studies demonstrate the correlation of male factor infertility and the consanguineous marriages (Inhorn & Patrizio, 2015; Inhorn et al., 2009; Tadmouri et al., 2009).

9.5 Diagnostic criteria and medical conditions as set by WHO criteria for infertility diagnosis

The WHO International Committee for Monitoring Assisted Reproductive Technology has defined infertility as the inability of a couple within the reproductive age to conceive after 12 months or more of regular unprotected intercourse. The reproductive age in females varies than in males – in females it is considered to be between 15 and 49 years, whereas in males the reproductive age seems to be remarkably longer in which sperm production starts from puberty and persists throughout their lives. Male factor infertility contributes to 20%–30% of infertility cases, which means almost 30 million males could be infertile (Agarwal et al., 2015).

Male factor infertility refers to the health complications in the male reproductive system that prevent pregnancy in healthy female (Poongothai et al., 2009). Male infertility is influenced by several factors as hormonal abnormalities, erectile dysfunction, infections, antisperm antibodies, exposure to chemical agents and radiations, testicular cancer, varicose, and most importantly, genetic abnormalities, therefore categorized as multifactorial syndrome (Bonde, 2013; Check, 2007; Jarow et al., 2013; O'Flynn O'Brien et al., 2010), leading to a marked reduction in the male fertility rates more particularly over the age of 40 years.

9.6 Types of microdeletions in the azoospermia factor gene cluster of Y chromosome

Using the multiplex PCR with the respective primers for each sequence of the AZF gene cluster, microdeletions are diagnosed by testing the complete panel, which identifies which one is absent: AZFa (the most proximal segment), AZFb (middle), and AZFc (distal); in addition, to the AZFd and AZFe, which have been recently discovered and verified from their overlapping with AZFb.

The association of Yq deletion and abnormal spermatogenesis in six azoospermic infertile males who lacked mature sperm in their ejaculate was reported by Vogt et al. (1996). On the basis of this finding and other significant efforts, scientists announced the presence of spermatogenesis factor (AZF region) in proximal, middle, and distal Yq11 chromosome. Studies reported AZF region on Y chromosome to be important for spermatogenesis and male reproductive system.

Early deletion analysis studies subdivided the three AZF domains into nonoverlapping regions considering AZFb as intimidate interval located between 5 M and 6 B subintervals (Vogt et al., 1996). Despite the initial efforts considering AZFb as a nonoverlapping interval, high-resolution breakpoint mapping and deletion-junction amplification and sequencing revealed otherwise. Repping et al. established results that AZFb does not exist as a distinct domain. Subsequently, Ferlin et al. used the chromosome - fluorescence *in situ* hybridization (BAC-) clones to sequence the complete map of AZFb to confirm its extension over 3.5 Mb. These reports identified the overlap of AZFb distal portion with AZFc interval through molecular breakpoint characterizations. Moreover, the "Best Practice" meeting on guidelines for the molecular diagnosis of Y chromosome microdeletions did not agree on distinguishing between distinct AZFb interval model and the overlapping AZFb/AZFc model. Thus according to various molecular characterization of AZF region, no absolute finalization has been confirmed to distinguish between the two models. At the same time, localization of AZFd subdivision between AZFb and AZFc regions remains a controversial issue. Some reports associate AZFd deletion to complications within male reproductive system through the use of multiplex PCR, whereas other studies reject the existence of AZFd interval within AZFb and AZFc subdivisions. Unlike AZFb and AZFc, AZFa is identified as a distinct interval located on proximal region of Yq11.21 (Fortesa et al., 2001; Lahn & Page, 1997).

The Y chromosome, particularly AZF region, is composed of highly repetitive sequences, amplicons, and massive palindromes allowing for intrachromosomal recombination to occur more commonly (Kuroda-Kawaguchi et al., 2001; Vogt, 2005). The intrachromosomal recombination in this region thus provokes partial or complete microdeletions in the AZF region in the Y chromosome (Rozen et al., 2003; Sun et al., 2000; Vogt, 2005). As a result, the deletion of candidate genes from AZF subdivision is associated with varying degrees of clinical consequences.

As an example, patients diagnosed with the deletion of entire AZFa region will certainly suffer from severe azoospermia and Sertoli-cell-only syndrome (Foresta et al., 2000; Hopps et al., 2003; Zhu et al., 2017). The AZFa sequence is important in spermatogenic process in which it regulates the early stage of spermatogonial proliferation and is also involved in the survival of germ cells (Gueler et al., 2012). Hence, clearly patients with entire AZFa deletion will not benefit from the assisted productive treatment of intracytoplasmic sperm injection (ICSI; Liu et al., 2017), while patients diagnosed with AZFb deletion would suffer from the absence of postmeiotic germ cells at the spermatocyte stage (Hopps et al., 2003; Soares et al., 2012). Thus ICSI can play an important role in overcoming the obstacles of male infertility. However, ICSI would not be useful for patients with complete AZFb microdeletion due to the absence of mature spermatozoa (Kleiman et al., 2011). Moreover, AZFc region is required to complete the spermatogenic processes, which in turn hypospermatogenesis is resulted in case of AZfc deficiency (Skaletsky et al., 2003; Song et al., 2016). Patients diagnosed with AZFc deletion may have sperm in ejaculate, though with inadequate quantity and quality (Fu et al., 2012; Krausz & Forti, 2006). Screening for the type of AZF microdeletion can manage in effective diagnosis and appropriate medical and surgical treatments for infertile males (Ferlin et al., 2007). Accordingly, AZFc deletion is most commonly detected among infertile males, probably be due to the presence of high repetitive sequences compared to other intervals (Kuroda-Kawaguchi et al., 2001).

9.7 Genetic diagnosis of azoospermia factor microdeletion by multiplex polymerase chain reaction technology

Classical cytogenetic techniques and the digital karyotyping used for diagnosis have limited applications in testing for microdeletions. Fortunately enough, however, the recent advancements in multiplex PCR method has made it possible for highly accurate detection of these microdeletions in a relatively short period of time. For instance, in the recent years, screening for Y chromosome microdeletion as highly attractive technology has received global interest in the clinics and the diagnostic laboratory since it is strongly related to the diagnosis of oligospermia and azoospermia. Among the several factors inducing male infertility, genetic abnormalities of the Y chromosome play a critical role in influencing male reproductive health, while about 40% of male infertility cases are idiopathic (Hamada et al., 2013). Chromosomal abnormalities are reported be about 10 times higher in infertile males than in the general population (Ceylan et al., 2009). Around 10% of male infertility is detected to be due to genetic causes including Y chromosome microdeletions (Mirfakhraie et al., 2011; Yousefi-Razin et al., 2016).

9.7.1 Clinical conditions

Analysis of the patients hormonal profiles were carried out in the laboratories of the Dubai Fertility Center according to the standard method using the normal ranges reference as set in the latest (5th Edition) of WHO manual for examination and processing of human hormonal profiling: testosterone (300–1010 ng/dL), LH (1–19 mIU/mL), FSH (1–19 mIU/ mL), and inhibin B (92–316 pg/mL) (Cooper, Noonan, von Eckardstein, Auger, et al., 2010).

9.7.2 Multiplex polymerase chain reaction protocol to be used in diagnosis of the azoospermia factor microdeletions of Y chromosome

The multiplex PCR technology was used for diagnosis of the microdeletions of AZFa, AZFb, AZFc, AZFd, AZFe gene cluster of the Y chromosome to determine any missing segment of the 20 STSs markers as described by manufacturer instructions (Promega, United States). The STS markers to be tested are:

1. AZFa (SY81, SY86, SY84, SY182),
2. AZFb (SY121, SYPR3, SY124, SY127, SY128, SY130, SY133, SY134),
3. AZFc (SY242, SY208, SY254, SY255, SY157),
4. AZFd (SY145, SY152 (proximal AZFc, referred as AZFd),
5. AZFe (SY242, SY208, SY254, SY255, SY157),
6. SY14 (SRY).
7. Internal controls included SMCX locus and ZFX/ZFY loci.

The procedure was carried out with accordance of the recommendations of European Academy of Andralogy (EAA) and the European Molecular Genetics Quality Network (EMQN) (Krausz et al., 2014). Along with the multiplex PCR run for each sample, two control treatments must be prepared; the first control with a fertile male DNA and the second control without DNA (−DNA).

The optimization of multiplex PCR was performed in accordance with the recommendations of EAA and the EMQN (Krausz et al., 2014). Then, appropriate PCR thermal cycler machine such as or equivalent to Applied Biosystem 9700 or Biorad S-1000 must be used with the following cycling program:

1. Set the program on an initial denaturation step at 94°C for 2 min;
2. Set the program for 35 cycles of denaturation at 94°C for 1 min;
3. Set the program for annealing step at 56°C/57°C for 30 s;
4. Set the program for an extension step at 72°C for 1 min;
5. Set the program for a final extension step at 72°C for 5 min.

The optimum electrophoresis protocol of the PCR products was run at 80 V for 1 h and 30 min on a 3% agarose gel, as it was prepared in 1 X TAE buffer containing 2 μg/mL ethidium bromide. The generated electrophoretic bands on the gel were visualized and analyzed using Biorad Gel Doc EZ and Image-Lab software for picture documentation.

9.7.3 Ethical criteria and consideration adopted for blood samples and YDNA

Following ethical principles as described above, a total of 50 blood samples were collected from different Arab populations for this study using the standard materials and methods for such purpose. For inclusion samples, fresh blood samples of the tested males stored in EDTA tube with utmost sample priority to azoospermia and severe oligospermia, and the least sample priority was suggested for mild and moderate oligospermia.

9.7.4 Clinical criteria and the practical cut-off value for azoospermia factor testing

Azoospermia is a medical condition where there is a complete absence of sperms in the semen sample of a male, given the sample is centrifuged. It affects about 1% of male population and accounts for 20% of male infertility cases, and at least four semen samples should be examined before diagnosing a male with azoospermia. For oligospermia, because the cut-off value set by WHO is 20 million sperms per milliliter, any sperm count less than this value is labeled as oligospermia. It is the most common cause of decreased chances of conception and infertility in men; therefore we should select the lowest count in severe oligospermia as recommended by international sources (Padubidri & Daftary, 2014).

In the absence of clinical intervention, successful fertilization is rare in both azoospermia and severe oligospermia, a condition where the number of sperms required in a male's ejaculate to conceive is less than the minimum requirement for conception.

9.7.5 Practical recommendations for inclusion criteria and stratification of Azoospermia

We recommend dividing the selected samples to be AZF-tested according to the severity into Five groups in addition, to the control group; with the suggested number of samples for statistical purposes to be at least ($n = 5$) per group as in Table 9.1.

TABLE 9.1 The inclusion criteria that we recommend for azoospermia factor testing in various ethnic groups are set in five groups.

Patient group of the medical condition	Minimum number of samples
Patients showing chromosomal abnormalities and azoospermia	Five representative samples of the group
Patients showing azoospermia	Five representative samples of the group
Patients showing mild oligospermia (10–15 million sperm/mL)	Five representative samples of the group
Patients showing moderate oligospermia (10–15 million sperm/mL)	Five representative samples of the group
Patients showing severe oligospermia (10–15 million sperm/mL)	Five representative samples of the group
Control (fertile males)	Five control samples after medical check

9.7.6 Commercial kits available in the market to be used

The most accurate commercial kits available for testing the AZF were optimized to verify the accuracy and to ensure that the most proper kit was used in this study; these are:

9.7.6.1 Promega kit for DNA extraction from blood samples

According to manufacturer protocol to extract DNA, we added appropriate volume of cell lysis solution in respect to blood sample size, then incubated for 10 min and centrifuged. We then discarded the supernatant, vortexed the pellet and then added appropriate volume of nuclei lysis solution. Then we added protein precipitation solution, centrifuged, and transferred the supernatant to a new tube containing appropriate amount of isopropanol. We then centrifuged, discarded the supernatant, and added ethanol and centrifuged again. Finally, we aspirated ethanol, airdried the pellet, and rehydrated DNA.

9.7.6.2 Devyser azoospermia factor 2 for azoospermia factor microdeletion detection

This molecular diagnostic application consisted of two kits Devyser AZF v2 and Devyser AZF Extension kits relying on PCR amplification of STS in the AZFa, AZFb, AZFc regions of the Y chromosome. Deletion was detected through absence of PCR amplification of an STS marker, whereas successful amplification indicates presence. The kit includes all of the STS markers, and control sequences recommended by the EAA and the EMQN for basic and extended molecular diagnosis of Y chromosome microdeletions in the AZFa, AZFb, and AZFc regions are included in the kit. Devyser kit makes microdeletion analysis easier since it requires only one tube per sample without the need of sample splitting and at the same time detects all markers needed for basic and extended AZF deletion screening. Devyser AZF can also perform automatic identification of STS markers, so no subjective data interpretation is required (Fig. 9.2).

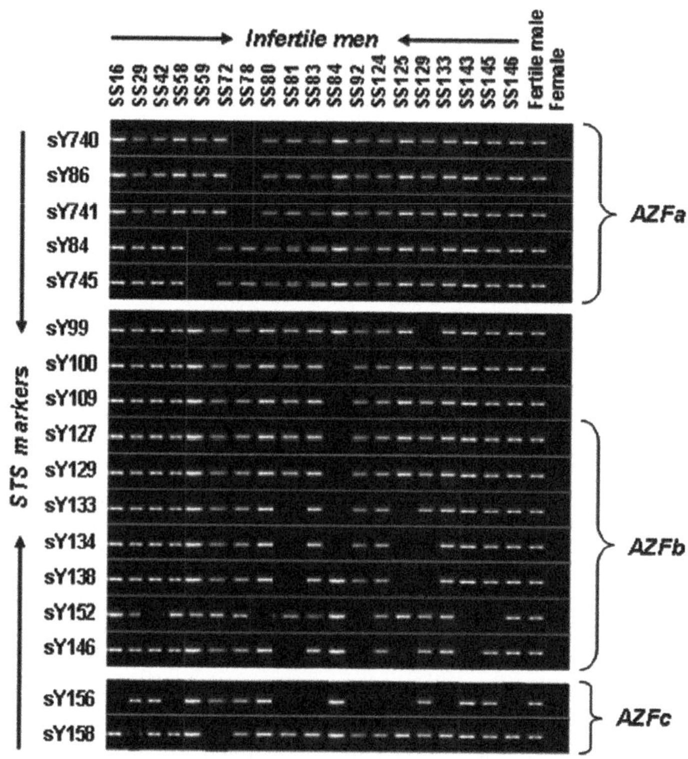

FIGURE 9.2 Promega results as in the kit protocol of the azoospermia factor diagnosis using the master mix multiplex polymerase chain reaction gel run in single electrophoresis try. Lanes 1–4 show the amplification products from reactions using multiplex master mix A with male DNA (lanes 1 and 2), female DNA (lane 3), and no DNA (lane 4). Lanes 5–8 show the amplification products from reactions using multiplex master mix B with male DNA (lanes 5 and 6), female DNA (lane 7), and no DNA (lane 8). Lanes 9–12 show the amplification products from reactions using multiplex master mix C with male DNA (lanes 9 and 10), female DNA (lane 11), and no DNA (lane 12). Lanes 13–16 show the amplification products from reactions using multiplex master mix D with male DNA (lanes 13 and 14), female DNA (lane 15), and no DNA (lane 16). Markers (M) are the 50 base pair DNA step ladder. The gel is 4% NuSieve 3:1 agarose. *Figure source: https://www.promega.com.*

9.8 Influence of the use of in vitro fertilization technology

Although the risk of genetic abnormality transmission is increased by the technique of assisted reproductive techniques such as ICSI and testicular sperm extraction, genetic counseling for AZF microdeletion is of importance to be performed prior to any of the listed techniques (Check, 2007). Moreover, the literature on male infertility factor still has several gaps and limited knowledge where some studies reveal the high prevalence risk of chromosomal disorders, especially in populations with consanguineous marriages due to ethnic or tribal concerns (Brugh & Lipshultz, 2004; Poongothai et al., 2009; Abu-Elmagd et al., 2015; Baschat et al., 1996). The high incidence of young age consanguinity initiates the frequency of both known and novel homozygous recessive disorders that would have adverse effects on some reproductive and developmental health parameters, therefore leading to infertility-related disorders (Baschat et al., 1996; Brugh & Lipshultz, 2004; Tadmouri et al., 2009) (Figs. 9.3 and 9.4).

9.9 Gene therapy application of azoospermia factor gene in different genealogical lineages of the Y-chromosome

The gene therapy technology provides the alternative pioneering future platform for infertility treatment. There must be further research on various

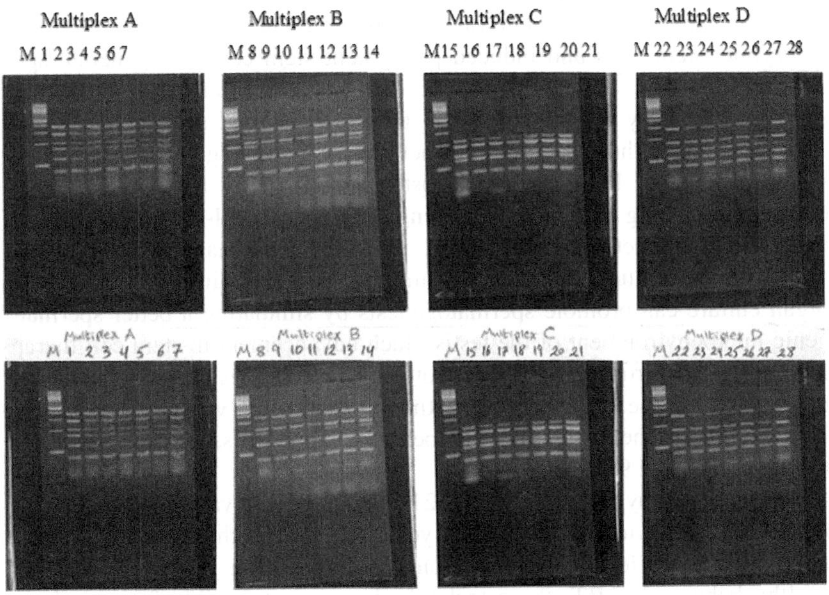

FIGURE 9.3 Our results of the azoospermia factor diagnosis using the master mix multiplex polymerase chain reaction gel run in multiple electrophoresis try.

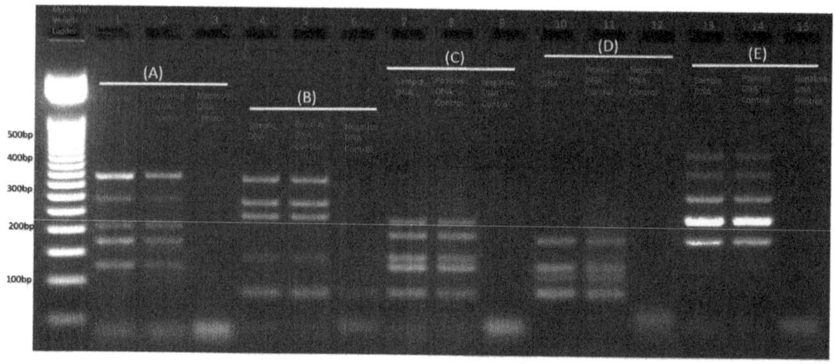

FIGURE 9.4 Our results of the azoospermia factor (AZF) diagnosis using the master mix multiplex polymerase chain reaction (PCR) gel run in one single electrophoresis try. Five multiplex PCR amplification on 3% agarose gel using the following STS markers (SY14, SY81, SY86, SY84, SY182, SY121, SYPR3, SY124, SY127, SY128, SY130, SY133, SY134, SY145, SY152, SY242, SY208, SY254, SY255, and SY157). The presence of electrophoretic bands determines the amplification of AZFa, AZFb, and AZFc intervals indicating no Deletion in AZFa, AZFb, and AZFc regions.

approaches for gene therapy of the human male infertility. Such approaches must be explored using the available technology including viral vector, IVF, human artificial chromosome (HAC), and stem cell technology. The stem cell therapy for NOA has been already explored with highly promising future. Despite the ethical constraints and the risk of tumorigenesis, stem cells are capable of self-renewal and multidirectional differentiation, and embryonic stem cells and induced pluripotent stem cells can generate spermatozoa through differentiation. Several successful attempts have been explored by many researchers using the mesenchymal stem cells promote spermatogenesis through paracrine activity, and Leydig stem cells act on sperm production by secreting testosterone (Abbas et al., 2020; Agarwal et al., 2020; Deng & Liu, 2020; Deng et al., 2019; El-Toukhy, 2019; Liu et al., 2020; Qian et al., 2020; Sara et al., 2018; Zhankina et al., 2021). Two-dimensional coculture of multiple stem cells and three-dimensional testicular organ culture can promote spermatogenesis by simulating a better spermatogenic microenvironment of the testis. Such advancement in stem cell therapy for application prospects will promote relevant studies and application. In the near future, the gene therapy treatment of infertility will have tremendous implications for the health and well-being of individuals, families, and societies (Figs. 9.5 and 9.6).

As indicated by Thoma et al. (2021), the cryopreservation technology has been used worldwide for the last 50 years to maintain the mature sperm as a method for male fertility preservation and for enabling the conception of a healthy baby with ART; these technologies are not feasible for prepubertal boys and men with spermatogenic failure.

Multiplex A Master Mix				Samples (+/-)						
STS	Locus	Product Size (bp)	Map Position							
SY254	*DAZ*	380	18							
SY157	DYS240	290	20							
SY81	DYS271	209	2							
SY130	DYS221	173	11							
SY182	*KAL-Y*	125	5							
	SMCX	83	Control							

Multiplex B Master Mix				Samples (+/-)						
STS	Locus	Product Size (bp)	Map Position							
SYPR3	*SMCY*	362	7							
SY127	DYS218	274	9							
SY242	*DAZ*	233	16							
SY208	*DAZ*	140	17							
	SMCX	83	Control							

Multiplex C Master Mix				Samples (+/-)						
STS	Locus	Product Size (bp)	Map Position							
SY128	DYS219	228	10							
SY121	DYS212	190	6							
SY145	DYF51S1	143	14							
SY255	*DAZ*	124	19							
	SMCX	83	Control							

Multiplex D Master Mix				Samples (+/-)						
STS	Locus	Product Size (bp)	Map Position							
SY133	DYS223	177	12							
SY152	DYS236	125	15							
SY124	DYS215	109	8							
	SMCX	83	Control							

Multiplex E Master Mix				Samples (+/-)						
STS	Locus	Product Size (bp)	Map Position							
	ZFX/ZFY	496	Control							
SY14	*SRY*	400	1							
SY134	DYS224	303	13							
SY86	DYS148	232	3							
SY84	DYS273	177	4							

FIGURE 9.5 Polymerase chain reaction amplification product profile for test samples. The presence (+) or absence (−) of the PCR amplification products for each sample was recorded. *Figure source: https://www.promega.com.*

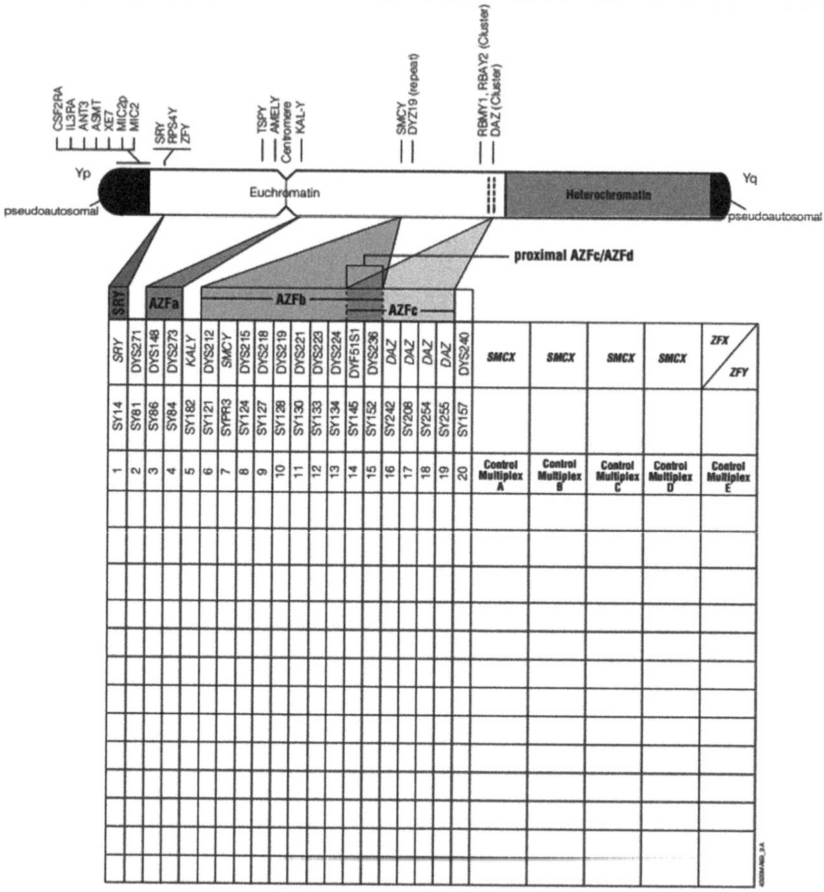

FIGURE 9.6 Y Chromosome Map Worksheet. For more detailed information, see supplemental fig. 9.2 of reference 8. Palindromes 8, 7, 6, 5, and 4 map in the proximal direction of SY121 and in the distal direction of SY182 (1). SY121 is located at the distal boundary of P4 (8). AZFb extends from P5 to proximal P1 (8). AZFc includes P1 and P2 (8). At least one copy of SY157 maps outside the AZFc boundary. Note: A positive SY133 signal has been observed in some individuals with confirmed AZFb deletion, suggesting that the SY133 locus may be present elsewhere in the chromosome for those individuals. *Figure source: https://www.promega.com.*

One of the pioneering approaches tested by Qain et al. is the transplantation of mesenchymal stem cells has exhibited successful therapeutic benefits in restoring spermatogenesis via gonadal graft angiogenesis, transplanted cell clonogenesis, and disordered somatic compartment recovery. This study aimed to elucidate the fertility protective effects and the underlying mechanisms of human amnion mesenchymal stem cells (hAMSCs) against busulfan-induced testis toxicity. This spiritual journey can involve delays and uncertainty related to childbearing; complicated health conditions and diagnoses;

and mental, physical, financial, and emotional strains related to the experience of infertility and its care and treatment.

Another important factor we have to consider for any further development and progress in gene therapy of infertility are the data collection considerations, that is, where and how we collect reproductive health data, which also impact our understanding and future perspective. Therefore survey data can provide an important complementary source of information for monitoring infertility globally and on any national level.

Recently, there has been a worldwide growing interest on gene therapy as the most sustainable therapeutic approach for cancers as well as genetic diseases. Currently, the research outcomes, using the latest technology such as next-generation sequencing and biochip microarray, have shown conclusively that the epidemiology of cancers is correlated to the genealogy and ethnicity of the population clusters around the world. Therefore, the genealogical profiling of the infertility of AZF azoospermia and cancers will be a vital and valuable tool to enhance the diagnosis, therapy, and thus the overall managements of the familial infertility and cancer disease in the region. The genealogical lifestyle of Arabs is the driving force for the high consanguinity, which continues to cause the high prevalence of genetic diseases.

We have conducted a genealogical genetic mapping of 2000 samples of Y chromosome of the Arabian populations using the STR DNA analysis. The results have been registered and deposited in the International DNA Gene Bank of Y-Chromosome Haplotype Reference Database (YHRD), University of Medicine in Berlin, Germany, YA003523 (http://www.yhrd.org).

Our results on the most common clads and subclads of the genealogical haplogroups and haplotypes show that the homogeneity of the Arabian genetic pool is a conserved one and thus the gene-flow is limited (when present). These results have been correlated to the online analysis of the WHO data (http://www.who.int) for Arabian populations. The statistics outcomes show the five most common cancers for male (bladder, prostate, colorectum, non-Hodgkin lymphoma, and lung) and women (breast, thyroid, cervix uteri, ovary, and corpus uteri), and the same order applies for the UAE. This represents a marked contrast as compared to United States where the five most common cancers for men (prostate, lung, colorectal, bladder, and skin) and for women (breast, ovary, pancreas, lung, and colon) show a different profile.

As expected, these cancer incidences will continue to increase among Arabian populations and thus double during the next few decades, leading to doubling the treatment expenses from \$50 billion now to \$100 billion in the future. Therefore the most vital, plausible, and sustainable solution is to focus our research efforts to determine the single-nucleotide polymorphism haplotypes variants of five top cancers and thus establish the gene therapy platform as a strategic therapeutic approach for UAE population, which could be then adopted by other Arabian populations. The importance of these data on the prevalence of genealogical cancers and the future gene therapy are discussed herein.

More recently, we have reported the genealogical genetic map of the Y chromosome and the genography of Arabian population (Mahasneh et al., 2021). The genealogical lifestyle of Arabs (0.5 billion) is the driving force for the high consanguinity, which continue to cause a high prevalence of genetic diseases including various types of cancers. The online analysis of the WHO data (http://www.who.int) shows conclusively that cancer, as all other genetic diseases, is correlated to the genealogical background and thus varies according to the ethnicity of population worldwide.

In conclusion, our long-standing research on the AZF gene cluster and the microsatellite STRs as correlated with prostate cancer and the haplogroups and haplotypes of Y chromosome support the theme that infertility is correlated to the male genealogical lineage and that the gene therapy technology provides the alternative pioneering platform for infertility treatment. There must be further research on various approaches for gene therapy of the human male infertility. The national programs for genealogical profiling of AZF will be a vital and valuable tool to promote our understanding the infertility complexity with the prostate cancer and haplogroups of genealogical lineages worldwide to enhance the health awareness of human societies and ultimately to facilitate gene therapy practices and thus the overall management of the familial cancer disease in the region.

References

Abbas, A. M., Hussein, R. S., Elsenity, M. A., Samaha, I. I., El Etriby, K. A., & Abd El-Ghany, Khodry, M. M. (2020). Higher clinical pregnancy rate with in-vitro fertilization vs intracytoplasmic sperm injection in treatment of non-male factor infertility: Systematic review and meta-analysis. *Journal of Gynecology Obstetrics and Human Reproduction*, *49*(6), Article 101706.

Abu-Elmagd, M., Assidi, M., Schulten, H. J., Dallol, A., Pushparaj, P., Ahmed, F., Scherer, S. W., & Al-Qahtani, M. (2015). Individualized medicine enabled by genomics in Saudi Arabia. *BMC Medical Genomics*, *8*(Suppl 1), S3. Available from https://doi.org/10.1186/1755-8794-8-S1-S3.

Agarwal, S., Agarwal, A., Khanna, A., & Singh, K. (2015). Microdeletion of Y chromosome as a cause of recurrent pregnancy loss. *Journal of Human Reproductive Sciences*, *8*(3), 159–164. Available from https://doi.org/10.4103/0974-1208.165145.

Agarwal, A., Majzoub, A., Parekh, N., & Henkel, R. (2020). A schematic overview of the current status of male infertility practice. *The World Journal of Men's Health*, *38*(3), 308–322.

AlGazali, L. I., Bener, A., Abdulrazzaq, Y. M., Micallef, R., al-Khayat, A. I., & Gaber, T. (1997). Consanguineous marriages in the United Arab Emirates. *Journal of Biosocial Science*, *29*, 491–497. Available from https://doi.org/10.1017/S0021932097004914.

Alkhalaf, M., & Al-Shoumer, K. (2010). Cytogenetic abnormalities and azoospermia factor (AZF) microdeletions in infertile men from Kuwait. *Journal of Molecular and Genetic*

Medicine: An International Journal of Biomedical Research, *4*, 232–234. Available from https://doi.org/10.4172/1747-0862.1000040.

Arafa, M. M., Majzoub, A., AlSaid, S. S., El Ansari, W., Al Ansari, A., Elbardisi, Y., & Elbardisi, H. T. (2017). Chromosomal abnormalities in infertile men with azoospermia and severe oligozoospermia in Qatar and their association with sperm retrieval intracytoplasmic sperm injection outcomes. *Arab Journal of Urology*, *16*(1), 132–139. Available from https://doi.org/10.1016/j.aju.2017.11.009.

Baschat, A. A., Küpker, W., Al Hasani, S., Diedrich, K., & Schwinger, E. (1996). Results of cytogenetic analysis in men with severe subfertility prior to intracytoplasmic sperm injection. *Human Reproduction (Oxford, England)*, *11*(2), 330–333. Available from https://doi.org/10.1093/humrep/11.2.330.

Ben-Halim, N., Ben Alaya Bouafif, N., Romdhane, L., Kefi Ben Atig, R., Chouchane, I., Bouyacoub, Y., Arfa, I., Cherif, W., Nouira, S., Talmoudi, F., Lasram, K., Hsouna, S., Ghazouani, W., Azaiez, H., El Matri, L., Abid, A., Tebib, N., Ben Dridi, M. F., Kachboura, S., Amouri, A., & Abdelhak, S. (2013). Consanguinity, endogamy, and genetic disorders in Tunisia. *Journal of Community Genetics*, *4*(2), 273–284. Available from https://doi.org/10.1007/s12687-012-0128-7.

Bonde, J. P. (2013). Occupational causes of male infertility. *Current Opinion in Endocrinology, Diabetes, and Obesity*, *20*(3), 234–239. Available from https://doi.org/10.1097/MED.0b013e32835f3d4b.

Brugh, V. M., 3rd, & Lipshultz, L. I. (2004). Male factor infertility: Evaluation and management. *The Medical Clinics of North America*, *88*(2), 367–385. Available from https://doi.org/10.1016/S0025-7125(03)00150-0.

Ceylan, G. G., Ceylan, C., & Elyas, H. (2009). Genetic anomalies in patients with severe oligozoospermia and azoospermia in eastern Turkey: A prospective study. *Genetics and Molecular Research: GMR*, *8*(3), 915–922. Available from https://doi.org/10.4238/vol8-3gmr616.

Check, J. H. (2007). Treatment of male infertility. *Clinical and Experimental Obstetrics & Gynecology*, *2007*(34), 201–206.

Cocuzza, M., Alvarenga, C., & Pagani, R. (2013). The epidemiology and etiology of azoospermia. *Clinics (Sao Paulo, Brazil)*, *68*(S1), 15–26. Available from https://doi.org/10.6061/clinics/2013(Sup01).

Cooper T.G., Noonan E., von Eckardstein S. et al. editor. 2010. WHO laboratory manual for the examination and processing of human semen. 5th ed. World Health Organization.

Cooper, T. G., Noonan, E., von Eckardstein, S., Auger, J., Baker, H. W., Behre, H. M., Haugen, T. B., Kruger, T., Wang, C., Mbizvo, M. T., & Vogelsong, K. M. (2010). World health organization reference values for human semen characteristics. *Human Reproduction Update*, *16*(3), 231–245. Available from https://doi.org/10.1093/humupd/dmp048.

Deng, C., Xie, Y., Zhang, C., Ouyang, B., Chen, H., Lv, L., Yao, J., Liang, X., Zhang, Y., Sun, X., Deng, C., & Liu, G. (2019). Urine-derived stem cells facilitate endogenous spermatogenesis restoration of busulfan-induced nonobstructive azoospermic mice by paracrine exosomes. *Stem Cells and Development*, *28*(19), 1322–1333. Available from https://doi.org/10.1089/scd.2019.0026.

Deng, C. C., & Liu, G. H. (2020). Stem cell therapy for non-obstructive azoospermia. *National Journal of Andrology*, *26*(4), 351–356.

El-Toukhy, T. (2019). Reproductive medicine in 2020 and beyond. *BJOG: An International Journal of Obstetrics and Gynaecology*, *126*(2), 133–134.

Ferlin, A., Arredi, B., Speltra, E., et al. (2007). Molecular and clinical characterization of Y chromosome microdeletions in infertile men: A 10-year experience in Italy. *The Journal of Clinical Endocrinology and Metabolism, 2007*(92), 762–770.

Foresta, C., Ferlin, A., & Moro, E. (2000). Deletion and expression analysis of AZFa genes on the human Y chromosome revealed a major role for DBY in male infertility. *Human Molecular Genetics, 2000*(9), 1161–1169.

Fortesa, C., Moro, E., & Ferlin, A. (2001). Y chromosome microdeletions and alterations of spermatogenesis. *Endocrine Reviews, 22*(2), 226–239.

Fu, L., Xiong, D. K., Ding, X. P., et al. (2012). Genetic screening for chromosomal abnormalities and Y chromosome microdeletions in Chinese infertile men. *Journal of Assisted Reproduction and Genetics, 2012*(29), 521–527.

Ghorbel, M., Gargouri Baklouti, S., Ben Abdallah, F., et al. (2012). Chromosomal defects in infertile men with poor semen quality. *Journal of Assisted Reproduction and Genetics, 29*(5), 451–456.

Gueler, B., Sonne, S. B., Zimmer, J., et al. (2012). AZFa protein DDX3Y is differentially expressed in human male germ cells during development and in testicular tumours: New evidence for phenotypic plasticity of germ cells. *Human Reproduction (Oxford, England), 27*, 1547–1555.

Hamada, A. J., Esteves, S. C., & Agarwal, A. (2013). A comprehensive review of genetics and genetic testing in azoospermia. *Clinics (Sao Paulo), 68*(Suppl 1), 39–60.

Hellani, A., Al-Hassan, S., Iqbal, M. A., & Coskun, S. (2006). Y chromosome microdeletions in infertile men with idiopathic oligo- or azoospermia. *Journal of Experimental & Clinical Assisted Reproduction, 3*, 1.

Hopps, C. V., Mielnik, A., Goldstein, M., et al. (2003). Detection of sperm in men with Y chromosome microdeletions of the AZFa, AZFb and AZFc regions. *Human Reproduction (Oxford, England), 18*, 1660–1665.

Hotaling, J., & Carrell, D. T. (2014). Clinical genetic testing for male factor infertility: Current applications and future directions. *Andrology, 2*(3), 339–350. Available from https://doi.org/10.1111/j.2047-2927.2014.00200.x.

Inhorn, M. C., Kobeissi, L., Nassar, Z., Lakkis, D., & Fakih, M. H. (2009). Consanguinity and family clustering of male factor infertility in Lebanon. *Fertility and Sterility, 91*, 1104–1109. Available from https://doi.org/10.1016/j.fertnstert.2008.01.008.

Inhorn, M. C., & Patrizio, P. (2015). Infertility around the globe: New thinking on gender, reproductive technologies and global movements in the 21st century. *Human Reproduction Update, 21*(4), 411–426.

Jarow, J. P., Troiani, J., McNellis, D., Wiederhorn, R., Fang, G., & Handelsman, H. (2013). Use of biomarkers to assess tissue specific androgen adequacy: Defining male hypogonadism. *The Journal of Urology, 189*, 633–637.

Jégou, B., & Skinner, M. K. (2018). Male reproduction. In K. Skinner Michael (Ed.), *Encyclopedia of reproduction* (2nd ed.). Pullman, WA: Center for Reproductive Biology, School of Biological Sciences, Washington State University, ISBN: 978-0-12-815145-7.

Khabour, O. F., Fararjeh, A. S., & Alfaouri, A. A. (2014). Genetic screening for AZF Y chromosome microdeletions in Jordanian azoospermic infertile men. *International Journal of Molecular Epidemiology and Genetics, 5*(1), 47–50.

Kleiman, S. E., Yogev, L., Lehavi, O., et al. (2011). The likelihood of finding mature sperm cells in men with AZFb or AZFb-c deletions: Six new cases and a review of the literature (1994–2010). *Fertility and Sterility, 95*, 2005–2012.

Krausz, C., & Forti, G. (2006). Sperm cryopreservation in male infertility due to genetic disorders. *Cell and Tissue Banking*, *7*, 105–112.

Krausz, C., Hoefsloot, L., Simoni, M., & Tüttelmann, F.European Academy of Andrology, & European Molecular Genetics Quality Network. (2014). EAA/EMQN best practice guidelines for molecular diagnosis of Y-chromosomal microdeletions: State-of-the-art 2013. *Andrology*, *2*(1), 5–19. Available from https://doi.org/10.1111/j.2047-2927.2013.00173.x.

Kumar, N., & Singh, A. (2015). Trends of male factor infertility, an important cause of infertility: A review of literature. *Journal of Human Reproductive Sciences*, *8*(4), 191. Available from https://doi.org/10.4103/0974-1208.170370.

Kuroda-Kawaguchi, K., Skaletsky, H., Brown, L. G., Minx, P. J., Cordum, H. S., Waterston, R. H., Wilson, R. K., Silber, S., Oates, R., Rozen, S., & Page, D. C. (2001). The AZFc region of the Y chromosome features massive palindromes and uniform recurrent deletions in infertile men. *Nature Genetics*, *29*(3), 279–286. Available from https://doi.org/10.1038/ng757.

Lahn, B. T., Pearson, N. M., & Jegalian, K. (2001). The human Y chromosome, in the light of evolution. *Nature Reviews. Genetics*, *2*, 207–216.

Lahn, B. T., & Page, D. C. (1997). Functional coherence of the human Y chromosome. *Sceince*, *278*(5338), 675–680. Available from https://doi.org/10.1126/science.278.5338.675.

Liu, H. C., Xie, Y., Deng, C. H., & Liu, G. H. (2020). Stem cell-based therapies for fertility preservation in males: Current status and future prospects. *World J Stem Cells*, *12*(10), 1097–1112. Available from https://doi.org/10.4252/wjsc.v12.i10.1097.

Liu, X. Y., Wang, R. X., Fu, Y., et al. (2017). Outcomes of intracytoplasmic sperm injection in oligozoospermic men with Y chromosome AZFb or AZFc microdeletions. *Andrologia*, *49*, 12602–12607.

Liu, X. G., Hu, H. Y., Guo, Y. H., & Sun, Y. P. (2016). Correlation between Y chromosome microdeletion and male infertility. *Genetics and Molecular Research: GMR*, *15*(2). Available from https://doi.org/10.4238/gmr.15028426, 10.4238/gmr.15028426.

Mahasneh, I. (2016). Will molecular biology reshape our near future on 2050 & beyond as we are picking up the needle from the straw? *International Journal of Molecular Biology Open Access*, *1*(1), 1–2. Available from http://medcraveonline.com/openacess.

Mahasneh, I. (2018). Genetic profiling of the 5-top cancers prevalence among Arabian populations in relation to their genealogical landscape as a cause to establish gene therapy platform in the region. *International Journal of Molecular Biology Open Access*, *3*(2), 54–56. Available from http://medcraveonline.com/openacess.

Mahasneh I., Zuriegat Q.H. (2020). Genetic profiling of the short tandem repeats (STRs) of Y-chromosome of populations of South Jordan. Journal of Forensic Medicine; 4(1), 1-16. <http://www.hilarispublisher.com>.

Mahasneh, I., Abumsimir, B., & Ennaji, M. M. (2018). DNA sequencing and genotyping profile of the microsatellites of Y-STRs of the Beer-Alsabaa Bedouins of Jordan as part of the Arabian genome project. *International Journal of Molecular Biology Open Access*, *3*(3), 149–152. Available from http://medcraveonline.com/openacess.

Mahasneh, I., Moulay Mustapha Ennaji, B., & Abumsimir, Y. K. (2021). Presence of G84E allelic heterogeneity of the European prostate cancer SNP mutation of HOX13B-G84E associated with the European R-haplogroup of Y-chromosome and absence of gene flow into moroccans patients. *Journal of Biosciences and Medicine*, *9*(5), 50–61. Available from https://doi.org/10.4236/jbm.2021.95006, https://www.scirp.org/journal/jbm.

Mirfakhraie, R., Kalantar, S. M., Mirzajani, F., et al. (2011). A novel mutation in the transactivation-regulating domain of the androgen receptor in a patient with azoospermia. *Journal of Andrology*, *32*, 367–370.

Naasse, Y., Charoute, H., El Houate, B., et al. (2010). Chromosomal abnormalities and Y chromosome microdeletions in infertile men from Morocco. *BMC Urology*, *15*, 95.

Navarro-Costa, P., Plancha, C. E., & Goncalves, J. (2010). Genetic dissection of the AZF regions of the human Y chromosome: Thriller or filler for male (in) fertility? *Journal of Biomedicine & Biotechnology*, *2010*, 936569.

O'Flynn O'Brien, K. L., Varghese, A. C., & Agarwal, A. (2010). The genetic causes of male factor infertility: A review. *Fertility and Sterility*, *93*, 1–12.

Padubidri, V. G., & Daftary, S. (2014). In V. G. Padubidri Shirish Daftary (Ed.), *Shaw's textbook of gynecology* (16th ed., p. 596). India: Elsevier, eBook ISBN: 9788131238721, Paperback ISBN: 9788131236727.

Poongothai, J., Gopenath, T. S., & Manonayaki, S. (2009). Genetics of human male infertility. *Singapore Medical Journal*, *50*, 336–347.

Qian, C., Meng, Q., Lu, J., Zhang, L., Li, H., & Huang, B. (2020). Human amnion mesenchymal stem cells restore spermatogenesis in mice with busulfan-induced testis toxicity by inhibiting apoptosis and oxidative stress. *Stem Cell Researc & Therapy*, *11*(1), 290.

Quintana-Murci, L., & Fellous, M. (2001). The human Y chromosome: The biological role of a "functional wasteland". *Journal of Biomedicine & Biotechnology*, *1*(1), 18–24. Available from https://doi.org/10.1155/S1110724301000080.

Rabinowitz, M. J., Huffman, P. J., Haney, N., & Kohn, T. P. (2021). Y-chromosome microdeletions: A review of prevalence, screening, and clinical considerations. *The Application of Clinical Genetics*, *2021*(14), 51–59.

Rozen, S., Skaletsky, H., Janet, D., Marszalek., Patrick, J. M., et al. (2003). Abundant gene conversion between arms of palindromes in human and ape Y chromosomes. *Nature*, *423*, 873–876.

Rutstein S.O., Shah I.H. 2004. Infecundity, Infertility, and Childlessness in Developing Countries: Demographic and Health Surveys (DHS) Comparative reports No. 9. ORC Macro and the World Health Organization, Calverton, MD.

Sara, C. V., Sabanegh, E., & Ashok Agarwal, A. (2018). Biological therapy for non-obstructive azoospermia. *Expert Opinion on Biological Therapy*, *18*(1), 19–23. Available from https://doi.org/10.1080/14712598.2018.1380622.

Shafae, M. M. E., Sabry, J. H., Behiry, E. G., Sabry, H. H., Salim, M. A., & Fayez, A. G. (2018). Independent of DAZL-T54A variant and AZF microdeletion in a sample of Egyptian patients with idiopathic non-obstructed azoospermia. *The Application of Clinical Genetics*, *2018*(11), 81–87.

Skaletsky, H., Kuroda-Kawaguchi, T., Minx, P. J., et al. (2003). The male-specific region of the human Y chromosome is a mosaic of discrete sequence classes. *Nature*, *423*, 825–837.

Soares, A. R., Costa, P., Silva, J., et al. (2012). AZFb microdeletions and oligozoospermia – Which mechanisms? *Fertility and Sterility*, *97*, 858–863.

Song, S. H., Chiba, K., Ramasamy, R., et al. (2016). Recent advances in the genetics of testicular failure. *Asian Journal of Andrology*, *18*, 350–355.

Sun, C., Skaletsky, H., Rozen, S., Gromoll, J., Nieschlag, E., Oates, R., & Page, D. C. (2000). Deletion of azoospermia factor a (AZFa) region of human Y chromosome caused by recombination between HERV15 proviruses. *Human Molecular Genetics*, *9*(15), 2291–2296. Available from https://doi.org/10.1093/oxfordjournals.hmg.a018920.

Tadmouri, G. O., Nair, P., Obeid, T., Al Ali, M. T., Al Khaja, N., & Hamamy, H. A. (2009). Consanguinity and reproductive health among Arabs. *Reproductive Health*, *6*, 17.

Thoma, M., Fledderjohann, J., Cox, C., & Adageba, R. K. (2021). Biological and social aspects of human infertility: A global perspective. *Global Public Health*. Available from https://doi.org/10.1093/acrefore/9780190632366.013.184.

Vogt, P. H. (2005). AZF deletions and Y chromosomal haplogroups: History and update based on sequence. *Human Reproduction Update*, *11*(4), 319–336. Available from https://doi.org/10.1093/humupd/dmi017.

Vogt, P. H., Edelmann, A., Kirsch, S., et al. (1996). Human Y chromosome azoospermia factors (AZF) mapped to different subregions in Yq11. *Human Molecular Genetics*, *5*, 933–943.

Yousefi-Razin, E., Nasiri, M. J., & Omrani, M. D. (2016). Frequency of Y chromosome microdeletions among Iranian infertile men with azoospermia and severe oligozoospermia: A meta-analysis. *Journal of Reproduction & Infertility*, *17*, 208–212.

Yu, X. W., Wei, Z. T., Jiang, Y. T., & Zhang, S. L. (2015). Y chromosome azoospermia factor region microdeletions and transmission characteristics in azoospermic and severe oligozoospermic patients. *International Journal of Clinical and Experimental Medicine*, *8*(9), 14634–14646.

Zhankina, R., Baghban, N., Askarov, M., Saipiyeva, D., Ibragimov, A., Kadirova, B., Khoradmehr, A., Nabipour, I., Shirazi, R., Zhanbyrbekuly, U., & Tamadon, A. (2021). Mesenchymal stromal/stem cells and their exosomes for restoration of spermatogenesis in non-obstructive azoospermia: A systemic review. *Stem Cell Res Therapy*, *12*(1), 229. Available from https://doi.org/10.1186/s13287-021-02295-9. Available from 33823925.

Zhu, X. B., Gong, Y. H., He, J., et al. (2017). Multicentre study of Y chromosome microdeletions in 1,808 Chinese infertile males using multiplex and real-time polymerase chain reaction. *Andrologia*, *49*, 12726–12732.

Chapter 10

Recent advances in high-risk human papillomavirus genotype relationship with bladder cancer tumor genesis

Said Abdallah Nabil[2], Berjas Abumsimir[2,3], Yassine Kasmi[2], Mohammed Mrabti[5], Abdelilah Laraqui[4] and Moulay Mustapha Ennaji[1]

[1]Group Leader Research team of Virology, Oncology, and Biotechnologies, Head of Laboratory of Virology, Oncology, Biosciences, Environment and New Energies (LVO-BEEN), Faculty of Sciences and Techniques Mohammedia, University Hassan II of Casablanca, Casablanca, Morocco, [2]Team of Virology, Oncology, and Biotechnologies, Laboratory of Virology, Oncology, Biosciences, Environment and New Energies (LVO-BEEN), Faculty of Sciences and Techniques Mohammedia, University Hassan II of Casablanca, Casablanca, Morocco, [3]Pharmacological and Diagnostic Research Centre (PDRC), Department of Medical Laboratory Sciences, Faculty of Allied Medical Sciences, Al-Ahliyya Amman University (AAU), Amman, Jordan, [4]Laboratory of Human Pathologies Biology, Faculty of Sciences, and Genomic Center of Human Pathologies, Faculty of Medicine and Pharmacy, Bio-Path Laboratory, Faculty of sciences-Agdal, Mohammed V University, Rabat, Morocco, [5]Research and Biosafety Laboratory, Mohammed V Construction Teaching Hospital, Mohammed V University, Rabat, Morocco

10.1 Introduction

Bladder cancer is a malignant tumor that commonly develops in the bladder's urothelium. It is ranked sixth in the world in terms of incidence and 12th in terms of mortality. This disease is increasingly diagnosed around the world (Sung et al., 2021).

The growth of bladder tumors has long been associated with exposure to a certain abiotic environmental factor, namely, aniline. In 1985, Dr. Ludwig Rehn hypothesized that the etiological factor involved in the development of bladder tumors in workers of the aniline dye industry in Germany is aniline (Dietrich & Dietrich, 2001). Although the role of aniline is still being discussed in the occurrence of bladder tumor, other environmental etiological factors are already

Immunological Implications and Molecular Diagnostics of Genitourinary Cancer.
DOI: https://doi.org/10.1016/B978-0-323-85496-2.00016-6

established, such as exposure to aromatic amines, ionizing radiation, and cyclophosphamide (Abol-Enein, 2008; García-Pérez et al., 2009; Ho et al., 2015).

Beyond the abiotic factors, the infection by pathogens such as parasitic agents (*Schistosoma*), bacterial agents, and other viruses is also associated with the development of bladder cancers. Among the viruses, high-risk human papillomavirus (HR-HPV), which was first detected in 1988, is also a potential bladder carcinogen (Kitamura et al., 1988). Indeed, the HR-HPV is linked to more than 10% of cancers worldwide, especially in the anogenital region, where their involvement is already proven. However, in the case of bladder cancer, studies concerning the molecular association between the presence of HR-HPV and the occurrence of bladder cancer, the invasiveness of the process and/or its recurrence are, on the other hand, contradictory and highly controversial, despite the detection of its oncogenic E6 and E7 viral mRNAs and proteins in bladder tumor tissues (Volgareva et al., 2009).

This chapter aims to provide an overview of the prevalence of HR-HPV and its potential molecular link in bladder tumorigenesis.

10.2 Human papillomaviruses

HPVs are a large family of small, nonenveloped viruses with a capsid having icosahedral symmetry. Currently 118 genotypes have been identified, of which 35 infect the genitourinary tract of humans (Bernard et al., 2010). The viral genome is a circular double-stranded DNA molecule made up of 8000 base pairs divided into three regions, as can be seen in Fig. 10.1 (Bernard et al., 2010).

1. The late region L (late) encodes the major proteins of the L1 and L2 capsids;
2. The long control region is a non-coding region that contains promoters for the early genes and the regulatory sequences for replication and transcription;
3. The early region E (early) comprises the genes (E1, E2, E4, E5A, E5B, E6, E7) that code for the so-called functional nonstructural proteins. They play different roles in viral DNA replication and cell transformation.

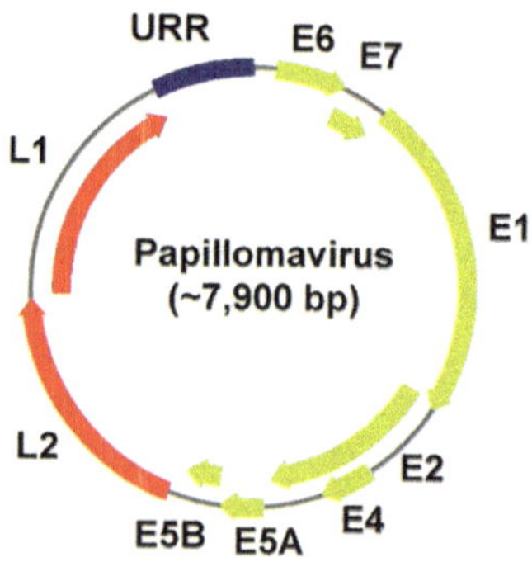

FIGURE 10.1 Genomic organization of human papillomaviruses.

In cells infected with HPV, the viral genome can exist in two forms: episomal and integrated. The episomal form results in a specific cytopathogenic effect: koilocytosis. It results from the complete replication of DNA and the viral capsid's protein synthesis (Mougin et al., 2008). While the integration of the viral genome is specific to HR-HPV, which is accompanied by a partial loss of the viral genome and the ability to replicate completely, there is no production of the virions (Mougin et al., 2008). This integration process leads to overexpression of E6 and E7 proteins, which can interfere with cell cycle regulatory proteins (Mougin et al., 2008; Shukla et al., 2014).

The product of the E7 gene binds to the pRb protein, cyclin E complexes, cyclin A complexes, the activity of cyclin complexes, histone deacetylases, as well as other proteins linked to the cell cycle (Münger et al., 2004). The direct consequence of the formation of the E7−Rb complex is the release of the E2F transcription factor complex from Rb, inducing the passage of cells into S phase and therefore maintaining replication, even if the cell does not have sufficient resources (Münger et al., 2004).

The oncoprotein E6 can interact with p53, which leads to the degradation of the complex via the ubiquitin pathway. In addition, the E6 protein also directly suppresses the transcription of p53 (Münger et al., 2004). This degradation of the p53 protein leads to a decrease in the expression of DNA repair enzymes, which leads to an increase in uncontrolled proliferation and mutation accumulation in the cells (Münger et al., 2004).

The coupling of E1 protein with the E2 protein initiates the replication of extra-chromosomal viral DNA and its transcription. The E4 protein binds to cytokeratins and promotes destruction of the cytoskeleton. It also plays an important role in virion maturation. The E3 and E8 proteins have no known role at this time. Finally, the E5, E6 and E7 proteins are involved jointly in immortalization and cell transformation processes.

10.3 Epidemiology of bladder cancer

A total of 573,278 new cases of bladder cancer have been reported in 2020, which represents more than 3% of the global cancer burden (Sung et al., 2021). The International Agency for Research on Cancer ranks this neoplasm 10th in terms of cancer incidence and third in urogenital cancer, behind uterine cancer and prostate cancer (Sung et al., 2021). The average age for the diagnosis of bladder cancer ranges from 65 to 70 years (Bray et al., 2018). The incidence rate is four times higher in men (9.6/100,000) than in women (2.4/100,000) (Sung et al., 2021). However, the incidence rate distribution is very heterogeneous across different regions of the world. The highest impact largely correlates with Southern Europe and North America, that is, the regions where the human development index is above average, probably due to higher exposure to industrial chemical carcinogens, easy access to tobacco, an aging population, and better cancer diagnosis. In addition, the incidence is also very high in the areas where *Schistosoma haematobium* is endemic, such as Egypt, the Middle East (Bray et al., 2018; Wong et al., 2018). On the other hand, the lowest rate is in Central Africa, Central America, and West Africa (Bray et al., 2018; Sung et al., 2021).

In terms of mortality, bladder cancer is the 13th leading cause of cancer death with 212,536 fatalities reported in 2020 (Sung et al., 2021). The variation in mortality between the sexes also reflects the incidence of bladder cancer. The mortality rate is also approximately four times higher in men (3.2/100,000) than in women (0.9/100,000) (Sung et al., 2021). The highest mortality rate has been reported in North and East Africa and the Middle East in part due to infection with schistosomiasis. The highest mortality is in Egypt, at 6.6/100,000. Fig. 10.2 presents data on age-standardized incidence rates by region for bladder cancer in 2020.

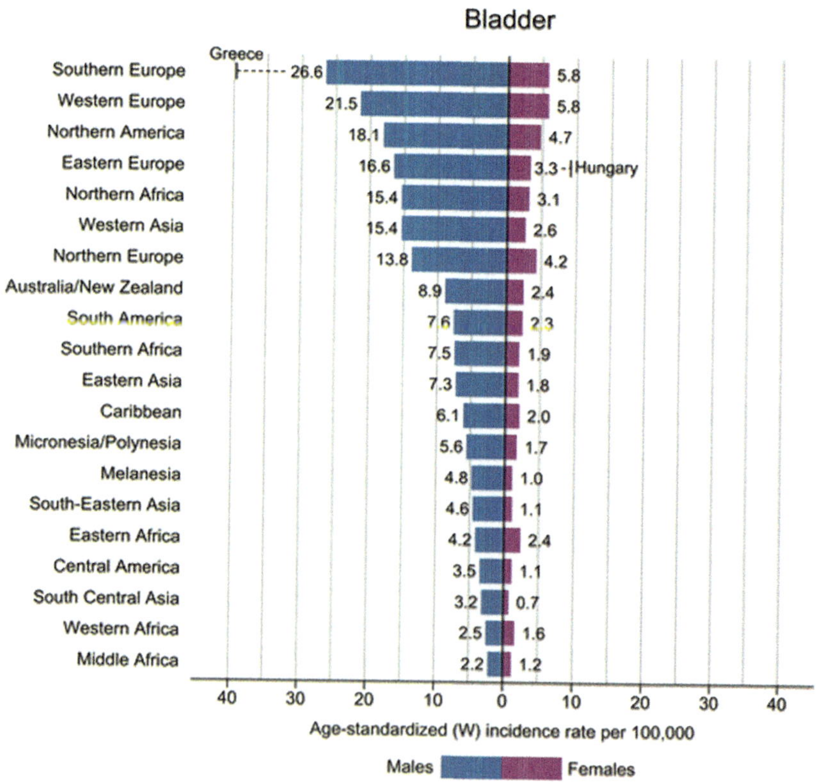

FIGURE 10.2 Age-standardized incidence rates by region for bladder cancer in 2020. *From GLOBOCAN 2020.*

10.4 Global prevalence of human papillomavirus in bladder cancer

Since the first detection by Kitamura et al. (1988) in cancerous bladder tissue, the prevalence of infection of different genotypes of HPV has been documented worldwide and ranges on average from 0% to 80% (Jimenez-Pacheco et al., 2012; Khaled et al., 2001). Furthermore, this distribution differs according to histological types, geographic location, and the detection method used. The highest distribution is observed in Asia (24.25%), followed by Africa (19.40%), North America (13.49%), and Europe (13.11%), regardless of the histological type according to recent metaanalysis (Li et al., 2011). In studies HPV-6, HPV-11, HPV-16, HPV-18, HPV-31, HPV-33, HPV-35, HPV-39, HPV-45, HPV-51, HPV-52, HPV-56, HPV-58, HPV-59, and HPV-68 are the most frequently detected genotypes (Li et al., 2011).

At the same time, in terms of distribution, oncogenic HPVs are more common in ureteral tumor cells than low-risk HPVs (Li et al., 2011). The detection of HR-HPV represents 10.8% to 36% of HPV in bladder tumor tissue, the most frequent being HPV-16,18,6,11,33. The HPV-16 type is by far the most frequent oncogenic genotype detected in the blood and tumor cells of bladder cancer patients (Li et al., 2011; Ohadian Moghadam et al., 2020).

Although HPV is usually transmitted sexually, and the incidence of bladder cancer is four times higher in men than women, the majority of current findings have not found a significant association between age/sex and HPV infection in urothelial cancer (Li et al., 2011; Shigehara et al., 2013).

10.4.1 Prevalence of high-risk human papillomavirus by histological type

10.4.1.1 Transitional cell carcinoma or urothelial carcinoma

Transitional cell carcinoma represents 90% of superficial bladder cancers that are diagnosed. It develops at the expense of the epithelium lining the bladder. This is the histological type that has been reported to have a high distribution of HR-HPV, that is, between 2% to 81.3% (Barghi et al., 2012; Shigehara et al., 2014). In terms of prevalence, the oncogenic genotypes 18, 16, 33, 31, and 51 are the most detected, particularly in low-grade than high-grade tumors.

10.4.1.2 Squamous cell carcinomas

Squamous cell carcinomas make up about 2%–5% of the total number of bladder tumors (Boyle et al., 2010). However, it is the first histological type in certain regions where bilharzia is endemic (Near East, Egypt, Sahel) (Boyle et al., 2010; Rundle et al., 1982). In these regions, the distribution of

HR-HPV in squamous cell carcinoma is generally associated with infection with bilharzia. In Egypt, HPV-18/16 DNA is found 22%–50% in the case of squamous cell carcinoma caused by bilharzia (Khaled et al., 2001). On the other hand, in nonbilharzial squamous cell carcinomas, HR-HPV is rarely detected (Collins et al., 2020).

10.4.1.3 Other histological types of bladder cancer

Regarding the other histological types, which represent only less than 5% of tumors, data relating the presence of HR- HPV are insufficient in the literature.

10.5 Recent evidence for high-risk human papillomavirus involvement in bladder cancer

10.5.1 Integration of human papillomavirus DNA

Integration of HPV DNA into the host genome is considered a critical step in the process of carcinogenesis (McBride & Warburton, 2017). This integration of HPV DNA is already formally identified as an etiological cause in cervical cancer (Vinokurova et al., 2008).

In the case of bladder cancer, sequencing identified the DNA of the HR-HPVs integrated into several genes of the cell chromosome mainly in the intergenic regions, followed by the intronic regions, upstream/downstream of the noncoding RNA–exon genes and intronic region. A large number of integration genes identified (AFAP1, RAP2A, UBE3D, P3H2, NF1P2, etc.) have only undergone an integration event on an ad hoc basis because the integration of the viral genome is carried out randomly (Yan et al., 2021). However, another site such as the tumor suppressor gene TP63 is already identified as one of the HPV hotspot genes in cervical cancer (Li et al., 2018) and related squamous cell carcinoma of the head and neck (Walline et al., 2017). This TP63 gene is also frequently integrated by HR-HPV in vulvar cancer. The integration in viral DNA in tumor suppressor genes (TP63 and BCL2L1) has the power to confer selective growth advantages to tumor cells, which leads to an increased cellular proportion of these integrations (TCGA, 2014).

10.5.2 Human papillomavirus and p16 overexpression status in bladder cancer

P16 is a regulator of the phosphorilization of the Rb gene product (retinoblastoma) in cell cycle pathways. This pRb protein allows the passage of cells in S phase and to carry out DNA replication for cell division, and inactivation of HPV by the E7 protein (Mougin et al., 2008). The formation of the pRb–E7 complex of HPVs causes a positive feedback loop with p16 leading to protein buildup without the ability to stop the cell cycle (Zhao et al., 2012). This subsequent p16 overexpression is well known to be associated with HR-HPV infection in cervical cancer, where it was considered an indirect biomarker to identify biologically active HPV infection (Alexander et al., 2014).

In bladder cancer, p16 overexpression is frequently expressed particularly in primary adenocarcinomas (Alexander et al., 2014). Recent studies have found a significant correlation between HR-HPV and p16 overexpression (Alexander et al., 2014). Overall, however, the current evidence is insufficient to classify p16 overexpression as a potent biomarker of HPV infection due to p16 overexpression that is frequently observed in a few negative HR-HPV bladder tumors (Kim et al., 2014). Thus, it remains difficult at the moment to bind this protein to any of the oncogenic activity of HR-HPV in the bladder.

10.5.3 Pathological clinical course

10.5.3.1 Passage of a guard and upper stage

Bladder tumor can have over 300 exonic mutations, over 200 segmental alterations in genomic copy number, and over 22 genomic rearrangements (TCGA, 2014). The presence of HR-HPV in tumor cells of the bladder is an additional biological factor, which may promote deeper penetration of the already existing mutation into the DNA of the infected cells. In fact, the comparison of the degree of anaplasia of the ureteral tumor cells showed that the HR-HPV-positive group has high anaplasia (G2 + G3), while the HR-HPV-negative group often has low degrees of anaplasia (G1). For example, Ohadian Moghadam et al. (2020) detected more DNA of HR-HPV in stages (T2–T4) than in lower stages (Ta-T1). In another study of Golovina and colleagues, HR-HPV viral DNA was detected in 42% of high-grade anaplasia and 8% of low-grade tumors (Golovina et al., 2016). Even if Badawi et al. (2008) and Shigehara et al. (2013) and other studies found more HR-HPV in tumor cells with weak anaplasia than in cells with stronger anaplasia, it is suggested that the oncogenic HPV seems to play an important role in the progression of tumors to more advanced stages and grades through the inactivation of tumor suppressors (p53 and pRb) and other unknown mechanisms (Badawi et al., 2008; Shigehara et al., 2013; Youshya et al., 2005).

10.5.3.2 Human papillomavirus status and bladder cancer recurrence

The HR-HPV infection is believed to be one of the biological factors for urological cancer relapse after treatment (Alibek et al., 2012). In the case of superficial urethral carcinoma, certain studies have established a direct correlation between tumor recurrence and the rate of prevalence of oncogenic HPVs, in particular HPV-16. A serological study focusing mainly on HPV-16 also showed a significant relationship between the tumor recurrence rate and the presence of anti-HPV antibodies and anti-HPV-16 antibodies (Badawi et al., 2008).

In another study, Golovina and colleagues detected HR-HPV DNA in 47% of primary tumors ($n = 71$) and 17% in recurrent tumors. They argued that HR-HPV (particularly type 16) is often involved in the genesis of bladder cancer. The HR-HPV-positive tumor cells affect the microenvironment of bladder cancer before being eliminated by the various treatments (surgery, chemotherapy, etc.). However, the already altered microenvironment acquires the ability to accelerate the emergence of new HPV-negative tumor cells from adjacent conventionally normal urothelium cells and cause recurrent bladder cancer (Golovina et al., 2014).

10.6 Detection of human papillomavirus infection in bladder cancer

Several techniques have been proposed to detect the presence of HPV infection. The gold standard for the diagnosis of HPV in tissue is polymerase chain reaction (PCR) test, which makes it possible to detect the presence of HPV and to determine its genotype in cancer. This technique is performed on frozen tissue samples or on paraffin-embedded tumor chips. This technique can readily discriminate between HPVs of high or low oncogenic risk.

HR-HPV can also be detected by the in-situ hybridization method. This method uses a probe directed specifically against a specific sequence of oncogenic HPV DNA. This technique is highly reliable and sensitive, but it is expensive and requires certain technicality.

Immunohistochemistry technique is based on the use of antibodies for protein localization. The use of anti-HPV antibodies is rare due to their low sensitivities and specificity. On the other hand, the anti-P16 antibody is frequently used, making it possible to know the distribution of expression in the tissue. The p16 protein, as described above, is more strongly expressed in HPV-positive than HPV-negative carcinoma because of the formation of the bonding of E7 with pRb, which no longer blocks the transcription of the p16 gene (Münger et al., 2004). Therefore this p16 protein is regarded as an indirect marker of HR-HPV infection (Roussel et al., 2010).

10.7 Human papillomavirus treatment and prevention

At present, there is no specific antiviral therapy to control HPV infection. However, there are already prophylactic anti-HPV vaccines administered preferentially to young girls aged 11–14 years to fight against cancer of the cervix of the uterus in many countries. At present, some countries like France and England have extended the vaccination coverage to both genders, especially before the first sexual intercourse, to prevent anogenital infections. If the etiological role of oncogenic HPVs was to be proven in tumorigenesis of the bladder, it would support the advantages of vaccination and therefore facilitate acceptance of the vaccine by men.

The design of these HPV vaccines is based on the self-assembly properties of the L1 capsid protein within eukaryotic cells (cells yeast or insect), resulting in the production of viral particles with a strong immunogenic potential but not infectious because they are without genetic material (Athanasiou et al., 2020). Three main vaccines are there on the market:

1. The Gardasil vaccine (SanofiPasteur—MSD), which is tetravalent: it was designed to protect against genotypes 6 and 11 of low oncogenic risk and genotypes 16 and 18, corresponding to the two subtypes most frequently found in carcinomatous lesions.
2. Cervarix (GSK) is bivalent, and it is effective against genotypes 16 and 18 of the HPV virus.
3. The Gardasil9 vaccine, released in 2014, protects against HPV-6, HPV-11, HPV-16, HPV-18, HPV-31, HPV-33, HPV-45, HPV-52, and HPV-58.

Clinical trials have shown 100% efficacy against vaccine-specific HPV infection and protection against precancerous lesion development (Malagón et al., 2012). However, these vaccines do not provide protection when an individual is already infected.

10.8 Conclusion

In difference to cervical cancer, the role of HR-HPV in the bladder has not been demonstrated heretofore. Research has not yet provided clear and definitive evidence of its involvement in the genesis or progression to higher grades/stages in bladder cancer because of the variation in study results probably due to the sensitivity of detection systems, geographic variation, distribution of HPV in tumor tissue, and study size. However, overall, HR- HPV infection appears to play a role in the development of a small percentage of urothelial tumors.

References

Abol-Enein, H. (2008). Infection: Is it a cause of bladder cancer? *Scandinavian Journal of Urology and Nephrology*, *42*, 79–84. Available from https://doi.org/10.1080/03008880802325309.

Alexander, R. E., Williamson, S. R., Richey, J., Lopez-Beltran, A., Montironi, R., Davidson, D. D., Idrees, M. T., Jones, C. L., Zhang, S., Wang, L., Rao, Q., Pedrosa, J. A., Kaimakliotis, H. Z., Monn, M. F., Koch, M. O., & Cheng, L. (2014). The expression patterns of p53 and p16 and an analysis of a possible role of HPV in primary adenocarcinoma of the urinary bladder. *PLoS One*, *9*, e95724. Available from https://doi.org/10.1371/journal.pone.0095724.

Alibek, K., Karatayeva, N., & Bekniyazov, I. (2012). The role of infectious agents in urogenital cancers. *Infectious Agents and Cancer*, *7*, 35. Available from https://doi.org/10.1186/1750-9378-7-35.

Athanasiou, A., Bowden, S., Paraskevaidi, M., Fotopoulou, C., Martin-Hirsch, P., Paraskevaidis, E., & Kyrgiou, M. (2020). HPV vaccination and cancer prevention. *Best Practice & Research Clinical Obstetrics & Gynaecology, Advances in Screening and Prevention of Women's Cancers*, *65*, 109–124. Available from https://doi.org/10.1016/j.bpobgyn.2020.02.009.

Badawi, H., Ahmed, H., Ismail, A., Diab, M., Moubarak, M., Badawy, A., & Saber, M. (2008). Role of human papillomavirus types 16, 18, and 52 in recurrent cystitis and urinary bladder cancer among Egyptian patients. *Medscape Journal of Medicine*, *10*, 232.

Barghi, M. R., Rahjoo, T., Borghei, M., Hosseini-Moghaddam, S. M., Amani, D., & Farrokhi, B. (2012). Association between the evidence of human papilloma virus infection in bladder transitional cell carcinoma in men and cervical dysplasia in their spouses. *Archives of Iranian Medicine*, *15*, 572–574.

Bernard, H.-U., Burk, R. D., Chen, Z., Van Doorslaer, K., Zur Hausen, H., & de Villiers, E.-M. (2010). Classification of papillomaviruses (PVs) based on 189 PV types and proposal of taxonomic amendments. *Virology*, *401*, 70–79.

Boyle, H., Fléchon, A., & Droz, J.-P. (2010). Tumeurs rares de la vessie. *Bulletin du Cancer*, *97*, S51–S57. Available from https://doi.org/10.1684/bdc.2010.1097.

Bray, F., Ferlay, J., Soerjomataram, I., Siegel, R. L., Torre, L. A., & Jemal, A. (2018). Global cancer statistics 2018: GLOBOCAN estimates of incidence and mortality worldwide for 36 cancers in 185 countries. *CA: A Cancer Journal for Clinicians*, *68*, 394–424. Available from https://doi.org/10.3322/caac.21492.

Collins, K., Hwang, M., Hamza, A., & Rao, P. (2020). Prevalence of high-risk human papillomavirus in primary squamous cell carcinoma of urinary bladder. *Pathology - Research and Practice*, *216*, 153084. Available from https://doi.org/10.1016/j.prp.2020.153084.

Dietrich, H., & Dietrich, B. (2001). Ludwig Rehn (1849–1930)–Pioneering findings on the aetiology of bladder tumours. *World Journal of Urology*, *19*, 151–153. Available from https://doi.org/10.1007/s003450100211.

García-Pérez, J., Pollán, M., Boldo, E., Pérez-Gómez, B., Aragonés, N., Lope, V., Ramis, R., Vidal, E., & López-Abente, G. (2009). Mortality due to lung, laryngeal and bladder cancer in towns lying in the vicinity of combustion installations. *The Science of the Total Environment*, *407*, 2593–2602. Available from https://doi.org/10.1016/j.scitotenv.2008.12.062.

Golovina, D. A., Ermilova, V. D., Zavalishina, L. E., Andreeva, Y. Y., Matveev, V. B., Frank, G. A., & Volgareva, G. M. (2016). Loss of cell differentiation in HPV-associated bladder cancer. *Bulletin of Experimental Biology and Medicine*, *161*, 96–98. Available from https://doi.org/10.1007/s10517-016-3354-x.

Golovina, D. A., Trofimova, O. B., Ermilova, V. D., Matveev, V. B., & Volgareva, G. M. (2014). Complex of molecular genetic and immunohistochemical methods for detection of human papillomavirus in the bladder cancer epithelium. *Bulletin of Experimental Biology and Medicine*, *157*, 70–73. Available from https://doi.org/10.1007/s10517-014-2494-0.

Ho, C.-H., Sung, K.-C., Lim, S.-W., Liao, C.-H., Liang, F.-W., Wang, J.-J., & Wu, C.-C. (2015). Chronic indwelling urinary catheter increase the risk of bladder cancer, even in patients without spinal cord injury. *Medicine*, *94*, e1736. Available from https://doi.org/10.1097/MD.0000000000001736.

Jimenez-Pacheco, A., Exposito-Ruiz, M., Arrabal-Polo, M. A., & Lopez-Luque, A. J. (2012). *Meta*-analysis of studies analyzing the role of human papillomavirus in the development of bladder carcinoma. *Korean Journal of Urology*, *53*, 240.

Khaled, H. M., Raafat, A., Mokhtar, N., Zekri, A. R. N., & Gaballah, H. (2001). Human papilloma virus infection and overexpression of P53 protein in Bilharzial Bladder Cancer. *Tumori*, *87*, 256–261. Available from https://doi.org/10.1177/030089160108700409.

Kim, S. H., Joung, J. Y., Chung, J., Park, W. S., Lee, K. H., & Seo, H. K. (2014). Detection of human papillomavirus infection and p16 immunohistochemistry expression in bladder cancer with squamous differentiation. *PLoS One*, *9*, e93525. Available from https://doi.org/10.1371/journal.pone.0093525.

Kitamura, T., Yogo, Y., Ueki, T., Murakami, S., & Aso, Y. (1988). Presence of human papillomavirus type 16 genome in bladder carcinoma in situ of a patient with mild immunodeficiency. *Cancer Research*, *48*, 7207–7211.

Li, N., Yang, L., Zhang, Y., Zhao, P., Zheng, T., & Dai, M. (2011). Human papillomavirus infection and bladder cancer risk: A *meta*-analysis. *Journal of Infectious Diseases*, *204*, 217–223.

Li, W., Qi, Y., Cui, X., Huo, Q., Zhu, L., Zhang, A., Tan, M., Hong, Q., Yang, Y., Zhang, H., Liu, C., Kong, Q., Geng, J., Tian, Y., Kong, F., & Man, D. (2018). Characteristic of HPV integration in the genome and transcriptome of cervical cancer tissues. *BioMed Research International*, *2018*, e6242173. Available from https://doi.org/10.1155/2018/6242173.

Malagón, T., Drolet, M., Boily, M.-C., Franco, E. L., Jit, M., Brisson, J., & Brisson, M. (2012). Cross-protective efficacy of two human papillomavirus vaccines: A systematic review and *meta*-analysis. *The Lancet Infectious Diseases*, *12*, 781–789. Available from https://doi.org/10.1016/S1473-3099(12)70187-1.

McBride, A. A., & Warburton, A. (2017). The role of integration in oncogenic progression of HPV-associated cancers. *PLoS Pathogens*, *13*, e1006211. Available from https://doi.org/10.1371/journal.ppat.1006211.

Mougin, C., Nicolier, M., & Decrion-Barthod, A.-Z. (2008). HPV et cancers: Mécanismes de l'oncogenèse. *Revue Francophone des Laboratoires*, *2008*, 35–42.

Münger, K., Baldwin, A., Edwards, K. M., Hayakawa, H., Nguyen, C. L., Owens, M., Grace, M., & Huh, K. (2004). Mechanisms of human papillomavirus-induced oncogenesis. *Journal of Virology*, *78*, 11451–11460.

Myandina, G. I., & Itkes, A. V. (2003). The Detection of the genome of human papillomavirus type 16 tumour cells in peripheral blood of patients with cancer of the bladder. Vestn. People's friendship University. *Series Medicine*, *5*(24), 29–32.

Ohadian Moghadam, S., Mansori, K., Nowroozi, M. R., Afshar, D., Abbasi, B., & Nowroozi, A. (2020). Association of human papilloma virus (HPV) infection with oncological outcomes in urothelial bladder cancer. *Infectious Agents and Cancer*, *15*. Available from https://doi.org/10.1186/s13027-020-00318-3.

Roussel, H., Rodriguez, C., Thariat, J., & Badoual, C. (2010). La protéine p16 dans des lésions autres que gynécologiques. *Annales de Pathologie, Carrefour Pathologie 2010 Congrès scientifique - Formation Médicale Continue 22 au 26 Novembre 2010*, *30*, 109–111. Available from https://doi.org/10.1016/j.annpat.2010.07.018.

Rundle, J. S. H., Hart, A. J. L., McGeorge, A., Smith, J. S., Malcolm, A. J., & Smith, P. M. (1982). Squamous cell carcinoma of bladder. A review of 114 patients. *British Journal of Urology*, *54*, 522–526.

Shigehara, K., Kawaguchi, S., Sasagawa, T., Nakashima, K., Nakashima, T., Shimamura, M., & Namiki, M. (2013). Etiological correlation of human papillomavirus infection in the development of female bladder tumor. *APMIS: Acta Pathologica, Microbiologica, et Immunologica Scandinavica*, *121*, 1169–1176. Available from https://doi.org/10.1111/apm.12070.

Shigehara, K., Sasagawa, T., & Namiki, M. (2014). Human papillomavirus infection and pathogenesis in urothelial cells: A mini-review. *Journal of Infection and Chemotherapy*, *20*, 741–747. Available from https://doi.org/10.1016/j.jiac.2014.08.033.

Shukla, S., Mahata, S., Shishodia, G., Pande, S., Verma, G., Hedau, S., Bhambhani, S., Kumari, A., Batra, S., Basir, S. F., Das, B. C., & Bharti, A. C. (2014). Physical state & copy number of high risk human papillomavirus type 16 DNA in progression of cervical cancer. *The Indian Journal of Medical Research*, *139*, 531–543.

Sung, H., Ferlay, J., Siegel, R. L., Laversanne, M., Soerjomataram, I., Jemal, A., & Bray, F. (2021). Global Cancer Statistics 2020: GLOBOCAN estimates of incidence and mortality worldwide for 36 cancers in 185 countries. *CA: A Cancer Journal for Clinicians*, *71*, 209–249. Available from https://doi.org/10.3322/caac.21660.

TCGA. (2014). Comprehensive molecular characterization of urothelial bladder carcinoma. *Nature*, *507*, 315–322. Available from https://doi.org/10.1038/nature12965.

Vinokurova, S., Wentzensen, N., Kraus, I., Klaes, R., Driesch, C., Melsheimer, P., Kisseljov, F., Dürst, M., Schneider, A., & von Knebel Doeberitz, M. (2008). Type-dependent integration frequency of human papillomavirus genomes in cervical lesions. *Cancer Research*, *68*, 307–313. Available from https://doi.org/10.1158/0008-5472.CAN-07-2754.

Volgareva, G. M., Zavalishina, L. E., Golovina, D. A., Andreeva, I. I., Ermilova, V. D., Cheban, N. L., Kuevda, D. A., Trofimova, O. B., Shipulina, O. I., Pavlova, L. S., Petrov, A. N., Matveev, V. B., Shtil', A. A., & Frank, G. A. (2009). Detection of oncoprotein E7 HPV16 in the cancer and normal urinary bladder urothelium. *Arkhiv Patologii*, *71*, 29–30.

Walline, H. M., Goudsmit, C. M., McHugh, J. B., Tang, A. L., Owen, J. H., Teh, B. T., McKean, E., Glover, T. W., Graham, M. P., Prince, M. E., Chepeha, D. B., Chinn, S. B., Ferris, R. L., Gollin, S. M., Hoffmann, T. K., Bier, H., Brakenhoff, R., Bradford, C. R., & Carey, T. E. (2017). Integration of high-risk human papillomavirus into cellular cancer-related genes in head and neck cancer cell lines. *Head & Neck*, *39*, 840–852. Available from https://doi.org/10.1002/hed.24729, The University of Michigan Head and Neck Specialized Program of Research Excellence (SPORE) Program.

Wong, M. C. S., Fung, F. D. H., Leung, C., Cheung, W. W. L., Goggins, W. B., & Ng, C. F. (2018). The global epidemiology of bladder cancer: A joinpoint regression analysis of its incidence and mortality trends and projection. *Scientific Reports*, *8*, 1129. Available from https://doi.org/10.1038/s41598-018-19199-z.

Yan, Y., Zhang, H., Jiang, C., Ma, X., Zhou, X., Tian, X., Song, Y., Chen, X., Yu, J., Li, R., Chen, H., Wang, X., Liu, T., He, Z., & Li, H. (2021). Human papillomavirus prevalence and integration status in tissue samples of bladder cancer in the Chinese population. *The Journal of Infectious Diseases*, *224*, 114–122. Available from https://doi.org/10.1093/infdis/jiaa710.

Youshya, S., Purdie, K., Breuer, J., Proby, C., Sheaf, M. T., Oliver, R. T. D., & Baithun, S. (2005). Does human papillomavirus play a role in the development of bladder transitional cell carcinoma? A comparison of PCR and immunohistochemical analysis. *Journal of Clinical Pathology*, *58*, 207–210. Available from https://doi.org/10.1136/jcp.2004.017152.

Zhao, W., Huang, C. C., Otterson, G. A., Leon, M. E., Tang, Y., Shilo, K., & Villalona, M. A. (2012). Altered p16(INK4) and RB1 expressions are associated with poor prognosis in patients with nonsmall cell lung cancer. *Journal of Clinical Oncology*, *2012*, 957437. Available from https://doi.org/10.1155/2012/957437.

Chapter 11

Tumor-associated macrophages in prostate cancer: role in progression and therapy

Arundhati Mehta[1,*], Shiv Govind Rawat[2,*], Yashwant Ratre (Kumar)[1], Vivek Soni (Kumar)[1,3], Dhananjay Shukla[1], Ajay Kumar[2] and Naveen Vishvakarma (Kumar)[1]

[1]*Department of Biotechnology, Guru Ghasidas Vishwavidyalaya, Bilaspur, Chhattisgarh, India,*
[2]*Department of Zoology, Banaras Hindu University, Varanasi, Uttar Pradesh, India,*
[3]*Trivitron Healthcare, Vishakhapatnam, Andhra Pradesh, India*

11.1 Introduction

Immune response has been sought as a foremost and frontline strategic dimension to counter the various ailments associated with health. Not only do immune cells eliminate and neutralize the pathogenic body invaders, but they also have the responsibility to obviate the development of defective (neoplastic) self-cells. During the earlier events of oncogenesis even in the prostate, transforming cells need to evade elimination by the immune system (Bonollo et al., 2020; Chen et al., 2018; Chung et al., 2005; Coussens & Werb, 2002). Over the course of oncogenic transformation, tumor cells that are able to thwart the antitumor immune response survive. As tumor grows, cells of the immune system infiltrate the tumor tissue to combat the transformed cells (Bingle et al., 2002; Chen et al., 2014; Crusz & Balkwill, 2015; Dai et al., 2017; De Visser et al., 2006). Cells of both lymphoid (T, B, and NK cells) and myeloid origins (granulocytes and macrophages) work in a concerted manner to safeguard host health in a diverse range of pathophysiological conditions. However, established prostate tumors withstand this large army of immune cells through their microenvironment and prevent their antitumor activation (Bingle et al., 2002; Gollapudi et al., 2013; Gomes et al., 2013; Hagemann et al., 2005). Rather, immune cells start cooperating with the progression of tumor cells under the influence of immunosuppressive

*Arundhati Mehta and Shiv Govind Rawat contributed equally as the first authors.

Immunological Implications and Molecular Diagnostics of Genitourinary Cancer.
DOI: https://doi.org/10.1016/B978-0-323-85496-2.00028-2

setup prevalent in the tumor microenvironment (TME) (Afik et al., 2016; Badawi et al., 2015; Chen et al., 2014; Escamilla et al., 2015; Fan et al., 2017; Hao et al., 2012). Derived from myelopoietic differentiation of hematopoietic stem cells, macrophages play an indispensable role in immune response owing to their remarkable abilities in antigen presentation, phagocytosis, production of cytokines, etc. As an integral part, macrophages hold promising activities in antitumor immune response (Yang & Zhang, 2017; Yin et al., 2013; Zheng et al., 2009; Zhou et al., 2020). However, this versatile cell of the immune system is also no exception to tumor-induced immunosuppression. Along with macrophages, other cells of the immune system also infiltrate tumor tissues including those of prostate origin. These are collectively known as tumor-infiltrating immune cells. As per the dual association with tumor cells and subsequent outcome of this host–tumor interaction, macrophages that infiltrate into and populate the TME are termed tumor-associated macrophages (TAMs).

Experimental evidence has confirmed a strong alliance of TAMs and tumor cells in maintaining the various hallmarks of cancer in prostatic malignancies (Bingle et al., 2002; Bonollo et al., 2020; Chen et al., 2014; Gollapudi et al., 2013). Under the influence of tumor-derived factors, macrophages of tumor tissues TAMs forget their capabilities as M1 phenotype to counter neoplastic cells' proliferation and serve to help transformed cells' progression (characteristic of M2 phenotype). TAMs have been shown to promote prostate cancer progression through various routes. The role of TAMs in maintaining the surrounding of the tumor cells, that is, TME is also confirmed (Cao et al., 2017; Hagemann et al., 2005; Krzyszczyk et al., 2018; Lissbrant et al., 2000). The contribution of TAM in promoting prostate tumor progression is not limited to various growth factors, but it also encompasses the production of factors for angiogenesis (Badawi et al., 2015; Chen et al., 2014; Ly et al., 2010; Riabov et al., 2014; Wang et al., 2016). Metastatic events in many tumor types, including prostate cancers, are also served by TAMs as an underwriter through the production of proteolytic enzymes for matrix remodeling (Gupta & Massagué, 2006; Hu et al., 2015; Kaplan et al., 2005; Lo & Lynch, 2018). TAMs are also known for their role in the onset of resistance against chemotherapeutic interventions and radiotherapy (Escamilla et al., 2015; Guan et al., 2019). Recently, cancer stem cells (CSCs) are also linked with the manifestation of the therapy-resistant phenotype of malignancies (Cao et al., 2017; Kreso & Dick, 2014; Phi et al., 2018). Interestingly, the degree of TAM infiltration in tumor tissues associates with stem cell-like characters in cancer cells (Cao et al., 2017; Plaks et al., 2015; Sainz et al., 2016). The pro-tumor M2 phenotype of TAM is an outcome of tumor-induced immunosuppression to prevent macrophage-mediated tumor cytotoxicity. Moreover, these M2-polarized TAM favor the suppression of other cells of the immune system like T cells (Erlandsson et al., 2019; Lu et al., 2011). Taken together, tumors cells impede the antitumor activity of macrophages and influence this versatile cell of immune cells to work in their own favor. However, this strong association of tumor cells of TAMs is also targeted for the therapeutic management of cancers. Preventing the support from macrophages to tumor cells can be drawn by restricting their recruitment to tumor tissues and their subsequent M2 polarization (Comito et al., 2017; Escamilla et al., 2015; Mitchem et al., 2013; Shen & Pili, 2019; Vishvakarma, 2014; Vishvakarma & Singh, 2010, 2011). Most interestingly, TAMs exhibit pro-tumor phenotype functionality in tumor tissues, but they can be reverted to antitumor M1 activation upon required stimulation. Nevertheless, genetic manipulations of TAMs are also underway as a strategic intervention for malignancies and improving the antitumor immune response (Escamilla et al., 2015; Franco & Hayward, 2012; Mitchem et al., 2013; Quail & Joyce, 2017).

Collectively, it is quite concrete that macrophages have a bidirectional association with tumors for their progression and regression. The multifaceted outcome of entangled association with tumor demonstrates the indispensability of TAMs for malignant progression in prostate tissue. Further deciphering the mechanistic connotation for the consequence of TAMs in prostate cancers will aid identification and/or designing of therapeutic interventions. This chapter aims to elaborate on the connection of TAMs and tumor cells and their consequences with special emphasis on prostate cancer. Furthermore, targeting TAMs for therapeutic intervention of prostate cancer is also discussed.

11.2 Prostate cancer initiation, progression, and immunity

The GLOBOCON reported 1,276,106 new cases in 2018 for prostate malignancies, the second most widely recognized noncutaneous ailment among males and the fifth major cause of mortality. Prostate cancer can be premature (early-stage) asymptomatic and sometimes even lead to a feckless path demanding active supervision (Bray et al., 2018). Several investigations have been conducted on the etiology of prostate cancer and are relatively unidentified, especially when collated with others. Progressive age, race, genetic factors, and family history are ingrained prostate cancer threat variables (Bostwick et al., 2004; Dagnelie et al., 2004). Other attributes that have a significant impact on PC include diet (enhanced saturated fat and red food consumption, less fruit, vegetable, vitamins, and coffee intake), overweight and sedentary lifestyle, inflammation, elevated blood sugar level, sepsis, etc. (Dagnelie et al., 2004; Markozannes et al., 2016). The key dietary mechanism that contributes to the incidence of prostate cancer is a persistent decline in androgen infusion and oxidative stress regression. Bearing extremely pervasive hereditary "risk" alleles may enhance the prevalence of prostate cancer manifold in hereditary prostate cancer (HPC). During position cloning, the genetic sources of HPC are efficiently reported but are not really beneficial for sporadic tumors, as cancer alleles are poorly penetrated, and thus the investigation needs to count Single nucleotide polymorphisms (SNPs) and Genome-Wide Association Studies (GWAS) analyst data for a better understanding of linkage of cancer risk with genes (Xu et al., 2009).

To discover the precise identity of the cells that can undergo carcinogenesis for a better understanding of the cellular origin of prostate cancer, it is likely that terminally differentiated luminal cells are transmogrified to produce provisional de-differentiation and transcendence acquisition. An additional option is to turn the prostate stem cells that are supposed to reside inside the basal cells into oncogenic ones (Knudsen & Vasioukhin, 2010). Novel research displaying the detection of castration-resistant Nkx3.1-CARNs expressing cells (stem cells) in the luminal cell chamber questioned the idea of prostate cancer in the basal cells (Wang et al., 2009). Though prostate cancer is an epithelial neoplasm, stroma cells also play a vital role in the induction and advancement of cancer. The development of proliferative inflammatory atrophy (PIA) domains of epithelial cells that are aligned with the inflammatory response in the stromal chamber is a major shift that occurs early on in prostate cancer startup (Knudsen & Vasioukhin, 2010). Reactive stroma is mainly carcinoma-associated fibroblasts (CAFs), also called myofibroblasts, in prostate cancer. The amount of CAF has escalated with the proliferation of tumors to upgraded ailments and has been found in premalignant PIN, that is, prostatic intraepithelial neoplasia (Ayala et al., 2003). Nevertheless, CAFs may not prevail in seclusion, and growing research demonstrates that the inflammatory response of the immune system is primarily attributable to carcinogenesis, partly through the effect of fibroblast programming. Both the promoters of cancer, namely, cancer inflammation and stimulation of the tumor stroma coexist and flourish with the progression of malignancy. It influences one another via a dynamic network of interactions comprising inflammatory, tumor, and stromal cells (Shiao et al., 2016).

11.3 Cancer and macrophage

Cancer is a chronic disorder that is usually triggered by acquired alterations in cell divisions that bypass cellular aging or programmed demise contributing to malignancy or neoplastic proliferation. TME is a significant arbitrator of tumor growth, upkeeping, penetration, and metastasis, which is secondary to these genetic amendments (Chung et al., 2005). The factors liable for this intervention comprise vessel stimulant factors, growth factors, cytokines, in addition, to other factors. These elements assist in the deployment of different cell clusters, which encompass immunocytes, mural cells (contributing to blood and lymphatic vasculature), endothelial cells, and fibroblast cells (Rajput & Wilber, 2010).

The inflammatory response is deeply related to prostatitis or prostate malignancy, and both benign and malevolent prostate tumor tissue have been identified for systemic inflammation (Hussein et al., 2009). Histopathological studies found that 80%–90% of prostate cancer cases had an immune invasion sign and that elevated diagnosis was linked to escalated inflammation (Gurel et al., 2014). Chronic inflammation is believed to contribute to the emergence and evolution of several forms of cancer including prostate cancer with its persistent immune response (Crusz & Balkwill, 2015; De Visser et al., 2006). It also induces PIA (De Marzo et al., 2007), which might lead to a notable prelude PIN (De Marzo et al., 2003). The immunologic infiltrator composition ranges broadly with the phase and recipient age of illness; however, cells of the innate and adaptive immune systems in prostate stroma have been defined. The bulk of immune cells that penetrate tumor tissue predominantly comprises (70%–80%) $CD3^+$ T cells and approximately 10%–15% $CD4^+$ T cells, macrophages, and $CD20^+$ B cells. Innate immune system cells are the ones that are capable of reacting with alien antigens yet do not acquire antigen-specific receptor recognition as with T and B receptors (Shiao et al., 2016).

Macrophages are typically recorded as the most dominant tenants of leukocytes (~30%) in the TME as opposed to other constituents such as mast cells and cells of stroma (Coussens & Werb, 2002; Quail & Joyce, 2017; Van Dalen et al., 2019). Macrophages are APCs (antigen presenting cells) within myeloid lineage prominently functioning in tissue development, homeostatic equilibrium, and immune tracking. By identifying the trend of Th1/Th2 lymphocytes, macrophages can be divided into two divisive appendices including conventionally induced macrophages as M1 and alternatively configured macrophages as M2 phenotype (Van Dalen et al., 2019).

11.4 Tumor-associated macrophages and prostate cancer

Macrophages that invade cancerous tissues are known as "tumor-associated macrophages." Historically, only in the TME, macrophages were believed to perform an antitumor role (Wu et al., 2019). TAMs form a significant section of the stromal portion of many rigid tumors and, as both tumor-promoting and tumor-inhibiting effects have been proposed, they serve as a dynamic character in commanding neoplasm development, progression, and tumor emergence (Lissbrant et al., 2000). Few studies have stated that TAMs, according to their various stimulation routes, could be segregated into M1 type (classical activation) and M2 type (alternative activation) macrophages (Takeya & Komohara, 2016; Weigert et al., 2016). M1-type macrophages are commonly assumed to facilitate inflammatory response, whereas M2-type macrophages encourage tissue regeneration/wound healing by triggering angiogenesis and matrix protein production (Takeya & Komohara, 2016). Elevated TAMs in prostate cancer tissues have been shown to forecast

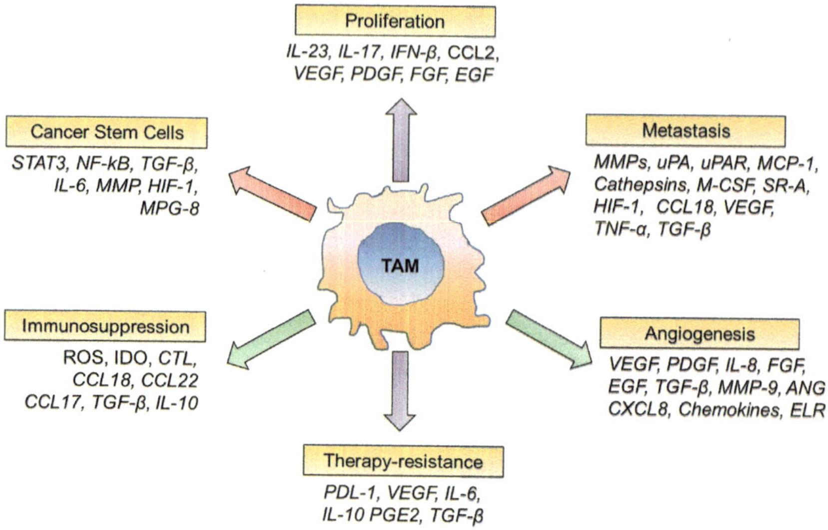

FIGURE 11.1 Contributions of tumor-associated macrophages in tumor progression. TAMs contribute to the onset and maintenance of various factors essential for the progression and aggressiveness of cancer cells. They directly produce or favor the production of mediators that support cell proliferation, stem cell behavior, angiogenesis, immunosuppression, metastasis, as well as resistance against therapy.

inadequate biochemical relapse following radical prostatectomy in prostate cancer patients, and M2-type macrophages are correlated with an additional prostate cancer intrusion (Lanciotti et al., 2014). In progressed prostate cancer patients, remote metastasis is a frequent and convoluted issue. Certain reports have assessed a rise in metastatic prostate cancer in the total number of TAMs, particularly the number of invaded M2-type macrophages, indicating that TAM incursion is a threat indicator for distinct prostate cancer metastasis (Hu et al., 2015; Sagnak et al., 2011). As summarized in Fig. 11.1, TAMs contribute at various fronts in the progression of tumor such as supporting their proliferation, assisting them in immunosuppression, promoting metastasis, driving angiogenesis, strengthening stemness in cancer to cells, and maintaining therapy resistance.

11.4.1 Prostate cancer progression and tumor-associated macrophage

TAMs offer a mutational history through the creation of reactive nitrogen (RNI), reactive oxygen species (ROSs), and the release of numerous growth factors (Meira et al., 2008; Pang et al., 2007; Van Dalen et al., 2019). The tissue-resident macrophage characteristic is passed to an immunosuppressive subsegment affected by cytokines (i.e., interleukin [IL] 4, IL10, and IL13) extracted from the tumor trailed by the development of the intraepithelial abscess/lesion. Colony-stimulating factor 1 (CSF1) and CCL2 or monocyte chemoattractant protein 1 (MCP1) secretion assigns monocytes derived from bone marrow cells to the tumor (Curiel et al., 2004; Van Dalen et al., 2019).

The rise in TAMs in prostate cancer can be facilitated by the parathyroid hormone–related protein (PTHrP) derived from prostate tumors, which has been demonstrated to mobilize myeloid lineage cells through chemokine (C–C motif) ligand 2 (CCL2) yielded by osteoblast (Li et al., 2009). Macrophages play a critical role in phagocytosis amid bacterial infectious disease (Hume, 2008), though phagocytosis, in contrast, is invariably neglected in tumor development (Danilin et al., 2012). An essential process, namely, efferocytosis in inflammation, autoimmunity, and tissue homeostasis corresponds to the tangible phagocytosis of an apoptotic cell (Mevorach et al., 2010). It is a physiological operation, like several tumor-promoting activities, that can be exploited by tumors to sustain their formation and advancement (Dai et al., 2017).

In controlling tumor initiation and progression of prostate cancer, the inherent pathways of TAMs are complicated. In particular, TAMs affect the proliferation and migration of cancer cells through overt communication with tumor cells or passively through cytokine sequestration, which supplies mechanical scope and takes part in every leap of the tumorigenesis (Wu et al., 2019). Researchers have decoded that the secretions (NOV/CCN3) from prostate cancer cells stimulate TAMs to express CD204, then trigger the NF-kB signaling cascade, facilitating VEGF secretion through M2 form of TAMs, and encouraging angiogenesis in tumor (Chen et al., 2014). Furthermore, Soki et al. revealed that TAMs in the microenvironment of prostate cancer with the condition of bone metastasis foster tumorigenesis by encounters with apoptotic cells via the MFG-E8 pathway. New and novel concepts for the therapy of prostate cancer may be established by closer investigation of possible pathways and immune checkpoints of TAMs in the prostate TME (Soki et al., 2015).

11.4.2 Tumor-associated macrophages as mediators of immunosuppression in prostate cancer

TAMs are the main immunoregulating players in the TME and participate in the repression of cytotoxic T lymphocytes (CTL) owing to their cytotoxic involvement in the tumor. The depletion of $CD8^+$ T population proliferation by TAM in the murine model of cancer was observed to be based on L-arginine metabolic processes via either the arginase-I or inducible synthase-nitric oxide (iNOS), leading to ROS production (Lu et al., 2011). IL-10 generated by TAMs elicit expression of the costimulatory molecule PD-L1 on myeloid lineage monocytes and impose suppression of the CTL action (Kuang et al., 2009). In addition, PGE2, IL-10, and TAM-derived indoleamine 2,3-dioxygenase (IDO) occupy an important position in the stimulation of Tregs and TAM-inferred initiation of chemotactic factors such as CCL17, CCL18, and CCL22. Cumulatively, these have contributed to the persecution of T cells' antitumor function in TME (Yang & Zhang, 2017).

Through discrete receptor signal transduction, macrophages conduct efferocytosis (Rothlin & Lemke, 2010). Unique "eat me" signal compounds are released by triggered macrophages; and link apoptotic cells and macrophages, like milk fat globule-E8 (MFG-E8), to promote efferocytosis (Aziz et al., 2011). TAMs are polarized for communication with tumor cells undergoing programmed cell death (apoptosis) in an MFG-E8-dependent pattern that endorses tumor propagation in the sense of prostate cancer bone metastasis (Soki et al., 2015). Attributes emitted by efferocytotic macrophages in the bone microenvironment might boost the tolerance of bone malignancies to cancer therapies, leading to a failure of treatment outcomes or diminished period of response (Dai et al., 2017).

Inflammatory immune cells and bone cells (osteoblasts) generate IL-6 and have sufficient potential for communication with prostate cancer cells (Ershler et al., 1997). Antiinflammatory strategies have been proven effective against a variety of malignancies (Kumar et al., 2012; Soni et al., 2020). A large number of studies and clinical data prove that IL-6 facilitates the development of prostate cancer (Culig & Puhr, 2012). In order to decide whether these levels could be utilized to anticipate biochemical relapse in patients receiving radical prostatectomy, Alcover and the team measured IL-6 serum levels along with its soluble receptor and noticed that preoperative IL-6 concentration greater than 1.2 pg/mL were linked with an elevated incidence of biochemical chronicity in men with prostate cancer (Alcover et al., 2010).

11.4.3 Prostate cancer stem cells and tumor-associated macrophage

A biological distinct group of stem-like cells, inside the mass of the tumor cell population, are CSCs, also known as tumor-initiating cells or tumor-propagating cells. Such cells are presumed to be the main operators of the oncogenesis multistage scheme, providing access to the clonogenic tumor tissue center (Kreso & Dick, 2014; Patrawala et al., 2006). CSCs reside in a cellular domain, like somatic stem cells, that supplies crucial transmissions of self-renewal and tumor progression (Plaks et al., 2015). Quite precisely, CSCs are shielded from immunosurveillance, cell death (apoptosis), and chemotherapeutic agents by the TME, and, above all, the premalignant niche offers CSCs with attributes that sustain, propel, and encourage their stemness (Sainz et al., 2016). Owing to TAM-mediated paracrine signals, which have macrophage-derived components stimulating CSC interface, fostering stem-like CSC characteristics, aggravated tumor progression, metastases, and even CSC chemotherapeutic resistance, the association has been observed for decades amongst elevated numbers of TAMs, greater prevalence, and poor patient results (Bingle et al., 2002; Qian & Pollard, 2010). Posterior research indicated that NF-kB upregulation in macrophages results in IL-6 generation and STAT3 signaling in adjacent neighboring cells supports the in vivo premalignant intestinal epithelial cell survival and CSC expansion (Kortylewski et al., 2009).

11.4.4 Tumor-associated macrophages and angiogenesis in prostate cancer

The production of cancer is a complex, multiphase phenomenon in which blended diverse genetic variants contribute to specific abilities, the traits of cancer. Angiogenesis has to be critically activated as the shape of blood vessels internally depends on the size, penetration on, and metastasis of the development of the tumor (Badawi et al., 2015). Angiogenesis is a crucial mechanism for delivering oxygen and vital nutrients to exponentially developing cancerous tissues. An angiogenic signup helps cancer cells to thrive and expand, providing them with the access to metastatic disease vasculature (Riabov et al., 2014). Through upregulation of expression and release of a number of pro-angiogenic variables, TAMs have the capacity to exacerbate the vessels' development. The TME polarizes M into M2 form or a blended M1/M2 phenotype, which has a significant pro-angiogenic expression (Ly et al., 2010).

The reverse polarization of TAM form into M1 indicates pro-angiogenic activity suppression and an increase in an antiangiogenic expression such as CXC-chemokine ligand 9 (CXCL9) and IFN-β. VEGF-A is referred to as the leading TAM secreting pro-angiogenic cytokine. The TAM levels of many forms of human cancer contribute to TAM density (Shieh et al., 2009). Via different complex strategies, macrophages are allocated to these hypoxic TME niches. The hypoxic factor 1 (HIF-1α), reported to increase in TAMs and other tumor-infiltration cells, administer the transcription gene that conforms itself with angiogenesis in hypoxic sites. TAMs discharge TNF-α, VEGF, IL-13β, FGF, MMPs, phosphorylase thymidine, a plasminogen activator-type urokinase (uPA), and other molecules. The angiogenic development of new blood vessels, which inevitably provides the tumor with nutrient resources, flourishes along with growth factors derived from platelets (Yang & Zhang, 2017). The evidence supporting the fact that macrophages are concurrently responsible for both angiogenesis and lymphangiogenesis has accumulated over the last few years via VEGF-A and MMP9 development. The excessively generated cytokines by TAM subgroups have been demonstrated to induce blood and lymph vessel growth (Gomes et al., 2013).

11.4.5 Role of tumor-associated macrophages in Extracellular matrix (ECM) remodeling, invasion, and metastasis

Numerous metabolites, other factors such as IL1, IL6, TNF, and macrophages have intensified neoplastic incidents for a considerable time, and innovative authentications have recently been provided by neoteric breakthroughs. In general, the location and status of the premetastatic regions are found to be cells of hematopoietic descent, especially monocytic cells of myeloid lineage (Hagemann et al., 2005; Kim et al., 2009; Mantovani et al., 2008). During tumor growth, the cells will obtain intrusion and metastatic spread to flee from the existing tumor location and resettle at the new nutrient-rich area (Erler et al., 2009; Gupta & Massagué, 2006; Hanahan & Weinberg, 2000). The emergence of premetastatic zones in secondary lesion target organs made up of BMDCs (bone marrow–derived clusters) facilitates the metastasis of the cancerous cells by encoding CD34, CD133, and c-kit (Kaplan et al., 2005).

Macrophages mobilized to TME prevail in tumor stroma at all stages of cancer advancement, which promote tumor proliferation, infiltration, and dissemination through a variety of techniques (Afik et al., 2016). Cancers are characterized by high levels of proteolytic deterioration of cellular and structural boundaries. An unnaturally articulated or conversely configured protein can lead to disruption, revamping, and ECM dissolution owing to the peculiar proteolytic linkage enzymes (Gilkes et al., 2014). Induction of TWIST, SNAIL, ZEB1, ZEB2, and several more transcription factors activates epithelial–mesenchymal transition. These expression factors inhibit the epithelial cell form and facilitate mesenchymal motility, BM, and ECM depletion traits (Vandewalle et al., 2009). ZEB-1 and -2 specifically tie down the transcription of epithelial cadherin (E cadherin marker) and provoke vimentin (mesenchymal marker) expression with the utilization of conserved zinc finger proteins (mesenchymal marker). ZEB-1 also strengthened relocation by an extracellular barrier of PC-3 human prostate cancer cells and enhanced metastatic invasion (Drake et al., 2009).

11.4.6 Chemo- and radio-resistance in prostate cancer and tumor-associated macrophage

Resistance to chemotherapy is one of the few main problems in the field of therapies for cancer and involves relapse in most cancer victims. It is also usually linked with cancer lesions that become more assertive and/or neoplastic (Holohan et al., 2013; Ireland et al., 2016; Phi et al., 2018). Therefore the underpinning biological mechanisms and strategies through which cancer cells turn resistant to therapy are essential to understand for developing/innovating sustainable treatment interventions. The resistance networks to "conventional" topical and molecular therapies have distinct traits, such as drug-goal alterations, pro-survival agitation, and insufficient cell death ablation. The recent past has seen a substantial increase with the increasing variety of anticancer drugs, powerful pharmacological prototype systems, and the advent of reliable high-performance evaluation methods. This will also allow patient division through the clinical assessment of therapeutic formulations and the application of diagnostic markers and unprecedented pathways to pinpoint and overcome drug resistance (Holohan et al., 2013).

Androgen deprivation treatment is often inadequate for males with CRPC, which includes the addition of docetaxel as an efficient chemical treatment. TAMs are known to have a pro-tumorigenic effect that leads to failure of treatment. Moreover, a decrease in metabolites polarizing macrophages toward the M2 phenotype circumvent the resistance against standard anticancer drugs (Soni et al., 2020; Vishvakarma et al., 2013). This indicates that chemoresistance and macrophage polarization exist in a collaborative manner.

11.4.7 Therapeutic implication of macrophages in prostate cancer

Macrophages, one of the major infiltrating immune cells of the TME, play an indispensable role in the development and progression of prostate cancer by altering various vital processes, including adaptive immunity, tumor cell survival, angiogenesis, invasion and metastasis, and chemoresistance (Lo & Lynch, 2018). The extant literature strongly suggests a correlation between the abundance of TAMs and poor survival and prognosis of prostate cancer patients (Lissbrant et al., 2000). Like other cancers, TAMs are also found in the M2-polarized state (alternatively activated or antiinflammatory macrophages) in the vicinity of prostate cancer. The alternatively polarized macrophages are one of the major altered components of immune cells, which help in the creation of a favorable microenvironment with respect to the uninterrupted growth of various cancers, including prostate cancer (Hu et al., 2015). Hence, TAMs have emerged as one of the potent and promising therapeutic targets for designing effective and safer immunotherapeutic strategies against prostate cancer.

11.4.8 Macrophage-mediated prostate cancer cytotoxicity

Usually, macrophages act as a barrier for the initiation and development of cancer either by directly killing neoplastic cells or via activating the cellular immunity. As stated earlier, macrophages display two different types of phenotypes, namely M1 and M2 phenotypes. M1 macrophages (classically activated macrophages or proinflammatory macrophages) exhibit tumoricidal activity by secreting various cytokines such as IL-12, IL-1β, IL-23, and RNI and ROS production (Zhou et al., 2020). On the other hand, M2 macrophages play an essential role in wound healing, tissue remodeling, and immunosuppression (Krzyszczyk et al., 2018). Interestingly, TAMs usually exhibit the M2 phenotype and are identified as one of the vital tumor-promoting cellular components of TME.

Accumulating evidence suggests that TAMs in the TME of prostate cancer mainly display the M2 phenotype. Thus TAMs present in the vicinity of prostate cancer do not exert cytotoxic action against prostate cancer cells. Interestingly, the enhancement of the tumoricidal activity of TAMs has been reported in the suppression of prostate cancer growth (Martinez-Marin et al., 2017). A study has shown the role of STAT3 in the immunophenotypic switch from tumoricidal M1 to tumor-promoting M2 macrophages by the cell-culture supernatant of prostate cancer (Solis-Martinez et al., 2018). Furthermore, this study reported the reversal of suppressed cytotoxic action of macrophages against prostate cancer cells by blockade of STAT3-mediated signaling through Stattic (6-nitrobenzo[b]thiophene-1, 1-dioxide), an inhibitor that inhibits activation, dimerization, and nuclear translocation of STAT3. Recently, in a study, Lee et al. demonstrated macrophage activating action of dihydrotestosterone (DHT) (Lee et al., 2019). In this study, they observed that DHT treatment increased the cytotoxic ability of macrophages against prostate cancer cells in a dose-dependent manner through TNF-related apoptosis-inducing ligand (TRAIL). Another recent report has shown the recovery of antitumor activity of TAMs against advanced prostate cancer cells by the inhibition of C-X-C chemokine receptor type 2 (CXCR2) (Di Mitri et al., 2019). This investigation reported the dramatically increased number of CXCR2 expressing TAMs in PTEN-null mutant prostate tumors and suggested the crucial role of CXCL2 in eliciting the tumor-promoting activity in TAMs through CXCR2 activation. Interestingly, this study showed that pharmacological blockade of CXCR2 receptor by AZD5069 augmented antitumor activity of TAMs against prostate cancer by inducing TNF-α production.

11.4.8.1 Regulation of macrophage polarization

The polarization of prostate cancer-associated macrophages toward tumor-promoting M2 phenotype has been observed as a critical immunosuppressive phenomenon during the initiation and development of various cancers (Erlandsson et al., 2019; Hao et al., 2012). Notably, prostate cancer-associated macrophages also display M2 phenotypes (Erlandsson et al., 2019), and thus various approaches are being tested in search of the most effective therapeutic targets to develop an immunotherapeutic strategy for the inhibition of prostate cancer via reversing the tumor-promoting (M2 phenotype) to tumor eliminating phenotype (M1 phenotype) of macrophages.

As noted earlier, CAFs, one of the most abundant cellular components of tumor stroma, have been recognized in the facilitation of the development and progression of prostate cancer (Franco & Hayward, 2012). CAFs promote prostate cancer progression either directly or indirectly through inducing angiogenesis or modulating immune responses (Franco & Hayward, 2012). Interestingly, studies have shown the involvement of CAFs in switching macrophage polarization from M1 to M2 in various cancers including prostate (Comito et al., 2014; Zhang et al., 2017). In a study, Comito et al. showed the tumor-promoting action of CAFs against prostate cancer owing to its modulatory action on the recruitment and differentiation of monocytes in tumor stroma (Comito et al., 2014). In this study, they demonstrated the role of CAF-secreted stromal-derived growth factor-1 (SDF-1) in the increased recruitment as well as their differentiation into pro-tumoral macrophages. Hence, owing to their immunomodulatory activity, CAFs are identified as potential therapeutic targets for the improvement of antitumor immunity and immunotherapeutic efficacy.

Phosphatidylserine, a phospholipid, has been reported as one of the contributors to the immunosuppressed microenvironment of prostate cancer (Birge et al., 2016). In a study, Yin et al. suggested that phosphatidylserine could be a useful therapeutic target for the reversal of immunosuppressed TME or re-activation of suppressed antitumor immune responses (Yin et al., 2013). As in their study, they noticed delayed tumor progression with concomitant polarization of TAMs toward M1 phenotype in prostate tumor-bearing mice administered with docetaxel in combination with antiphosphatidylserine-targeting antibody 2aG4. Furthermore, their findings suggested the repolarization of M2-like TAMs into M1-like TAMs by 2aG4 because of their binding with TAM membrane-associated phosphatidylserine. The in vitro experiments of this study also stated the immunostimulatory action of 2aG4 against TAMs. Overall, their findings confirmed the indispensable role of phosphatidylserine in TAM polarization in prostate cancer. Therefore targeting of phosphatidylserine by antiphosphatidylserine neutralizing antibody may improve the host antitumor immunity by reversing the immunosuppressive effects of phosphatidylserine in the TME.

Milk fat globule EGF factor 8 (MFG-E8) is another factor that induces M2 polarization in macrophages. MFG-E8 is a secreted protein, produced by a variety of cells, including activated macrophages, which binds to phosphatidylserine residue of apoptotic cells and $\alpha_v\beta_3/\alpha_v\beta_5$ integrin of macrophages and promotes efferocytosis (Aziz et al., 2009). Several studies have suggested the role of MFG-E8-mediated efferocytosis in the suppression of antitumor immunity (Jinushi et al., 2009). As stated earlier, Soki et al. showed a significantly elevated level of MFG-E8 in the serum and tissue exosomes of prostate cancer patients compared to patients with benign tumors or tumor-free healthy individuals (Soki et al., 2014). Furthermore, coculturing of macrophages with apoptotic prostate cancer cells induced the expression of MFG-E8 in macrophages, which consequently polarized the macrophages into M2 phenotype. This study also confirmed the direct involvement of MFG-E8 into M2 polarization of macrophages by examining the effect of recombinant MFG-E8 on the bone marrow-derived macrophages. Thereafter, they reconfirmed this by observing the reversal effect of MFG-E8 neutralization (by using antiMFG-E8 antibody) on the MFG-E8-mediated M2 polarization. More importantly, this study demonstrated the role of the STAT3 pathway in the MFG-E8-mediated M2 polarization. Hence, this study suggested the therapeutic values of MFG-E8 in designing the immunotherapeutic regimens against prostate cancer.

The controversial role of protein kinase C zeta (PKCζ) has been reported in prostate cancer (Garg et al., 2014). However, recent findings suggest the tumor-suppressive nature of PKCζ (Kim et al., 2013). In this context, a study by Fan et al. demonstrated the role of prostate cancer-associated PKCζ in the regulation of chemotaxis and polarization of TAMs (Fan et al., 2017). In this study, they observed a negative correlation between the PKCζ expression in prostate cancer and recruitment and M2 polarization of macrophages in the TME possibly by suppressing IL-4 and IL-10 production. Another study by Liu et al. elucidated that miR-148a induces migration of prostate cancer cells by promoting M2 polarization of macrophages by suppressing PKCζ expression (Liu et al., 2019). Furthermore, this study also reported PKCζ as a target gene of miR-148a. Both these studies suggested the pivotal role of PKCζ in the M2 polarization of TAMs in prostate cancer. The role of miRNA let-7b has also been reported in the regulation of TAM-mediated angiogenesis and mobility of prostate cancer (Wang et al., 2016). The expression of miRNA let-7b is found markedly high in prostate cancer-associated macrophages compared to their normal counterparts and its inhibition is reported in the suppression of pro-tumoral activities of prostatic TAMs. Hence, miR-148a and miRNA let-7b might be potential therapeutic targets for the development of immunotherapeutic approaches against prostate cancer.

11.4.8.2 Strategies modulating macrophage recruitment

Prostate cancer cells and other noncancerous cellular components present in their surroundings secrete numerous factors that attract monocytes from the circulation or macrophages from the surrounding tissues (Bonollo et al., 2020). These factors include CCL2, CSF1, CCN3, LL-37, and IL-6, which are implicated in the recruitment and differentiation of monocyte/macrophage in primary and metastatic tumors (Cao et al., 2017).

Convincing reports suggest a correlation between the numbers of TAMs and poorer prognosis and decreased overall survival in prostate cancer patients (Lissbrant et al., 2000). Gollapudi et al. demonstrated the tumor-supportive action of TAMs in the growth and development of prostate cancer as they detected a markedly higher number of TAMs in prostate cancer compared to prostatic intraepithelial neoplasia and benign tissue (Gollapudi et al., 2013). Furthermore, in an investigation, Hu et al. noticed a significantly increased number of TAMs, particularly alternatively activated macrophages in metastatic prostate cancer compared to nonmetastatic cancer (Hu et al., 2015).

CCL-2 has been reported as a potential regulator of prostate cancer progression (Loberg et al., 2006). Moreover, the high level of CCL-2 is widely detected in the TME of several cancers, including prostate cancer (Hao et al., 2020). Studies suggest the direct implication of CCL-2 in the induction of proliferation and migration of prostate cancer cells (Loberg et al., 2006). Furthermore, reports also indicate the vital role of CCL-2 in the infiltration of macrophages to tumor sites (Loberg et al., 2007). Interestingly, a study by Mizutani et al. has explored the crucial regulatory action of CCL-2 in the metastasis of prostate cancer by affecting the infiltration of macrophages (Mizutani et al., 2009). This study showed that neutralization of CCL2 led to inhibition of prostate cancer growth by interfering with the recruitment of macrophages at the tumor site. The role of tumor-derived macrophage colony-stimulating factor 1 (M-CSF1or CSF1) has also been reported in the infiltration/recruitment of TAMs into tumor sites in prostate cancer as well as in their polarization toward M2 phenotype through the colony-stimulating factor-1 receptor (CSF1R) (Mizutani et al., 2009). Furthermore, a study has shown the possible role of disrupted TAM recruitment in the retardation of prostate cancer growth by the inhibition of CSF1R (Escamilla et al., 2015). Therefore targeting of CSF1–CSF1R axis has emerged as one of the potential therapeutic approaches for the treatment of prostate cancer via interfering with the infiltration or polarization of TAMs.

The CCN3/nephroblastoma overexpressed (NOV), a member of the CCN family of matrix proteins, is reported in the tumorigenesis of prostate cancer (Schmitz et al., 2013). It is found to be involved in the regulation of numerous cellular processes, including cell adhesion, migration, proliferation, differentiation, and survival (Ellis et al., 2003; Lin et al., 2003). Interestingly, in a study, Chen et al. reported the upregulated expression of CCN3 in prostate cancer cells and their role in the recruitment and M2 polarization of TAMs (Chen et al., 2014). Moreover, they also demonstrated the role of CCN3-induced M2 polarization of TAMs in prostate cancer angiogenesis via focal adhesion kinase (FAK)/Akt/NF-κB signaling. A study by Cha et al. showed the implication of prostate cancer-derived cathelicidin-related antimicrobial peptide (CRAMP) in the infiltration of immature myeloid progenitors as well as their differentiation and polarization into tumor-promoting M2 macrophages at the tumor sites (Cha et al., 2016). Hence, prostate cancer-derived CCN3 and CRAMP can be targeted to restrict TAM-mediated growth of prostate cancer.

Taken together, the above-mentioned studies indicate the potential role of TAMs in the growth and development of prostate cancer. Therefore blockade of TAMs infiltration or recruitment of monocytes might be a promising immunotherapeutic approach for the treatment of prostate cancer.

11.4.8.3 Inhibitory strategies against tumor-associated macrophage

Tasquinimod, a quinolone-3-carboxamide derivative, has emerged as a potential therapeutic drug for the treatment of castration-resistant prostate cancer (Mehta & Armstrong, 2016). It targets inflammatory protein S100A9 and has been reported in the reversal of suppressed TME of prostate cancer by impairing the accumulation and function of suppressive myeloid cells, namely, myeloid-derived suppressor cells and TAMs in the tumor milieu (Shen et al., 2015; Shen & Pili, 2019). Hence, tasquinimod has tremendous potential for the improvement of the effectiveness of immunotherapy.

PTEN (phosphatase and tensin homolog deleted on chromosome 10) is a lipid phosphatase that inhibits PI3K-mediated signaling pathways by dephosphorylating phosphatidylinositol 3,4,5-trisphosphate (PIP3) into phosphatidylinositol 4,5-bisphosphate (PIP2) and hence modulates various cellular processes such as survival, proliferation, apoptosis, cell motility, and angiogenesis (Chalhoub & Baker, 2009). It is a well-known tumor suppressor and found to be downregulated in numerous cancers (Chen et al., 2018). Remarkably, a study has shown the implication of PTEN inhibition-mediated CCL2 and VEGF expression in the M2 polarization macrophages and thus suggested PI3K as a therapeutic target for the repolarization of M2 into M1 (Li et al., 2015).

Zoledronic acid (ZA) is a nitrogen-containing bisphosphonate and has been reported as an effective therapeutic drug for the reduction of bone pain in metastatic prostate cancer (McKeage & Plosker, 2008). A recent study by Comito et al. have unraveled the role of ZA-altered TAM polarization in the inhibition of growth and metastasis of prostate cancer (Comito et al., 2017). Remarkably, this study showed attenuation of invasive and angiogenic properties of TAMs by ZA through an immunophenotypic switch from M2 to M1 phenotype.

CCL2 is an inflammatory chemokine that facilitates the recruitment of monocytes from bone marrow to inflammatory sites through interaction with C-C motif chemokine receptor 2 (CCR2) (Hao et al., 2020).

C-X-C motif chemokine receptor 2 (CXCR2) is a seven transmembrane-domain G protein-coupled receptor (GPCR), and its activation through its ligands plays an important role in the chemotaxis of leukocytes at inflammatory sites (Zhu et al., 2012). Interestingly, in a recent study, the role of CXCR2 was observed in the M2 polarization of TAMs in PTEN-null prostate tumors. Further, this study showed the shift in the polarization of TAMs from M2 to M1 phenotype by the inhibition of CXCR2 with the help of its antagonist AZD5069 (Di Mitri et al., 2019).

Another recent study by Guan et al. showed that inhibition of TAMs recruitment by the blockade of colony-stimulating factor-1 (CSF-1) or macrophage-colony stimulating factor (M-CSF) signaling through its antagonist PLX3397 significantly enhanced the therapeutic efficacy of docetaxel against castration-resistant prostate cancer (Guan et al., 2019).

Altogether, in this section, we have discussed the molecular targets of TAMs, which can be harnessed for enhancing the therapeutic efficacy of anticancer drugs or for designing novel immunotherapeutic regimens against prostate cancer.

11.4.8.4 Gene modification in macrophage

A number of strategies have been developed to combat the tumor-promoting nature of TAMs. These strategies include reducing the number of TAMs or altering their functional activities within the TME. In the last few years, enhancement of the antitumor activity of TAMs by gene modification has emerged as one of the effective treatment modalities to inhibit the growth of several deadly cancers, including prostate cancer.

IL-12 is a proinflammatory cytokine and plays an inevitable role in inducing antitumor immunity (Nguyen et al., 2020). The immunotherapeutic potential of IL-12 is tested against various cancers owing to its ability to activate tumoricidal activities of immune cells, namely, macrophages, Tc, and NK cells (Nguyen et al., 2020). In a study, Satoh et al. tried a novel approach to prostate cancer therapy that involves the genetic modification in macrophages to express the high level of IL-12 (Satoh et al., 2003). They selected macrophages for their study as they are found in their suppressed state in the TME as well as these are the cells that play a key role in the activation of antitumor immunity due to various properties such as tumor-killing ability, antigen-presenting activity, ability to activate cytotoxic lymphocytes. In this study, they noticed inhibition of tumor growth and metastasis along with prolonged survival of metastatic prostate cancer-bearing mice after the injection of macrophages transduced with murine IL-12 recombinant adenoviral vector (AdmIL-12). Furthermore, they explored that tumor inhibition by the intratumoral injection of AdmIL-12-transduced macrophages occurs possibly because of increased infiltration of $CD4^+$ and $CD8^+$ T cells and NK cell activity (Satoh et al., 2003).

In a similar kind of study, Tabata et al. showed that like AdmIL-12, intratumor injection of AdGlipr1-transduced macrophages also decelerated the growth and metastasis of prostate cancer via activating NK, and cytotoxic T cell activities (Tabata et al., 2011). In this study, they also observed increased cell surface expression of MHC II, CD40, and CD80 molecules in macrophages transduced with murine Glipr1 recombinant adenoviral vector. GLIPR1 is a downstream target of p53 and has proapoptotic activities in various cancer cell lines, including prostate cancer (Tabata et al., 2011).

Convincing reports indicate that hypoxia acts as a crucial player in providing the chemo-resistant property to tumor cells present in the core region (Doktorova et al., 2015). Therefore targeting hypoxic tumor cells has emerged as one of the potential therapeutic approaches for the treatment of various cancers. As macrophages are one of the major infiltrating cells at the site of hypoxic regions, macrophages are identified as the best source for delivering the therapeutic genes or viruses at the hypoxic areas to restrict the growth of cancer. In a study, Muthana et al. exploited this property of macrophages and delivered oncolytic adenovirus to hypoxic prostate tumors (Muthana et al., 2011). In this study, systemic injection of macrophages cotransduced with hypoxia response element-regulated E1A/B construct and E1A-dependent oncolytic adenovirus into the prostate tumor-bearing mice impeded the tumor growth owing to selective killing of prostate tumor cells by adenovirus released from macrophages at the hypoxic tumor areas (Muthana et al., 2011).

11.5 Conclusion

Prostate cancers have multidimensional implications for macrophages to play in. Although an association between prostate cancer onset and progression with macrophage phenotypic activation in TME is established, further mechanistic exploration on the acquaintance is expected to provide further delineation. Based on available facts, targets have been identified to break the contributions of macrophages in the progression of prostate cancer. Attempts to repolarize these myeloid cells or to make them more tumoricidal have shown success in preclinical evaluations. Further assessment of macrophage behavior in TME and identification of key factors underlying their unusual functionality will assist the development of a therapeutic regimen pursuing the bond of TAM and tumor cells.

Acknowledgment

Fellowship supports to AM, and YKR [GGU-VRET Fellowship], SGR, and VKS [UGC-SRF; F.16–6(Dec.2016)/2017(NET)] are duly acknowledged here. The authors also acknowledge the supports received from DBT-GOI [BT/PR7020/INF/22/172/ 2012] and the Special Assistance Program at the Department of Biotechnology [GGU].

References

Afik, R., Zigmond, E., Vugman, M., Klepfish, M., Shimshoni, E., Pasmanik-Chor, M., Shenoy, A., Bassat, E., Halpern, Z., Geiger, T., Sagi, I., & Varol, C. (2016). Tumor macrophages are pivotal constructors of tumor collagenous matrix. *Journal of Experimental Medicine, 213* (11), 2315–2331. Available from https://doi.org/10.1084/jem.20151193.

Alcover, J., Filella, X., Luqué, P., Molina, R., Izquierdo, L., Augé, J. M., & Alcaraz, A. (2010). Prognostic value of IL-6 in localized prostatic cancer. *Anticancer Research, 30*(10), 4369–4372.

Ayala, G., Tuxhorn, J. A., Wheeler, T. M., Frolov, A., Scardino, P. T., Ohori, M., Wheeler, M., Spitler, J., & Rowley, D. R. (2003). Reactive stroma as a predictor of biochemical-free recurrence in prostate cancer. *Clinical Cancer Research*, *9*(13), 4792–4801.

Aziz, M., Ishihara, S., Mishima, Y., Oshima, N., Moriyama, I., Yuki, T., Kadowaki, Y., Rumi, M. A. K., Amano, Y., & Kinoshita, Y. (2009). MFG-E8 attenuates intestinal inflammation in murine experimental colitis by modulating osteopontin-dependent αvβ3 integrin signaling. *Journal of Immunology*, *182*(11), 7222–7232. Available from https://doi.org/10.4049/jimmunol.0803711.

Aziz, M., Jacob, A., Matsuda, A., & Wang, P. (2011). Review: Milk fat globule-EGF factor 8 expression, function and plausible signal transduction in resolving inflammation. *Apoptosis: An International Journal on Programmed Cell Death*, *16*(11), 1077–1086. Available from https://doi.org/10.1007/s10495-011-0630-0.

Badawi, M. A., Abouelfadl, D. M., El-Sharkawy, S. L., Abd El-Aal, W. E., & Abbas, N. F. (2015). Tumor-associated macrophage (TAM) and angiogenesis in human colon carcinoma. *Macedonian Journal of Medical Sciences*, *3*(2), 209–214. Available from https://doi.org/10.3889/oamjms.2015.044.

Bingle, L., Brown, N. J., & Lewis, C. E. (2002). The role of tumour-associated macrophages in tumour progression: Implications for new anticancer therapies. *Journal of Pathology*, *196*(3), 254–265. Available from https://doi.org/10.1002/path.1027.

Birge, R. B., Boeltz, S., Kumar, S., Carlson, J., Wanderley, J., Calianese, D., Barcinski, M., Brekken, R. A., Huang, X., Hutchins, J. T., Freimark, B., Empig, C., Mercer, J., Schroit, A. J., Schett, G., & Herrmann, M. (2016). Phosphatidylserine is a global immunosuppressive signal in efferocytosis, infectious disease, and cancer. *Cell Death and Differentiation*, *23*(6), 962–978. Available from https://doi.org/10.1038/cdd.2016.11.

Bonollo, F., Thalmann, G. N., Julio, M. K. D., & Karkampouna, S. (2020). The role of cancer-associated fibroblasts in prostate cancer tumorigenesis. *Cancers*, *12*(7), 1–28. Available from https://doi.org/10.3390/cancers12071887.

Bostwick, D. G., Burke, H. B., Djakiew, D., Euling, S., Ho, S. M., Landolph, J., Morrison, H., Sonawane, B., Shifflett, T., Waters, D. J., & Timms, B. (2004). Human prostate cancer risk factors. *Cancer*, *101*(10), 2371–2490. Available from https://doi.org/10.1002/cncr.20408.

Bray, F., Ferlay, J., Soerjomataram, I., Siegel, R. L., Torre, L. A., & Jemal, A. (2018). Global cancer statistics 2018: GLOBOCAN estimates of incidence and mortality worldwide for 36 cancers in 185 countries. *CA Cancer Journal for Clinicians*, *68*(6), 394–424. Available from https://doi.org/10.3322/caac.21492.

Cao, J., Liu, J., Xu, R., Zhu, X., Zhao, X., & Qian, B. Z. (2017). Prognostic role of tumour-associated macrophages and macrophage scavenger receptor 1 in prostate cancer: A systematic review and meta-analysis. *Oncotarget*, *8*(47), 83261–83269. Available from https://doi.org/10.18632/oncotarget.18743.

Cha, H. R., Lee, J. H., Hensel, J. A., Sawant, A. B., Davis, B. H., Lee, C. M., Deshane, J. S., & Ponnazhagan, S. (2016). Prostate cancer-derived cathelicidin-related antimicrobial peptide facilitates macrophage differentiation and polarization of immature myeloid progenitors to protumorigenic macrophages. *The Prostate*, *76*(7), 624–636. Available from https://doi.org/10.1002/pros.23155.

Chalhoub, N., & Baker, S. J. (2009). PTEN and the PI3-kinase pathway in cancer. *Annual Review of Pathology: Mechanisms of Disease*, *4*, 127–150. Available from https://doi.org/10.1146/annurev.pathol.4.110807.092311.

Chen, C. Y., Chen, J., He, L., & Stiles, B. L. (2018). PTEN: Tumor suppressor and metabolic regulator. *Frontiers in Endocrinology*, 9. Available from https://doi.org/10.3389/fendo.2018.00338.

Chen, P. C., Cheng, H. C., Wang, J., Wang, S. W., Tai, H. C., Lin, C. W., & Tang, C. H. (2014). Prostate cancer-derived CCN3 induces M2 macrophage infiltration and contributes to angiogenesis in prostate cancer microenvironment. *Oncotarget*, *5*(6), 1595–1608. Available from https://doi.org/10.18632/oncotarget.1570.

Chung, L. W. K., Baseman, A., Assikis, V., & Zhau, H. E. (2005). Molecular insights into prostate cancer progression: The missing link of tumor microenvironment. *Journal of Urology*, *173*(1), 10–20. Available from https://doi.org/10.1097/01.ju.0000141582.15218.10.

Comito, G., Giannoni, E., Segura, C. P., Barcellos-De-Souza, P., Raspollini, M. R., Baroni, G., Lanciotti, M., Serni, S., & Chiarugi, P. (2014). Cancer-associated fibroblasts and M2-polarized macrophages synergize during prostate carcinoma progression. *Oncogene*, *33*(19), 2423–2431. Available from https://doi.org/10.1038/onc.2013.191.

Comito, G., Segura, C. P., Taddei, M. L., Lanciotti, M., Serni, S., Morandi, A., Chiarugi, P., & Giannoni, E. (2017). Zoledronic acid impairs stromal reactivity by inhibiting M2-macrophages polarization and prostate cancer-associated fibroblasts. *Oncotarget*, *8*(1), 118–132. Available from https://doi.org/10.18632/oncotarget.9497.

Coussens, L. M., & Werb, Z. (2002). Inflammation and cancer. *Nature*, *420*(6917), 860–867. Available from https://doi.org/10.1038/nature01322.

Crusz, S. M., & Balkwill, F. R. (2015). Inflammation and cancer: Advances and new agents. *Nature Reviews Clinical Oncology*, *12*(10), 584–596. Available from https://doi.org/10.1038/nrclinonc.2015.105.

Culig, Z., & Puhr, M. (2012). Interleukin-6: A multifunctional targetable cytokine in human prostate cancer. *Molecular and Cellular Endocrinology*, *360*(1–2), 52–58. Available from https://doi.org/10.1016/j.mce.2011.05.033.

Curiel, T. J., Coukos, G., Zou, L., Alvarez, X., Cheng, P., Mottram, P., Evdemon-Hogan, M., Conejo-Garcia, J. R., Zhang, L., Burow, M., Zhu, Y., Wei, S., Kryczek, I., Daniel, B., Gordon, A., Myers, L., Lackner, A., Disis, M. L., Knutson, K. L., & Zou, W. (2004). Specific recruitment of regulatory T cells in ovarian carcinoma fosters immune privilege and predicts reduced survival. *Nature Medicine*, *10*(9), 942–949. Available from https://doi.org/10.1038/nm1093.

Dagnelie, P. C., Schuurman, A. G., Goldbohm, R. A., & Van Den Brandt, P. A. (2004). Diet, anthropometric measures and prostate cancer risk: A review of prospective cohort and intervention studies. *BJU International*, *93*(8), 1139–1150. Available from https://doi.org/10.1111/j.1464-410X.2004.04795.x.

Dai, J., Lu, Y., Roca, H., Keller, J. M., Zhang, J., McCauley, L. K., & Keller, E. T. (2017). Immune mediators in the tumor microenvironment of prostate cancer. *Chinese Journal of Cancer*, *36*(1). Available from https://doi.org/10.1186/s40880-017-0198-3.

De Marzo, A. M., Meeker, A. K., Zha, S., Luo, J., Nakayama, M., Platz, E. A., Isaacs, W. B., & Nelson, W. G. (2003). Human prostate cancer precursors and pathobiology. *Urology*, *62*(5), 55–62. Available from https://doi.org/10.1016/j.urology.2003.09.053.

De Marzo, A. M., Platz, E. A., Sutcliffe, S., Xu, J., Grönberg, H., Drake, C. G., Nakai, Y., Isaacs, W. B., & Nelson, W. G. (2007). Inflammation in prostate carcinogenesis. *Nature Reviews. Cancer*, *7*(4), 256–269. Available from https://doi.org/10.1038/nrc2090.

De Visser, K. E., Eichten, A., & Coussens, L. M. (2006). Paradoxical roles of the immune system during cancer development. *Nature Reviews. Cancer*, *6*(1), 24–37. Available from https://doi.org/10.1038/nrc1782.

Di Mitri, D., Mirenda, M., Vasilevska, J., Calcinotto, A., Delaleu, N., Revandkar, A., Gil, V., Boysen, G., Losa, M., Mosole, S., Pasquini, E., D'Antuono, R., Masetti, M., Zagato, E., Chiorino, G., Ostano, P., Rinaldi, A., Gnetti, L., Graupera, M., & Alimonti, A. (2019).

Re-education of tumor-associated macrophages by CXCR2 blockade drives senescence and tumor inhibition in advanced prostate cancer. *Cell Reports*, *28*(8), 2156–2168.e5. Available from https://doi.org/10.1016/j.celrep.2019.07.068.

Danilin, S., Merkel, A. R., Johnson, J. R., Johnson, R. W., Edwards, J. R., & Sterling, J. A. (2012). Myeloid-derived suppressor cells expand during breast cancer progression and promote tumor-induced bone destruction. *OncoImmunology*, *1*(9), 1484–1494. Available from https://doi.org/10.4161/onci.21990.

Doktorova, H., Hrabeta, J., Khalil, M. A., & Eckschlager, T. (2015). Hypoxia-induced chemoresistance in cancer cells: The role of not only HIF-1. *Biomedical Papers*, *159*(2), 166–177. Available from https://doi.org/10.5507/bp.2015.025.

Drake, J. M., Strohbehn, G., Bair, T. B., Moreland, J. G., & Henry, M. D. (2009). ZEB1 enhances transendothelial migration and represses the epithelial phenotype of prostate cancer cells. *Molecular Biology of the Cell*, *20*(8), 2207–2217. Available from https://doi.org/10.1091/mbc.E08-10-1076.

Ellis, P. D., Metcalfe, J. C., Hyvönen, M., & Kemp, P. R. (2003). Adhesion of endothelial cells to NOV is mediated by the integrins αvβ3 and α5β1. *Journal of Vascular Research*, *40*(3), 234–243. Available from https://doi.org/10.1159/000071887.

Erlandsson, A., Carlsson, J., Lundholm, M., Fält, A., Andersson, S. O., Andrén, O., & Davidsson, S. (2019). M2 macrophages and regulatory T cells in lethal prostate cancer. *The Prostate*, *79*(4), 363–369. Available from https://doi.org/10.1002/pros.23742.

Erler, J. T., Bennewith, K. L., Cox, T. R., Lang, G., Bird, D., Koong, A., Le, Q. T., & Giaccia, A. J. (2009). Hypoxia-induced lysyl oxidase is a critical mediator of bone marrow cell recruitment to form the premetastatic niche. *Cancer Cell*, *15*(1), 35–44. Available from https://doi.org/10.1016/j.ccr.2008.11.012.

Ershler, W. B., Harman, S. M., & Keller, E. T. (1997). Immunologic aspects of osteoporosis. *Developmental and Comparative Immunology*, *21*(6), 487–499. Available from https://doi.org/10.1016/S0145-305X(97)00029-3.

Escamilla, J., Schokrpur, S., Liu, C., Priceman, S. J., Moughon, D., Jiang, Z., Pouliot, F., Magyar, C., Sung, J. L., Xu, J., Deng, G., West, B. L., Bollag, G., Fradet, Y., Lacombe, L., Jung, M. E., Huang, J., & Wu, L. (2015). CSF1 receptor targeting in prostate cancer reverses macrophage-mediated resistance to androgen blockade therapy. *Cancer Research*, *75*(6), 950–962. Available from https://doi.org/10.1158/0008-5472.CAN-14-0992.

Fan, H. H., Li, L., Zhang, Y. M., Yang, J., Li, M. C., Zeng, F. Y., & Deng, F. (2017). PKCζ in prostate cancer cells represses the recruitment and M2 polarization of macrophages in the prostate cancer microenvironment. *Tumor Biology*, *39*(6). Available from https://doi.org/10.1177/1010428317701442.

Franco, O. E., & Hayward, S. W. (2012). *Targeting the tumor stroma as a novel therapeutic approach for prostate cancer. Advances in Pharmacology* (Vol. 65, pp. 267–313). Academic Press Inc. Available from https://doi.org/10.1016/B978-0-12-397927-8.00009-9.

Garg, R., Benedetti, L. G., Abera, M. B., Wang, H., Abba, M., & Kazanietz, M. G. (2014). Protein kinase C and cancer: What we know and what we do not. *Oncogene*, *33*(45), 5225–5237. Available from https://doi.org/10.1038/onc.2013.524.

Gilkes, D. M., Semenza, G. L., & Wirtz, D. (2014). Hypoxia and the extracellular matrix: Drivers of tumour metastasis. *Nature Reviews Cancer*, *14*(6), 430–439. Available from https://doi.org/10.1038/nrc3726.

Gollapudi, K., Galet, C., Grogan, T., Zhang, H., Said, J. W., Huang, J., Elashoff, D., Freedland, S. J., Rettig, M., & Aronson, W. J. (2013). Association between tumor-associated macrophage infiltration, high grade prostate cancer, and biochemical recurrence after radical prostatectomy. *American Journal of Cancer Research, 3*(5), 523–529.

Gomes, F. G., Nedel, F., Alves, A. M., Nör, J. E., & Tarquinio, S. B. C. (2013). Tumor angiogenesis and lymphangiogenesis: Tumor/endothelial crosstalk and cellular/microenvironmental signaling mechanisms. *Life Sciences, 92*(2), 101–107. Available from https://doi.org/10.1016/j.lfs.2012.10.008.

Guan, W., Hu, J., Yang, L., Tan, P., Tang, Z., West, B. L., Bollag, G., Xu, H., & Wu, L. (2019). Inhibition of TAMs improves the response to docetaxel in castration-resistant prostate cancer. *Endocrine-Related Cancer, 26*(1), 131–140. Available from https://doi.org/10.1530/ERC-18-0284.

Gupta, G. P., & Massagué, J. (2006). Cancer metastasis: Building a framework. *Cell, 127*(4), 679–695. Available from https://doi.org/10.1016/j.cell.2006.11.001.

Gurel, B., Lucia, M. S., Thompson, I. M., Goodman, P. J., Tangen, C. M., Kristal, A. R., Parnes, H. L., Hoque, A., Lippman, S. M., Sutcliffe, S., Peskoe, S. B., Drake, C. G., Nelson, W. G., De Marzo, A. M., & Platz, E. A. (2014). Chronic inflammation in benign prostate tissue is associated with high-grade prostate cancer in the placebo arm of the prostate cancer prevention trial. *Cancer Epidemiology Biomarkers and Prevention, 23*(5), 847–856. Available from https://doi.org/10.1158/1055-9965.EPI-13-1126.

Hagemann, T., Wilson, J., Kulbe, H., Li, N. F., Leinster, D. A., Charles, K., Klemm, F., Pukrop, T., Binder, C., & Balkwill, F. R. (2005). Macrophages induce invasiveness of epithelial cancer cells via NF-κB and JNK. *Journal of Immunology, 175*(2), 1197–1205. Available from https://doi.org/10.4049/jimmunol.175.2.1197.

Hanahan, D., & Weinberg, R. A. (2000). The hallmarks of cancer. *Cell, 100*(1), 57–70. Available from https://doi.org/10.1016/S0092-8674(00)81683-9.

Hao, N. B., Lü, M. H., Fan, Y. H., Cao, Y. L., Zhang, Z. R., & Yang, S. M. (2012). Macrophages in tumor microenvironments and the progression of tumors. *Clinical and Developmental Immunology*, 2012. Available from https://doi.org/10.1155/2012/948098.

Hao, Q., Vadgama, J. V., & Wang, P. (2020). CCL2/CCR2 signaling in cancer pathogenesis. *Cell Communication and Signaling, 18*(1). Available from https://doi.org/10.1186/s12964-020-00589-8.

Holohan, C., Van Schaeybroeck, S., Longley, D. B., & Johnston, P. G. (2013). Cancer drug resistance: An evolving paradigm. *Nature Reviews. Cancer, 13*(10), 714–726. Available from https://doi.org/10.1038/nrc3599.

Hu, W., Qian, Y., Yu, F., Liu, W., Wu, Y., Fang, X., & Hao, W. (2015). Alternatively activated macrophages are associated with metastasis and poor prognosis in prostate adenocarcinoma. *Oncology Letters, 10*(3), 1390–1396. Available from https://doi.org/10.3892/ol.2015.3400.

Hume, D. A. (2008). Differentiation and heterogeneity in the mononuclear phagocyte system. *Mucosal Immunology, 1*(6), 432–441. Available from https://doi.org/10.1038/mi.2008.36.

Hussein, M. R. A., AL-Assiri, M., & Musalam, A. O. (2009). Phenotypic characterization of the infiltrating immune cells in normal prostate, benign nodular prostatic hyperplasia and prostatic adenocarcinoma. *Experimental and Molecular Pathology, 86*(2), 108–113. Available from https://doi.org/10.1016/j.yexmp.2008.11.010.

Ireland, L., Santos, A., Ahmed, M. S., Rainer, C., Nielsen, S. R., Quaranta, V., Weyer-Czernilofsky, U., Engle, D. D., Perez-Mancera, P. A., Coupland, S. E., Taktak, A., Bogenrieder, T., Tuveson, D. A., Campbell, F., Schmid, M. C., & Mielgo, A. (2016). Chemoresistance in pancreatic cancer is driven by stroma-derived insulin-like growth factors. *Cancer Research, 76*(23), 6851–6863. Available from https://doi.org/10.1158/0008-5472.CAN-16-1201.

Jinushi, M., Sato, M., Kanamoto, A., Itoh, A., Nagai, S., Koyasu, S., Dranoff, G., & Tahara, H. (2009). Milk fat globule epidermal growth factor-8 blockade triggers tumor destruction through coordinated cell-autonomous and immune-mediated mechanisms. *Journal of Experimental Medicine*, *206*(6), 1317–1326. Available from https://doi.org/10.1084/jem.20082614.

Kaplan, R. N., Riba, R. D., Zacharoulis, S., Bramley, A. H., Vincent, L., Costa, C., MacDonald, D. D., Jin, D. K., Shido, K., Kerns, S. A., Zhu, Z., Hicklin, D., Wu, Y., Port, J. L., Altorki, N., Port, E. R., Ruggero, D., Shmelkov, S. V., Jensen, K. K., & Lyden, D. (2005). VEGFR1-positive haematopoietic bone marrow progenitors initiate the pre-metastatic niche. *Nature*, *438*(7069), 820–827. Available from https://doi.org/10.1038/nature04186.

Kim, J. Y., Valencia, T., Abu-Baker, S., Linares, J., Lee, S. J., Yajima, T., Chen, J., Eroshkin, A., Castilla, E. A., Brill, L. M., Medvedovic, M., Leitges, M., Moscat, J., & Diaz-Meco, M. T. (2013). C-Myc phosphorylation by PKCζ represses prostate tumorigenesis. *Proceedings of the National Academy of Sciences of the United States of America*, *110*(16), 6418–6423. Available from https://doi.org/10.1073/pnas.1221799110.

Kim, S., Takahashi, H., Lin, W. W., Descargues, P., Grivennikov, S., Kim, Y., Luo, J. L., & Karin, M. (2009). Carcinoma-produced factors activate myeloid cells through TLR2 to stimulate metastasis. *Nature*, *457*(7225), 102–106. Available from https://doi.org/10.1038/nature07623.

Knudsen, B. S., & Vasioukhin, V. (2010). *Mechanisms of prostate cancer initiation and progression. Advances in Cancer Research* (Vol. 109, C, pp. 1–50). Academic Press Inc. Available from https://doi.org/10.1016/B978-0-12-380890-5.00001-6.

Kortylewski, M., Xin, H., Kujawski, M., Lee, H., Liu, Y., Harris, T., Drake, C., Pardoll, D., & Yu, H. (2009). Regulation of the IL-23 and IL-12 balance by Stat3 signaling in the tumor microenvironment. *Cancer Cell*, *15*(2), 114–123. Available from https://doi.org/10.1016/j.ccr.2008.12.018.

Kreso, A., & Dick, J. E. (2014). Evolution of the cancer stem cell model. *Cell Stem Cell*, *14*(3), 275–291. Available from https://doi.org/10.1016/j.stem.2014.02.006.

Krzyszczyk, P., Schloss, R., Palmer, A., & Berthiaume, F. (2018). The role of macrophages in acute and chronic wound healing and interventions to promote pro-wound healing phenotypes. *Frontiers in Physiology*, *9*. Available from https://doi.org/10.3389/fphys.2018.00419.

Kuang, D. M., Zhao, Q., Peng, C., Xu, J., Zhang, J. P., Wu, C., & Zheng, L. (2009). Activated monocytes in peritumoral stroma of hepatocellular carcinoma foster immune privilege and disease progression through PD-L1. *Journal of Experimental Medicine*, *206*(6), 1327–1337. Available from https://doi.org/10.1084/jem.20082173.

Kumar, A., Vishvakarma, N. K., Bharti, A. C., & Singh, S. M. (2012). Gender-specific antitumor action of aspirin in a murine model of a T-cell lymphoma bearing host. *Blood Cells, Molecules and Diseases*, *48*(2), 137–144. Available from https://doi.org/10.1016/j.bcmd.2011.10.006.

Lanciotti, M., Masieri, L., Raspollini, M. R., Minervini, A., Mari, A., Comito, G., Giannoni, E., Carini, M., Chiarugi, P., & Serni, S. (2014). The role of M1 and M2 macrophages in prostate cancer in relation to extracapsular tumor extension and biochemical recurrence after radical prostatectomy. *BioMed Research International*, 2014. Available from https://doi.org/10.1155/2014/486798.

Lee, G. T., Kim, J. H., Kwon, S. J., Stein, M. N., Hong, J. H., Nagaya, N., Billakanti, S., Kim, M. M., Kim, W. J., & Kim, I. Y. (2019). Dihydrotestosterone increases cytotoxic activity of macrophages on prostate cancer cells via trail. *Endocrinology*, *160*(9), 2049–2060. Available from https://doi.org/10.1210/en.2019-00367.

Li, N., Qin, J., Lan, L., Zhang, H., Liu, F., Wu, Z., Ni, H., & Wang, Y. (2015). PTEN inhibits macrophage polarization from M1 to M2 through CCL2 and VEGF-A reduction and NHERF-1 synergism. *Cancer Biology and Therapy*, *16*(2), 297–306. Available from https://doi.org/10.1080/15384047.2014.1002353.

Li, X., Loberg, R., Liao, J., Ying, C., Snyder, L. A., Pienta, K. J., & McCauley, L. K. (2009). A destructive cascade mediated by CCL2 facilitates prostate cancer growth in bone. *Cancer Research*, *69*(4), 1685–1692. Available from https://doi.org/10.1158/0008-5472.CAN-08-2164.

Lin, C. G., Leu, S. J., Chen, N., Tebeau, C. M., Lin, S. X., Yeung, C. Y., & Lau, L. F. (2003). CCN3 (NOV) is a novel angiogenic regulator of the CCN protein family. *Journal of Biological Chemistry*, *278*(26), 24200–24208. Available from https://doi.org/10.1074/jbc.M302028200.

Lissbrant, I. F., Stattin, P., Wikstrom, P., Damber, J. E., Egevad, L., & Bergh, A. (2000). Tumor associated macrophages in human prostate cancer: Relation to clinicopathological variables and survival. *International Journal of Oncology*, *17*(3), 445–451. Available from https://doi.org/10.3892/ijo.17.3.445.

Liu, J., Ding, D., Jiang, Z., Du, T., Liu, J., & Kong, Z. (2019). Long non-coding RNA CCAT1/miR-148a/PKCζ prevents cell migration of prostate cancer by altering macrophage polarization. *The Prostate*, *79*(1), 105–112. Available from https://doi.org/10.1002/pros.23716.

Lo, C. H., & Lynch, C. C. (2018). Multifaceted roles for macrophages in prostate cancer skeletal metastasis. *Frontiers in Endocrinology*, *9*. Available from https://doi.org/10.3389/fendo.2018.00247.

Loberg, R. D., Day, L. S. L., Harwood, J., Ying, C., St., John, L. N., Giles, R., Neeley, C. K., & Pienta, K. J. (2006). CCL2 is a potent regulator of prostate cancer cell migration and proliferation. *Neoplasia (New York, N.Y.)*, *8*(7), 578–586. Available from https://doi.org/10.1593/neo.06280.

Loberg, R. D., Ying, C., Craig, M., Yan, L., Snyder, L. A., & Pienta, K. J. (2007). CCL2 as an important mediator of prostate cancer growth in vivo through the regulation of macrophage infiltration. *Neoplasia (New York, N.Y.)*, *9*(7), 556–562. Available from https://doi.org/10.1593/neo.07307.

Lu, T., Ramakrishnan, R., Altiok, S., Youn, J. I., Cheng, P., Celis, E., Pisarev, V., Sherman, S., Sporn, M. B., & Gabrilovich, D. (2011). Tumor-infiltrating myeloid cells induce tumor cell resistance to cytotoxic T cells in mice. *Journal of Clinical Investigation*, *121*(10), 4015–4029. Available from https://doi.org/10.1172/JCI45862.

Ly, L. V., Baghat, A., Versluis, M., Jordanova, E. S., Luyten, G. P. M., Van Rooijen, N., Van Hall, T., Van Der Velden, P. A., & Jager, M. J. (2010). In aged mice, outgrowth of intraocular melanoma depends on proangiogenic M2-type macrophages. *Journal of Immunology*, *185*(6), 3481–3488. Available from https://doi.org/10.4049/jimmunol.0903479.

Mantovani, A., Allavena, P., Sica, A., & Balkwill, F. (2008). Cancer-related inflammation. *Nature*, *454*(7203), 436–444. Available from https://doi.org/10.1038/nature07205.

Markozannes, G., Tzoulaki, I., Karli, D., Evangelou, E., Ntzani, E., Gunter, M. J., Norat, T., Ioannidis, J. P., & Tsilidis, K. K. (2016). Diet, body size, physical activity and risk of prostate cancer: An umbrella review of the evidence. *European Journal of Cancer*, *69*, 61–69. Available from https://doi.org/10.1016/j.ejca.2016.09.026.

Martinez-Marin, D., Jarvis, C., Nelius, T., De Riese, W., Volpert, O. V., & Filleur, S. (2017). PEDF increases the tumoricidal activity of macrophages towards prostate cancer cells in vitro. *PLoS One*, *12*(4). Available from https://doi.org/10.1371/journal.pone.0174968.

McKeage, K., & Plosker, G. L. (2008). Zoledronic acid: A pharmacoeconomic review of its use in the management of bone metastases. *Pharmacoeconomics*, *26*(3), 251–268. Available from https://doi.org/10.2165/00019053-200826030-00007.

Mehta, A. R., & Armstrong, A. J. (2016). Tasquinimod in the treatment of castrate-resistant prostate cancer – current status and future prospects. *Therapeutic Advances in Urology*, *8* (1), 9–18. Available from https://doi.org/10.1177/1756287215603558.

Meira, L. B., Bugni, J. M., Green, S. L., Lee, C. W., Pang, B., Borenshtein, D., Rickman, B. H., Rogers, A. B., Moroski-Erkul, C. A., McFaline, J. L., Schauer, D. B., Dedon, P. C., Fox, J. G., & Samson, L. D. (2008). DNA damage induced by chronic inflammation contributes to colon carcinogenesis in mice. *Journal of Clinical Investigation*, *118*(7), 2516–2525. Available from https://doi.org/10.1172/JC135073.

Mevorach, D., Trahtemberg, U., Krispin, A., Attalah, M., Zazoun, J., Tabib, A., Grau, A., & Verbovetski-Reiner, I. (2010). What do we mean when we write \senescence,\\apoptosis,\ \necrosis,\ or \clearance of dying cells\? *Annals of the New York Academy of Sciences*, *1209* (1), 1–9. Available from https://doi.org/10.1111/j.1749-6632.2010.05774.x.

Mitchem, J. B., Brennan, D. J., Knolhoff, B. L., Belt, B. A., Zhu, Y., Sanford, D. E., Belaygorod, L., Carpenter, D., Collins, L., Piwnica-Worms, D., Hewitt, S., Udupi, G. M., Gallagher, W. M., Wegner, C., West, B. L., Wang-Gillam, A., Goedegebuure, P., Linehan, D. C., & DeNardo, D. G. (2013). Targeting tumor-infiltrating macrophages decreases tumor-initiating cells, relieves immunosuppression, and improves chemotherapeutic responses. *Cancer Research*, *73*(3), 1128–1141. Available from https://doi.org/10.1158/0008-5472.CAN-12-2731.

Mizutani, K., Sud, S., McGregor, N. A., Martinovski, G., Rice, B. T., Craig, M. J., Varsos, Z. S., Roca, H., & Pienta, K. J. (2009). The chemokine CCL2 increases prostate tumor growth and bone metastasis through macrophage and osteoclast recruitment. *Neoplasia (New York, N. Y.)*, *11*(11), 1235–1242. Available from https://doi.org/10.1593/neo.09988.

Muthana, M., Giannoudis, A., Scott, S. D., Fang, H. Y., Coffelt, S. B., Morrow, F. J., Murdoch, C., Burton, J., Cross, N., Burke, B., Mistry, R., Hamdy, F., Brown, N. J., Georgopoulos, L., Hoskin, P., Essand, M., Lewis, C. E., & Maitland, N. J. (2011). Use of macrophages to target therapeutic adenovirus to human prostate tumors. *Cancer Research*, *71*(5), 1805–1815. Available from https://doi.org/10.1158/0008-5472.CAN-10-2349.

Nguyen, K. G., Vrabel, M. R., Mantooth, S. M., Hopkins, J. J., Wagner, E. S., Gabaldon, T. A., & Zaharoff, D. A. (2020). Localized interleukin-12 for cancer immunotherapy. *Frontiers in Immunology*, 11. Available from https://doi.org/10.3389/fimmu.2020.575597.

Pang, B., Zhou, X., Yu, H., Dong, M., Taghizadeh, K., Wishnok, J. S., Tannenbaum, S. R., & Dedon, P. C. (2007). Lipid peroxidation dominates the chemistry of DNA adduct formation in a mouse model of inflammation. *Carcinogenesis*, *28*(8), 1807–1813. Available from https://doi.org/10.1093/carcin/bgm037.

Patrawala, L., Calhoun, T., Schneider-Broussard, R., Li, H., Bhatia, B., Tang, S., Reilly, J. G., Chandra, D., Zhou, J., Claypool, K., Coghlan, L., & Tang, D. G. (2006). Highly purified CD44 + prostate cancer cells from xenograft human tumors are enriched in tumorigenic and metastatic progenitor cells. *Oncogene*, *25*(12), 1696–1708. Available from https://doi.org/10.1038/sj.onc.1209327.

Phi, L. T. H., Sari, I. N., Yang, Y. G., Lee, S. H., Jun, N., Kim, K. S., Lee, Y. K., & Kwon, H. Y. (2018). Cancer stem cells (CSCs) in drug resistance and their therapeutic implications in cancer treatment. *Stem Cells International*, 2018. Available from https://doi.org/10.1155/2018/5416923.

Plaks, V., Kong, N., & Werb, Z. (2015). The cancer stem cell niche: How essential is the niche in regulating stemness of tumor cells? *Cell Stem Cell, 16*(3), 225–238. Available from https://doi.org/10.1016/j.stem.2015.02.015.

Qian, B. Z., & Pollard, J. W. (2010). Macrophage diversity enhances tumor progression and metastasis. *Cell, 141*(1), 39–51. Available from https://doi.org/10.1016/j.cell.2010.03.014.

Quail, D. F., & Joyce, J. A. (2017). Molecular pathways: Deciphering mechanisms of resistance to macrophage-targeted therapies. *Clinical Cancer Research, 23*(4), 876–884. Available from https://doi.org/10.1158/1078-0432.CCR-16-0133.

Rajput, S., & Wilber, A. (2010). Roles of inflammation in cancer initiation, progression, and metastasis. *Frontiers in Bioscience - Scholar, 2*(1), 176–183. Available from http://www.bioscience.org/fbs/getfile.php?FileName = /2010/v2s/af/55/55.pdf.

Riabov, V., Gudima, A., Wang, N., Mickley, A., Orekhov, A., & Kzhyshkowska, J. (2014). Role of tumor associated macrophages in tumor angiogenesis and lymphangiogenesis. *Frontiers in Physiology*, 5. Available from https://doi.org/10.3389/fphys.2014.00075.

Rothlin, C. V., & Lemke, G. (2010). TAM receptor signaling and autoimmune disease. *Current Opinion in Immunology, 22*(6), 740–746. Available from https://doi.org/10.1016/j.coi.2010.10.001.

Sagnak, L., Topaloglu, H., Ozok, U., & Ersoy, H. (2011). Prognostic significance of neuroendocrine differentiation in prostate adenocarcinoma. *Clinical Genitourinary Cancer, 9*(2), 73–80. Available from https://doi.org/10.1016/j.clgc.2011.07.003.

Sainz, B., Carron, E., Vallespinós, M., & Machado, H. L. (2016). Cancer stem cells and macrophages: Implications in tumor biology and therapeutic strategies. *Mediators of Inflammation*, 2016. Available from https://doi.org/10.1155/2016/9012369.

Satoh, T., Saika, T., Ebara, S., Kusaka, N., Timme, T. L., Yang, G., Wang, J., Mouraviev, V., Cao, G., Fattah, E. M. A., & Thompson, T. C. (2003). Macrophages transduced with an adenoviral vector expressing interleukin 12 suppress tumor growth and metastasis in a preclinical metastatic prostate cancer model. *Cancer Research, 63*(22), 7853–7860.

Schmitz, P., Gerber, U., Juügel, E., Schuťze, N., Blaheta, R., & Bendas, G. (2013). Cyr61/CCN1 affects the integrin-mediated migration of prostate cancer cells (PC-3) in vitro. *International Journal of Clinical Pharmacology and Therapeutics, 51*(1), 47–50. Available from https://doi.org/10.5414/CPP51047.

Shen, L., & Pili, R. (2019). Tasquinimod targets suppressive myeloid cells in the tumor microenvironment. *OncoImmunology, 8*(10). Available from https://doi.org/10.1080/2162402X.2015.1072672.

Shen, L., Sundstedt, A., Ciesielski, M., Miles, K. M., Celander, M., Adelaiye, R., Orillion, A., Ciamporcero, E., Ramakrishnan, S., Ellis, L., Fenstermaker, R., Abrams, S. I., Eriksson, H., Leanderson, T., Olsson, A., & Pili, R. (2015). Tasquinimod modulates suppressive myeloid cells and enhances cancer immunotherapies in murine models. *Cancer Immunology Research, 3*(2), 136–148. Available from https://doi.org/10.1158/2326-6066.CIR-14-0036.

Shiao, S. L., Chu, G. C. Y., & Chung, L. W. K. (2016). Regulation of prostate cancer progression by the tumor microenvironment. *Cancer Letters, 380*(1), 340–348. Available from https://doi.org/10.1016/j.canlet.2015.12.022.

Shieh, Y. S., Hung, Y. J., Hsieh, C. B., Chen, J. S., Chou, K. C., & Liu, S. Y. (2009). Tumor-associated macrophage correlated with angiogenesis and progression of mucoepidermoid carcinoma of salivary glands. *Annals of Surgical Oncology, 16*(3), 751–760. Available from https://doi.org/10.1245/s10434-008-0259-6.

Soki, F. N., Cho, S. W., Kim, Y. W., Jones, J. D., Park, S. I., Koh, A. J., Entezami, P., Daignault-Newton, S., Pienta, K. J., Roca, H., & McCauley, L. K. (2015). Bone marrow macrophages support prostate cancer growth in bone. *Oncotarget*, *6*(34), 35782–35796. Available from https://doi.org/10.18632/oncotarget.6042.

Soki, F. N., Koh, A. J., Jones, J. D., Kim, Y. W., Dai, J., Keller, E. T., Pienta, K. J., Atabai, K., Roca, H., & McCauley, L. K. (2014). Polarization of prostate cancer-associated macrophages is induced by milk fat globule-EGF factor 8 (MFG-E8)-mediated efferocytosis. *Journal of Biological Chemistry*, *289*(35), 24560–24572. Available from https://doi.org/10.1074/jbc.M114.571620.

Soni, V. K., Shukla, D., Kumar, A., & Vishvakarma, N. K. (2020). Curcumin circumvent lactate-induced chemoresistance in hepatic cancer cells through modulation of hydroxycarboxylic acid receptor-1. *The International Journal of Biochemistry & Cell Biology*, *123*, 105752. Available from https://doi.org/10.1016/j.biocel.2020.105752.

Tabata, K., Kurosaka, S., Watanabe, M., Edamura, K., Satoh, T., Yang, G., Abdelfattah, E., Wang, J., Goltsov, A., Floryk, D., & Thompson, T. C. (2011). Tumor growth and metastasis suppression by Glipr1 gene-modified macrophages in a metastatic prostate cancer model. *Gene Therapy*, *18*(10), 969–978. Available from https://doi.org/10.1038/gt.2011.51.

Takeya, M., & Komohara, Y. (2016). Role of tumor-associated macrophages in human malignancies: Friend or foe? *Pathology International*, *66*(9), 491–505. Available from https://doi.org/10.1111/pin.12440.

Van Dalen, F. J., Van Stevendaal, M. H. M. E., Fennemann, F. L., Verdoes, M., & Ilina, O. (2019). Molecular repolarisation of tumour-associated macrophages. *Molecules (Basel, Switzerland)*, *24*(1). Available from https://doi.org/10.3390/molecules24010009.

Vandewalle, C., Van Roy, F., & Berx, G. (2009). The role of the ZEB family of transcription factors in development and disease. *Cellular and Molecular Life Sciences*, *66*(5), 773–787. Available from https://doi.org/10.1007/s00018-008-8465-8.

Vishvakarma, N. K. (2014). Novel antitumor mechanisms of curcumin: Implication of altered tumor metabolism, reconstituted tumor microenvironment and augmented myelopoiesis. *Phytochemistry Reviews*, *13*(3), 717–724. Available from https://doi.org/10.1007/s11101-014-9364-2.

Vishvakarma, N. K., Kumar, A., Singh, V., & Singh, S. M. (2013). Hyperglycemia of tumor microenvironment modulates stage-dependent tumor progression and multidrug resistance: Implication of cell survival regulatory molecules and altered glucose transport. *Molecular Carcinogenesis*, *52*(12), 932–945. Available from https://doi.org/10.1002/mc.21922.

Vishvakarma, N. K., & Singh, S. M. (2010). Immunopotentiating effect of proton pump inhibitor pantoprazole in a lymphoma-bearing murine host: Implication in antitumor activation of tumor-associated macrophages. *Immunology Letters*, *134*(1), 83–92. Available from https://doi.org/10.1016/j.imlet.2010.09.002.

Vishvakarma, N. K., & Singh, S. M. (2011). Augmentation of myelopoiesis in a murine host bearing a T cell lymphoma following in vivo administration of proton pump inhibitor pantoprazole. *Biochimie*, *93*(10), 1786–1796. Available from https://doi.org/10.1016/j.biochi.2011.06.022.

Wang, Q., Li, W., Zhang, Y., Yuan, X., Xu, K., Yu, J., Chen, Z., Beroukhim, R., Wang, H., Lupien, M., Wu, T., Regan, M. M., Meyer, C. A., Carroll, J. S., Manrai, A. K., Jänne, O. A., Balk, S. P., Mehra, R., Han, B., & Brown, M. (2009). Androgen receptor regulates a distinct transcription program in androgen-independent prostate cancer. *Cell*, *138*(2), 245–256. Available from https://doi.org/10.1016/j.cell.2009.04.056.

Wang, Z., Xu, L., Hu, Y., Huang, Y., Zhang, Y., Zheng, X., Wang, S., Wang, Y., Yu, Y., Zhang, M., Yuan, K., & Min, W. (2016). MiRNA let-7b modulates macrophage polarization and enhances tumor-associated macrophages to promote angiogenesis and mobility in prostate cancer. *Scientific Reports*, 6. Available from https://doi.org/10.1038/srep25602.

Weigert, A., Mora, J., Sekar, D., Syed, S., & Brüne, B. (2016). Killing is not enough: How apoptosis hijacks tumor-associated macrophages to promote cancer progression. *Advances in Experimental Medicine and Biology*, *930*, 205–239. Available from https://doi.org/10.1007/978-3-319-39406-0_9.

Wu, S. Q., Su, H., Wang, Y. H., & Zhao, X. K. (2019). Role of tumor-associated immune cells in prostate cancer: Angel or devil. *Asian Journal of Andrology*, *21*(5), 433–437. Available from https://doi.org/10.4103/aja.aja_47_19.

Xu, J., Sun, J., Kader, A. K., Lindström, S., Wiklund, F., Hsu, F. C., Johansson, J. E., Zheng, S. L., Thomas, G., Hayes, R. B., Kraft, P., Hunter, D. J., Chanock, S. J., Isaacs, W. B., & Grönberg, H. (2009). Estimation of absolute risk for prostate cancer using genetic markers and family history. *The Prostate*, *69*(14), 1565–1572. Available from https://doi.org/10.1002/pros.21002.

Yang, L., & Zhang, Y. (2017). Tumor-associated macrophages: From basic research to clinical application. *Journal of Hematology & Oncology*, *10*(1), 58. Available from https://doi.org/10.1186/s13045-017-0430-2.

Yin, Y., Huang, X., Lynn, K. D., & Thorpe, P. E. (2013). Phosphatidylserine-targeting antibody induces M1 macrophage polarization and promotes myeloid-derived suppressor cell differentiation. *Cancer Immunology Research*, *1*(4), 256–268. Available from https://doi.org/10.1158/2326-6066.CIR-13-0073.

Zhang, A., Qian, Y., Ye, Z., Chen, H., Xie, H., Zhou, L., Shen, Y., & Zheng, S. (2017). Cancer-associated fibroblasts promote M2 polarization of macrophages in pancreatic ductal adenocarcinoma. *Cancer Medicine*, *6*(2), 463–470. Available from https://doi.org/10.1002/cam4.993.

Zheng, Y., Cai, Z., Wang, S., Zhang, X., Qian, J., Hong, S., Li, H., Wang, M., Yang, J., & Yi, Q. (2009). Macrophages are an abundant component of myeloma microenvironment and protect myeloma cells from chemotherapy drug-induced apoptosis. *Blood*, *114*(17), 3625–3628. Available from https://doi.org/10.1182/blood-2009-05-220285.

Zhou, J., Tang, Z., Gao, S., Li, C., Feng, Y., & Zhou, X. (2020). Tumor-associated macrophages: Recent insights and therapies. *Frontiers in Oncology*, 10. Available from https://doi.org/10.3389/fonc.2020.00188.

Zhu, Q., Han, X., Peng, J., Qin, H., & Wang, Y. (2012). The role of CXC chemokines and their receptors in the progression and treatment of tumors. *Journal of Molecular Histology*, *43*(6), 699–713. Available from https://doi.org/10.1007/s10735-012-9435-x.

Chapter 12

Emerging therapeutic targets of genitourinary tumors

Pramodkumar Pyarelal Gupta[1] and Yassine Kasmi[2]
[1]*School of Biotechnology and Bioinformatics, D Y Patil Deemed to be University, Navi Mumbai, Maharashtra, India,* [2]*Team of Virology, Oncology, and Biotechnologies, Laboratory of Virology, Oncology, Biosciences, Environment and New Energies (LVO-BEEN), Faculty of Sciences and Techniques Mohammedia, University Hassan II of Casablanca, Casablanca, Morocco*

12.1 Introduction

Genitourinary (GU) systems consist of kidneys, ureters, bladder, urethra, and genital organs. A huge mass of patients suffer from a large variety of GU system-based disease and injuries that include many congenital abnormalities, iatrogenic injuries, and disorders such as cancer, trauma, infection, and inflammation. These abnormal causes often implicate or result in the loss of tissue structure or function (Kim et al., 2000).

GU malignancies cover a diverse group of cancers pertaining to a specific anatomical and physiological function (Zarrabi et al., 2019). Renal cell carcinoma (RCC), urothelial carcinoma of the bladder, ureter, and renal pelvis (UC), and prostate adenocarcinoma (PC) are the most commonly encountered histological subtypes within this group (Zarrabi et al., 2019).

The respective number of cases reported for cancer globally for prostate cancer, kidney cancer, bladder cancer, testicular cancer, and penile cancer as per the GLOBOCAN database in 2020 are given in Fig. 12.1.

Metastasis is one of the major obstacles to effective treatment of GU cancers. GU cancer metastases are important targets for scientists and clinicians to drive the discovery of new therapies. Recently, the race to develop new therapeutic solutions, including molecularly targeted agents and immune checkpoint inhibitors, has introduced a radical shift in therapeutic choices for the metastatic stage.

12.2 PD-1

PD-1 is a receptor expressed on the surface of activated T cells, B cells, NKT cells, and dendritic cells, but not on resting T cells (Agata et al., 1996).

Immunological Implications and Molecular Diagnostics of Genitourinary Cancer.
DOI: https://doi.org/10.1016/B978-0-323-85496-2.00005-1

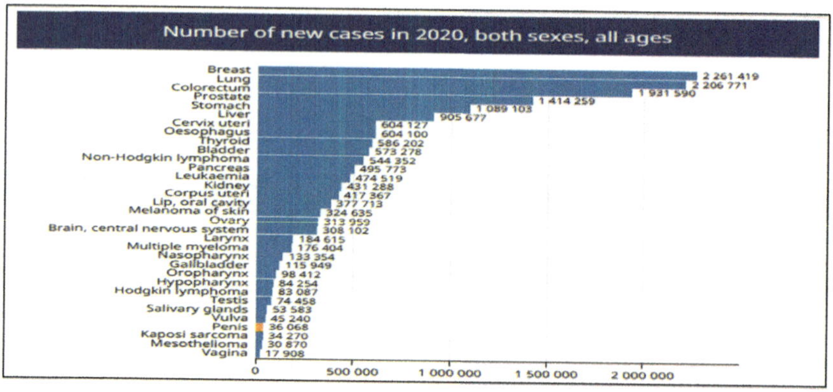

FIGURE 12.1 Global cancer statistics (https://gco.iarc.fr/).

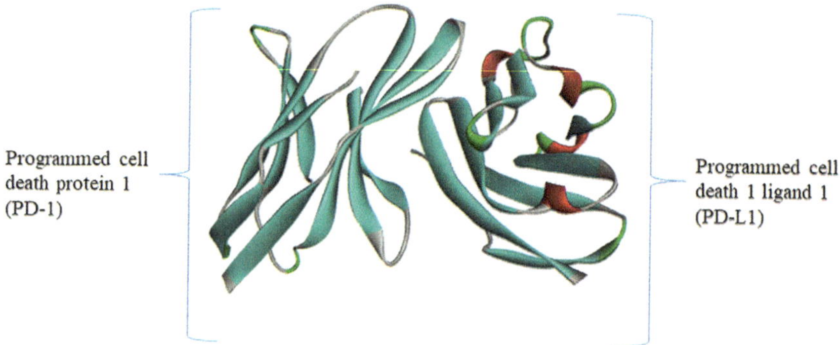

FIGURE 12.2 PD-1and PD-L-1 complex 4ZQK.pdb.

The link between the PD-1 receptor with ligands PD-L1, Fig. 12.2 (also called B7-H1 and CD274) and PD-L2 (also B7-DC and CD273) introduces inhibition of T-cell function. PD-L1 is also a ligand for CD80. Unlike PD-L2, PD-L1 is constitutively expressed and can be further upregulated by inflammatory mediators such as IFN-α,-β, and -γ (Butte et al., 2007; Keir et al., 2007). The proportion of PD-1 positive immune cells in the tumor environment varies from 0% in chondrosarcoma to 93% in ovarian tumors.

A pair of receptor-ligands, PD-1/PD-L1 and CD137/CD137L, have recently emerged because of promising results. Through intracellular signaling pathways, these two receptors regulate the activity of T cells, and thus they are involved in the immune response (Driessens et al., 2009). Recent studies by Ostroumov et al. (2018) have shown that the expression of PD-L1 leads to the introduction of apoptosis of cytotoxic T cells and the increase of regulatory T cells in favor of cancer cells (Ostroumov et al., 2018). In the same context, Chalfin et al. (2021) showed that shorter survival may be associated with a high number of CTCs at baseline, the presence of specific morphological subtypes of CTCs, PD-L1þ CTCs, and a low percentage of CD4/8 T cells in patients with metastatic GU cancer.

The PD-L1 antibody avelumab (Bavencio, Merck KgaA) (Dirix et al., 2018; Kim, 2017; Shirley, 2018) received accelerated US-FDA approval in spring 2017 after significant success in the JAVELIN solid tumor trial (Heery et al., 2017; Kaufman et al., 2016). Anti-CD137 antibodies such as urelumab (Bristol-Myers Squibb) (Segal et al., 2017; Timmerman et al., 2020) and utomilumab (Pfizer) (Chiappori et al., 2020; Gopal et al., 2020) are in clinical trials.

Although there have been significant results of the PD-L1 antibody avelumab (Bavencio, Merck KgaA) in several tumor types, including melanoma, nonsmall cell lung cancer, bladder cancer, kidney cancer, etc., the results of the PD-L1 antibody have not been conclusive (Haffner et al., 2018). The therapeutic effect of PD-1/PD-L1 antibodies in prostate cancer remain controversial (Li et al., 2019). The low efficacy of anti-PD-1 immunotherapy can be explained by the prevalence of PD-L1, which varied considerably (between 0% and 92%) in prostate cancer patients (Calagua et al., 2017; Gatalica et al., 2014; Gevensleben et al., 2016).

Analysis of the EspaceNET patent database shows that more than 500 patent applications related to the application of PD-1 in prostate cancer have been filed and validated in the last three years. This explains the importance of this target in the development of inhibitors and diagnostic kits for prostate cancer specifically and for GU cancer in general, especially concerning the metastatic stages. The US has filed over 50% of these patents.

12.3 Von Hippel–Lindau tumor suppressor/HIF2-vascular endothelial growth factor

The von Hippel–Lindau (VHL) gene is located on chromosome 3p25, a region of the genome that is frequently deleted or altered in RCC, linked to VHL disease, Fig. 12.3, and is at increased risk of developing clear cell carcinoma of the kidney, which is the most common histological type of kidney cancer (Maher & Kaelin, 1997). Studies have shown that biallelic mutations in VHL characterize sporadic clear cell renal carcinomas (Kim & Kaelin, 2004).

The VHL protein (pVHL) functions as part of an E3 ubiquitin ligase that ubiquitylates a family of HIF proteins (Iwai et al., 1999). Inhibition or inactivation of pVHL allows HIF to accumulate and move to the nucleus where it acts as a transcription factor and then plays a pro-tumorigenic role (Wiesener et al., 2001).

As shown in the previous paragraph, inactivation of VHL leads to an increase in HIF protein, and thus another target is the HIF gene itself. Multiple Vascular endothelial growth factor (VEGF) inhibitors are now approved for the treatment of RCC, including an HIF2α inhibitor, which has

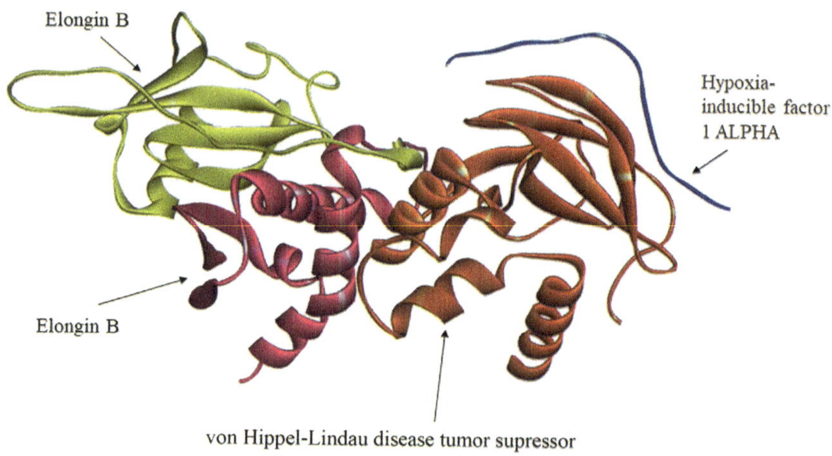

FIGURE 12.3 von Hippel–Lindau protein 1LQB.pdb.

entered the third phase of development for this disease (Choueiri & Kaelin, 2020). Liu et al.'s (2020) menu studies revealed significantly increased expression of SMYD3, SET (suppressor of variegation, enhancer of zeste, trithorax) and MYND (myeloid-Nervy-DEAF-1) domain-containing protein 3 of Epidermal Frowth Factor Receptor (EGFR) in renal cell tumors carrying VHL loss-of-function mutations, of which they showed that HIF-2α has the ability to bind directly to the SMYD3 promoter, which subsequently induces SMYD3 transcription and expression causing and explaining the VHL/HIF-2α/SMYD3 cascade-mediated EGFR hyperactivity through which SMYD3 promotes RCC progression (Liu et al., 2020). Analysis of the EspaceNET patent database shows that more than 500 patent applications relating to the application of PD-1 in prostate cancer have been filed and validated in the last five years. The bulk of the patents essentially deal with the issue of developing antibodies for the induction of metastasis activity in GU cancers. In terms of patent location, the US is in the first place with over 60% of the valid patents, followed by South Korea with 20%.

12.4 Vascular endothelial growth factor receptor

VEGF inhibitors and mTOR inhibitors have been introduced as molecularly targeted drugs in recent years, and drug therapy has changed considerably. An accumulation of HIF-1α leads to an overproduction of VEGF and platelet-derived growth factor (PDGF), which in turn leads to angiogenesis and tumor cell proliferation. This makes targeting VEGF an important pathway in clear cell RCC.

Vascular endothelial growth factor receptor (VEGFR) is a type of receptor tyrosine kinase and is a ligand for VEGFR. VEGFR-1 promotes vascular

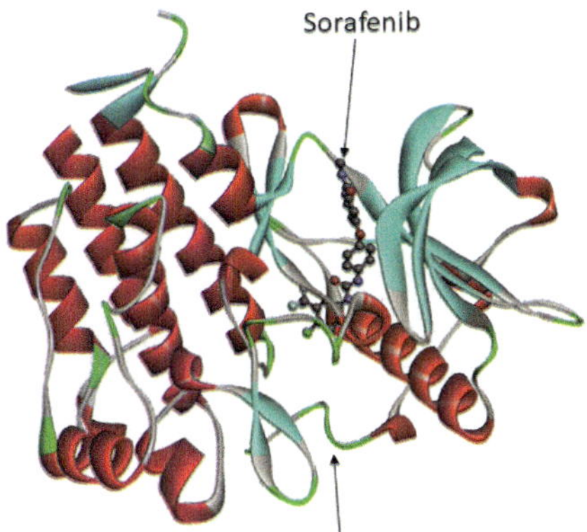

FIGURE 12.4 Vascular endothelial growth factor receptor-2 in complex with Sorafenib, 4ASD.pdb.

endothelial cell proliferation and migration, enhances vascular permeability, activates monospheres, and macrophages, etc., and VEGFR is involved in the expression of these actions. VEGFR-1 and VEGF-2 Fig. 12.4 are expressed in vascular endothelial cells and play a central role in the process of angiogenesis, while VEGF-3 is expressed in lymphatic vessels and is involved in their development. It has also been reported that neurophyllin, a cell membrane protein, has the ability to bind to VEGF165, another splice product of VEGF-A (Soker et al., 1998).

According to Dudek et al. (2020), pembrolizumab + is an anti-VEGF antibody, which is an anti-PD-1 antibody for patients with metastatic clear cell RCC (Dudek et al., 2020). According to the KEYNOTE-427 study, the objective response rate (ORR) of KEYTRUDA alone for untreated metastatic RCC was 33.6%, but the combination with an anti-VEGF antibody is an additional tumor suppressor. The results of this study for patients with the above background are as follows. The ORR of the primary endpoint Phase 1b 41.7% are (95% confidence interval: 15.2%−72.3%) 60.9% in the second phase (95% confidence interval: 45.4%−74.9%) showed that in addition, the distribution of response was partial response (PR) 5 people, stable disease (SD) 6 people in phase 1b, complete response (CR) 1 person, partial response (PR) 25 people, stable disease (SD) in phase 2. There were 18 people.

Currently approved VEGF inhibitors include sorafenib (Nexavar) Fig. 12.3, sunitinib (Sutent), and axitinib (Inwriter), and mTOR inhibitors include everolimus (Affinitol) and temsirolimus (Torisel). Sorafenib is the first targeted drug introduced for kidney cancer, but not only confined to the

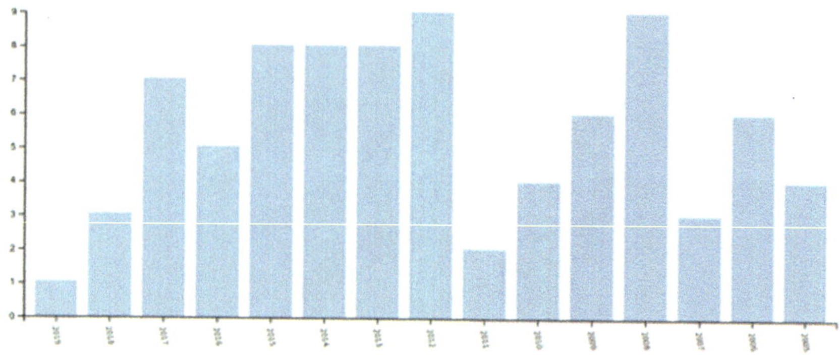

FIGURE 12.5 Evolution of paper published on vascular endothelial growth factor and metastasis in urinary cancers in the Web of Sciences.

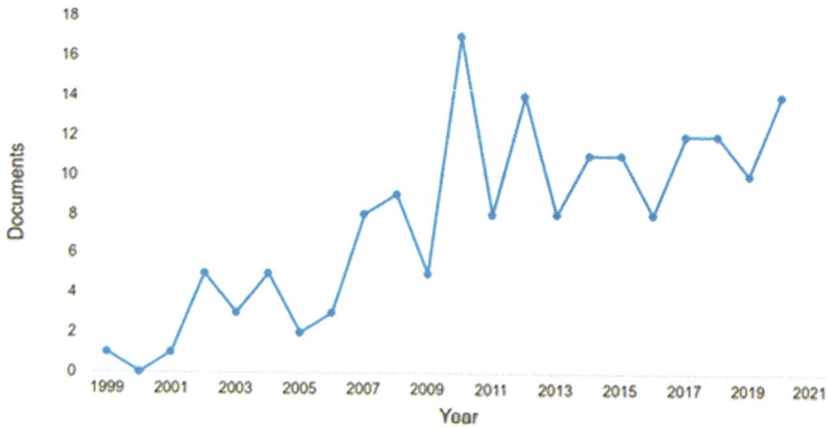

FIGURE 12.6 Evolution of paper published on vascular endothelial growth factor and metastasis in urinary cancers in scopus.

VEGFR and PDGF receptor (PDGFR), but it also shows an potent activity against the Raf kinase, stem cell factor receptor (KIT) and fms-type tyrosine.

Analysis of Scopus and the Web of Sciences databases (see Figs. 12.5 and 12.6) shows that the evolution of VEGD receptor studies in metastatic prostate cancer has been recognized as a significant evolution over the last 5 years, of which the US invariably occupies the first position with over 50% of the publications.

12.5 Indoleamine-2,3-dioxygenase

Indoleamine-2,3-dioxygenase (IDO) Fig. 12.7 is a rate-determining enzyme of tryptophan metabolism in the kynurenine pathway, causing depletion of tryptophan and suppression of microbial and T-cell proliferation. It is an

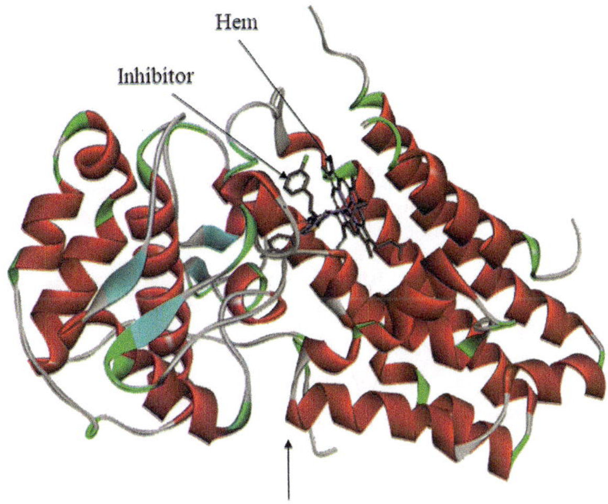

FIGURE 12.7 Indoleamine-2,3-dioxygenase-1 in complex with an inhibitor, 4PK6.pdb.

immunomodulatory enzyme produced by alternatively activated macrophages and other immunomodulatory cells and is also used in immune evasion strategies in many tumors (Jiang et al., 2015). It is known that tumor cells use IDO to affect immune evasion by local depletion of L-tryptophan. Human IDO (hIDO) is overexpressed in various human cancers such as prostate, large intestine, pancreatic, gastric, ovarian, brain, and lung cancer (Uyttenhove et al., 2003). Norharman has neuroprotective properties as it suppresses neurotoxic kynurenine metabolites such as kynurenic acid, 3-hydroxy-quinurenine and nitric oxide synthase through inhibition of IDO. Rosmarinic acid inhibits the expression of IDO via inhibition of cyclooxygenase (COX) (Chiarugi et al., 2000). COX-2 inhibitors reduce IDO, thereby reducing inflammatory cytokine activity and leading to lower kynurenine levels. α-Methyl-tryptophan also inhibits indoleamine dioxygenase (Lee et al., 2007).

12.6 Androgen receptor

The androgen receptor Fig. 12.8, also known as nuclear receptor subfamily 3 group C member 4, is a well-known steroid hormone receptor and is a ligand-activated transcription factor that controls the eukaryotic gene expression and plays a role in cellular proliferation, differentiation, multiple cellular events, apoptosis, and invasion in the target tissues (Yang et al., 2009). As AR is a ligand-induced transcription factor, it is widely expressed in primary prostate cancer and in metastases. The expression levels of AR in prostate cancer are regulated by peptide hormones and steroids. A total of 71

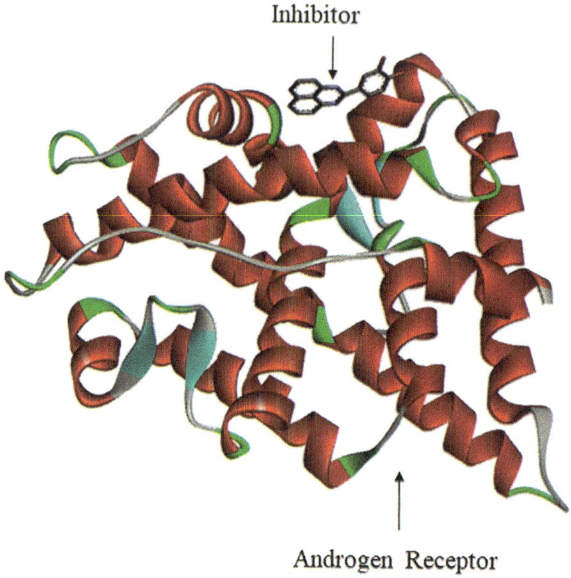

FIGURE 12.8 Androgen receptor with an inhibitor, 2YHD.pdb.

unique miRNA regulate the expression of AR in prostate cancer cells, whereas miRNA-34a and miRNA-34c are downregulated by androgen, which reported the causative effect as p53 suppression, thus inhibiting the doxorubicin-induced apoptosis (Culig & Santer, 2014). Numerous AR mutations have been noted and reported by a number of scientific groups. These mutations have been discovered in the prostate cancer and may increase with tumor progression. Mutations such as Thr877 Ala in LNCaP cells, Leu701 His, and Thr877 Ala in MDA PCa 2b cell line, Val715 Met in a patient sample and other drug-induced mutations have also been reported. The AR mutations and overexpressions of selected coactivators contribute to the agonistic properties of antiandrogen as certain coactivator's expression is enhanced during androgen ablation. AR activity is regulated by peptides such as cytokines or growth factors, which reduce the concentration of androgen required for maximal stimulation of the receptor. In prostate cancer, variant Ars, which exhibit constitutive activity, were detected. Novel therapies that interfere with intracrine synthesis of androgens or inhibit nuclear translocation of the AR have been introduced in the clinic. The downregulation of AR is carried out by numerous compounds present in vegetables and fruits (Culig & Santer, 2014). Therapies such as drug Hydroxyflutamide acting as a competitive AR binding, Bicaluatamide acting as a competitive AR binding, Enzalutamide acting as a competitive AR binding, have been approved. The inhibition of nuclear AR translocation is an approved castration-resistant prostate cancer (CRPC) after chemotherapy (Culig & Santer, 2014).

12.7 Conclusion

The identified drug target GU cancers and tumors are well studied for their therapeutic use in the treatment. Many more are in pipeline to be identified in due course and explored for their use as biomarkers in diagnosis or therapeutic application.

References

Agata, Y., Kawasaki, A., Nishimura, H., Ishida, Y., Tsubat, T., Yagita, H., et al. (1996). Expression of the PD-1 antigen on the surface of stimulated mouse T and B lymphocytes. *International Immunology*, *8*(5), 765–772. Available from https://academic.oup.com/intimm/article-lookup/doi/10.1093/intimm/8.5.765.

Butte, M. J., Keir, M. E., Phamduy, T. B., Sharpe, A. H., & Freeman, G. J. (2007). Programmed death-1 ligand 1 interacts specifically with the B7-1 costimulatory molecule to inhibit T cell responses. *Immunity*, *27*(1), 111–122. Available from https://linkinghub.elsevier.com/retrieve/pii/S1074761307003287.

Calagua, C., Russo, J., Sun, Y., Schaefer, R., Lis, R., Zhang, Z., et al. (2017). Expression of PD-L1 in hormone-naïve and treated prostate cancer patients receiving neoadjuvant abiraterone acetate plus prednisone and leuprolide. *Clinical Cancer Research*, *23*(22), 6812–6822. Available from http://clincancerres.aacrjournals.org/lookup/doi/10.1158/1078-0432.CCR-17-0807.

Chalfin, H. J., Pramparo, T., Mortazavi, A., Niglio, S. A., Schonhoft, J. D., Jendrisak, A., et al. (2021). Circulating tumor cell subtypes and T-cell populations as prognostic biomarkers to combination immunotherapy in patients with metastatic genitourinary cancer. *Clinical Cancer Research*, *27*(5), 1391–1398. Available from http://clincancerres.aacrjournals.org/lookup/doi/10.1158/1078-0432.CCR-20-2891.

Chiappori, A., Thompson, J., Eskens, F., Spano, J.-P., Doi, T., Hamid, O., et al. (2020). P860 results from a combination of OX40 (PF-04518600) and 4–1BB (utomilumab) agonistic antibodies in melanoma and non-small cell lung cancer in a phase 1 dose expansion cohort. *Journal for ImmunoTherapy of Cancer*, *8*(Suppl 1), A9–A10. Available from https://jitc.bmj.com/lookup/doi/10.1136/LBA2019.14.

Chiarugi, A., Dello Sbarba, P., Paccagnini, A., Donnini, S., Filippi, S., & Moroni, F. (2000). Combined inhibition of indoleamine 2,3-dioxygenase and nitric oxide synthase modulates neurotoxin release by interferon-gamma-activated macrophages. *Journal of Leukocyte Biology*, *68*(2), 260–266. Available from http://www.ncbi.nlm.nih.gov/pubmed/10947071.

Choueiri, T. K., & Kaelin, W. G. (2020). Targeting the HIF2–VEGF axis in renal cell carcinoma. *Nature Medicine*, *26*(10), 1519–1530. Available from http://www.nature.com/articles/s41591-020-1093-z.

Culig, Z., & Santer, F. R. (2014). Androgen receptor signaling in prostate cancer. *Cancer and Metastasis Reviews*, *33*(2–3), 413–427. Available from http://link.springer.com/10.1007/s10555-013-9474-0.

Dirix, L. Y., Takacs, I., Jerusalem, G., Nikolinakos, P., Arkenau, H.-T., Forero-Torres, A., et al. (2018). Avelumab, an anti-PD-L1 antibody, in patients with locally advanced or metastatic breast cancer: a phase 1b JAVELIN solid tumor study. *Breast Cancer Research and Treatment*, *167*(3), 671–686. Available from http://link.springer.com/10.1007/s10549-017-4537-5.

Driessens, G., Kline, J., & Gajewski, T.F. (2009). Costimulatory and coinhibitory receptors in anti-tumor immunity. *Immunological Reviews, 229*(1), 126-144. Available from http://link.springer.com/10.1111/j.1600-065X.2009.00771.x.

Dudek, A. Z., Liu, L. C., Gupta, S., Logan, T. F., Singer, E. A., Joshi, M., et al. (2020). Phase Ib/II clinical trial of pembrolizumab with bevacizumab for metastatic renal cell carcinoma: BTCRC-GU14-003. *Journal of Clinical Oncology*, *38*(11), 1138–1145. Available from https://ascopubs.org/doi/10.1200/JCO.19.02394.

Gatalica, Z., Snyder, C., Maney, T., Ghazalpour, A., Holterman, D. A., Xiao, N., et al. (2014). Programmed cell death 1 (PD-1) and its ligand (PD-L1) in common cancers and their correlation with molecular cancer type. *Cancer Epidemiology, Biomarkers & Prevention*, *23*(12), 2965–2970. Available from http://cebp.aacrjournals.org/lookup/doi/10.1158/1055-9965.EPI-14-0654.

Gevensleben, H., Dietrich, D., Golletz, C., Steiner, S., Jung, M., Thiesler, T., et al. (2016). The immune checkpoint regulator PD-L1 is highly expressed in aggressive primary prostate cancer. *Clinical Cancer Research*, *22*(8), 1969–1977. Available from http://clincancerres.aacrjournals.org/lookup/doi/10.1158/1078-0432.CCR-15-2042.

Gopal, A. K., Levy, R., Houot, R., Patel, S. P., Popplewell, L., Jacobson, C., et al. (2020). First-in-human study of utomilumab, a 4-1BB/CD137 agonist, in combination with rituximab in patients with follicular and other CD20 + non-hodgkin lymphomas. *Clinical Cancer Research*, *26*(11), 2524–2534. Available from http://clincancerres.aacrjournals.org/lookup/doi/10.1158/1078-0432.CCR-19-2973.

Haffner, M. C., Guner, G., Taheri, D., Netto, G. J., Palsgrove, D. N., Zheng, Q., et al. (2018). Comprehensive evaluation of programmed death-ligand 1 expression in primary and metastatic prostate cancer. *American Journal of Pathology*, *188*(6), 1478–1485. Available from https://linkinghub.elsevier.com/retrieve/pii/S0002944017311793.

Heery, C. R., O'Sullivan-Coyne, G., Madan, R. A., Cordes, L., Rajan, A., Rauckhorst, M., et al. (2017). Avelumab for metastatic or locally advanced previously treated solid tumours (JAVELIN Solid Tumor): a phase 1a, multicohort, dose-escalation trial. *The Lancet Oncology*, *18*(5), 587–598. Available from https://linkinghub.elsevier.com/retrieve/pii/S1470204517302395.

Iwai, K., Yamanaka, K., Kamura, T., Minato, N., Conaway, R. C., Conaway, J. W., et al. (1999). Identification of the von Hippel-Lindau tumor-suppressor protein as part of an active E3 ubiquitin ligase complex. *Proceedings of the National Academy of Sciences of the United States of America*, *96*(22), 12436–12441. Available from http://www.pnas.org/cgi/doi/10.1073/pnas.96.22.12436.

Jiang, T., Sun, Y., Yin, Z., Feng, S., Sun, L., & Li, Z. (2015). Research progress of indoleamine 2,3-dioxygenase inhibitors. *Future Medicinal Chemistry*, *7*(2), 185–201. Available from http://www.ncbi.nlm.nih.gov/pubmed/25686005.

Kaufman, H. L., Russell, J., Hamid, O., Bhatia, S., Terheyden, P., D'Angelo, S. P., et al. (2016). Avelumab in patients with chemotherapy-refractory metastatic Merkel cell carcinoma: a multicentre, single-group, open-label, phase 2 trial. *The Lancet Oncology*, *17*(10), 1374–1385. Available from https://linkinghub.elsevier.com/retrieve/pii/S1470204516303643.

Keir, M., Francisco, L., & Sharpe, A. (2007). PD-1 and its ligands in T-cell immunity. *Current Opinion in Immunology*, *19*(3), 309–314. Available from https://linkinghub.elsevier.com/retrieve/pii/S0952791507000647.

Kim, B.-S., Mooney, D. J., & Atala, A. (2000). *Genitourinary system. Principles of Tissue Engineering* (pp. 655–667). Elsevier. Available from https://linkinghub.elsevier.com/retrieve/pii/B9780124366305500507.

Kim, E. S. (2017). Avelumab: First global approval. *Drugs, 77*(8), 929–937. Available from http://link.springer.com/10.1007/s40265-017-0749-6.

Kim, W. Y., & Kaelin, W. G. (2004). Role of VHL gene mutation in human cancer. *Journal of Clinical Oncology, 22*(24), 4991–5004. Available from http://ascopubs.org/doi/10.1200/JCO.2004.05.061.

Lee, H. J., Jeong, Y.-I., Lee, T.-H., Jung, I. D., Lee, J. S., Lee, C.-M., et al. (2007). Rosmarinic acid inhibits indoleamine 2,3-dioxygenase expression in murine dendritic cells. *Biochemical Pharmacology, 73*(9), 1412–1421. Available from http://www.ncbi.nlm.nih.gov/pubmed/17229401.

Li, Y., Huang, Q., Zhou, Y., He, M., Chen, J., Gao, Y., et al. (2019). The clinicopathologic and prognostic significance of programmed cell death ligand 1 (PD-L1) expression in patients with prostate cancer: A systematic review and *meta*-analysis. *Frontiers in Pharmacology, 9*. Available from https://www.frontiersin.org/article/10.3389/fphar.2018.01494/full.

Liu, C., Liu, L., Wang, K., Li, X.-F., Ge, L.-Y., Ma, R.-Z., et al. (2020). VHL-HIF-2α axis-induced SMYD3 upregulation drives renal cell carcinoma progression via direct trans-activation of EGFR. *Oncogene, 39*(21), 4286–4298. Available from http://www.ncbi.nlm.nih.gov/pubmed/32291411.

Maher, E. R., & Kaelin, W. G. (1997). von Hippel-Lindau disease. *Medicine (Baltimore), 76*(6), 381–391. Available from http://journals.lww.com/00005792-199711000-00001.

Ostroumov, D., Fekete-Drimusz, N., Saborowski, M., Kühnel, F., & Woller, N. (2018). CD4 and CD8 T lymphocyte interplay in controlling tumor growth. *Cellular and Molecular Life Sciences, 75*(4), 689–713. Available from http://link.springer.com/10.1007/s00018-017-2686-7.

Segal, N. H., Logan, T. F., Hodi, F. S., McDermott, D., Melero, I., Hamid, O., et al. (2017). Results from an integrated safety analysis of urelumab, an agonist anti-CD137 monoclonal antibody. *Clinical Cancer Research, 23*(8), 1929–1936. Available from http://clincancerres.aacrjournals.org/lookup/doi/10.1158/1078-0432.CCR-16-1272.

Shirley, M. (2018). Avelumab: A review in metastatic merkel cell carcinoma. *Targeted Oncology, 13*(3), 409–416. Available from http://link.springer.com/10.1007/s11523-018-0571-4.

Soker, S., Takashima, S., Miao, H. Q., Neufeld, G., & Klagsbrun, M. (1998). Neuropilin-1 is expressed by endothelial and tumor cells as an isoform-specific receptor for vascular endothelial growth factor. *Cell, 92*(6), 735–745. Available from http://www.ncbi.nlm.nih.gov/pubmed/9529250.

Timmerman, J., Herbaux, C., Ribrag, V., Zelenetz, A. D., Houot, R., Neelapu, S. S., et al. (2020). Urelumab alone or in combination with rituximab in patients with relapsed or refractory B-cell lymphoma. *American Journal of Hematology, 95*(5), 510–520. Available from https://onlinelibrary.wiley.com/doi/10.1002/ajh.25757.

Uyttenhove, C., Pilotte, L., Théate, I., Stroobant, V., Colau, D., Parmentier, N., et al. (2003). Evidence for a tumoral immune resistance mechanism based on tryptophan degradation by indoleamine 2,3-dioxygenase. *Nature Medicine, 9*(10), 1269–1274. Available from http://www.ncbi.nlm.nih.gov/pubmed/14502282.

Wiesener, M. S., Münchenhagen, P. M., Berger, I., Morgan, N. V., Roigas, J., Schwiertz, A., Jürgensen, J. S., Gruber, G, Maxwell, P. H., Löning, S. A., Frei, U, Maher, E. R., Gröne, H. J., & Eckardt, K. U. (2001). Constitutive activation of hypoxia-inducible genes related to overexpression of hypoxia-inducible factor-1alpha in clear cell renal carcinomas. *Cancer*

Research, *61*(13), 5215–5222. Available from http://www.ncbi.nlm.nih.gov/pubmed/11431362.

Yang, J., Zhao, Y.-L., Wu, Z.-Q., Si, Y.-L., Meng, Y.-G., Fu, X.-B., et al. (2009). The single-macro domain protein LRP16 is an essential cofactor of androgen receptor. *Endocrine-Related Cancer*, *16*(1), 139–153. Available from http://www.ncbi.nlm.nih.gov/pubmed/19022849.

Zarrabi, K., Paroya, A., & Wu, S. (2019). Emerging therapeutic agents for genitourinary cancers. *Journal of Hematology & Oncology*, *12*(1), 89. Available from https://jhoonline.biomedcentral.com/articles/10.1186/s13045-019-0780-z.

Chapter 13

Cell–cell differentiation induction: model for cervical cancer

Moulay Mustapha Ennaji[1], Kaoutar Anouar Tadlaoui[2] and Ikram Tiabi[2]
[1]Group Leader Research team of Virology, Oncology, and Biotechnologies, Head of Laboratory of Virology, Oncology, Biosciences, Environment and New Energies (LVO-BEEN), Faculty of Sciences and Techniques Mohammedia, University Hassan II of Casablanca, Casablanca, Morocco, [2]Team of Virology, Oncology, and Biotechnologies, Laboratory of Virology, Oncology, Biosciences, Environment and New Energies (LVO-BEEN), Faculty of Sciences and Techniques Mohammedia, University Hassan II of Casablanca, Casablanca, Morocco

13.1 Introduction

Cervical cancer (CC) is a primary or secondary malignant proliferation of cells in the cervix. CC is the second most common cancer among females worldwide. The World Health Organization (WHO) reported 500,000 new cases diagnosed each year, 83% of which are observed in developing countries (Santé, 2017). In Morocco, it remains a real public health problem with an estimate of around 6000 new cases and around 3000 deaths per year (Bezad, 2013). CC particularly affects young women and is most often not discovered until an advanced stage.

It is currently well established that the human papillomavirus (HPV) is the primary pathogen causing CC. Thus other sexual and nonsexual factors are involved as cofactors in the progression of HPV infection to CC (Arbyn, 2013, 2009).

CC is preceded by a precancerous phase, which can last for several years before the onset of clinical symptoms, the major sign of which is genital hemorrhage (Kamina, 1979).

Regular Pap smear screening can help detect precancerous lesions and treat them at an early stage. The cervical–vaginal smear remains a simple, inexpensive, harmless, and painless test that can be carried out anywhere in the doctor's office.

The diagnosis is based on the cyto-colpo-histology tripod, where the anatomopathological study remains essential either to confirm the diagnosis,

Immunological Implications and Molecular Diagnostics of Genitourinary Cancer.
DOI: https://doi.org/10.1016/B978-0-323-85496-2.00001-4

assess the degree of malignancy, provide the elements conditioning the prognosis or provide the theranostic elements.

The cervix arises from the fusion of the middle part of the Mullerian ducts. It has two anatomical parts: the ectocervix and the endocervix. In the former, certain undifferentiated cells, called reserve cells, may exhibit squamous or columnar differentiation. The external channel of mesonephrosis can persist in the form of remnants of Wolff in the cervix, which explains the presence of certain cervical tumors (Laffargue & Giacalone, 1992).

Cell differentiation can lead to numerous changes in the physiological aspect of the cell: its size, shape, polarity, metabolic activity, sensitivity to certain signals, and expression of genes. In cytopathology, the level of cell differentiation is used as a measure of cancer progression (malignancy, type, and grade) (Alberts et al., 2002).

The tumor grade is established on several microscopic criteria in the examination of the cancer cell including differentiation. Thus the resemblance level of cancer cells to their tissue of origin defines differentiation.

13.2 Cervical cancer

13.2.1 Epidemiology of cervical cancer

Globally, CC is the fourth most common cancer in women. In 2012 its death rate was up to 52% per year, of which more than 85% occurred in developing countries (L'OMS, 2013). The net survival of CC between 1989 and 2004 was 66% 5 years after diagnosis and 59% 10 years after diagnosis (Duport et al., 2014).

According to the WHO, the incidence of CC in Morocco in 2012 was 2258, and the death rate accounted for 10.3% of cancer deaths in women, or 10,712 deaths (OMS, 2014).

13.2.2 Anatomopathology of the cervix

The uterus (Fig. 13.1) is a hollow, inverted triangle–shaped muscular organ, approximately 10 cm in length, located in the lower part of a woman's abdomen, between the bladder and the rectum. The upper part of the uterus, which is larger, is called the uterine body. The upper right and left extremities of the body clear the fallopian tubes, which carry away the ovaries, whereas, the lower part, which is the most constricted, opening up the vagina, is called the cervix (Balaya et al., 2016). It is a dense muscle tissue made up of two parts.

The endocervix, which is the inner part of the cervix that starts from the isthmus and continues to the opening that opens into the vagina (Balaya et al., 2016). The exocervix is the outer part of the cervix and is located in the upper part of the vagina (Balaya et al., 2016).

CC develops precisely in the lower, narrow part of the uterus. The most common form of these cancers (around 80% of cases) develops from cells of

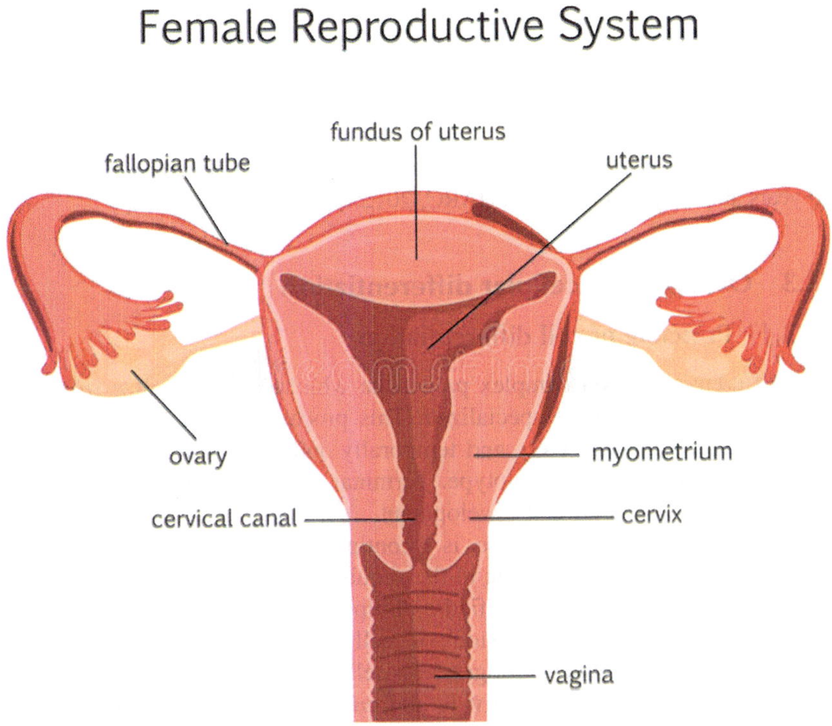

FIGURE 13.1 Female reproductive system. *From https://www.freepik.com/free-vector/female-reproductive-system-scientific_10156137.htm#page = 1&position = 8&from_view = detail#&position = 8&from_view = detail The 5 main anatomically female's internal reproductive organs are the vagina, uterus, fallopian tubes, cervix, and ovary. The uterus is the predominant organ in it.*

the Malpighian epithelium: these are squamous cell carcinomas (SCs), whereas cancers that develop from the glandular epithelium are called adenocarcinomas (Pointreau et al., 2010). Treated early according to a specific protocol, these tumors provide a good prognosis.

13.2.3 Risk factors of cervical cancer

Sexually transmitted infections, including HPV, are an important factor in the development of CC. The HPV genital infection is highly persistent, especially with HPV high oncogenic risk (HPV16 and HPV18), involved in 82% of cancers and precancerous lesions of the cervix (Ronco et al., 2010; Tadlaoui et al., 2020).

Other factors also increase the risk of developing CC, such as overweight and obesity, multiparity, early sexual intercourse, precocious puberty (before age 12 years), late menopause, alcohol or tobacco consumption, having multiple sexual partners, as well as certain genital infections like chlamydia or herpes (Tranbaloc, 2008).

Additionally, prolonged use of hormonal contraceptives in pill, implant, patch, or hormonal intrauterine device form also impacts the risk of developing CC. The latter increases with the extension of the duration of treatment with oral contraceptives. This risk decreases when the contraceptive pill is stopped to almost zero 10 years after stopping treatment (IARC, 2012; Tadlaoui et al., 2020).

13.3 Overview of cellular differentiation

13.3.1 Principle of cell differentiation

Cell differentiation is a complex process in which cells specialize from one cell type to another more specialized. This process is usually due to genes that are expressed selectively and temporally and whose products allow the cell to express a distinct phenotype. Terminal differentiation, therefore constitutes the final stage of cell development.

Cell differentiation, otherwise, is a continuous process of developing cell specificity from the zygote stage to the acquisition of a specific cell type and tissue system. A zygote is qualified as totipotent because it gives rise to an entire organism by a succession of cell divisions and specializations. Gradually as development progresses, cell differentiation continues into adulthood as adult stem cells divide and create well-differentiated daughter cells. However, the number and type of cells that a parent cell can form are increasingly limited. Stem cells from two or three lineages are called pluripotent cells. Pluripotency refers to the ability to become any type of cell. This is in the stem or progenitor cells at the start of the differentiation process. As the cell differentiates and acquires specialized functions, pluripotency is gradually lost (Ng et al., 2019). Finally, cells intended to develop a single cell type, although they are still embryonic, are called unipotent.

The degree of cell differentiation can be assessed by the expression of certain markers during the program of differentiation of a given cell type. It is possible to distinguish two main groups of cell differentiation markers:

- Universal cell differentiation markers
- Specific cell differentiation markers

13.3.1.1 Universal cell differentiation markers

These are proteins normally expressed in all cells, hence the name universal cell marker, the typical example of which is actin. In further detail, skeletal muscle actin is only one of six different types of actin synthesized in vertebrate cells. All but the most primitive eukaryotic species have multiple actin genes encoding slightly different proteins, expressed in different tissues of development. Actin genes are extremely conserved. Actin molecules of radically different origin are functionally interchangeable. The main properties of actin molecules extracted from skeletal muscle are therefore shared by actin molecules from all other tissues, hence the qualification of actin as a universal differentiation marker (Franke et al., 1978; Huxley, 1969).

13.3.1.2 Specific cell differentiation markers

These are cell differentiation markers expressed differentially during the differentiation program or specific to a cell type. For example, keratin is specific for epithelial cells, myosin for muscle cells, and neurofilaments (Vielkind & Swierenga, 1989) for neural cells. Among the proteins present in most cells and differentially expressed during the differentiation program, are fibronectin (Hynes, 1982), vimentin (Franke et al., 1979), and N-CAM (Moore et al., 1987).

- Fibronectin

  Fibronectin is a major component of the extracellular matrix found in all tissues (Hay, 1981). It is a 450–500 kDa glycoprotein, which is found in the form of large fibrillary aggregates in the extracellular matrix and in a form soluble in physiological fluids such as blood plasma (Poulouin et al., 1997). Most of the protein is not directly bound to cells; a fraction attaches to the surface of fibroblasts and other cells when cultured. Fibronectin began to attract attention as soon as it was discovered to be present in trace amounts on the surface of fibroblasts derived from tumors in contrast to a high level in normal fibroblasts (Hynes, 1982; Ruoslahti et al., 1981; Yamada & Olden, 1978).
- Vimentin

  Vimentin is a component of the family of intermediate filaments, with a molecular mass of 55 kDa (Franke et al., 1979). It is one of the main components of the cytoskeletal structure, which could be copolymerized with other cell-type-specific subunits. It is a protein found in fibroblasts and many other cell types (Franke et al., 1979), such as mesenchymal cells and cell types derived from mesoderm. It is expressed during cell development and differentiation of the latter (Massiere, 2011).

  Vimentin plays an essential role in the integrity of the cell cytoplasm and the stability of the cytoskeleton (Goldman et al., 1996). In addition, it is a useful control marker for appropriate tissue processing (Dauphin et al., 2012; Massiere, 2011; Schwarz et al., 2002).
- N-CAM

  N-CAMs are intercellular adhesion molecules originally identified in neural cells (N-CAM) and in endothelial cells almost 30 years ago (Covault et al., 1986; Foets et al., 1992; Moore et al., 1987). These are glycoproteins with a molecular mass of 145 kDa responsible for links between cells. N-CAMs are also expressed in myoblasts (Covault et al., 1986; Moore et al., 1987).

Because of its strong expression, especially its characteristic pattern similar to that of CD166, some researchers proposed it as a specific marker of CE (He et al., 2016).

- Cytokeratin

Cytokeratin is an insoluble fibrous protein expressed in epithelial cells. It is a polymer of keratin. There are many different types of keratins encoded by an important family of genes, which probably evolved through duplications and mutations from an ancestral gene. Different types of cytokeratin are produced in different layers of the epidermis. They are therefore a function of the degree of differentiation of the epithelial cells (Fuchs & Green, 1980).

Their specific localization in epithelial tissues allows the identification of cancer cells of epithelial origin thanks to immunohistochemical techniques using anticytokeratin antibodies. Cytokeratin, therefore constitutes a histochemical marker of the differentiation of epithelial cells (Moll et al., 1992; Scott & Helm, 1999).

The qualitative and quantitative evaluation of the expression products of these cell differentiation markers constitutes a good indication of the state of the cell.

13.3.2 Correlation between cell growth and cell differentiation

Traditionally, growth and differentiation have been considered to be mutually exclusive. At the start of embryogenesis, cell growth is intense, but later, at the time of differentiation, cells do not divide as frequently. The terminally differentiated cells tend to lose their potential for replication. A good example is that of skin cells, namely, keratinocytes. This negative relationship between growth and differentiation can also be observed in cells in in vitro culture. For example, myoblasts continue to grow in cell culture in vitro, but when subjected to certain conditions reducing their growth, terminal differentiation into syncytium and then into myocytes occurs (Yaffe, 1968). The terminal state of differentiation is clearly incompatible with cell growth and division (Cheng & Leblond, 1974).

13.3.3 Cellular models for the study of proliferation and differentiation

13.3.3.1 Myoblasts

In in vitro cell culture, myoblasts retain their capacity for proliferation and their capacity to fuse and differentiate into myotubes in response to an appropriate change in the culture conditions (Yaffe, 1969). This cell culture model of myoblasts was notably used by Kubo in 1991 (Kubo, 1991).

13.3.3.2 Differentiation of myoblasts

Myoblasts in vitro culture differentiate synchronously if the culture medium is appropriately modified (e.g., substituting horse serum for bovine serum). They, therefore represent a practical model for the molecular study of the control of gene expression during differentiation.

Differentiation of myoblasts requires coordinated changes in the expression of many genes. In the proliferative state, the product of these genes is absent or present in very small quantities. However, once differentiation is induced, a large number of characteristic proteins appear such as the acetylcholine receptors (Merlie et al., 1977). The synthesis of these proteins becomes detectable just before fusion (Yaffe, 1969).

13.3.4 Virus interaction and cell proliferation/differentiation

Several mechanisms have been proposed in order to test the cell transformation, which results in the stimulation of proliferation and the inhibition of differentiation (Reiss et al., 1989). The polypeptides encoded by oncogenic viruses can alter a unique cellular component that in turn affects a wide variety of cellular functions to give rise to the neoplastic phenotype, or the oncogene product itself may directly alter different components of the cell. Many researchers believe that the second alternative is more plausible (Band et al., 1991; Inoue et al., 1992; Shay et al., 1993).

Even though the translation products of many oncogenes appear to affect different cellular functions, it is possible that only a few of these effects are necessary for oncogenesis (Shay et al., 1993). If an anarchical division is at the heart of the neoplastic phenotype, the fundamental difference distinguishing a cancer cell from a normal cell could be its inability to stop at the restriction (R) point of the cycle under conditions that inhibit normal cell proliferation.

Few or no neoplastic cells cultured in vitro are preferentially arrested at the point R (Shay et al., 1993). Instead, they stop growing at a wide variety of points in the cell cycle, especially when starved or subjected to toxic conditions. A way for oncogenes to disrupt the normal mechanism of growth regulation is to prevent normal cell differentiation in a cell, which thus retains unlimited growth potential.

In fact, many tumor cells are less well-differentiated than their normal counterparts (Smith et al., 1979). Cancer cells are immortalized, and unlike normal cells, they do not have a limited lifespan in culture. Many viruses associated with oncogenesis can confer immortality on their host cell (Auersperg & Roskelley, 1991; Rochford et al., 1993).

Furthermore, a tumor virus can simply overload the host cell with the product of a normal cellular gene involved in the control of cell division (or not). It seems that it is only because of the excessive presence of this product that the transformed cell proliferates in an anarchic manner. Therefore this engages the cell on a pathway of malignancy and inhibits its evolutionary potential in its differentiation program (Bishop, 1981; Oskarsson et al., 1980).

13.4 Cell differentiation study methods

There are several lines of poorly differentiated embryonic cells such as rat L6 myoblasts (Kidokoro, 1975; Yaffe, 1968, 1969), mouse C2 caff (Caffrey et al., 1989), which make it possible to follow certain stages of differentiation. Primary cultures of several types of animals such as chickens (Hume & Thomas, 1989; Kano et al., 1987, 1989), rats (Beam & Knudson, 1988; Cognard et al., 1986; Weiss & Horn, 1986), mice (Beam & Knudson, 1988; Gonoi & Hasegawa, 1988), and also humans (Trautmann et al., 1986) are also used for this purpose. All of the studies cited above have focused on the morphological changes that accompany the different stages of differentiation. Each stage is associated with the genetic expression of specific markers.

There are different techniques that use differentiation markers. They are linked to either specific antigens or enzymatic reactions that are also specific, such as transglutaminase for keratinocytes (Lichti & Yuspa, 1988).

Electronic or optical microscopy makes it possible to follow the product of a given gene by immunological labeling. (Abercrombie et al., 1971; Goldman & Knipe, 1973; Izzard & Lochner, 1976; McNutt et al., 1971, 1973).

Fluorescence microscopy analyses are however most often used (Ali et al., 1977; Hynes, 1973; Hynes & Bye, 1974; Mautner & Hynes, 1977; Vaheri & Mosher, 1978). The qualitative and quantitative analysis of antigens is often done by immunological labeling in flow cytometry (Hand et al., 1978; Horan et al., 1975; Leary et al., 1976; McSharry et al., 1988). The genetic expression can also be studied at the level of the transcript. Its evaluation using standard hybridization techniques is often limited owing to its lack of sensitivity (Singer-Sam et al., 1990; Thomas et al., 1989).

For this reason, several groups have preferred the polymerase chain reaction test for the detection of specific messenger RNAs after reverse transcription into DNA (Becker-André & Hahlbrock, 1989; Doherty et al., 1989; Harbarth & Vosberg, 1988; Murakawa et al., 1988; Rappolee et al., 1989; Singer-Sam et al., 1990).

A currently widely used technique is immunohistochemistry, which allows the detection of antigens, or epitopes characteristic of a tissue type in tumor cells:

- Expression of cytokeratins by epithelial tumors (Moll, 1993);
- Expression of vimentin by connective tumors (Satelli & Li, 2011);
- Expression of the common leukocyte antigen in leukocyte differentiation tumors (Zhang et al., 2018).

13.5 Tumor differentiation: case of cervical cancer

13.5.1 Generality of tumor differentiation

Tumor tissue most often tends to reproduce the structural aspect of normal tissue: the appearance of tissue originating from tumor cells. It is rarely when the tumor tissue is different, and in this case, the tumor is termed "metaplastic" (Duyckaerts et al., 2003).

We speak of tumor differentiation when there is a tendency for a tumor to reproduce the structure of normal adult or embryonic tissue. The differentiation of a tumor is one of the very important elements in classifying tumors into defined categories called histological types of tumors.

When tumor cells clearly and homogeneously resemble normal tissue cells, cell differentiation is good; we speak of a well-differentiated tumor. On the other hand, when the resemblance is low or focal, we speak of a poorly or moderately differentiated tumor.

In general, benign tumors are well-differentiated, while malignant tumors can be well or poorly differentiated. Tumor differentiation of malignant tumors is frequently reduced to the presence of a few microscopic characters. As a result, it is sometimes difficult to establish the differentiation of a malignant tumor and, therefore its presumed origin (Duyckaerts et al., 2003).

Furthermore, there are undifferentiated or anaplastic tumors (Duyckaerts et al., 2003).

Anaplastic cancer refers to malignant tumor without any differentiation.

Undifferentiated carcinoma refers to malignant tumor with epithelial differentiation without the possibility of determining squamous or glandular differentiation.

However, CCs can be tumors with glandular differentiation (cylindrical or glandular epithelium), or metaplastic tumors with squamous differentiation, which tend to reproduce more or less perfectly the structure of the squamous epithelium: case of invasive SC carcinoma of the cervix (Duyckaerts et al., 2003).

13.5.2 Cell differentiation of cervical carcinoma

The cervix arises from the fusion of the middle part of the Mullerian ducts. The squamous epithelium of the ectocervix arises from the epithelium of the primary birth canal. The columnar epithelium becomes muciparous by metaplasia of this same primary epithelium. Certain undifferentiated cells, called reserve cells present in the endocervix, can manifest squamous or cylindrical differentiation. The outer channel of mesonephrosis can persist in the form of Wolffian remains in the cervix, which explains the presence of certain cervical tumors (Laffargue & Giacalone, 1992).

The appearance of these carcinomas also varies depending on the degree of differentiation (mitotic activity and cytological atypia):

- Grade 1: well-differentiated SC carcinoma;
- Grade 2: moderately differentiated SC carcinoma;
- Grade 3: poorly differentiated SC carcinoma;
- Grade 4: undifferentiated carcinoma.

13.6 Conclusion

In the field of surgical pathology, the concept of cell differentiation is used as a prognostic parameter, which is different from its use in developmental biology. The stage of tumor differentiation is a major aspect of the histopathological classification of solid cancers. The stage of differentiation is strongly related to tumor behavior, and generally, an undifferentiated immature tumor is more aggressive than its well-differentiated counterpart.

However, the contribution of gene expression related to the differentiation of tumor cells is often overlooked in the experimental framework of the biology of carcinogenesis. Thus the mechanisms of alteration of the differentiation stages of cancer cells are little studied, but recently, it has been demonstrated with the introduction of the concept of tumor stem cells. Although tumor development biologists view differentiation as a unidirectional event, tumor pathologists and biologists have introduced the concept of dedifferentiation to explain the phenotypic changes involved in solid cancers (Jögi et al., 2012).

Acknowledgment

I would like to extend my deep thanks and gratitude for support, encouragement, and contribution by Faculty of Sciences and Techniques of Mohammedia, University Hassan II of Casablanca, Morocco, my Professor My Mustapha ENNAJI and my team research of Virology, Oncology, Total Quality and Medical Biotechnology.

References

Abercrombie, M., Heaysman, J. E. M., & Pegrum, S. M. (1971). The locomotion of fibroblasts in culture. IV. Electron microscopy of the leading lamella. *Experimental Cell Research, 67*(2), 359–367. Available from https://doi.org/10.1016/0014-4827(71)90420-4.

Alberts, B., Johnson, A., Lewis, J., Raff, M., Roberts, K., & Walter, P. (2002). An overview of gene control. *Molecular Biology of the Cell.*

Ali, I. U., Mautner, V., Lanza, R., & Hynes, R. O. (1977). Restoration of normal morphology, adhesion and cytoskeleton in transformed cells by addition of a transformation-sensitive surface protein. *Cell, 11*(1), 115–126. Available from https://doi.org/10.1016/0092-8674(77)90322-1.

Arbyn, M. (2013). *Epidémiologie du cancer du col utérin dans le monde; Symposium international sur la prévention du cancer du col utérin teDépistage, Vaccination et Perspectives pour les Pays en Développement* (pp. 15–16).

Auersperg, N., & Roskelley, C. (1991). Retroviral oncogenes: Interrelationships between neoplastic transformation and cell differentiation. *Critical Reviews in Oncogenesis*, *2*(2), 125–160.

Balaya, V., Ngo, C., Rossi, L., Cornou, C., Bensaid, C., Douard, R., Bats, A. S., & Lecuru, F. (2016). Bases anatomiques et principe du nerve-sparing au cours de l'hystérectomie radicale pour cancer du col utérin. *Gynécologie Obstétrique & Fertilité*, *44*(9), 517–525. Available from https://doi.org/10.1016/j.gyobfe.2016.07.009.

Band, V., De Caprio, J. A., Delmolino, L., Kulesa, V., & Sager, R. (1991). Loss of p53 protein in human papillomavirus type 16 E6-immortalized human mammary epithelial cells. *Journal of Virology*, *65*(12), 6671–6676. Available from https://doi.org/10.1128/jvi.65.12.6671-6676.1991.

Beam, K. G., & Knudson, C. M. (1988). Effect of postnatal development on calcium currents and slow charge movement in mammalian skeletal muscle. *Journal of General Physiology*, *91*(6), 799–815. Available from https://doi.org/10.1085/jgp.91.6.799.

Becker-André, M., & Hahlbrock, K. (1989). Absolute mRNA quantification using the polymerase chain reaction (PCR). A novel approach by a PCR aided transcipt titration assay (PATTY). *Nucleic Acids Research*, *17*(22), 9437–9446. Available from https://doi.org/10.1093/nar/17.22.9437.

Bezad, R. (2013). *Prévention et dépistage du cancer du col utérin au Maroc; Symposium international sur la prévention du cancer du col utérin: Dépistage, Vaccination et Perspectives pour les Pays en Développement* (pp. 15–16).

Bishop, J. M. (1981). Enemies within: The genesis of retrovirus oncogenes.

Caffrey, J. M., Brown, A. M., & Schneider, M. D. (1989). Ca2 + and Na + currents in developing skeletal myoblasts are expressed in a sequential program: Reversible suppression by transforming growth factor beta-1, an inhibitor of the myogenic pathway. *Journal of Neuroscience*, *9*(10), 3443–3453. Available from https://doi.org/10.1523/jneurosci.09-10-03443.1989.

Cheng, H., & Leblond, C. P. (1974). Origin, differentiation and renewal of the four main epithelial cell types in the mouse small intestine V. Unitarian theory of the origin of the four epithelial cell types. *American Journal of Anatomy*, *141*(4), 537–561. Available from https://doi.org/10.1002/aja.1001410407.

Cognard, C., Lazdunski, M., & Romey, G. (1986). Different types of Ca2 + channels in mammalian skeletal muscle cells in culture. *Proceedings of the National Academy of Sciences*, *83*(2), 517–521. Available from https://doi.org/10.1073/pnas.83.2.517.

Covault, J., Merlie, J. P., Goridis, C., & Sanes, J. R. (1986). Molecular forms of N-CAM and its RNA in developing and denervated skeletal muscle. *Journal of Cell Biology*, *102*(3), 731–739. Available from https://doi.org/10.1083/jcb.102.3.731.

Dauphin, M., Barbe, C., Lemaire, S., Lagonotte, E., Delepine, G., Birembaut, P., Gilles, C., & Polette, M. (2012). Rôle pronostique de la vimentine comme marqueur de transition épithélio-mésenchymateuse dans les carcinomes non à petites cellules du poumon. *Annales de Pathologie*, S157. Available from https://doi.org/10.1016/j.annpat.2012.09.038.

Doherty, P. J., Huesca-Contreras, M., Dosch, H. M., & Pan, S. (1989). Rapid amplification of complementary DNA from small amounts of unfractionated RNA. *Analytical Biochemistry*, *177*(1), 7–10. Available from https://doi.org/10.1016/0003-2697(89)90003-1.

Duport, N., Heard, I., Barré, S., & Woronoff, A. S. (2014). *Le cancer du col de l'utérus: état des connaissances en 2014*. Coordination Scientifique.

Duyckaerts, C., Fouret., & Hauw, J. J. (2003). *Anathomie Pathologique: Pathologie Tumorale*. Médecine Sorbonne Université.

Foets, B., van den Oord, J., Engelmann, K., & Missotten, L. (1992). A comparative immunohistochemical study of human corneotrabecular tissue. *Graefe's Archive for Clinical and Experimental Ophthalmology*, *230*(3), 269–274. Available from https://doi.org/10.1007/BF00176303.

Franke, W. W., Schmid, E., Osborn, M., & Weber, K. (1978). Different intermediate-sized filaments distinguished by immunofluorescence microscopy. *Proceedings of the National Academy of Sciences*, *75*(10), 5034–5038. Available from https://doi.org/10.1073/pnas.75.10.5034.

Franke, W. W., Schmid, E., Winter, S., Osborn, M., & Weber, K. (1979). Widespread occurrence of intermediate-sized filaments of the vimentin-type in cultured cells from diverse vertebrates. *Experimental Cell Research*, *123*(1), 25–46. Available from https://doi.org/10.1016/0014-4827(79)90418-X.

Fuchs, E., & Green, H. (1980). Changes in keratin gene expression during terminal differentiation of the keratinocyte. *Cell*, *19*(4), 1033–1042. Available from https://doi.org/10.1016/0092-8674(80)90094-X.

Goldman, R. D., Khuon, S., Chou, Y. H., Opal, P., & Steinert, P. M. (1996). The function of intermediate filaments in cell shape and cytoskeletal integrity. *Journal of Cell Biology*, *134*(4), 971–983. Available from https://doi.org/10.1083/jcb.134.4.971.

Goldman, R. D., & Knipe, D. M. (1973). Functions of cytoplasmic fibers in non-muscle cell motility. *Cold Spring Harbor Symposia on Quantitative Biology*, 523–534. Available from https://doi.org/10.1101/SQB.1973.037.01.063.

Gonoi, T., & Hasegawa, S. (1988). Post-natal disappearance of transient calcium channels in mouse skeletal muscle: Effects of denervation and culture. *The Journal of Physiology*, *401*(1), 617–637. Available from https://doi.org/10.1113/jphysiol.1988.sp017183.

Hand, R. E., Tennant, R. W., Yang, W. K., & Lavelle, G. C. (1978). Immunofluorescent analysis of murine leukemia virus-infected cells by flow microfluorometry. *Journal of Immunological Methods*, *23*(1–2), 175–186. Available from https://doi.org/10.1016/0022-1759(78)90121-7.

Harbarth, P., & Vosberg, H. P. (1988). Enzymatic amplification of myosin heavy-chain mRNA sequences in vitro. *DNA (Mary Ann Liebert, Inc.)*, *7*(4), 297–306. Available from https://doi.org/10.1089/dna.1988.7.297.

Hay, E. D. (1981). Extracellular matrix. *Journal of Cell Biology*, *91*(3). Available from https://doi.org/10.1083/jcb.91.3.205s.

He, Z., Forest, F., Gain, P., Rageade, D., Bernard, A., Acquart, S., Peoc'h, M., Defoe, D. M., & Thuret, G. (2016). 3D map of the human corneal endothelial cell. *Scientific Reports*, 6. Available from https://doi.org/10.1038/srep29047.

Horan, M., Horan, P. K., & Williams, C. A. (1975). Quantitative measurement of SV40 T-antigen production. *Experimental Cell Research*, *91*(2), 247–252. Available from https://doi.org/10.1016/0014-4827(75)90101-9.

Hume, R. I., & Thomas, S. A. (1989). A calcium- and voltage-dependent chloride current in developing chick skeletal muscle. *The Journal of Physiology*, *417*(1), 241–261. Available from https://doi.org/10.1113/jphysiol.1989.sp017799.

Huxley, H. E. (1969). The mechanism of muscular contraction. *Science (New York, N.Y.)*, *164*(3886), 1356–1366. Available from https://doi.org/10.1126/science.164.3886.1356.

Hynes, R. O. (1973). Alteration of cell-surface proteins by viral transformation and by proteolysis. *Proceedings of the National Academy of Sciences*, *70*(11), 3170–3174. Available from https://doi.org/10.1073/pnas.70.11.3170.

Hynes, R. O. (1982). Fibronectin and its relation to cellular structure and behavior. *Cell Biology of the Extracellular Matrix*, 295–334.

Hynes, R. O., & Bye, J. M. (1974). Density and cell cycle dependence of cell surface proteins in hamster fibroblasts. *Cell*, *3*(2), 113–120. Available from https://doi.org/10.1016/0092-8674(74)90114-7.

IARC. (2012). *Combined estrogen-progestogen contraceptivescancer of the cervix. IARC Monograph A Review of Human Carcinogens: Pharmaceuticals* (Vol. 100, pp. 292–293).

Inoue, H., Kondoh, G., Mirawati Sudiro, T., & Hakura, A. (1992). Stability of p53 protein in rat cells transformed by various viral transforming genes. *Virology*, *187*(1), 343–347. Available from https://doi.org/10.1016/0042-6822(92)90325-J.

Izzard, C. S., & Lochner, L. R. (1976). Cell to substrate contacts in living fibroblasts. An interference reflexion study with an evaluation of the technique. *Journal of Cell Science*, *21*(1), 129–159.

Jögi, A., Vaapil, M., Johansson, M., & Påhlman, S. (2012). Cancer cell differentiation heterogeneity and aggressive behavior in solid tumors. *Upsala Journal of Medical Sciences*, *117*(2), 217–224. Available from https://doi.org/10.3109/03009734.2012.659294.

Kamina, P. (1979). Anatomie gynecologique et obstetricale.

Kano, M., Wakuta, K., & Satoh, R. (1987). Calcium channel components of action potential in chick skeletal muscle cells developing in culture. *Developmental Brain Research*, *32*(2), 233–240. Available from https://doi.org/10.1016/0165-3806(87)90103-9.

Kano, M., Wakuta, K., & Satoh, R. (1989). Two components of calcium channel current in embryonic chick skeletal muscle cells developing in culture. *Developmental Brain Research*, *47*(1), 101–112. Available from https://doi.org/10.1016/0165-3806(89)90112-0.

Kidokoro, Y. (1975). Sodium and calcium components of the action potential in a developing skeletal muscle cell line. *The Journal of Physiology*, *244*(1), 145–159. Available from https://doi.org/10.1113/jphysiol.1975.sp010788.

Kubo, Y. (1991). Comparison of initial stages of muscle differentiation in rat and mouse myoblastic and mouse mesodermal stem cell lines. *The Journal of Physiology*, *442*(1), 743–759. Available from https://doi.org/10.1113/jphysiol.1991.sp018817.

Laffargue, F., & Giacalone, P. L. (1992). Cancer du col de l'utérus. Epidémiologie, anatomie pathologique, dépistage, diagnostic, évolution, pronostic, traitement. *Revue du Praticien*, *42* (20), 2615–2620.

Leary, J. F., Notter, M. F., & Todd, P. (1976). Lasar flow cytophotometric immunoperoxidase detection of herpes simplex virus type 2 antigens in infected cultured human cells. *Journal of Histochemistry & Cytochemistry*, *24*(12), 1249–1257. Available from https://doi.org/10.1177/24.12.187690.

Lichti, U., & Yuspa, S. H. (1988). Modulation of tissue and epidermal transglutaminases in mouse epidermal cells after treatment with 12-o-tetradecanoylphorbol-13-acetate and/or retinoic acid in vivo and in culture. *Cancer Research*, *48*(1), 74–81.

L'OMS. (2013). Approche globale de prévention et de lutte contre le cancer du col de l'utérus: Vers une meilleure santé pour les femmes et les jeunes filles.

Massiere, J. (2011). *La transition épithélio-mésenchymateuse dans les cellules épithéliales gastriques: Rôle des microARN régulés par Helicobacter pylori* (Doctoral dissertation) (Vol. 2).

Mautner, V., & Hynes, R. O. (1977). Surface distribution of lets protein in relation to the cytoskeleton of normal and transformed cells. *Journal of Cell Biology*, *75*(3), 743–768. Available from https://doi.org/10.1083/jcb.75.3.743.

McNutt, N. S., Culp, L. A., & Black, P. H. (1971). Contact-inhibited revertant cell lines isolated from SV40-transformed cells. *Journal of Cell Biology*, *50*(3), 691–708. Available from https://doi.org/10.1083/jcb.50.3.691.

McNutt, N. S., Culp, L. A., & Black, P. H. (1973). Contact-Inhibited revertant cell lines isolated from SV40-transformed cells. *Journal of Cell Biology*, 412–428. Available from https://doi.org/10.1083/jcb.56.2.412.

McSharry, J., Laffin, J., Fogleman, D., Lehman, J. M., & Elmendorf, S. (1988). Detection of an early cytomegalovirus antigen with two-color quantitative flow cytometry. *Cytometry*, *9*(3), 254–260. Available from https://doi.org/10.1002/cyto.990090311.

Merlie, J. P., Buckingham, M. E., & Whalen, R. G. (1977). Molecular aspects of myogenesis. *Current Topics in Developmental Biology*, *11*(C), 61–114. Available from https://doi.org/10.1016/S0070-2153(08)60743-7.

Moll, R. (1993). Cytokeratine als differenzierungsmarker. expressionsprofile von epithelien und epithelialen tumoren. *Veröffentlichungen aus der Pathologie*, *142*, 1–197.

Moll, R., Lowe, A., Laufer, J., & Franke, W. W. (1992). Cytokeratin 20 in human carcinomas: A new histodiagnostic marker detected by monoclonal antibodies. *American Journal of Pathology*, *140*(2), 427–447.

Moore, S. E., Thompson, J., Kirkness, V., Dickson, J. G., & Walsh, F. S. (1987). Skeletal muscle neural cell adhesion molecule (N-CAM): Changes in protein and mRNA species during myogenesis of muscle cell lines. *Journal of Cell Biology*, *105*(3), 1377–1386. Available from https://doi.org/10.1083/jcb.105.3.1377.

Murakawa, G. J., Zaia, J. A., Spallone, P. A., Stephens, D. A., Kaplan, B. E., Wallace, R. B., & Rossi, J. J. (1988). Direct detection of HIV-1 RNA from AIDS and ARC patient samples. *DNA (Mary Ann Liebert, Inc.)*, *7*(4), 287–295. Available from https://doi.org/10.1089/dna.1988.7.287.

Ng, I. C., Pawijit, P., Tan, J., & Yu, H. (2019). *Anatomy and physiology for biomaterials research and development. Encyclopedia of Biomedical Engineering* (Vols. 1–3, pp. 225–236). Elsevier. Available from https://doi.org/10.1016/B978-0-12-801238-3.99876-3.

Oskarsson, M., Mcclements, W. L., Blair, D. G., Maizel, J. V., & Vande Woude, G. F. (1980). Properties of a normal mouse cell DNA sequence (sarc) homologous to the src sequence of Moloney sarcoma virus. *Science (New York, N.Y.)*, *207*(4436), 1222–1224. Available from https://doi.org/10.1126/science.6243788.

Pointreau, Y., Ruffier Loubière, A., Denis, F., & Barillot, I. (2010). Cancer du col utérin. *Cancer/Radiothérapie*, S147–S153. Available from https://doi.org/10.1016/s1278-3218(10)70018-4.

Poulouin, L., Gallet, O., & Imhoff, J. M. (1997). La fibronectine: Propriétés et fonctions de la molécule native et de ses fragments.

Rappolee, D. A., Wang, A., Mark, D., & Werb, Z. (1989). Novel method for studying mRNA phenotypes in single or small numbers of cells. *Journal of Cellular Biochemistry*, *39*(1), 1–11. Available from https://doi.org/10.1002/jcb.240390102.

Reiss, M., DiMaio, D., & Zibello, T. A. (1989). Bovine papillomavirus type I induces resistance to Ca + (+)-induced terminal differentiation in murine keratinocytes. *Cancer Communications*, *1*(2), 75–82. Available from https://doi.org/10.3727/095535489820875318.

Rochford, R., Hobbs, M. V., Garnier, J. L., Cooper, N. R., & Cannon, M. J. (1993). Plasmacytoid differentiation of Epstein-Barr virus-transformed B cells in vivo is associated with reduced expression of viral latent genes. *Proceedings of the National Academy of Sciences*, *90*(1), 352–356. Available from https://doi.org/10.1073/pnas.90.1.352.

Ronco, G., Giorgi-Rossi, P., Carozzi, F., Confortini, M., Palma, P. D., Del Mistro, A., Ghiringhello, B., Girlando, S., Gillio-Tos, A., De Marco, L., Naldoni, C., Pierotti, P., Rizzolo, R., Schincaglia, P., Zorzi, M., Zappa, M., Segnan, N., & Cuzick, J. (2010). Efficacy of human papillomavirus testing for the detection of invasive cervical cancers and cervical intraepithelial neoplasia: A randomised controlled trial. *The Lancet Oncology*, *11*(3), 249–257. Available from https://doi.org/10.1016/S1470-2045(09)70360-2.

Ruoslahti, E., Hayman, E. G., Engvall, E., Cothran, W. C., & Butler, W. T. (1981). Alignment of biologically active domains in the fibronectin molecule. *Journal of Biological Chemistry*, *256*(14), 7277–7281.

Santé, M. de la. (2017). La lutte contre le cancer du col de l'utérus: Guide des pratiques essentielles.

Satelli, A., & Li, S. (2011). Vimentin in cancer and its potential as a molecular target for cancer therapy. *Cellular and Molecular Life Sciences*, *68*(18), 3033–3046. Available from https://doi.org/10.1007/s00018-011-0735-1.

Schwarz, A., Mengel, M., Gwinner, W., Eisenberger, U., Hiss, M., Radermacher, J., Fiebeler, A., Abou-Rebyeh, F., & Haller, H. (2002). Protocol biopsy program after renal transplantation: Structure and first results. *Transplantation Proceedings*, *34*(6), 2238–2239. Available from https://doi.org/10.1016/S0041-1345(02)03286-4.

Scott, M. P., & Helm, K. F. (1999). Cytokeratin 20: A marker for diagnosing merkel cell carcinoma. *American Journal of Dermatopathology*, *21*(1), 16–20. Available from https://doi.org/10.1097/00000372-199902000-00003.

Shay, J. W., Wright, W. E., Brasiskyte, D., & Van der Hagen, B. A. (1993). E6 of human papillomavirus type 16 can overcome the M1 stage of immortalization in human mammary epithelial cells but not in human fibroblasts. *Oncogene*, *8*(6), 1407–1413.

Singer-Sam, J., Robinson, M. O., Bellvé, A. R., Simon, M. L., & Riggs, A. D. (1990). Measurement by quantitative PCR of changes in HPRT, PGK-1, PGK-2, APRT, MTase, and Zfy gene transcripts during mouse spermatogenesis. *Nucleic Acids Research*, *18*(5), 1255–1259. Available from https://doi.org/10.1093/nar/18.5.1255.

Smith, A. E., Smith, R., & Paucha, E. (1979). Characterization of different tumor antigens present in cells transformed by simian virus 40. *Cell*, *18*(2), 335–346. Available from https://doi.org/10.1016/0092-8674(79)90053-9.

Tadlaoui, K. A., Hassou, N., Bennani, B., & Ennaji, M. M. (2020). *Emergence of oncogenic high-risk human papillomavirus types and cervical cancer. Emerging and Reemerging Viral Pathogens: Volume 1: Fundamental and Basic Virology Aspects of Human, Animal and Plant Pathogens* (pp. 539–570). Elsevier. Available from http://www.sciencedirect.com/science/book/9780128194003.

Thomas, K. H., Wilkie, T. M., Tomashefsky, P., Bellve, A. R., & Simon, M. I. (1989). Differential gene expression during mouse spermatogenesis. *Biology of Reproduction*, *41*(4), 729–739. Available from https://doi.org/10.1095/biolreprod41.4.729.

Tranbaloc, P. (2008). Histoire naturelle des lésions précurseurs du cancer du col utérin. *Gynécologie Obstétrique & Fertilité*, *36*(6), 650–655. Available from https://doi.org/10.1016/j.gyobfe.2008.03.016.

Trautmann, A., Delaporte, C., & Marty, A. (1986). Voltage-dependent channels of human muscle cultures. *Pflügers Archiv European Journal of Physiology*, *406*(2), 163–172. Available from https://doi.org/10.1007/BF00586678.

Vaheri, A., & Mosher, D. F. (1978). High molecular weight, cell surface-associated glycoprotein (fibronectin) lost in maglinant transformation. *Biochimica et Biophysica Acta (BBA) – Reviews on Cancer*, *516*(1), 1–25. Available from https://doi.org/10.1016/0304-419x(78)90002-1.

Vielkind, U., & Swierenga, S. H. (1989). A simple fixation procedure for immunofluorescent detection of different cytoskeletal components within the same cell. *Histochemistry*, *91*(1), 81–88. Available from https://doi.org/10.1007/BF00501916.

Weiss, R. E., & Horn, R. (1986). Functional differences between two classes of sodium channels in developing rat skeletal muscle. *Science (New York, N.Y.)*, *233*(4761), 361–364. Available from https://doi.org/10.1126/science.2425432.

Yaffe, D. (1968). Retention of differentiation potentialities during prolonged cultivation of myogenic cells. *Proceedings of the National Academy of Sciences of the United States of America, 61*(2), 477–483. Available from https://doi.org/10.1073/pnas.61.2.477.

Yaffe, D. (1969). Chapter 2 cellular aspects of muscle differentiation in vitro. *Current Topics in Developmental Biology, 4*(C), 37–77. Available from https://doi.org/10.1016/S0070-2153(08)60480-9.

Yamada, K. M., & Olden, K. (1978). Fibronectins—adhesive glycoproteins of cell surface and blood. *Nature*, 179–184. Available from https://doi.org/10.1038/275179a0.

Zhang, Y., Yu, S., Han, Y., Wang, Y., & Sun, Y. (2018). Human leukocyte antigen-G expression and polymorphisms promote cancer development and guide cancer diagnosis/treatment (Review). *Oncology Letters, 15*(1), 699–709. Available from https://doi.org/10.3892/ol.2017.7407.

Chapter 14

The clinical significance of long noncoding RNAs expression in cervical cancers

Maryame Lamsisi[3], Amal Bouziyane[2,3], Berjas Abumsimir[3,4], Oubaida ElBiad[5,6], Youssef Ennaji[2], Abdelilah Laraqui[7], Mohammed El Mzibri[8,10], Hicham Benaguida[9], Mustapha Benhessou[3,9], Mohammed Ennachit[9], Mohamed El Karroumi[9] and Moulay Mustapha Ennaji[1]

[1]*Group Leader Research team of Virology, Oncology, and Biotechnologies, Head of Laboratory of Virology, Oncology, Biosciences, Environment and New Energies (LVO-BEEN), Faculty of Sciences and Techniques Mohammedia, University Hassan II of Casablanca, Casablanca, Morocco,* [2]*University Mohammed VI of Health Science, Casablanca, Morocco,* [3]*Team of Virology, Oncology, and Biotechnologies, Laboratory of Virology, Oncology, Biosciences, Environment and New Energies (LVO-BEEN), Faculty of Sciences and Techniques Mohammedia, University Hassan II of Casablanca, Casablanca, Morocco,* [4]*Pharmacological and Diagnostic Research Centre (PDRC), Department of Medical Laboratory Sciences, Faculty of Allied Medical Sciences, Al-Ahliyya Amman University (AAU), Amman, Jordan,* [5]*Laboratory of Research and Biosafety L3, Military Teaching Hospital Mohammed V, Rabat, Morocco,* [6]*Sequencing Unit, Virology Laboratory, Center for Virology, Infectious and Tropical Diseases, Mohammed V Military Instruction Hospital, Faculty of Medicine and Pharmacy, Mohammed V University, Rabat, Morocco,* [7]*Laboratory of Human Pathologies Biology, Faculty of Sciences, and Genomic Center of Human Pathologies, Faculty of Medicine and Pharmacy, Bio-Path Laboratory, Faculty of sciences-Agdal, Mohammed V University, Rabat, Morocco,* [8]*Biology and Medical Research Unit, CNESTEN, Rabat, Morocco,* [9]*Mohammed VI Centre for Treatment of Cancer, University Hospital Ibn Rochd, Casablanca, Morocco,* [10]*Life Sciences Division CNESTEN, Rabat, Morocco*

14.1 Introduction

Cervical cancer is the fourth most commonly diagnosed cancer among females worldwide, representing a major global health issue (Bray et al., 2018). Squamous cell carcinoma (SCC) is the most common histological subtype of cervical cancer, representing 70% of all cases, while 25% are adenocarcinomas. Virtually all cervical cancers are caused by persistent infection with one or

Immunological Implications and Molecular Diagnostics of Genitourinary Cancer.
DOI: https://doi.org/10.1016/B978-0-323-85496-2.00013-0

multiple high-risk human papillomaviruses (HPVs). Despite the remarkable advances in prevention, screening, diagnosis, and treatment during the past decades, there are important disparities in cervical cancer outcomes, and the overall outcome of patients, especially with advanced disease, is still poor (Cohen et al., 2019). The available tools for screening and diagnosis encounter many challenges associated with their sensitivity, specificity, cost of implementation, and lack of trained personnel, while treatment is often challenged by resistance and severe side effects. Therefore more reliable test options need to be improved, and treatment needs to be targeted efficiently. More importantly, disease prevention and treatment strategies need to take into account the individual variability. This requires deciphering the aberrant genomic and epigenomic events underlying cervical cancer development (Goossens et al., 2015).

The remarkable advances in molecular biology and discovery of revolutionary technologies such as high-throughput sequencing has enabled the accumulation of substantial knowledge about the aberrant pathways and new molecular players in complex diseases, especially cancer. Long noncoding RNAs (lncRNAs) are a relatively new subclass of noncoding RNAs of more than 200 nt in size, which are aberrantly expressed in cancers. Although the observed evolutionary conservation of lncRNAs currently appears to be inferior to other RNAs, some secondary structures within many lncRNA orthologs are conserved and functional (Kopp & Mendell, 2018). After transcription, lncRNAs can act in *cis*, controlling nearby genes, or in *trans*, controlling distant genes, thus inducing or inhibiting their expression in a tissue-specific manner (Castro-Oropeza et al., 2018).

Several lncRNAs are directly involved in cancer as oncogenes or tumor suppressors. For instance, lncRNA H19 inhibited cells growth, mobility, and invasion in a mechanism involving the downregulation of insulin receptor substrate 1 (IRS-1) in thyroid cancer (Wang et al., 2017), and ZFAS1 acts as an oncogene in colorectal cancer through two mechanisms including the destabilization of p53 and its interaction with CDKl/cyclin B1, thus promoting cell cycle and inhibiting cell apoptosis (Thorenoor et al., 2016). Previous studies revealed that in cervical cancer, lncRNAs regulate genes related to cell proliferation, cell cycle arrest, apoptosis, epithelial to mesenchymal transition (EMT), metastasis, invasion, chemoresistance, and resistance to radiotherapy. Moreover, it has been found that the knockdown of certain oncogenic lncRNAs and the ectopic expression of tumor suppressor lncRNAs could reverse tumor aggressiveness. For example, the repression of lncRNA PCAT6 inhibited cell proliferation, migration, and invasion (Lv et al., 2019), while overexpression of WT1-AS attenuated cervical cancer progression in vitro and suppressed tumor growth in vivo (Dai et al., 2019). These findings indicated that lncRNAs could be potential targets for biomarker discovery of diagnosis, prognosis, and disease recurrence. In addition, targeting these molecules could constitute a new approach for cervical cancer treatment. In this chapter, we address the clinical significance of lncRNAs in cervical cancer screening, diagnosis, prognosis, and treatment.

14.2 Long noncoding RNAs as potential biomarker candidates

14.2.1 Long noncoding RNAs s as biomarkers for screening of cervical cancer

The current understanding of the role of persistent HPV infection in cervical cancer development has provided opportunities for preventive approaches. The transition of the initial cytological changes induced by HPV to malignant cancer takes several steps involving three grades of cervical intraepithelial neoplasia (CINs); If left untreated, CINs can progress to invasive cancer, in a process that can extend over many years. Screening of nonsymptomatologic patients using Pap tests and HPV detection has made it possible to detect and treat CINs and thus prevent invasive cervical cancers, and it has markedly reduced cervical cancer rates over the last decades.

Certain lncRNAs are exclusively expressed in precancerous lesions of the cervix. Gibb et al. found a total of 668 lncRNAs that were uniquely expressed in the cervix and had either minimal or no expression in other human tissues. They also found differential expression patterns of another set among these lncRNAs specific to CINs (Gibb et al., 2012). Wang et al. reported the differential expression of CCAT2 and LINC01133 levels between serums of patients with CINs and normal controls. These lncRNAs showed a significant ability to discriminate CIN groups from normal groups (AUC = 0.827 for CCAT2 and AUC = 0.823 for LINC01133), and the discriminatory value was further enhanced by the combination of both CCAT2 and LINC01133 (AUC = 0.894), achieving 96.1% specificity and 67.1% sensitivity (Wang et al., 2020). In another study, DLX6-AS1 expression in serum-derived exosomes was able to distinguish cervical cancer from CIN (AUC = 0.831) with 75.4% sensitivity and 71.8% specificity (Ding et al., n.d.). More studies are needed to further investigate their use in the triage of CINs during screening.

Assessing the risk of developing precancerous lesions of the cervix might also provide another preventive approach enabling the identification of women at risk. Single nucleotide polymorphisms (SNPs) are largely used in this context, and SNPs occurring in lncRNA genes have been reported to be correlated to the risk of developing diseases (Castellanos-Rubio & Ghosh, 2019). Wang et al. studied 12 SNPs in lncRNA MALAT1 and lncRNA THRIL in CINs vs controls, and they found that THRIL rs7133268 AG genotype was associated with decreased risk of developing cervical precancerous lesions (Wang et al., 2018). There are other studies investigating lncRNAs polymorphisms in relation to the diagnosis and prognosis of cervical cancers, which are discussed in the following sections. However, only a few reports are available regarding CINs.

14.3 Long noncoding RNAs as biomarkers for diagnosis and early detection of cervical cancers

It is well established that early detection of cervical cancer can reduce its related mortality. The survival rate of patients decreases as the stage of the disease progresses, reaching only 20% at stage IV of cervical cancer (Grigsby et al., 2020) Table 14.1. Also, surgical treatment is only effective in curing cervical cancer when it is detected in the early stages, which is attributable to the absence of effective therapeutic approaches for patients with advanced cervical cancer (Small et al., 2017).

The challenge of early diagnosis arises from the absence of symptoms specific to cervical cancer and the invasiveness of the currently available clinical diagnosis procedures. Most of the symptoms that may be presented for cervical cancer are nonspecific and most suggestive of advanced disease.

TABLE 14.1 Survival of cervical cancer patients according to FIGO stage.

FIGO stage (2018)	Five-year PFS (%)
Stage I	80
IA1	89
IA2	100
IB1	90
IB2	84
IB3	79
Stage II	59
IIA1	86
IIA2	N/A
IIB	72
Stage III	35
IIIA	46
IIIB	55
IIIC1	62
IIIC2	35
Stage IV	20
IVA	39
IVB	11

PFS, Progression free survival; *N/A*, not applicable.

These include postcoital or abnormal vaginal bleeding, pelvic or lower back pain, pelvic pressure, hematochezia, hematuria, or vaginal passage of urine or stool that indicate fistula formation (Cohen et al., 2019; Stumbar et al., 2019). However, there are no symptoms specific to early cervical cancer. Thus the clinical diagnosis of cervical cancer requires invasive procedures. Symptomatic patients must undergo pelvic examination, visualization of the cervix and vaginal mucosa using speculum examination, and cervical cytology. Colposcopy and biopsy are required when symptoms are presented, or when the cytology indicates invisible lesions (Cohen et al., 2019). Other noninvasive alternatives are used for the diagnosis of cervical cancer, including serum protein biomarkers such as squamous cell carcinoma antigen (SCC Ag) (Dasari et al., 2015). However, their unsatisfactory sensitivity and specificity limit their diagnosis benefit (Dasari et al., 2015).

Individual lncRNAs can be detected in tissues and minimally invasive samples such as sera and plasma and have shown satisfying ability to discriminate cervical cancer patients from normal patients (Table 14.2). In addition, multiple lncRNA signatures improve the diagnostic value of cervical cancer. Wang et al. analyzed the diagnostic value of three IncRNAs, namely, CCAT2, LINC00511, and LINC01133, in cervical squamous carcinoma. The combination of these three lncRNAs resulted in an improved AUC value of 0.868, with a sensitivity and specificity of 74.8% and 90.0%, respectively. They also found that the combination of the three lncRNAs with SCC further

TABLE 14.2 Diagnosis performance of long noncoding RNAs in cervical cancer.

LncRNA	Sample	AUC	SEN	SPE	References
GIHCG	Serum	0.9408	88.75%	87.50%	Zhang et al. (2019)
MEG3	Serum	0.844	82.76%	75.00%	Wan & Zhao (2020)
DLX6-AS1	Serum Exosomes	0.892	78.1%	88.2%	Ding et al. (n.d.)
XLOC_010588	Tissues	0.918	84.4%	86.7%	Liao et al. (2014)
FALEC	Plasma	0.91	–	–	Naizhaer et al. (2019)
LncRNA-EXOC7	Serum	0.9388	–	–	Guo et al. (2020)
	Serum Exosomes	0.8982			
SRA	Tissues	0.737	–	–	Kim et al. (2018)
GHET1	Tissues	0.874	–	–	Zhang et al. (2019)

improved the AUC value to 0.940 along with the sensitivity and specificity, which reached 81.6% and 97.1%, respectively (Wang et al., 2020).

However, owing to issues in study design, the variability of techniques, and the absence of standardization for biomarker research tools, the initial findings on lncRNAs related to their diagnosis performance often cannot be reproduced in subsequent studies, thus limiting the clinical implementation and validation of these biomarkers. As a result, among the several suggested ncRNAs by a large number of studies, only one ncRNA-based test, the (PROGENSA PCA3), which is a urinary test for the detection of lncRNA PCA3, has been successfully translated to clinical application with FDA approval (Durand et al., 2011).

14.4 Long noncoding RNAs as biomarkers of prognosis and survival

A growing number of studies have reported the differential expression of lncRNAs and their association with the clinicopathological features of cervical cancer patients and their survival (Table 14.3). Several lncRNAs were reported to be aberrantly expressed in cervical cancer. For example, HOTAIR expression was elevated in cervical cancer tissues and correlated with FIGO stage, tumor size; lymphatic metastasis, and depth of invasion, which suggest its involvement in cervical cancer progression and an independent predictor for overall survival (Huang et al., 2014). High levels of HOTAIR were associated with tumor recurrence and short overall survival (Li et al., 2015), suggesting circulating HOTAIR as a possible prognostic biomarker in cervical cancer, as well as a promising target for targeted therapy in cervical cancer.

On the contrary, tumor suppressor lncRNAs, such as growth arrest-specific transcript 5 (GAS5), WT1-AS, and XLOC_010588 were downregulated in cervical cancer tissues. In vitro assays suggested the knockdown of GAS5 promoted cell proliferation, invasion, and migration, which suggested GAS5 as a potential marker for cervical cancer. This was supported by the finding that low levels of GAS5 significantly correlated with advanced cancer progression (Cao et al., 2014). lncRNA XLOC_010588, also named tumor suppressor candidate 8 (TUSC8), regulates cell proliferation via c-Myc downregulation in cervical cancer (Liao et al., 2014). XLOC_010588 was significantly underexpressed in cervical cancer and linked to FIGO stage, tumor size, and SCC Ag (Liao et al., 2014). It implicated that TUSC8 could be an independent predictor of the overall survival of cervical cancer. Also, decreased expression of lncRNA LET was significantly correlated with FIGO stage, lymphatic metastasis, and depth of cervical invasion. In addition, cervical cancer patients with lower lncRNA LET had worse overall survival compared to those with higher expression levels of lncRNA LET

TABLE 14.3 Prognosis value of long noncoding RNAs in cervical cancer.

LncRNA	Expression Level	FIGO Stage	Tumor size	LNM	HPV	DM	Survival	References
UCA1	Upregulated	–	–	–	–	–	Low	Yang et al. (2020)
BLACAT1	Upregulated	Non significant(ns)	–	–	–	–	Low	Cheng et al. (2020)
FEZF1-AS1	Upregulated	+	ns	–	ns	+	Low	Zhang & Li (2018)
Loc554202	Upregulated	+	+	+	+	–	Low	Chen & Zhu (2017)
WT1-AS	Downregulated	+	ns	+	–	–	High	Dai et al. (2019)
CASC15	Upregulated	+	ns	+	ns	–	Low	Shan et al. (2019)
GAS5	Downregulated	+	ns	+	–	+	High	Li et al. (2018)
		+	ns	+	–	–	High	Cao et al. (2014)
PCAT6	Upregulated	+	ns	+	–	–	Low	Lv et al. (2019)
ROR1-AS1	Upregulated	+	ns	ns	–	+	Low	Zhang et al. (2020)
SNHG14	Upregulated	+	+	+	–	–	Low	Zhang et al. (2019)
SNHG7	Upregulated	+	ns	+	–	–	Low	Zeng et al. (2019)
RP11–396F22.1	Upregulated	+	+	+	ns	–	Low	Zhao et al. (2018)
LncRNA-IL7R	Upregulated	+	+	+	ns	–	Low	Fan et al. (2018)
GHET1	Upregulated	+	ns	+	–	+	Low	Zhang et al. (2019)
TCONS_00026907	Upregulated	+	+	+	ns	–	Low	Jin et al. (2017)
SPRY4-IT1	Upregulated	+	+	+	–	–	Low	Cao et al. (2016)

(Continued)

TABLE 14.3 (Continued)

LncRNA	Expression Level	FIGO Stage	Tumor size	LNM	HPV	DM	Survival	References
ZFAS1	Upregulated	+	ns	+	–	–	Low	Feng et al. (2019)
HOTAIR	Upregulated	+	+	+	–	–	Low	Huang et al. (2014)
		+	ns	+	–	–	Low	Li et al. (2015)
CCAT2	Upregulated	+	ns	+	–	–	Low	Chen et al. (2015)
XLOC_010588	Downregulated	+	+	ns	–	–	High	Liao et al. (2014)
FALEC	Upregulated	+	+	ns	–	–	Low	Naizhaer et al. (2019)
SRA	Upregulated	ns	ns	ns	–	–	Low	Kim et al. (2018)
CERNA2	Upregulated	+	ns	+	–	+	Low	Wang et al. (2019)
ANRIL	Upregulated	+	ns	+	–	–	Low	Zhang et al. (2017)
DLX6-AS1	Upregulated	+	ns	+	ns	–	Low	Ding et al. (n.d.)
LINC00662	Upregulated	+	ns	+	–	–	–	Wei et al. (2020)

(Jiang et al., 2015), suggesting the potential of lncRNA LET as a candidate biomarker for the prognosis of cervical cancer.

14.5 Long noncoding RNAs in cervical cancer treatment and therapy

14.5.1 Long noncoding RNAs in resistance to treatment of cervical cancer

The most used therapeutic approaches for cervical cancer include chemotherapy, radiotherapy, and surgery. Chemotherapy in cervical cancer relies mainly on cisplatin, which is a platinum-based drug that induces DNA platinum adducts to block the DNA repair process, thus arresting the cell cycle and promoting cell apoptosis (Peng et al., 2020). However, the multiple side effects and drug resistance are major challenges that limit the clinical benefit of chemotherapy.

A number of oncogenic lncRNAs are involved in the chemoresistance of cells and patients, and the inhibition of these lncRNAs, namely, NCK1-AS1 has been shown to improve the outcome of chemotherapy in vitro (Zhang et al., 2019). On the other hand, the induced expression of other lncRNAs such as CASC2 and miR503HG amplified cisplatin-induced cytotoxicity through different mechanisms that appear to involve their interaction with microRNAs such as miR-21 to modulate PTEN, or miR-155/Caspase-3, and Akt signaling pathway (Feng et al., 2017; Wen et al., 2017; Zhao et al., 2020). In radiotherapy, overexpression of HOTAIR could induce radioresistance in cells and enhance tumor growth after radiation in vivo (Li et al., 2018; Jing et al., 2015). The effect of HOTAIR in response to radiation was mediated by inhibiting p21 and upregulating HIF-1α (Jing et al., 2015; Li et al., 2018). In addition, knocking down HOTAIR upregulated p21 and sensitized cervical cancer to radiotherapy in vitro and in vivo (Jing et al., 2015). CeRNA seems to be a common mechanism involved in lncRNA-mediated radioresistance in cervical cancer. For instance, MALAT1 and SNHG6 were involved in radioresistance of cervical cancer through reciprocally sponging miR-145 expression and miR-485-3p, respectively (Lu et al., 2016) (Fig. 14.1). Table 14.4 summarizes lncRNA mechanisms in modulating the response of patients with cervical cancer to treatment.

Cancer stem cells (CSCs) are a subpopulation of cancer cells that have the capacity to unlimitedly self-renew and differentiate in addition, to a low pace of cellular division, allowing them to particularly resist chemotherapy (Barbato et al., 2019). It was reported that this aggressive subpopulation of cancer cells has a unique characteristic and deploys specific mechanisms to inactivate therapeutic agents (Barbato et al., 2019).

Studies have demonstrated that certain lncRNAs contributed to the response of cervical CSCs to chemotherapy. It was observed that CSCs

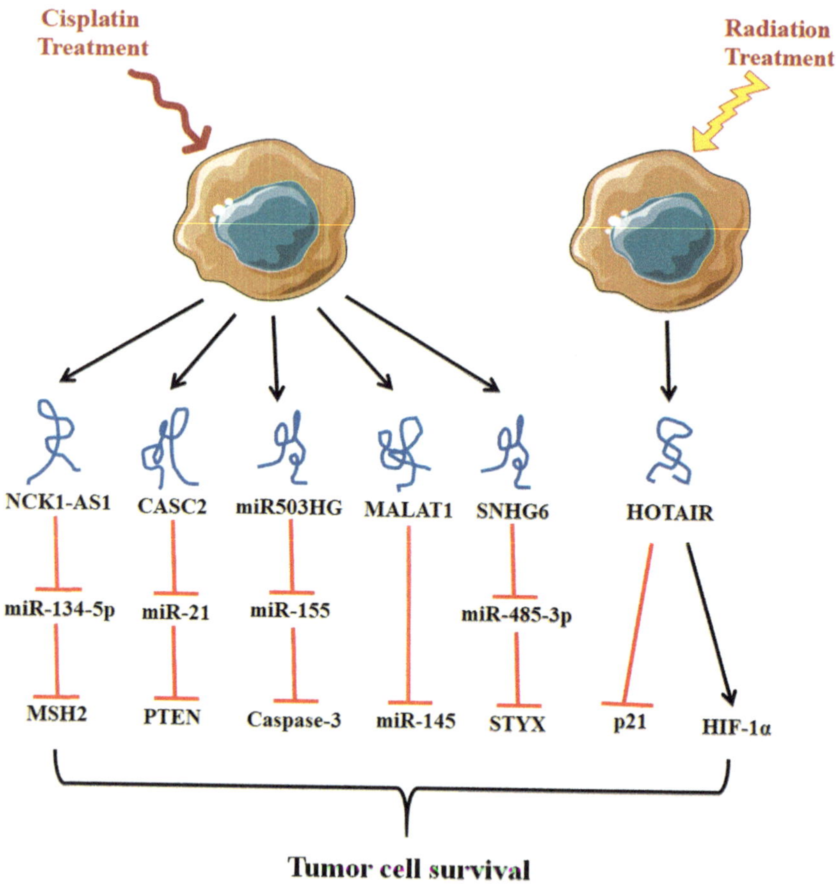

FIGURE 14.1 The mechanism of long noncoding RNAs in treatment resistance of cervical cancer. When tumor cells are subjected to radiation or chemotherapy, they express several lncRNAs that stimulate a regulation pathway leading to the blockade of tumor suppressors, thus leading to tumor cells' survival.

treated with cisplatin overexpressed six lncRNAs (HOXA-AS2, UCA1, HOTAIR, HIF1A-AS1, and IPW), and the inhibition of these lncRNAs inhibited CSC sphere formations (Li et al., 2019) (Fig. 14.2).

Therefore targeting these lncRNAs in a combination with radiotherapy or chemotherapy might provide new therapeutic options in cervical cancer treatment to improve patient outcomes.

14.5.2 Long noncoding RNAs in cervical cancer therapy

Fundamental studies on molecular mechanisms of lncRNAs in cervical cancer were important to understand the targeting of these molecules for more

TABLE 14.4 Roles of long noncoding RNAs in resistance to therapy of cervical cancer.

Impact	LncRNA	Samples	Mechanism	References
Chemoresistance to cisplatin	TUG1	Cells and patients	Activating the MAPK pathway	Wei et al. (2019)
	MALAT1	Cells	Activating the PI3K/AKT pathway	Wang et al. (2018)
	NNT-AS1	Cells and patients	Regulating NNT-AS1/miR-186/HMGB1 axis	Liu et al. (2020)
	PVT1	Cells	Epigenetically silencing miR-195	Shen et al. (2017)
	UCA1	Cells	Inhibiting apoptotic pathway and enhancing cell proliferation	Wang et al. (2017)
	HOXD-AS1	Cells	Modulating miR-130a-3p/ZEB1 axis	Chi et al. (2018)
	NCK1-AS1	Cells	Competitively binding to miR-134-5p	Zhang et al. (2019)
Chemosensitivity to cisplatin	miR503HG	Cells and patients	Regulating miR-155/Caspase-3	Zhao et al. (2020)
	GAS5	Cells	Regulating the phosphorylation of Akt	Wen et al. (2017)
	CASC2	Cells and patients	Modulating /miR-21/PTEN axis	Feng et al. (2017)
Radioresistance	SNHG6	Cells	Sponging miR-485-3p	Liu et al. (2020)
	SNHG12	Cells	Regulating miR-148a/CDK1 pathway	Wang et al. (2020)
	HOTAIR	Cells	Promoting HIF-1α expression	Li et al. (2019)
	LINC00662	Cells	Regulating miR-497−5p/CDC25A axis	Wei et al. (2020)
	UCA1	Cells	Through the glycolytic pathway by modulating HK2	Fan et al. (2018)
	NEAT1	Cells and nude mice	Regulating miR-193b-3p/CCND1 axis	Han et al. (2018)
	LINC00958	Cells, nude mice, and Patients	Interacting with the miR-5095/RRM2 axis	Zhao et al. (2019)

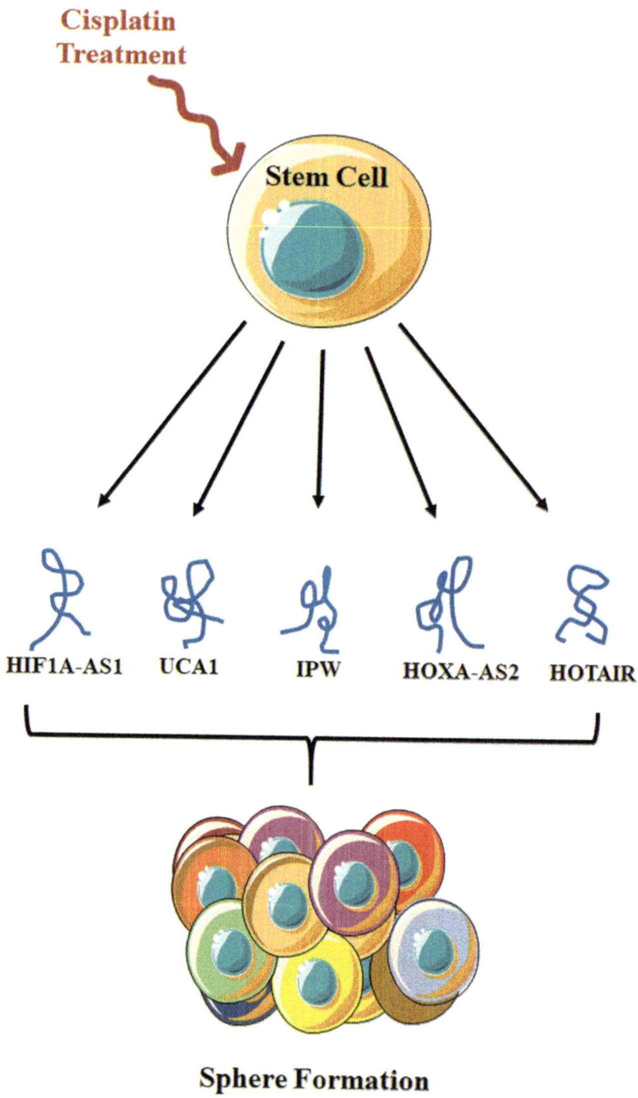

FIGURE 14.2 **Long noncoding RNAs are employed by stem cells to induce sphere formation.** In response to cisplatin treatment, CSCs overexpressed several lncRNAs that mediate sphere formation.

efficient and targeted therapies. For instance, silencing LINC0051 affected negatively the cell viability, proliferation, migration, invasion, and induced cell cycle arrest at G1 phase. Additionally, LINC0051 knockdown increased the levels of the mRNA and protein of proapoptotic genes, namely Bax and cleaved-caspase-3, while it decreased those of antiapoptotic Bcl-2 and invasion-related genes MMP2 and MMP-9. In addition, silencing of LINC00511 could inhibit resistance to paclitaxel (PTX) of PTX-resistant cells, and the inhibition of LINC00511 + PTX treatment enhanced cells sensitivity to PTX (Mao et al., 2019) (Fig. 14.3).

Codelivery of drugs with different natures and mechanisms, such as chemotherapy and gene therapy, improved the cytotoxicity and antitumor effects of these drugs. Ye et al. designed a liposome-based codelivery system that targets tumors by simultaneously delivering oxaliplatin and MDC1-AS mRNA. The latter is an antisense lncRNA to the MDC1 gene. MDC1 is a mediator of DNA damage response mechanism by regulating the checkpoint-mediated cell cycle arrest. MDC1-AS forms RNA-RNA dimers with MDC1 and protects it from RNase degradation, thereby increasing its stability and level of expression. On the other hand, OXA inhibits DNA replication and transcription by forming inter- and intrastrand platinum-DNA adducts. The combination of MDC1-AS and OXA promoted apoptosis and inhibited SIHA cells migration and invasion activities, as well as effectively inhibited tumor growth in vivo (Ye et al., 2021).

In another aspect, it was demonstrated that new molecules suggested for drug discoveries, such as Metformin, Baicalein, Propofol, and Artesunate (ART), mediate their cytotoxicity against cervical cancer cells through lncRNAs (He et al., 2020). For instance, the ART-based treatment of cervical

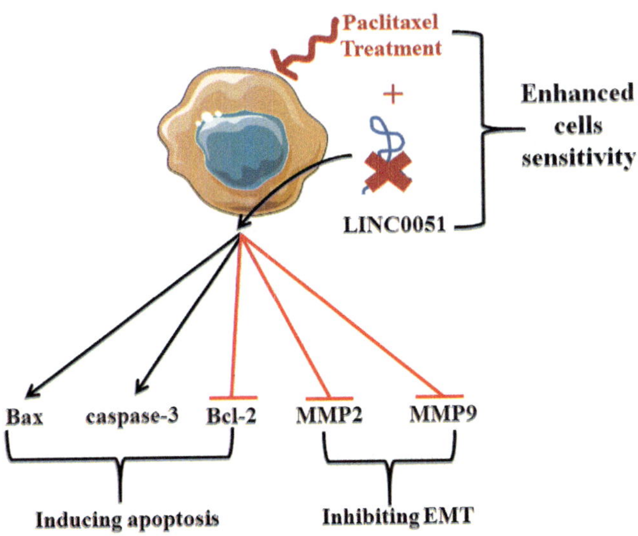

FIGURE 14.3 Paclitaxel treatment coupled with lncRNA LINC0051 inhibition enhanced cell sensitivity to treatment. The addition of LINC0051 inhibition to Paclitaxel treatment increased cell sensitivity to treatment by stimulating the expression of Bax and caspase-3 and inhibiting Bcl-2, thus promoting apoptosis on the one hand, and inhibiting MMP 2 and 9, leading to the blockade of EMT on the other hand.

cancer cells significantly reduced HOTAIR expression, and the overexpression of HOTAIR reversed the ART effect by mediating the expression of its downstream gene COX2 at a posttranscriptional level (Zhang et al., 2016).

14.6 Conclusions

LncRNAs are major players in cellular physiology and are responsible for gene regulation during transcription, translation, and posttranslational events. Understanding the molecular mechanisms of lncRNAs in specific tissues provided more insight and approaches to genetic diseases, such as cancer, from prevention to treatment. In cervical cancer, a growing body of evidence revealed the functional roles of several lncRNAs in controlling cell proliferation, cancer progression, and drug resistance in vitro and in vivo. The differential expression of lncRNAs and the possibility of detecting them noninvasively in body fluids such as blood, serum, and urine make them interesting candidates for new biomarker discovery for diagnosis, prognosis, and response to treatment. In addition, blockade of oncogenic lncRNAs and induced expression of tumor suppressor lncRNAs have reversed tumor aggressiveness and may be used for targeted therapy in cervical cancer. However, before any transition to clinical application, it is crucial to standardize techniques for detecting and quantifying lncRNAs in order to compare their performance and overcome the lack of reproducibility between studies, in addition, to improving delivery systems for targeting specific tissues in therapy.

Acknowledgment

The authors would like to acknowledge The Ministry of High Education of Morocco, the University Hassan II of Casablanca, and the Faculty of Sciences and Techniques, Mohammedia, for supporting this work, as well as the staff of the Laboratory of Virology, Microbiology, Quality and Biotechnologies/Ecotoxicology and Biodiversity for their technical assistance and support.

References

Barbato, L., Bocchetti, M., Di Biase, A., & Regad, T. (2019). Cancer stem cells and targeting strategies. *Cells*, *8*(8), 926. Available from https://doi.org/10.3390/cells8080926.

Bray, F., Ferlay, J., Soerjomataram, I., Siegel, R. L., Lindsey, A. T., & Jemal, A. (2018). Global Cancer Statistics 2018: GLOBOCAN Estimates of Incidence and Mortality Worldwide for 36 Cancers in 185 Countries. *CA: A Cancer Journal for Clinicians*, *68*, 394–424.

Cao, S., Liu, W., Li, F., Zhao, W., & Qin, C. (2014). Decreased expression of lncRNA GAS5 predicts a poor prognosis in cervical cancer. *International Journal of Clinical and Experimental Pathology*, *7*(10), 6776–6783. Available from http://www.ijcep.com/files/ijcep0001900.pdf.

Cao, Y., Liu, Y., Lu, X., Wang, Y., Qiao, H., & Liu, M. (2016). Upregulation of Long Noncoding RNA SPRY4-IT1 Correlates with Tumor Progression and Poor Prognosis in Cervical Cancer. *FEBS Open Bio*, *6*(9), 954–960.

Castellanos-Rubio, A., & Ghosh, S. (2019). Disease-associated SNPs in inflammation-related lncRNAs. *Frontiers in Immunology*, 10. Available from https://doi.org/10.3389/fimmu.2019.00420.

Castro-Oropeza, R., Melendez-Zajgla, J., Maldonado, V., & Vazquez-Santillan, K. (2018). The emerging role of lncRNAs in the regulation of cancer stem cells. *Cellular Oncology*, *41*(6), 585–603. Available from https://doi.org/10.1007/s13402-018-0406-4.

Chen, X., Liu, L., & Zhu, W. (2015). Up-Regulation of Long Non-Coding RNA CCAT2 Correlates with Tumor Metastasis and Poor Prognosis in Cervical Squamous Cell Cancer Patients. *International Journal of Clinical and Experimental Pathology*, *8*(10), 13261–13266.

Chen, J., & Zhu, J. (2017). Elevated Expression Levels of Long Non-Coding RNA, Loc554202, Are Predictive of Poor Prognosis in Cervical Cancer. *Tohoku Journal of Experimental Medicine*, *243*(3), 165–172.

Cheng, H., Tian, J., Wang, C., Ren, L., & Wang, N. (2020). LncRNA BLACAT1 Is Upregulated in Cervical Squamous Cell Carcinoma (CSCC) and Predicts Poor Survival. *Reproductive Sciences*, *27*(é), 585–591.

Chi, C., Mao, M., Shen, Z., Chen, Y., Chen, J., & Hou, W. (2018). HOXD-AS1 Exerts Oncogenic Functions and Promotes Chemoresistance in Cisplatin-Resistant Cervical Cancer Cells. *Human Gene Therapy*, *29*(12).

Cohen, P. A., Jhingran, A., Oaknin, A., & Denny, L. (2019). Cervical cancer. *The Lancet*, 169–182. Available from https://doi.org/10.1016/s0140-6736(18)32470-x.

Dai, S. G., Guo, L. L., Xia, X., & Pan, Y. (2019). Long non-coding RNA WT1-AS inhibits cell aggressiveness via miR-203a-5p/FOXN2 axis and is associated with prognosis in cervical cancer. *European Review for Medical and Pharmacological Sciences*, *23*(2), 486–495. Available from https://doi.org/10.26355/eurrev_201901_16860.

Dasari, S., Wudayagiri, R., & Valluru, L. (2015). Cervical cancer: Biomarkers for diagnosis and treatment. *Clinica Chimica Acta*, *445*, 7–11. Available from https://doi.org/10.1016/j.cca.2015.03.005.

Ding, X.-Z., Zhang, S.-Q., Deng, X.-L., & Qiang, J.-H. DLX6-AS1 is a promising biomarker for prognosis prediction of cervical cancer.

Durand, X., Moutereau, S., Xylinas, E., & Taille, A. D. L. (2011). ProgensaTM PCA3 test for prostate cancer. *Expert Review of Molecular Diagnostics*.

Fan, Y., Nan, Y., Huang, J., Zhong, H., & Zhou, W. (2018). Up-Regulation of Inflammation-Related LncRNA-IL7R Predicts Poor Clinical Outcome in Patients with Cervical Cancer. *Bioscience Reports*, *38*(3), 20180483.

Fan, L., Huang, C., Li, J., Gao, T., Lin, Z., & Yao, T. (2018). Long Non-Coding RNA Urothelial Cancer Associated 1 Regulates Radioresistance via the Hexokinase 2/Glycolytic Pathway in Cervical Cancer. *International Journal of Molecular Medicine*, *42*(4), 1875–1884.

Feng, L.-L., Shen, F.-R., Zhou, J.-H., & Chen, Y.-G. (2019). Expression of the LncRNA ZFAS1 in Cervical Cancer and Its Correlation with Prognosis and Chemosensitivity. *Gene*, *696*, 105–112.

Feng, Y., Zou, W., Hu, C., Li, G., Zhou, S., He, Y., Ma, F., Deng, C., & Sun, L. (2017). Modulation of CASC2/miR-21/PTEN pathway sensitizes cervical cancer to cisplatin. *Archives of Biochemistry and Biophysics*, *623–624*, 20–30. Available from https://doi.org/10.1016/j.abb.2017.05.001.

Gibb, E. A., Becker-Santos, D. D., Enfield, K. S. S., Guillaud, M., Niekerk, D., van, Matisic, J. P., MacAulay, C. E., & Lam, W. L. (2012). Aberrant expression of long noncoding RNAs in cervical intraepithelial neoplasia. *International Journal of Gynecological Cancer, 22*(9), 1557–1563. Available from https://doi.org/10.1097/igc.0b013e318272f2c9.

Goossens, N., Nakagawa, S., Sun, X., & Hoshida, Y. (2015). Cancer biomarker discovery and validation. *Translational Cancer Research.*

Grigsby, P. W., Leslie, S., Massad, D. G., Mutch, M. A., Powell, H., Thaker, C., McCourt, A., Hagemann, K., Fuh, L., Kuroki, J. K., Schwarz, S., Markovina, A. J., Lin., Dehdashti, F., & Siegel, B. A. (2020). FIGO 2018 staging criteria for cervical cancer: Impact on stage migration and survival. *Gynecologic Oncology.*

Guo, Y., Wang, X., Wang, K., & He, Y. (2020). Appraising the Value of Serum and Serum-Derived Exosomal LncRNA-EXOC7 as a Promising Biomarker in Cervical Cancer. *Clinical Laboratory, 66*(7), 1357–1363.

Han, D., Wang, J., & Cheng, G. (2018). LncRNA NEAT1 Enhances the Radio-Resistance of Cervical Cancer via MiR-193b-3p/CCND1 Axis. *Oncotarget, 9*(2), 2395–2409.

Huang, L., Liao, L.-M., Liu, A.-W., Wu, J.-B., Cheng, X.-L., Lin, J.-X., & Zheng, M. (2014). Overexpression of long noncoding RNA HOTAIR predicts a poor prognosis in patients with cervical cancer. *Archives of Gynecology and Obstetrics, 290*(4), 717–723. Available from https://doi.org/10.1007/s00404-014-3236-2.

Jiang, S., Wang, H. L., & Yang, J. (2015). Low expression of long non-coding RNA LET inhibits carcinogenesis of cervical cancer. *International Journal of Clinical and Experimental Pathology, 8*(1), 806–811. Available from http://www.ijcep.com/files/ijcep0003353.pdf.

Jin, X., Chen, X., Hu, Y., Ying, F., Zou, R., Lin, F., Shi, Z., Zhu, X., Yan, X., Li, S., & Zhu, H. (2017). LncRNA-TCONS_00026907 Is Involved in the Progression and Prognosis of Cervical Cancer through Inhibiting MiR-143-5p. *Cancer Medicine, 6*(6), 1409–1423.

Jing, L., Yuan, W., Ruofan, D., Jinjin, Y., & Haifeng, Q. (2015). HOTAIR enhanced aggressive biological behaviors and induced radio-resistance via inhibiting p21 in cervical cancer. *Tumor Biology, 36*(5), 3611–3619. Available from https://doi.org/10.1007/s13277-014-2998-2.

Kim, H. J., Kim, L. K., Lee, S. H., Park, S. A., Eoh, K. J., & Kim, Y. T. (2018). Expression Levels of the Long Noncoding RNA Steroid Receptor Activator Promote Cell Proliferation and Invasion and Predict Patient Prognosis in Human Cervical Cancer. *Oncology Letters, 16*(4), 5410–5418.

Kopp, F., & Mendell, J. T. (2018). Functional classification and experimental dissection of long noncoding RNAs. *Cell, 172*(3), 393–407. Available from https://doi.org/10.1016/j.cell.2018.01.011.

Li, Y., Wan, Y. P., & Bai, Y. (2018). Correlation between Long Strand Non-Coding RNA GASS Expression and Prognosis of Cervical Cancer Patients. *European Review for Medical and Pharmacological Sciences, 22*(4), 943–949.

Li, J., Wang, Y., Yu, J., Dong, R., & Qiu, H. (2015). A high level of circulating HOTAIR is associated with progression and poor prognosis of cervical cancer. *Tumor Biology, 36*(3), 1661–1665. Available from https://doi.org/10.1007/s13277-014-2765-4.

Li, M., Lu, B., Dong, X., Zhou, Y., He, Y., Zhang, T., & Bao, L. (2019). Enhancement of cisplatin-induced cytotoxicity against cervical cancer spheroid cells by targeting long non-coding RNAs. *Pathology – Research and Practice, 215*(11), 152653. Available from https://doi.org/10.1016/j.prp.2019.152653.

Li, N., Meng, D., Gao, L., Xu, Y., Liu, P., Tian, Y., Yi, Z., Zhang, Y., Tie, X., & Xu, Z. (2018). Overexpression of HOTAIR leads to radioresistance of human cervical cancer via promoting HIF-1α expression. *Radiation Oncology, 13*(1), 210. Available from https://doi.org/10.1186/s13014-018-1153-4.

Liao, L.-M., Sun, X.-Y., Liu, A.-W., Wu, J.-B., Cheng, X.-L., Lin, J.-X., Zheng, M., & Huang, L. (2014). Low expression of long noncoding XLOC_010588 indicates a poor prognosis and promotes proliferation through upregulation of c-Myc in cervical cancer. *Gynecologic Oncology*, *133*(3), 616–623. Available from https://doi.org/10.1016/j.ygyno.2014.03.555.

Liu, J., Liu, X., & Li, R. (2020). LncRNA SNHG6 Enhances the Radioresistance and Promotes the Growth of Cervical Cancer Cells by Sponging MiR-485-3p. *Cancer Cell International*, *21*(1).

Liu, Y., Guo, R., Qiao, Y., Han, L., & Liu, M. (2020). LncRNA NNT-AS1 Contributes to the Cisplatin Resistance of Cervical Cancer through NNT-AS1/MiR-186/HMGB1 Axis. *Cancer Cell International*, *20*(1), 190.

Lu, H., He, Y., Lin, L., Qi, Z., Ma, L., Li, L., & Su, Y. (2016). Long non-coding RNA MALAT1 modulates radiosensitivity of HR-HPV + cervical cancer via sponging miR-145. *Tumor Biology*, *37*(2), 1683–1691. Available from https://doi.org/10.1007/s13277-015-3946-5.

Lv, X. J., Tang, Q., Tu, Y. Q., Yan, D. D., & Wei, Q. C. (2019). Long noncoding RNA PCAT6 regulates cell growth and metastasis via Wnt/β-catenin pathway and is a prognosis marker in cervical cancer. *European Review for Medical and Pharmacological Sciences*, *23*(5), 1947–1956. Available from https://doi.org/10.26355/eurrev_201903_17233.

Mao, B.-D., Xu, P., Zhong, Y., Ding, W.-W., & Meng, Q.-Z. (2019). LINC00511 knockdown prevents cervical cancer cell proliferation and reduces resistance to paclitaxel. *Journal of Biosciences*, *44*(2). Available from https://doi.org/10.1007/s12038-019-9851-0.

Naizhaer, G., Kuerban, A., Meilipa., Kuerban, R., & Zhop, P. (2019). Up-Regulation of LncRNA FALEC Indicates Prognosis and Diagnosis Values in Cervical Cancer. *Pathology Research and Practice*, *215*(8), 152495.

Peng, Y., Tang, D., Zhao, M., Kajiyama, H., Kikkawa, F., & Kondo, Y. (2020). Long non-coding RNA: A recently accentuated molecule in chemoresistance in cancer. *Cancer and Metastasis Reviews*, *39*(3), 825–835. Available from https://doi.org/10.1007/s10555-020-09910-w.

Shan, S., Li, H. F., Yang, X. Y., Guo, S., Guo, Y., Chu, L., Xu, M. J., & Xin, D. M. (2019). Higher LncRNA CASC15 Expression Predicts Poor Prognosis and Associates with Tumor Growth in Cervical Cancer. *European Review for Medical and Pharmacological Sciences*, *23*(2), 507–512.

Shen, C. J., Cheng, Y. A., & Wang, C. L. (2017). LncRNA PVT1 Epigenetically Silences MiR-195 and Modulates EMT and Chemoresistance in Cervical Cancer Cells. *Journal of Drug Targeting*, *25*(7), 637–644.

Small, W., Bacon, M. A., Bajaj, A., Chuang, L. T., Fisher, B. J., Harkenrider, M. M., Jhingran, A., Kitchener, H. C., Mileshkin, L. R., Viswanathan, A. N., & Gaffney, D. K. (2017). Cervical cancer: A global health crisis. *Cancer*, *123*(13), 2404–2412. Available from https://doi.org/10.1002/cncr.30667.

Stumbar, S. E., Stevens, M., & Feld, Z. (2019). Cervical cancer and its precursors: A preventative approach to screening, diagnosis, and management. *Primary Care - Clinics in Office Practice*.

Thorenoor, N., Faltejskova-Vychytilova, P., Hombach, S., Mlcochova, J., Kretz, M., Svoboda, M., & Slaby, O. (2016). Long non-coding RNA ZFAS1 interacts with CDK1 and is involved in p53-dependent cell cycle control and apoptosis in colorectal cancer. *Oncotarget*, *7*(1), 622–637. Available from https://doi.org/10.18632/oncotarget.5807.

Wan, S., & Zhao, H. (2020). Analysis of Diagnostic and Prognostic Value of LncRNA MEG3 in Cervical Cancer. *Oncology Letters*, *20*(5), 183.

Wang, M., Ouyang, J., & Li, H. (2019). CERNA2: A Predictor for Clinical Progression and Poor Prognosis in Cervical Carcinoma. *Journal of Cellular Biochemistry, 120*(7), 11216–11221.

Wang, P., Liu, G., Xu, W., Liu, H., Bu, Q., & Sun, D. (2017). Long noncoding RNA H19 inhibits cell viability, migration, and invasion via downregulation of IRS-1 in thyroid cancer cells. *Technology in Cancer Research & Treatment, 16*(6), 1102–1112. Available from https://doi.org/10.1177/1533034617733904.

Wang, C., Shao, S., Deng, L., Wang, S., & Zhang, Y. (2020). LncRNA SNHG12 Regulates the Radiosensitivity of Cervical Cancer through the MiR-148a/CDK1 Pathway. *Cancer Cell International, 20*(1).

Wang, W.-J., Wang, D., Zhao, M., Sun, X.-J., Li, Y., Lin, H., Che, Y.-Q., & Huang, C.-Z. (2020). Serum lncRNAs (CCAT2, LINC01133, LINC00511) with squamous cell carcinoma antigen panel as novel non-invasive biomarkers for detection of cervical squamous carcinoma. *Cancer Management and Research, 12*, 9495–9502. Available from https://doi.org/10.2147/cmar.s259586.

Wang, B., Huang, Z., Gao, R., Zeng, Z., Yang, W., Sun, Y., Wei, W., Wu, Z., Yu, L., Li, Q., Zhang, S., Li, F., Liu, G., Liu, B., Leng, L., Zhan, W., Yu, Y., Yang, G., & Zhou, S. (2017). Expression of Long Noncoding RNA Urothelial Cancer Associated 1 Promotes Cisplatin Resistance in Cervical Cancer. *Cancer Biotherapy and Radiopharmaceuticals, 32*(3), 101–110.

Wang, N., Hou, M. S., Zhan, Y., Shen, X. B., & Xue, H. Y. (2018). MALAT1 promotes cisplatin resistance in cervical cancer by activating the PI3K/AKT pathway. *European Review for Medical and Pharmacological Sciences, 22*(22), 7653–7659. Available from https://doi.org/10.26355/eurrev_201811_16382.

Wang, Y., Liu, Y., Li, Z., Yan, X., Huang, C., Ye, X., Sun, X., Qin, S., Zhong, X., Zeng, C., Liu, D., Zou, X., Liu, Y., Wu, J., Wen, Z., Yang, G., Jing, C., & Wei, X. (2018). Association between MALAT1 and THRIL polymorphisms and precancerous cervical lesions. *Genetic Testing and Molecular Biomarkers, 22*(9), 509–517. Available from https://doi.org/10.1089/gtmb.2018.0097.

Wei, J., Wang, L., Sun, Y., & Bao, Y. (2020). LINC00662 Contributes to the Progression and the Radioresistance of Cervical Cancer by Regulating MiR-497-5p and CDC25A. *Cell Biochemistry and Function, 38*(8), 1139–1151.

Wei, X., Zhou, Y., Qiu, J., Wang, X., Xia, Y., & Sui, L. (2019). Low Expression of TUG1 Promotes Cisplatin Sensitivity in Cervical Cancer by Activating the MAPK Pathway. *Journal of B.U.ON., 24*(3), 1020–1026.

Wen, Q., Liu, Y., Lyu, H., Xu, X., Wu, Q., Liu, N., Yin, Q., Li, J., & Sheng, X. (2017). Long noncoding RNA GAS5, which acts as a tumor suppressor via microRNA 21, regulates cisplatin resistance expression in cervical cancer. *International Journal of Gynecologic Cancer, 27*(6), 1096–1108. Available from https://doi.org/10.1097/igc.0000000000001028.

Yang, T. J., Wang, L., Zhang, Y., Zheng, J. D., & Liu, L. (2020). LncRNA UCA1 Regulates Cervical Cancer Survival and EMT Occurrence by Targeting MiR-155. *European Review for Medical and Pharmacological Sciences, 24*(19), 9869–9879.

Ye, H., Chu, X., Cao, Z., Hu, X., Wang, Z., Li, M., Wan, L., Li, Y., Cao, Y., Diao, Z., Peng, F., Liu, J., & Xu, L. (2021). A novel targeted therapy system for cervical cancer: Co-delivery system of antisense LncRNA of MDC1 and oxaliplatin magnetic thermosensitive cationic liposome drug carrier. *International Journal of Nanomedicine, 16*, 1051–1066. Available from https://doi.org/10.2147/ijn.s258316.

Zeng, J., Ma, Y. X., Liu, Z. H., & Zeng, Y. L. (2019). LncRNA SNHG7 Contributes to Cell Proliferation, Invasion and Prognosis of Cervical Cancer. *European Review for Medical and Pharmacological Sciences*, *23*(21), 9277–9285.

Zhao, H., Zheng, G. H., Li, G. C., Xin, L., Wang, Y. S., Chen, Y., & Zheng, X. M. (2019). Long noncoding RNA LINC00958 regulates cell sensitivity to radiotherapy through RRM2 by binding to microRNA-5095 in cervical cancer. *Journal of cellular physiology*, *234*(12), 23349–23359. Available from https://doi.org/10.1002/jcp.28902.

Zhang, X., Mao, L., Li, L., He, Z., Wang, N., & Song, Y. (2019). Long Noncoding RNA GIHCG Functions as an Oncogene and Serves as a Serum Diagnostic Biomarker for Cervical Cancer. *Journal of Cancer*, *10*(3), 672–681.

Zhang, L., Qian, H., Sha, M., Luan, Z., Lin, M., Yuan, D., Li, X., Huang, J., Ye, L., & Zhang, Z. (2016). Downregulation of HOTAIR expression mediated anti-metastatic effect of artesunate on cervical cancer by inhibiting COX-2 expression. *PLoS One*, *11*(10), e0164838. Available from https://doi.org/10.1371/journal.pone.0164838.

Zhang, H. H., & Li, A. H. (2018). Long Non-Coding RNA FEZF1-AS1 Is up-Regulated and Associated with Poor Prognosis in Patients with Cervical Cancer. *European Review for Medical and Pharmacological Sciences*, *22*(11), 3357–3362.

Zhang, W., Liu, Y., He, Y., & Chen, P. (2019). Suppression of long noncoding RNA NCK1-AS1 increases chemosensitivity to cisplatin in cervical cancer. *Journal of Cellular Physiology*, *234*(4), 4302–4313. Available from https://doi.org/10.1002/jcp.27198.

Zhang, D., Sun, G., Zhang, H., Tian, J., & Li, Y. (2017). Long Non-Coding RNA ANRIL Indicates a Poor Prognosis of Cervical Cancer and Promotes Carcinogenesis via PI3K/Akt Pathways. *Biomedicine and Pharmacotherapy*, *85*, 511–516.

Zhang, L., Yao, H. R, Liu, S. K., & Song, L. L. (2020). Long Noncoding RNA ROR1-AS1 Overexpression Predicts Poor Prognosis and Promotes Etastasis by Activating Wnt/β-Catenin/EMT Signaling Cascade in Cervical Cancer. *European Review for Medical and Pharmacological Sciences*, *24*(6), 2928–2937.

Zhang, Q., Zhang, Y., & Wang, Y. (2019). GHET1 Acts as a Prognostic Indicator and Functions as an Oncogenic LncRNA in Cervical Cancer. *Bioscience Reports*, *39*(4), BSR20182506.

Zhao, Y., Huang, J., Liu, T., He, S., Shang, C., Guo, L., Du, Q., & Yao, S. (2018). Overexpression of Long Non-Coding RNA RP11-396F22.1 Correlates Poor Prognosis of Patients with Early-Stage Cervical Cancer. *American Journal of Translational Research*, *10*(3), 684.

Zhao, S., Yu, M., & Wang, L. (2020). LncRNA miR503HG regulates the drug resistance of recurrent cervical squamous cell carcinoma cells by regulating miR-155/caspase-3. *Cancer Management and Research*, *12*, 1579–1585. Available from https://doi.org/10.2147/cmar.s225489.

Chapter 15

Triple-negative breast cancer and its correlation with viral agents

Lamyae El Khalki[1,2,3], Moulay Mustapha Ennaji[4] and Abdelmajid Zyad[1]

[1]Team of Experimental Oncology and Natural Substances; Cellular and Molecular Immunopharmacology, Faculty of Sciences and Technology, University of Sultan Moulay Slimane, Beni Mellal, Morocco, [2]Department of Microbiology, Immunology, and Inflammation, Temple University, Philadelphia, PA, United States, [3]Center for Inflammation and Lung Research, Temple University, Philadelphia, PA, United States, [4]Group Leader Research team of Virology, Oncology, and Biotechnologies, Head of Laboratory of Virology, Oncology, Biosciences, Environment and New Energies (LVO-BEEN), Faculty of Sciences and Techniques Mohammedia, University Hassan II of Casablanca, Casablanca, Morocco

15.1 Introduction

Triple-negative breast cancer (TNBC) represents approximately 10%–20% of all breast cancer subtypes and it is an aggressive breast cancer subtype with no targeted therapy owing to the absence of estrogen and progesterone hormone receptors with the lack of human epidermal growth factor receptor-2/Neu overexpression (Kumar & Aggarwal, 2016). In 2018 an estimated effective of 2.1 million women were newly diagnosed with breast cancer, with approximately one new case diagnosed every 18 s; additionally, the number of death is estimated by 626,679 (Bray et al., 2018).

Although the risk factors for breast cancer are well established, namely, female gender, premenopausal status, shorter duration of breast feeding, African-American race, the underlying causes of TNBC continue to remain unknown (Lawson et al., 2018). It is therefore important to note that viral infections caused by viruses such as such as Epstein–Barr virus (EBV), mouse mammary tumor virus (MMTV), human papillomavirus (HPV), and bovine leukemia virus are crucial risk factors of TNBC (Lawson et al., 2018). Each of these viruses has their own oncogenic properties, and they will be discussed in this chapter. Since targeted therapy is not yet widely available for TNBC patients, cytotoxic chemotherapy remains the only available way for their treatment. Unfortunately, chemotherapy has extremely

Immunological Implications and Molecular Diagnostics of Genitourinary Cancer.
DOI: https://doi.org/10.1016/B978-0-323-85496-2.00019-1

serious adverse effects during and after the treatment, for example, high costs of the drugs, high incidence of systemic toxicity, and the development of resistances in tumor cells.

Considering the WHO's recommendations, the histological type and stage are critical parameters for the diagnosis and treatment of cancer; additionally, in the case of breast cancer, the molecular level is an important factor. Furthermore, breast cancer is considered to be a heterogeneous disease. Indeed, over the last decade, this heterogeneity was taken into account to define the treatment concept. In this report, we present the different type of breast cancer considering the histological form of tumor and the molecular signature with a special focus into the TNBC, which is one of the most aggressive form of breast cancer that cannot be treated by endocrine therapy (Anders & Carey, 2008).

15.2 Breast cancer presentation

15.2.1 Histological types of breast cancer

15.2.1.1 Ductal carcinoma in situ

It refers to the abnormal cells found in the milk ducts. These cells are described as noninvasive as they do not spread to nearby breast tissue. It is an early form of cancer that can sometimes become invasive and affect other tissues (Réseau canadien du cancer du sein—accueil).

15.2.1.2 Lobular carcinoma in situ

Lobular carcinoma in situ (LCIS) refers to the abnormal cells found in the lobules, the glands that produce milk in the breast. Although it is rare for an LCIS to turn into invasive cancer, it is linked to an increased risk of developing invasive breast cancer later in life (Réseau canadien du cancer du sein—accueil).

15.2.1.3 Invasive ductal carcinoma

It refers to the cancer that starts in the ducts (the ones that carry milk from the glands to the nipple) and spreads to the surrounding breast tissue.

Secretory mammary carcinoma: This is a cancer identified by too much mucin secretion in the tumor. It is considered to be an invasive ductal carcinoma subtype, which tends to lead to metastases and local recurrences. It proliferates slowly, but it is best to treat it vigorously. It accounts for less than 0.1% of all invasive breast cancer cases, and possible treatments include chemotherapy, radiation therapy, and mastectomy. The decision to choose one treatment or the other is made on a case-by-case basis given the rarity of this subtype of breast cancer (Réseau canadien du cancer du sein—accueil).

15.2.1.4 Invasive lobular carcinoma

Invasive lobular carcinoma is a cancer that arises in the lobules (groups of mammary glands) and invades nearby breast tissue.

15.2.1.5 Metaplastic carcinoma

It is an unusual type of cancer that is characterized by the change from one type of cancer cell to another. Less than 1% of breast cancer cases are metaplastic and can be treated with surgery, radiation therapy, and chemotherapy (Réseau canadien du cancer du sein—accueil).

15.2.1.6 Inflammatory breast cancer

It is a rare form of cancer that makes the breast red, swollen, and tender as if it were infected. This is an aggressive, locally advanced type of cancer (i.e., cancer that spreads to surrounding tissues or nodes but not to other organs) that blocks lymphatic vessels in the skin of the breast. Symptoms of inflammatory breast cancer can develop quickly and often resemble other health problems (Réseau canadien du cancer du sein—accueil).

15.2.1.7 Metastatic breast cancer

It is also known as advanced or stage IV breast cancer and can be defined as the spread of cancer cells from their place of origin to other parts of the body. Almost 1200 Canadian women are initially diagnosed with metastatic breast cancer each year. Some women who are initially diagnosed with early breast cancer will eventually develop metastatic breast cancer. The risk of this type of cancer depends on various clinical and pathological properties of the initial tumor. Unfortunately, there are no current statistics available in Canada today on the number of people whose cancer has progressed from early stage to stage IV (Réseau canadien du cancer du sein—accueil).

Metastasis (the spread of cancer to other parts of the body) can happen before or after treatment for cancer in the breast. They can be the result of recurrent breast cancer (i.e., breast cancer that comes back after it has been undetectable for a while). Although breast cancer cells can spread to almost any part of the body, they usually settle in the bones. They are also often found in the lungs, liver, brain, and skin (Réseau canadien du cancer du sein—accueil)

15.2.2 Stages of breast cancer

The stage of breast cancer is an important parameter in the pathology report. Staging takes into account the spread, the size of the tumor, and the spread to nearby lymph nodes and other parts of the body. It is generally used to guide treatment decision-making (Réseau canadien du cancer du sein—accueil).

The most common terms used to describe the stage of breast cancer are:

1. Local: cancer confined to the breast.
2. Regional: there is a spread to surrounding lymph nodes.
3. Distant: cancer that has spread to other parts of the body.

The staging of breast cancer uses the "TNM" system, which refers to tumor, nodes, and metastases (tumor, lymph nodes, and metastases). This classification takes into account the size of the tumor, the number of lymph nodes affected, and the existence of metastases. In accordance with these criteria, a stage between 0 and IV is assigned. For example, a T1N0M0 cancer refers to a small, early breast cancer without lymph node involvement and without metastasis (stage I). T4N3M1 cancer refers to advanced metastatic breast cancer with a large tumor in the breast and a large number of affected lymph nodes (stage IV) (Réseau canadien du cancer du sein—accueil).

1. Stage 0 means the cancer cells have not spread (they have not reached neighboring normal tissue).
2. Stage I refers to a small, local invasive tumor (which remains in the breast) that has not spread to the lymph nodes.
3. Stage II describes cancer with a larger, invasive tumor that may have spread to nearby lymph nodes.
4. Stage III invasive cancers present in the lymph nodes.
5. Stage IV is the metastatic stage

15.2.3 Molecular types of breast cancer

Given the gene expression profile, Perou et al. could identify four types of breast carcinoma by comparing them to normal tissue, RE + /luminal, basal-like, Erb-B2, and normal-like (Perou et al., 2000):

The two subtypes of luminal-like breast cancer are luminal A and luminal B group. They are characterized by the expression of the estrogen receptor and genes associated with the RE pathway. Subsequently, luminal class was divided into luminal A and luminal B classes, thereby resulting in addition of a fifth class of breast cancer (Carey et al., 2006);

HER-2-like breast cancer is characterized by the overexpression and amplification of the HER-2 gene on chromosome 17q12 and overexpression of the oncoprotein HER-2, a protein belonging to the epidermal growth factor receptor superfamily, which can also express estrogen and progesterone.

Cancers of the breast basal-like phenotype: cells from basal cell / myoepithelial express neither hormone receptors nor HER-2 oncoprotein and are often referred to as "triple negative." They express, however, a number of genes of the basal cells of the epithelium.

Breast cancers, known as normal breast-like, are characterized by a triple-negative profile and by the expression of genes observed in normal breast tissue and adipose tissue.

15.3 A focus on triple-negative breast cancer

The term "triple-negative breast cancer" appeared for the first time in the literature in 2005 (Brenton et al., 2005). "Triple negative" breast cancer represents nearly 20% of breast cancers and constitutes a heterogeneous group characterized by the absence of hormone receptors for estrogen and progesterone and the absence of overexpression of HER-2 growth factor. Lehmann et al. conducted a study involving 386 TNBC, characterized by the absence of the gene expressions of ER, PR, and HER-2, as well as that of the amplification of ERBB2/HER2; in their study, the existence of six molecular subtypes was highlighted (Lehmann et al., 2011).

1. Basal-like 1 (BL1): it is characterized by enrichment in genes involved in DNA damage response (DDR) and cell cycle, while BL2 shares part of the cell cycle genes with BL1, but it is not enriched in DDR genes.
2. Basal-like 2 (BL2): it is characterized by the overexpression of genes of the signaling pathway of the family of receptors for growth factors and myoepithelial differentiation.

Immunomodulatory (IM): it is enriched in genes responsible for the interactions between the host and cancer, that is to say, the antigens and immune genes involved in the transduction pathways of the immune signal.

Mesenchymal (M) and mesenchymal stem-like (MSL): MSL is characterized with the M subtype by an enrichment for the genes regulating cell motility, M invasion, and differentiation, but the MSL subtype is the most enriched in regulating genes of epithelial–M transition and cancer stem cells. The MSL subtype shares with the IM subtype many genes involved in the regulation of the immune response.

Luminal with androgen receptor (LAR): it is characterized by the overexpression of gene coding for luminal differentiation and for regulators of the androgen receptor (AR) signaling pathway.

15.4 Risk factors associated with triple-negative breast cancer

While early pregnancy has been recognized for the other subtypes of breast cancer (Luminal A, Luminal B, and HER-2) as a protective factor against BC, gestation appears to be an important risk factor in the development of the triple-negative phenotype. Indeed, it has been reported that women who had more children (three or more) had a higher risk (1.4 times) of TNBC (Phipps et al., 2011). Later, a study by Tamimi et al. (2012) reaffirmed that multiple pregnancies were associated with an increased risk of developing TNBC.

A link has also been established with racial ancestry since 21% of breast cancer cases among African-American population classified as TNBC (compared to 15% of the cases among Caucasian population) (Amirikia et al., 2011; Chlebowski et al., 2005). Also, a high incidence of this subtype of breast cancer has been observed among the Hispanic population, with a frequency of 21.3% in Peru (Vallejos et al., 2010), 27% in Brazil (Cintra et al., 2012), 24.1% in Venezuela (Fernandez & Reigosa, 2013), and 23.1% in Mexico (Lara-Medina et al., 2011).

15.5 Implications of viral agents in triple-negative breast cancer

The involvement of viral agents in cancers has been revealed through numerous studies carried out during the 20th century; in fact 15%–20% of cancer cases are associated with infectious agents. Viruses are at the top of the list as evidenced by various studies.

Previous studies have suggested the presence of herpesvirus, papillomavirus, polyomavirus, and MMTV-like sequences in breast cancer (Mazouni et al., 2011; Petropoulos, 1997).

Another study reported a much higher rate of human cytomegalovirus infection (97%) in biopsy specimens of breast cancer patients compared to controls by immunohistochemistry (Harkins et al., 2010).

Others have found EBV DNA in breast cancer samples and suggested an association of EBV with more severe forms of breast cancer (Alibek et al., 2013; Amarante & Watanabe, 2009; Harkins et al., 2010; Mazouni et al., 2011).

SV40 DNA was reported in 22% of 109 breast cancer samples as determined by PCR with confirmation by immunohistochemistry (Alibek et al., 2013).

One of the most frequent viruses in cancer—the HPV—has also been linked to breast carcinoma. Data obtained by a study showed the presence of high-risk HPVs (HR-HPVs) in 42% of breast tissues of which the viral activity was only confirmed in 5 out of 26 invasive carcinomas cases. This finding, the first to be reported in the United Kingdom, suggests that the selective expression of viral oncoprotein in invasive cases may propose a role for HR-HPVs in the development of certain types of breast cancer (Salman et al., 2017). Other studies have proposed an association between the beta-retrovirus human mammary tumor virus and breast cancer. This is due to the detection of MMTV-like sequences in breast cancer samples and not in normal tissues (Pogo & Holland, 1997).

15.6 The special case of triple-negative breast cancer

Banerjee et al. (2015) detected a signature of different microbial groups in a sample made of 100 CSTNs. The technique used was based on the PathoChip array, which contains a set of 60,000 probes that cover all known viral agents as well as human pathogenic bacterial, fungi, and parasites (Baldwin et al., 2014). Thus the genome of several microbial agents has been detected. In the group of bacteria, the PathoChip screen allowed to spot: *Brevundimonas diminuta, Arcanobacterium haemolyticum, Peptoniphilus indolicus, Prevotella nigrescens, Propiniobacterium jensenii*, and *Capnocytophaga canimorsus*. The fungal and parasitic pooled probes (P) captured targets that mapped to rRNA genes of the following fungal organisms: *Pleistophora mulleris, Piedraia hortae, Paecilomyces reniformis, Phialophora verrucosa*, and *Fonsecaea pedrosoi*; and the 18S rRNA regions following parasites: *Trichuris trichura, Thelazia gulosa*, and *Leishmania major*.

The MiSeq reads confirmed the presence of viral genomic regions of polyoma viruses (SV40, JC, MCPV); herpesviruses (HCMV); papilloma viruses (HPV16, HPV18, HPV2); retroviruses (HTLV1, MMTV), poxviruses (pseudo cowpox virus, bovine papular stomatitis virus, and orf virus) (Banerjee et al., 2015).

A study by Corbex et al. focusing on inflammatory and triple-negative breast tumors showed that the most prevalent viruses were EBV1 and HPV16. Inflammatory breast cancer carried significantly more viruses (any type) than nonIBC tumors (30% vs 13%, $p < 0.04$). Similarly, triple-negative tumors displayed higher virus-positivity than nontriple-negative tumors (44% vs 14%, $p < 0.009$) (Corbex et al., 2014).

Another study regarding the involvement of HPV in TNBC has shown that the prevalence of HPV-positivity in TNBC specimens was 15%. On the basis of its carcinogenetic ability, an etiological role in the pathogenesis of the cancer could be presumed (Piana et al., 2014).

Also, an investigation of human JC and BK polyomaviruses in breast carcinomas showed that JCV DNA presence also correlates with "triple negative" phenotype ($p = 0.021$). Moreover, significant correlation was found between multiple viral infection (JCV, and/or SV40, and/or MMTV-like in the same tumor) and "triple negative" phenotype ($p = 0.001$) and also with p53 accumulation ($p = 0.028$) (Hachana et al., 2012).

15.7 Treatment modalities of triple-negative breast cancer

15.7.1 Current treatment strategies and limitations

The choice of breast cancer treatment is based on tumor size, nodal status, histologic grade, and the presence of ER, PR, and HER-2 expression to predict the response to either hormone therapy and/or trastuzumab (for HER-2) (Society & Clinical, 2016). Now, because TNBC lacks ER, PR, and HER-2, the treatment used for other breast cancer types is not effective in this case. Generally, and depending on its tumor size and metastasis status, TNBC is treated with surgery (mastectomy or lympectomy), radiotherapy, and chemotherapy. To improve the prognosis and survival of patients with TNBC, some new treatments have been developed, such as targeted therapy and immunotherapy (Jia et al., 2016)

TNBC involves surgical excision of breast tumor mass by mastectomy or breast-conserving surgery by lympectomy, followed by adjuvant radiotherapy (Kumar & Aggarwal, 2016). However, surgery has some limitations; where 19%–30% of patients negatively rated their breast cosmetics, arm swelling/ pain, limitation of movement, loss of feeling in fingers, and breast sensitivity and tenderness, in 5 and 10 years after breast-conserving surgery and radiation (Hau et al., 2013). Furthermore, from a psychological perspective, a recent study found that women with pronounced breast asymmetry were much more likely to have negative psychological outcomes (Waljee et al., 2008).

Radiotherapy implies using high-energy rays to kill cancer cells and inhibit their growth. It was reported that radiotherapy is an essential component of breast-conserving treatment as shown in a previous study (Dragun et al., 2011). In addition to radiotherapy, many studies have shown that chemotherapy was beneficial for TNBC treatment (Wahba & El-Hadaad, 2015). Regimens based on Anthracycline (doxorubicin, epirubicin, etc.), taxane (paclitaxel, docetaxel, etc.), and platinum agents (cisplatin, carboplatin, etc.) represent the standard treatment strategies for breast cancer patients and have been shown to be highly active in TNBC subtype as well.

However, chemotherapy showed several side effects on TNBC patients, and a recent study found that the most common side effects mentioned by both patients and healthcare professionals were skin toxicity, tiredness, and breast deformity (Raphael et al., 2020), in addition to others related to neurotoxicity (Livshits et al., 2014), cardiovascular (Smith et al., 2010), hematopoietic and gastro-intestinal, and nephrotoxicity (Livshits et al., 2014).

Moreover, despite the anticancer effects of chemotherapy, cancer cells tend to escape apoptosis and maintain their viability through cellular senescence and cytoprotective autophagy (Reilly et al., 2015). Chemo-resistance accounts for 90% of drug failures in metastatic cancers (Abdullah & Chow, 2013). Understanding the mechanisms of chemo-resistance in TNBC has a potential to develop more effective drugs by not only targeting TNBC cancer cells but also targeting cellular chemo-resistance pathways.

There is no damage to the healthy cells by using targeted therapy compared with that of chemotherapy. Based on the type of TNBC and the components of their main pathways, some inhibitors have been developed and used to treat TNBC, for example:

PARP inhibitors: Poly (ADP-ribose) polymerase (e.g., olaparib) are used to work competitively with NAD + (nicotinamide adenine dinucleotide) to bind into PARP molecules and consequently inhibit DNA repair (Slade, 2020). Furthermore, adding a DNA-damaging agent (cisplatin) to PARP inhibitors therapy has given promising results for TNBC treatment (Chang-qing et al., 2019). In January 2018, the US Food and Drug Administration (FDA) approved Olaparib for the treatment of BRCA1/2 mutant metastatic breast cancers (McCann & Hurvitz, 2018). The most common adverse events of

PARP inhibitors are hematological (anemia), gastrointestinal (nausea), kidney insufficiency (increase in creatinine concentrations), and fatigue (LaFargue et al., 2019; Ruiz-Schutz et al., 2019).

Vascular endothelial growth factor (VEGF) inhibitors: Generally, VEGF inhibitors block the growth of tumor neovascularization; the antiVEGF monoclonal antibody, bevacizumab, has shown some promising results in patients with metastatic breast cancer when added to paclitaxel, a first line chemotherapy drug (Miller et al., 2007). However, bevacizumab in breast cancer and TNBC has not been approved by the FDA, owing to the lack of evidence regarding its efficacy and increased toxicity (D'Agostino, 2011).

Epithelial growth factor receptor (EGFR) inhibitors: A large proportion of TNBC tumors overexpress the EGFR, which is a negative prognostic factor in TNBC (Cheang et al., 2008). Interestingly, it was reported that the monoclonal antibody cetuximab, an EGFR inhibitor, has shown some interesting activity in TNBC patients when combined with carboplatin (Carey et al., 2012). One of the most occurred adverse events in patients treated with cetuximab or panitumumab is hypomagnesemia, which can change the duration of the treatment (Cosmai et al., 2015). In a previous study, ocular toxicities were reported to be the adverse effects of cetuximab and erlotinib (Borkar et al., 2013).

Src tyrosine kinase inhibitors: Src tyrosine kinase (Rous sarcoma virus) is overexpressed in TNBC and has been associated with metastatic disease progression (Finn et al., 2007). A previous study has shown that dasatinib, an Src tyrosine kinase inhibitor, inhibited the growth of TNBC and was synergistic when combined to cisplatin (Kim et al., 2013). Lehmann et al. demonstrated that M and MSL TNBC subtypes were sensitive to dasatinib (Lehmann et al., 2011), which was reported to be toxic on cardiovascular system, lungs, and bone marrow (Livshits et al., 2014).

PI3K/mTOR inhibitors: Aberrations in the phosphatidylinositol 3-kinase (PI3K)/protein kinase B/mammalian target of rapamycin (mTOR) pathway are common in TNBC. A previous study has shown that a patient-derived xenograft TNBC model when treated with the mTOR inhibitor exhibited 77%–99% tumor-growth inhibition (Zhang et al., 2014). Apitolisib is a PI3K inhibitor that also targets mTOR. In a cell-derived TNBC model (MDA-MB-231), mice treated with apitolisib achieved tumor-growth inhibition of over 50% (Wallin et al., 2011). Several studies are now supporting the entry of PI3K/Akt/mTOR inhibitors to early-phase clinical trials (Costa et al., 2018). Previous findings reported that gastrointestinal complications, thrombocytopenia, diarrhea, nausea, and asthenia are considered to be the dose-limiting effects of PI3K/mTOR inhibitor treatment (Antonuzzo et al., 2017).

ARs antagonists: In the LAR, TNBC subtype androgen hormone binds to ARs, which induces a translocation of the AR to the nucleus and activates genes transcription. AR antagonists such as enzalutamide and bicalutamide competitively target AR and consequently inhibit tumor growth. A study reported the most common adverse events related to AR antagonist treatment to be tremor (42%), nausea (42%), vomiting (37%), fatigue (37%), anemia, delirium, mental status change, and confused state in breast cancer patients (Bardia et al., 2018).

Immunotherapy: PD-L1 or programmed cell death ligand 1 is an immune checkpoint protein that can bind to receptor PD-1, which is located on T cells and then inhibits the activity of the T cell effectors in tissues, such that tumor cells can finally escape the T cell immune response (Chang-qing et al., 2019). PD-L1 in tumor cells or tumor microenvironment has been positively associated with TNBC (Pardoll, 2012). The key tools for cancer immunotherapy are the immune checkpoint inhibitors or antagonists such as immune checkpoint antagonists of the PD-1/PD-L1 (atezolizumab). In March 2019, the FDA approved the immunotherapy drug atezolizumab used in combination with the chemotherapy drug nab-paclitaxel in metastatic TNBC (FDA Approves Atezolizumab for Triple-Negative Breast, Cancer). However, a study reported that PD-L1 inhibitors are frequently associated with cutaneous side effects (Collins et al., 2017). Additionally, another recent study reported that problems in cutaneous, gastrointestinal, and pulmonary systems are common serious adverse events in the treatment with PD-L1 inhibitors (Yang et al., 2019).

To conclude, there are still big challenges for the treatment of TNBC, such as the lack of effective targets and the side effects of chemotherapy. However, it is mandatory to take into consideration the diversity of these adverse effects in making clinical decisions when treating patients. Therefore further trials are warranted for optimal use of such agents in the clinical practice.

15.8 Natural anticancer agents in triple-negative breast cancer

Humans have always depended on nature for their well-being since they discovered very early the therapeutic properties of certain natural products to overcome their suffering and improve their health. Today, in order to develop more effective drugs with low to no undesirable side effects, pharmaceutical industries and researchers are working on improving the current treatments and discovering new ones.

Natural product-derived drugs constitute a vast majority (more than 60%) of the chemotherapeutic agents (e.g., taxol, vinblastine, and doxorubicin) currently in use for all types of cancers (Gordaliza, 2007; Newman et al., 2003). For example, vinblastine and vincristine are vinca alkaloids isolated from the pink periwinkle plant *Catharantus rosea* and obtained by simple structural modifications (Efferth et al., 2007). Another example of the current chemotherapeutic agent, paclitaxel, which was first isolated from the bark of the Western yew trees *Taxus brevifolia* and *Taxus baccata* (Kingston, 2007).

These drugs are widely marketed and were successfully used as effective anticancer drugs.

Recently, several papers have analyzed and summarized the anticancer effect of many important natural compounds with different mechanisms on TNBC (Pandurangan & Mustafa, 2018; Varghese et al., 2018); For example, berberine, $C_{20}H_{18}NO_4^+$ (Fig. 15.1), is a natural isoquinoline alkaloid compound isolated from the stems and roots of several plants such as *Berberis vulgaris*, *Berberis aristata*, and *Coptidis rhizome*, with 23 new berberine semisynthesized derivatives in 2018 (Wang et al., 2018). It exhibits several pharmacological activities such as antiplatelet effect, antibacterial, antiinflammatory, IM, antioxidative, neuroprotective, hypolipidemic, antidiabetic, and anticancer activities (Imanshahidi, 2008). In addition to a previous study that reported that berberine killed MCF-7 breast cancer cells through apoptosis induction (El Khalki et al., 2018), several preclinical studies have also reported the anticancer effect of berberine, where it exhibited its inhibitory effects on a variety of tumors such as hepatoma, leukemia, lung, colon, ovarian, cervical, and breast cancer cells through apoptosis induction and cell cycle arrest, inhibition of migration and invasion, reduction of the expression of VEGF mRNA and inhibition of angiogenesis (El Khalki et al., 2018; Kim et al., 2008; Liu et al., 2019; Patil et al., 2010).

Moreover, we have reported that berberine has a cytotoxic activity against a large panel of TNBC cells, with three sensitive cell lines, namely, HCC70 (IC50 = 0.19 μM), BT-20 (IC50 = 0.23 μM), and MDA-MB-468 (IC50 = 0.48 μM) (El Khalki et al., 2020). Using flow cytometry techniques, berberine, at 0.5 and 1 μM for 120 and 144 h, not only induced cell cycle

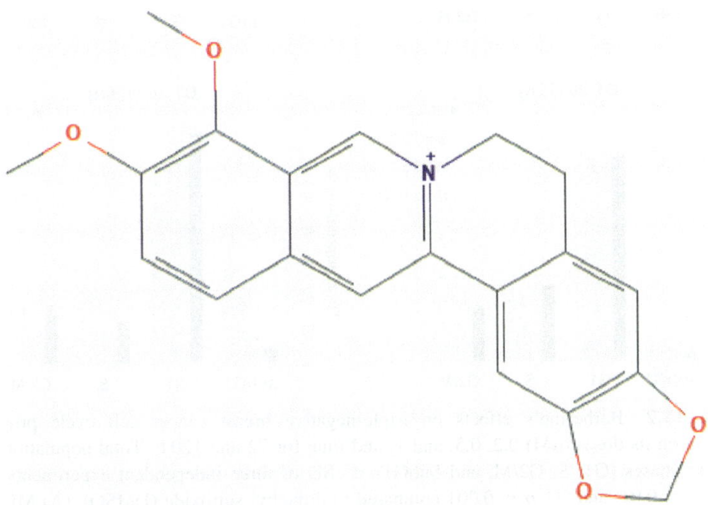

FIGURE 15.1 Chemical structure depiction of berberine $C_{20}H_{18}NO_4^+$ (Berberine).

arrest, at G1 and/or G2/M phases (Fig. 15.2 and Fig. 15.3), but it also triggered significant apoptosis (Fig. 15.4). At the molecular level, these results are consistent with the expression of their related proteins using Western blot assays (Fig. 15.3 and Fig. 15.4) (El Khalki et al., 2020). Interestingly,

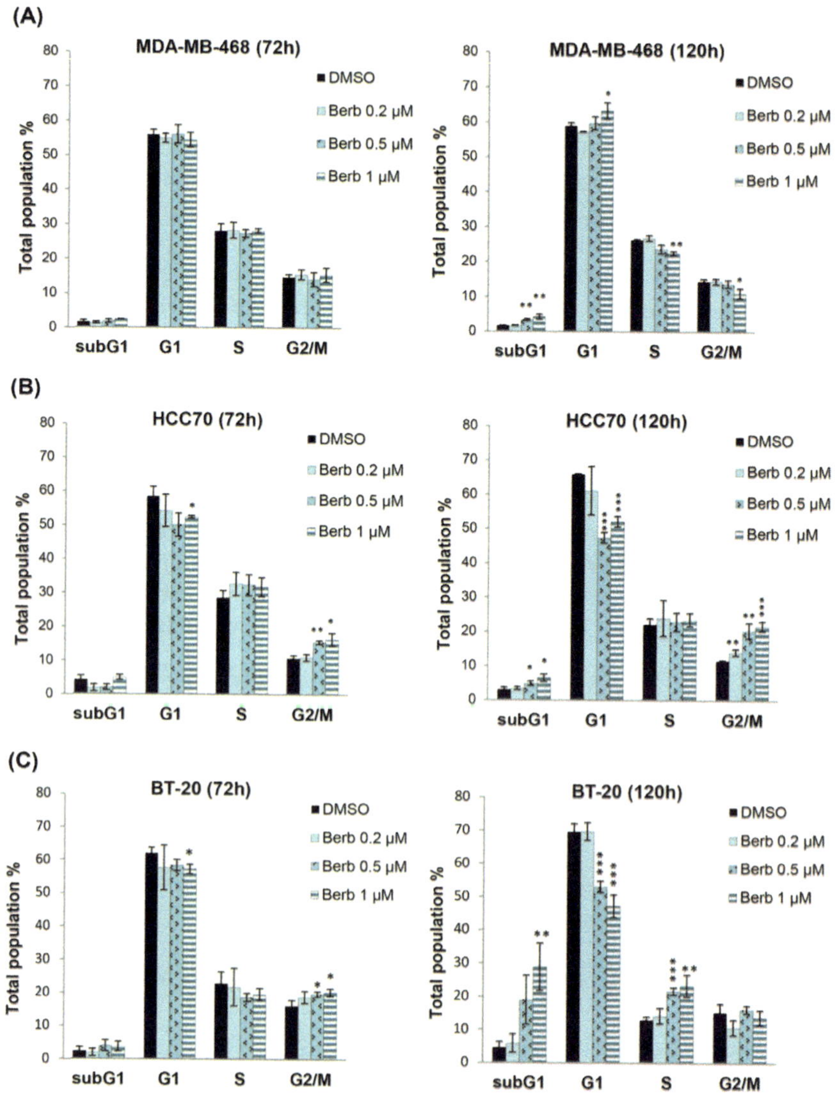

FIGURE 15.2 Berberine's effects on triple-negative breast cancer cell cycle progression depending on its doses (μM) 0.2, 0.5, and 1, and time for 72 and 120 h. Total population (%) of cell cycle phases (G1, S, G2/M, and SubG1) ± SD of three independent experiments, * $p < 0.05$, ** $p < 0.01$, and *** $p < 0.001$ compared to dimethyl sulfoxide (DMSO). (A) MDA-MB-468, (B) HCC70 and (C) BT-20. Berb—Berberine (El Khalki et al., 2020).

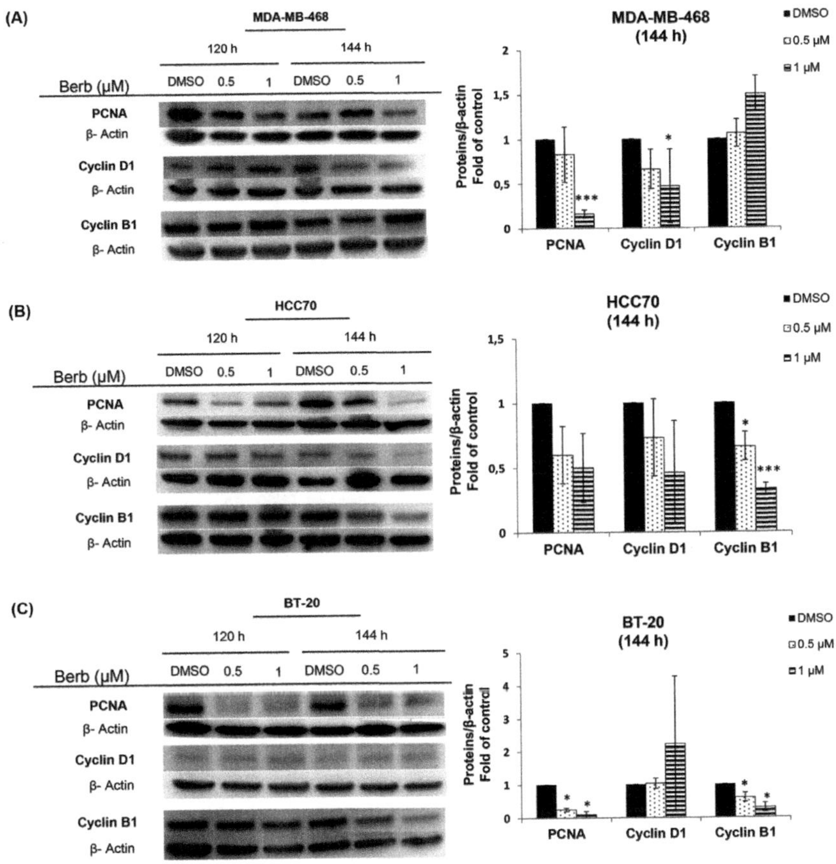

FIGURE 15.3 Representative Western blot results of the expression of cell cycle related proteins PCNA, Cyclin D1, and Cyclin B1 of (A) MDA-MB-468, (B) HCC70, and (C) BT-20 treated with berberine at 0.5 and 1 µM for 120 and 144 h. Results of three independent experiments ± SD, * $p < 0.05$, ** $p < 0.01$ and *** $p < 0.001$ compared to DMSO, Berb—Berberine (El Khalki et al., 2020).

while berberine showed a significant effect on the cell growth of TNBC cells, it did not show any toxic effect neither on the viability of normal human cells MCF-10A cultured in a 3D matrigel model nor on the survival of peripheral blood mononuclear cells from healthy donors (El Khalki et al., 2020). These results suggest that berberine may be a good potential candidate for TNBC drug development (El Khalki et al., 2020). In our laboratory, we had also tested artemisinin, thymoquinone, and carvacrol, other pure natural molecules, to assess the viability of TNBC cells. We found that thymoquinone and carvacrol were not as cytotoxic as berberine, although there are some previous studies that have been conducted in our laboratory, Jaafari et al. reported that carvacrol was cytotoxic against MCF-7 and P-815 cell

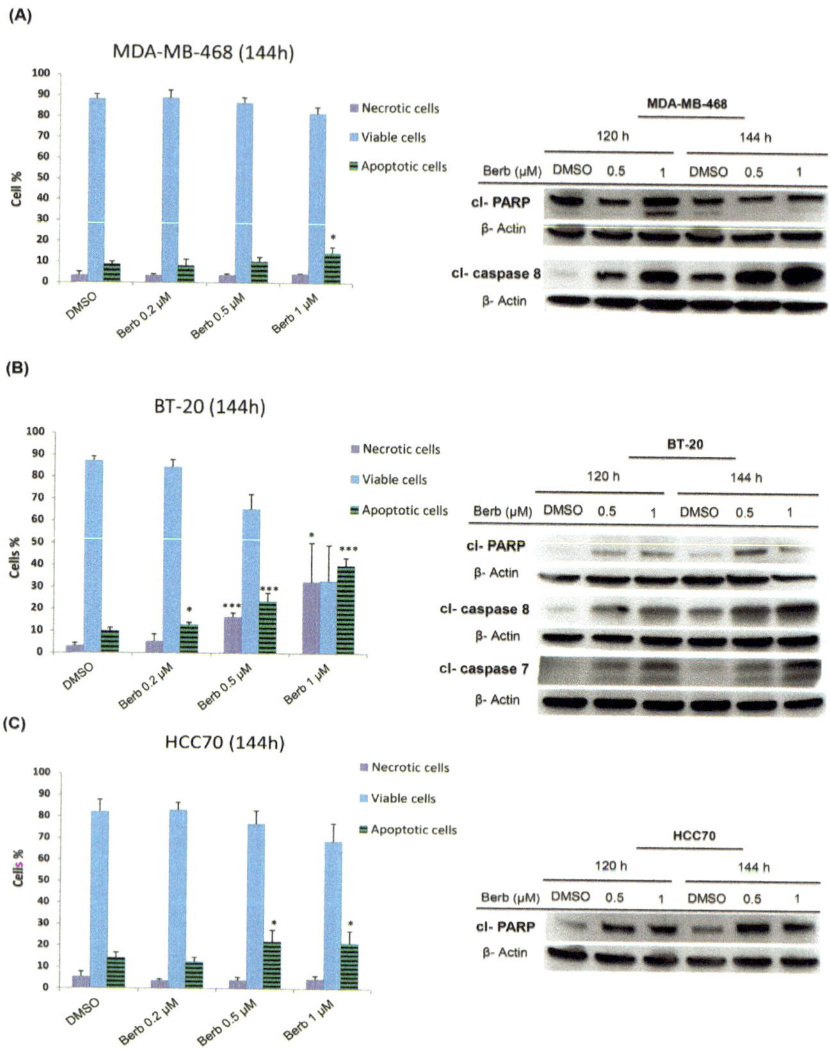

FIGURE 15.4 Berberine induced apoptosis in a dose- and time-dependent manner. Annexin-V and PI staining after 144 h of the treatment with berberine at 0.2, 0.5, and 1 μM. Western blot results of three independent experiments showing apoptosis-related protein expression upon berberine's treatment at 120 and 144 h. (A) MDA-MB-468, (B) BT-20, and (C) HCC70. ± SD of three independent experiments, * $p < 0.05$, ** $p < 0.01$, and *** $p < 0.001$ compared to DMSO. Berb—Berberine (El Khalki et al., 2020).

lines (Jaafari et al., 2012). On the other hand, artemisinin has shown a significant cytotoxic effect on TNBC cell lines: MDA-MB-468 (IC50 = 2.23 μM) and HCC38 (IC50 = 1.25 μM), with a significant synergistic effect when combined with cisplatin. However, its mechanism of action on TNBC cells still needs to be investigated in depth.

Furthermore, some clinical trials reported that berberine decreased the incidence and severity of radiation-induced lung injury and acute intestinal symptoms in cancer patients with radiotherapy (Li et al., 2010; Liu et al., 2008).

15.9 Conclusion

In conclusion the findings of different studies show that natural compounds may be promising new tools to develop more effective TNBC drugs by identifying their action pathway and targeted proteins. Furthermore, these observations may enable a better use of these natural compounds in combination with therapies to improve efficacy of the treatment with low to no side effects. Additionally, developing more effective prophylactic vaccines targeting infectious agents is highly recommended in order to prevent TNBC development and to reduce the risk of disease recurrence after the treatment.

Acknowledgments

The authors would like to express their gratitude to Dr. Thierry Dubois, Head of Breast Cancer Biology group laboratory, Curie Institute of Paris, and all the members of the laboratory, for their precious help and technical assistance.

References

Abdullah, L. N., & Chow, E. K.-H. (2013). Mechanisms of chemoresistance in cancer stem cells. *Clinical and Translational Medicine*, *2*(1), 3. Available from https://doi.org/10.1186/2001-1326-2-3.

Alibek, K., Kakpenova, A., Mussabekova, A., Sypabekova, M., & Karatayeva, N. (2013). Role of viruses in the development of breast cancer. *Infectious Agents and Cancer*, *8*(1). Available from https://doi.org/10.1186/1750-9378-8-32.

Amarante, M. K., & Watanabe, M. A. E. (2009). The possible involvement of virus in breast cancer. *Journal of Cancer Research and Clinical Oncology*, *135*(3), 329–337. Available from https://doi.org/10.1007/s00432-008-0511-2.

Amirikia, K. C., Mills, P., Bush, J., & Newman, L. A. (2011). Higher population-based incidence rates of triple-negative breast cancer among young African-American women. *Cancer*, *117*(12), 2747–2753. Available from https://doi.org/10.1002/cncr.25862.

Anders, C., & Carey, L. A. (2008). Understanding and treating triple-negative breast cancer. *Oncology*, *22*(11), 1233–1239. <https://www.ncbi.nlm.nih.gov/pmc/articles/PMC2868264/>. Accessed March 4, 2021.

Antonuzzo, L., Del Re, M., Barucca, V., et al. (2017). Critical focus on mechanisms of resistance and toxicity of m-TOR inhibitors in pancreatic neuroendocrine tumors. *Cancer Treatment Reviews*, *57*, 28–35. Available from https://doi.org/10.1016/j.ctrv.2017.05.001.

Baldwin, D. A., Feldman, M., Alwine, J. C., & Robertson, E. S. (2014). Metagenomic assay for identification of microbial pathogens in tumor tissues. *MBio*, *5*(5). Available from https://doi.org/10.1128/mBio.01714-14.

Banerjee, S., Wei, Z., Tan, F., et al. (2015). Distinct microbiological signatures associated with triple negative breast cancer. *Scientific Reports*, *5*(1), 1–14. Available from https://doi.org/10.1038/srep15162.

Bardia, A., Gucalp, A., DaCosta, N., et al. (2018). Phase 1 study of seviteronel, a selective CYP17 lyase and androgen receptor inhibitor, in women with estrogen receptor-positive or triple-negative breast cancer. *Breast Cancer Research and Treatment*, *171*(1), 111–120. Available from https://doi.org/10.1007/s10549-018-4813-z.

Berberine | C20H18NO4+ – PubChem. 2020 <https://pubchem.ncbi.nlm.nih.gov/compound/Berberine#section = 2D-Structure>. Accessed 01.10.20.

Borkar, D. S., Lacouture, M. E., & Basti, S. (2013). Spectrum of ocular toxicities from epidermal growth factor receptor inhibitors and their intermediate-term follow-up: A five-year review. *Supportive Care in Cancer: Official Journal of the Multinational Association of Supportive Care in Cancer*, *21*(4), 1167–1174. Available from https://doi.org/10.1007/s00520-012-1645-y.

Bray, F., Ferlay, J., Soerjomataram, I., Siegel, R. L., Torre, L. A., & Jemal, A. (2018). Global cancer statistics 2018: GLOBOCAN estimates of incidence and mortality worldwide for 36 cancers in 185 countries. *CA: A Cancer Journal for Clinicians*, *68*(6), 394–424. Available from https://doi.org/10.3322/caac.21492.

Brenton, J. D., Carey, L. A., Ahmed, A., & Caldas, C. (2005). Molecular classification and molecular forecasting of breast cancer: Ready for clinical application? *Journal of Clinical Oncology: Official Journal of the American Society of Clinical Oncology*, *23*(29), 7350–7360. Available from https://doi.org/10.1200/JCO.2005.03.3845.

Carey, L. A., Perou, C. M., Livasy, C. A., et al. (2006). Race, breast cancer subtypes, and survival in the carolina breast cancer study. *Journal of the American Medical Association*, *295*(21), 2492–2502. Available from https://doi.org/10.1001/jama.295.21.2492.

Carey, L. A., Rugo, H. S., Marcom, P. K., et al. (2012). TBCRC 001: Randomized phase II study of cetuximab in combination with carboplatin in stage IV triple-negative breast cancer. *Journal of Clinical Oncology: Official Journal of the American Society of Clinical Oncology*, *30*(21), 2615–2623. Available from https://doi.org/10.1200/JCO.2010.34.5579.

Chang-qing, Y., Jie, L., Shi-qi, Z., Kun, Z., Zi-qian, G., & Ran, X. (2019). Recent treatment progress of triple negative breast cancer. *Progress in Biophysics and Molecular Biology*. Available from https://doi.org/10.1016/j.pbiomolbio.2019.11.007.

Cheang, M. C. U., Voduc, D., Bajdik, C., et al. (2008). Basal-like breast cancer defined by five biomarkers has superior prognostic value than triple-negative phenotype. *Clinical Cancer Research: An Official Journal of the American Association for Cancer Research*, *14*(5), 1368–1376. Available from https://doi.org/10.1158/1078-0432.CCR-07-1658.

Chlebowski, R. T., Chen, Z., Anderson, G. L., et al. (2005). Ethnicity and breast cancer: Factors influencing differences in incidence and outcome. *Journal of the National Cancer Institute*, *97*(6), 439–447. Available from https://doi.org/10.1093/jnci/dji064.

Cintra, J. R., Teixeira, M. T., Diniz, R. W., et al. (2012). Immunohistochemical profile and clinical-pathological variables in breast cancer – PubMed. *Revista da Associacao Medica Brasileira*, *58*, 178–187. Available from https://pubmed.ncbi.nlm.nih.gov/22569612/, Accessed March 4, 2021.

Collins, L. K., Chapman, M. S., Carter, J. B., & Samie, F. H. (2017). Cutaneous adverse effects of the immune checkpoint inhibitors. *Current Problems in Cancer*, *41*(2), 125–128. Available from https://doi.org/10.1016/j.currproblcancer.2016.12.001.

Corbex, M., Bouzbid, S., Traverse-Glehen, A., et al. (2014). Prevalence of papillomaviruses, polyomaviruses, and herpesviruses in triple-negative and inflammatory breast tumors from algeria compared with other types of breast cancer tumors, Aguayo FR, (ed.)*PLoS One*, *9* (12), e114559. Available from https://doi.org/10.1371/journal.pone.0114559.

Cosmai, L., Gallieni, M., & Porta, C. (2015). Renal toxicity of anticancer agents targeting HER2 and EGFR. *Journal of Nephrology*, *28*(6), 647–657. Available from https://doi.org/10.1007/s40620-015-0226-9.

Costa, R. L. B., Han, H. S., & Gradishar, W. J. (2018). Targeting the PI3K/AKT/mTOR pathway in triple-negative breast cancer: A review. *Breast Cancer Research and Treatment*, *169*(3), 397–406. Available from https://doi.org/10.1007/s10549-018-4697-y.

D'Agostino, R. B. (2011). Changing end points in breast-cancer drug approval – The avastin story. *The New England Journal of Medicine*, *365*(2). Available from https://doi.org/10.1056/nejmp1106984.

Dragun, A. E., Pan, J., Rai, S. N., Kruse, B., & Jain, D. (2011). Locoregional recurrence in patients with triple-negative breast cancer: Preliminary results of a single institution study. *American Journal of Clinical Oncology: Cancer Clinical Trials*, *34*(3), 231–237. Available from https://doi.org/10.1097/COC.0b013e3181dea993.

Efferth, T., Li, P. C. H., Konkimalla, V. S. B., & Kaina, B. (2007). From traditional Chinese medicine to rational cancer therapy. *Trends in Molecular Medicine*, *13*(8), 353–361. Available from https://doi.org/10.1016/j.molmed.2007.07.001.

El Khalki, L., Maire, V., Dubois, T., & Zyad, A. (2020). Berberine impairs the survival of triple negative breast cancer cells: Cellular and molecular analyses. *Molecules (Basel, Switzerland)*, *25*(506), 1–18.

El Khalki, L., Tilaoui, M., Jaafari, A., Ait Mouse, H., & Zyad, A. (2018). Studies on the dual cytotoxicity and antioxidant properties of berberis vulgaris extracts and its main constituent berberine. *Advances in Pharmacological Science*, 2018. Available from https://doi.org/10.1155/2018/3018498.

FDA Approves Atezolizumab for Triple-Negative Breast Cancer – National Cancer Institute. <https://www.cancer.gov/news-events/cancer-currents-blog/2019/atezolizumab-triple-negative-breast-cancer-fda-approval>. Accessed 30.05.20.

Fernandez, A., & Reigosa, A. (2013). [Molecular classification of breast cancer patients obtained through the technique of chromogenic in situ hybridization (CISH)] – PubMed. *Investigative Clinical*, *54*, 406–416. Available from https://pubmed.ncbi.nlm.nih.gov/24502182/, Accessed March 4, 2021.

Finn, R. S., Dering, J., Ginther, C., et al. (2007). Dasatinib, an orally active small molecule inhibitor of both the src and abl kinases, selectively inhibits growth of basal-type/"triple-negative" breast cancer cell lines growing in vitro. *Breast Cancer Research and Treatment*, *105*(3), 319–326. Available from https://doi.org/10.1007/s10549-006-9463-x.

Gordaliza, M. (2007). Natural products as leads to anticancer drugs. *Clinical & Translational Oncology: Official Publication of the Federation of Spanish Oncology Societies and of the National Cancer Institute of Mexico*, *9*(12), 767–776. Available from https://doi.org/10.1007/s12094-007-0138-9.

Hachana, M., Amara, K., Ziadi, S., Gacem, R. Ben, Korbi, S., & Trimeche, M. (2012). Investigation of human JC and BK polyomaviruses in breast carcinomas. *Breast Cancer Research and Treatment*, *133*(3), 969–977. Available from https://doi.org/10.1007/s10549-011-1876-5.

Harkins, L. E., Matlaf, L. A., Soroceanu, L., et al. (2010). Detection of human cytomegalovirus in normal and neoplastic breast epithelium. *Herpesviridae*, *1*(1), 8. Available from https://doi.org/10.1186/2042-4280-1-8.

Hau, E., Browne, L., Capp, A., et al. (2013). The impact of breast cosmetic and functional outcomes on quality of life: Long-term results from the St. George and Wollongong randomized breast boost trial. *Breast Cancer Research and Treatment, 139*(1), 115–123. Available from https://doi.org/10.1007/s10549-013-2508-z.

Imanshahidi, M. (2008). Pharmacological and therapeutic effects of Berberis vulgaris and its active constituent, berberine. *Pharmacological Research, 22*, 999–1012. Available from https://doi.org/10.1002/ptr.2399.

Jaafari, A., Tilaoui, M., Mouse, H. A., et al. (2012). Comparative study of the antitumor effect of natural monoterpenes: Relationship to cell cycle analysis. *Brazilian Journal of Pharmacognosy, 22*(3), 534–540. Available from https://doi.org/10.1590/S0102-695X2012005000021.

Jia, L. Y., Shanmugam, M. K., Sethi, G., & Bishayee, A. (2016). Potential role of targeted therapies in the treatment of triple-negative breast cancer. *Anti-Cancer Drugs, 27*, 147–155. Available from https://doi.org/10.1097/CAD.0000000000000328.

Kim, E. M. H., Mueller, K., Gartner, E., & Boerner, J. (2013). Dasatinib is synergistic with cetuximab and cisplatin in triple-negative breast cancer cells. *The Journal of Surgical Research, 185*(1), 231–239. Available from https://doi.org/10.1016/j.jss.2013.06.041.

Kim, J., Lee, K.-M., Ko, E., et al. (2008). Berberine inhibits growth of the breast cancer cell lines MCF-7 and MDA-MB-231. *Planta Medica, 74*(1), 39–42. Available from https://doi.org/10.1055/s-2007-993779.

Kingston, D. G. I. (2007). The shape of things to come: Structural and synthetic studies of taxol and related compounds. *Phytochemistry, 68*(14), 1844–1854. Available from https://doi.org/10.1016/j.phytochem.2006.11.009.

Kumar, P., & Aggarwal, R. (2016). An overview of triple-negative breast cancer. *Archives of Gynecology and Obstetrics, 293*(2), 247–269. Available from https://doi.org/10.1007/s00404-015-3859-y.

LaFargue, C. J., Dal Molin, G. Z., Sood, A. K., & Coleman, R. L. (2019). Exploring and comparing adverse events between PARP inhibitors. *The Lancet Oncology, 20*(1), e15–e28. Available from https://doi.org/10.1016/S1470-2045(18)30786-1.

Lara-Medina, F., Pérez-Sánchez, V., Saavedra-Pérez, D., et al. (2011). Triple-negative breast cancer in Hispanic patients: High prevalence, poor prognosis, and association with menopausal status, body mass index, and parity. *Cancer, 117*(16), 3658–3669. Available from https://doi.org/10.1002/cncr.25961

Lawson, J. S., Salmons, B., & Glenn, W. K. (2018). Oncogenic viruses and breast cancer: Mouse mammary tumor virus (MMTV), bovine leukemia virus (BLV), human papilloma virus (HPV), and epstein-barr virus (EBV). *Frontiers in Oncology, 8*(JAN). Available from https://doi.org/10.3389/fonc.2018.00001.

Lehmann, B. D., Bauer, J. A., Chen, X., et al. (2011). Identification of human triple-negative breast cancer subtypes and preclinical models for selection of targeted therapies. *The Journal of Clinical Investigation, 121*(7), 2750–2767. Available from https://doi.org/10.1172/JCI45014.

Li, G. H., Wang, D. L., Hu, Y. De, et al. (2010). Berberine inhibits acute radiation intestinal syndrome in human with abdomen radiotherapy. *Medical Oncology (Northwood, London, England), 27*(3), 919–925. Available from https://doi.org/10.1007/s12032-009-9307-8.

Liu, D., Meng, X., Wu, D., Qiu, Z., & Luo, H. (2019). A natural isoquinoline alkaloid with antitumor activity: Studies of the biological activities of berberine. *Frontiers in Pharmacology, 10*(FEB). Available from https://doi.org/10.3389/fphar.2019.00009.

Liu, Y., Yu, H., Zhang, C., et al. (2008). Protective effects of berberine on radiation-induced lung injury via intercellular adhesion molecular-1 and transforming growth factor-beta-1 in patients with lung cancer. *European Journal of Cancer, 44*(16), 2425–2432. Available from https://doi.org/10.1016/j.ejca.2008.07.040.

Livshits, Z., Rao, R. B., & Smith, S. W. (2014). An approach to chemotherapy-associated toxicity. *Emergency Medicine Clinics of North America*, *32*(1), 167–203. Available from https://doi.org/10.1016/j.emc.2013.09.002.

Mazouni, C., Fina, F., Romain, S., et al. (2011). Epstein-Barr virus as a marker of biological aggressiveness in breast cancer. *British Journal of Cancer*, *104*(2), 332–337. Available from https://doi.org/10.1038/sj.bjc.6606048.

McCann, K. E., & Hurvitz, S. A. (2018). Advances in the use of PARP inhibitor therapy for breast cancer. *Drugs Context*, *7*, 212540. Available from https://doi.org/10.7573/dic.212540.

Miller, K., Wang, M., Gralow, J., et al. (2007). Paclitaxel plus bevacizumab vs paclitaxel alone for metastatic breast cancer. *The New England Journal of Medicine*, *357*(26), 2666–2676. Available from https://doi.org/10.1056/NEJMoa072113.

Newman, D. J., Cragg, G. M., & Snader, K. M. (2003). Natural products as sources of new drugs over the period 1981 – 2002. *Journal of Natural Products*, *66*(7), 1022–1037. Available from https://doi.org/10.1021/np030096l.

Pandurangan AK, Mustafa MR. (2018). Therapeutic strategies of natural agents 14 on triple-negative breast cancer. In: Anticancer plants: natural products and biotechnological implements. Vol 2. Springer Singapore; 321-341. http://doi.org/10.1007/978-981-10-8064-7_14.

Pardoll, D. M. (2012). The blockade of immune checkpoints in cancer immunotherapy. *Nature Reviews. Cancer*, *12*(4), 252–264. Available from https://doi.org/10.1038/nrc3239.

Patil, J. B., Kim, J., & Jayaprakasha, G. K. (2010). Berberine induces apoptosis in breast cancer cells (MCF-7) through mitochondrial-dependent pathway. *European Journal of Pharmacology*, *645*(1–3), 70–78. Available from https://doi.org/10.1016/j.ejphar.2010.07.037.

Perou, C. M., Sørile, T., Eisen, M. B., et al. (2000). Molecular portraits of human breast tumours. *Nature*, *406*(6797), 747–752. Available from https://doi.org/10.1038/35021093.

Petropoulos C. Retroviral Taxonomy, Protein Structures, Sequences, and Genetic Maps. 1997. https://www.ncbi.nlm.nih.gov/books/NBK19417/. Accessed March 4, 2021.

Phipps, A. I., Chlebowski, R. T., Prentice, R., et al. (2011). Reproductive history and oral contraceptive use in relation to risk of triple-negative breast cancer. *Journal of the National Cancer Institute*, *103*(6), 470–477. Available from https://doi.org/10.1093/jnci/djr030.

Piana, A. F., Sotgiu, G., Muroni, M. R., Cossu-Rocca, P., Castiglia, P., & De Miglio, M. R. (2014). HPV infection and triple-negative breast cancers: An Italian case-control study. *Virology Journal*, *11*(1), 190. Available from https://doi.org/10.1186/s12985-014-0190-3.

Pogo BGT, Holland JF. (1997). Possibilities of a viral etiology for human breast cancer: A review. In: Biological Trace Element Research. Vol 56. Humana Press Inc. 131-142. http://doi.org/10.1007/BF02778989.

Raphael, D. B., ter Stege, J. A., Russell, N. S., Boersma, L. J., & van der Weijden, T. (2020). What do patients and health care professionals view as important attributes in radiotherapy decisions? Input for a breast cancer patient decision aid. *The Breast*, *49*, 149–156. Available from https://doi.org/10.1016/j.breast.2019.11.005.

Reilly, E. A. O., Gubbins, L., Sharma, S., et al. (2015). The fate of chemoresistance in triple negative breast cancer (TNBC). *BBACLI*, *3*, 257–275. Available from https://doi.org/10.1016/j.bbacli.2015.03.003.

Réseau canadien du cancer du sein – accueil. 2021, <https://www.cbcn.ca/fr/>. Accessed 04.03.21.

Ruiz-Schutz, V. C., Gomes, L. M., Mariano, R. C., et al. (2019). Risk of fatigue and anemia in patients with advanced cancer treated with olaparib: A meta-analysis of randomized controlled trials. *Critical Reviews in Oncology/Hematology*, *141*, 163–173. Available from https://doi.org/10.1016/j.critrevonc.2019.06.012.

Salman, N. A., Davies, G., Majidy, F., et al. (2017). Association of high risk human papillomavirus and breast cancer: A UK based study. *Scientific Reports*, *7*, 43591. Available from https://doi.org/10.1038/srep43591.

Slade, D. (2020). PARP and PARG inhibitors in cancer treatment. *Genes & Development*, *34*(5), 360–394. Available from https://doi.org/10.1101/gad.334516.119.

Smith, L. A., Cornelius, V. R., Plummer, C. J., et al. (2010). Cardiotoxicity of anthracycline agents for the treatment of cancer: Systematic review and meta-analysis of randomised controlled trials. *BMC Cancer*, *10*(1), 337. Available from https://doi.org/10.1186/1471-2407-10-337.

Society, A., & Clinical, O. F. (2016). ASCO educational book. *ASCO Educational Book*, *2016* (34), 1–931.

Tamimi, R. M., Colditz, G. A., Hazra, A., et al. (2012). Traditional breast cancer risk factors in relation to molecular subtypes of breast cancer. *Breast Cancer Research and Treatment*, *131* (1), 159–167. Available from https://doi.org/10.1007/s10549-011-1702-0.

Vallejos, C., Gómez, H., Cruz, W., et al. (2010). Breast cancer classification according to immunohistochemistry markers: Subtypes and association with clinicopathologic variables in a peruvian hospital database. *Clinical Breast Cancer*, *10*(4), 294–300. Available from https://doi.org/10.3816/CBC.2010.n.038.

Varghese, E., Samuel, S. M., Abotaleb, M., Cheema, S., Mamtani, R., & Büsselberg, D. (2018). The "Yin and Yang" of natural compounds in anticancer therapy of triple-negative breast cancers. *Cancers (Basel)*, *10*(10). Available from https://doi.org/10.3390/cancers10100346.

Wahba, H. A., & El-Hadaad, H. A. (2015). Current approaches in treatment of triple-negative breast cancer. *Cancer Biology & Medicine*, *12*(2), 106–116. Available from https://doi.org/10.7497/j.issn.2095-3941.2015.0030.

Waljee, J. F., Hu, E. S., Ubel, P. A., Smith, D. M., Newman, L. A., & Alderman, A. K. (2008). Effect of esthetic outcome after breast-conserving surgery on psychosocial functioning and quality of life. *Journal of Clinical Oncology: Official Journal of the American Society of Clinical Oncology*, *26*(20), 3331–3337. Available from https://doi.org/10.1200/JCO.2007.13.1375.

Wallin, J. J., Edgar, K. A., Guan, J., et al. (2011). GDC-0980 is a novel class I PI3K/mTOR kinase inhibitor with robust activity in cancer models driven by the PI3K pathway. *Molecular Cancer Therapeutics*, *10*(12), 2426–2436. Available from https://doi.org/10.1158/1535-7163.MCT-11-0446.

Wang, Y. X., Yang, L., Wang, H. Q., et al. (2018). Synthesis and evolution of berberine derivatives as a new class of antiviral agents against enterovirus 71 through the MEK/ERK pathway and autophagy. *Molecules (Basel, Switzerland)*, *23*(8), 2084. Available from https://doi.org/10.3390/molecules23082084.

Yang, J., He, X., Lv, Q., Jing, J., & Shi, H. (2019). Management of adverse events in cancer patients treated with PD-1/PD-L1 blockade: Focus on asian populations. *Frontiers in Pharmacology*, *10*(726). Available from https://doi.org/10.3389/fphar.2019.00726.

Zhang, H., Cohen, A. L., Krishnakumar, S., et al. (2014). Patient-derived xenografts of triple-negative breast cancer reproduce molecular features of patient tumors and respond to mTOR inhibition. *Breast Cancer Research: BCR*, *16*(2), R36. Available from https://doi.org/10.1186/bcr3640.

Chapter 16

Role of exosomes in bladder cancer diagnosis and therapy

Ikram Tiabi[1], Maryame Lamsisi[1], Imane Saif[1], Youssef Ennaji[1], Soukayna Alaoui Sosse[1], Berjas Abumsimir[1,2], Thomas Bourlet[3], Guorong Li[3,4], Mohammed Mrabti[5,6], Abdelilah Laraqui[7] and Moulay Mustapha Ennaji[8]

[1]Team of Virology, Oncology, and Biotechnologies, Laboratory of Virology, Oncology, Biosciences, Environment and New Energies (LVO-BEEN), Faculty of Sciences and Techniques Mohammedia, University Hassan II of Casablanca, Casablanca, Morocco, [2]Pharmacological and Diagnostic Research Centre (PDRC), Department of Medical Laboratory Sciences, Faculty of Allied Medical Sciences, Al-Ahliyya Amman University (AAU), Amman, Jordan, [3]Laboratory of Infectious Agents and Hygiene (GIMAP), EA3064, University Hospital and University Jean Monnet, Saint-Etienne, France, [4]North Hospital, CHU Saint Etienne, Saint Etienne, France, [5]Urology Department, Mohammed V Military Hospital, Rabat, Morocco, [6]Research and Biosafety Laboratory, Mohammed V Construction Teaching Hospital. Mohammed V University, Rabat, Morocco, [7]Laboratory of Human Pathologies Biology, Faculty of Sciences, and Genomic Center of Human Pathologies, Faculty of Medicine and Pharmacy, Bio-Path Laboratory, Faculty of sciences-Agdal, Mohammed V University, Rabat, Morocco, [8]Group Leader Research team of Virology, Oncology, and Biotechnologies, Head of Laboratory of Virology, Oncology, Biosciences, Environment and New Energies (LVO-BEEN), Faculty of Sciences and Techniques Mohammedia, University Hassan II of Casablanca, Casablanca, Morocco

16.1 Introduction

Bladder cancer (BC) is a very common urologic malignancy, with 573,278 new cases and 212,536 deaths reported worldwide in 2020 (Sung et al., 2021). Recent scientific evidence shows that both normal and pathological cells routinely secrete a set of specific membrane vesicles carrying many components that represent parental cells (Soung et al., 2017). These extracellular vesicles (EVs) consist of small exosomes (40–120 nm) and large microvesicles (300–1000 nm); they are detected in many body fluids such as blood, saliva, and urine.

Exosomes are typically secreted by different cell types and are hypothesized to be mediators for communication between cells (Yáñez-Mó et al., 2015). The International Society for Extracellular Vesicles proposes to refer to "EVs" rather than exosomes or microvesicles and indicates terms for EV

Immunological Implications and Molecular Diagnostics of Genitourinary Cancer.
DOI: https://doi.org/10.1016/B978-0-323-85496-2.00027-0

subtypes owing to their physical characteristics. Recently, studies have shown that exosomes can provide novel noninvasive diagnostic and prognostic biomarkers in patients with cancers, including BC, and the structure of the lipid bilayer membrane makes exosomes promising carriers for therapeutic applications (Théry et al., 2018).

16.2 Exosomes: nanovesicles of endosomal origin

Cells produce vesicles in the extracellular medium. These vesicles are then delimited by a double lipidic layer. There are several types of vesicles whose origin, physical properties (size, density, sedimentation), and biochemical properties vary. It is possible to differentiate two categories of vesicles on the basis of their origin: vesicles derived from the budding of the plasma membrane and exosomes, which have an intracellular source. Exosomes are of endosomal origin and are released into secretion after fusion to the plasma membrane of a multivesicular endosome.

Exosome biogenesis starts with an endocytosis phase during which cells internalize different molecules. Subsequently, a second invasion of the membrane will take place in the endosomes, before their release by a mechanism of exocytosis (Kalluri, 2016). The first step corresponds to the invagination of the plasma membrane, which constitutes a structure containing membrane proteins and soluble extracellular medium proteins. This structural configuration will lead to the creation of a primitive endosome which, in some cases, will fuse with other primitive endosomes. It should be noted that the endoplasmic reticulum and the Golgi system are involved in the formation and content of these early endosomes (Mathieu et al., 2019). Subsequently, these early endosomes will mature and transform into late endosomes and then into multivesicular bodies (MVBs).

These MVBs are formed by the invagination of the late endosome membrane and give rise to small vesicles called intraluminal vesicles (ILVs): the future exosomes (Fig. 16.1). Finally, these ILVs can fuse with autophagosomes and/or lysosomes and thus be recycled and/or be degraded or fuse with the plasma membrane and give rise to exosomes (McAndrews & Kalluri, 2019). The specific mechanisms of exosome establishment are still poorly understood. However, many studies indicate the participation of different molecules, suggesting that there is no universal mechanism but rather different mechanisms (Bebelman et al., 2018), whose activity is dependent on many parameters such as the type of cell and its physiological state.

16.2.1 Exosome heterogeneity

Exosomes have a specific composition that characterizes them and distinguishes them from other EVs (Crescitelli et al., 2013; Kowal et al., 2016). This composition gives them specific roles that are controlled by the release dynamics of these nanovesicles. The Exocarta website references the contents of exosomes (http://www.exocarta.org/).

The diversity of signaling and pathways in exosome biogenesis, as well as the impact of the cellular environment, result in phenotypic diversity of

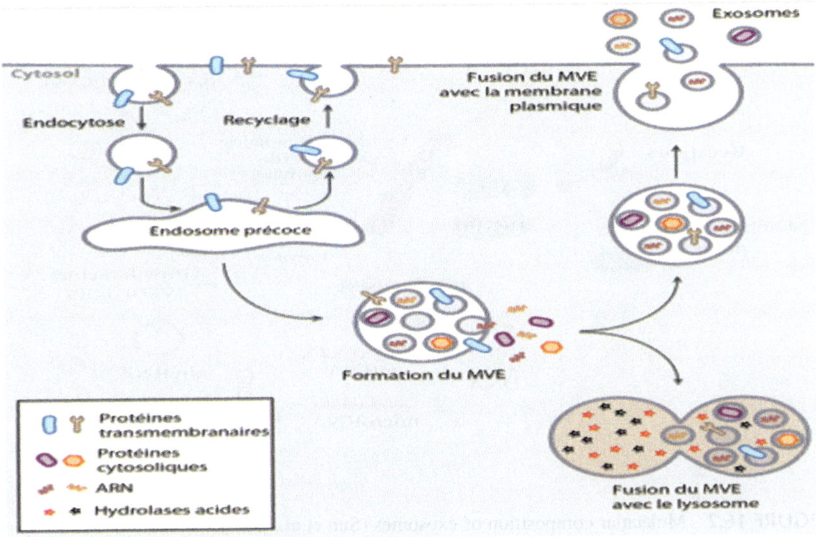

FIGURE 16.1 Exosome biosynthetic pathway (Javalet, 2016).

exosomes. In particular, there are subpopulations of different sizes, from different sources, with different content and therefore have a difference in role (Kalluri & LeBleu, 2020; Zhang et al., 2018). This heterogeneity has been highlighted in particular by proteomic analyses that have identified protein signatures of certain cell types, while sequencing analyses identified discrepancies with the parental cell, suggesting a highly specific sorting mechanism (Kowal et al., 2016). The roles of exosomes on target cells, therefore, vary with the size and the type of receptors represented on their surface, the quality and quantity of material they carry, and the way they are transmitted to the recipient cells (Jeppesen et al., 2019).

16.2.2 Functions of exosomes

Exosomes comprise a large number of biologically active substances, including proteins, mRNAs, and microRNAs, that are specifically equipped to facilitate cell-to-cell communication via the transfer of their cargo to recipient cells (Pitt et al., 2016; Zöller., 2016) (Fig. 16.2). After being released into the extracellular environment, exosomes can reach the recipient cells and release their contents, which will cause a functional response and alter their physiological state. They are likely to behave differently after binding to the membrane of the recipient cell, but these same mechanisms are still poorly understood. It remains unknown, for example, whether a different mode of operation affects the fate of the exosome (Kowal et al., 2016).

First, exosomes are likely to carry associations of ligands that are susceptible to different cell surface receptors simultaneously. This would be similar to

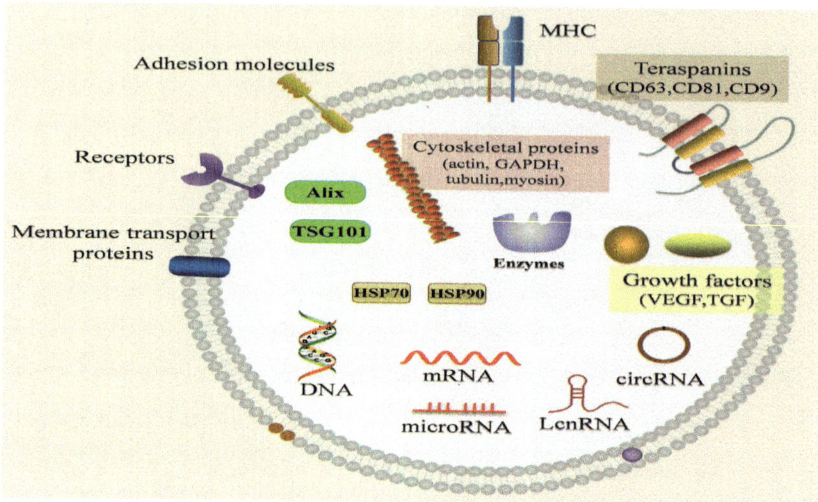

FIGURE 16.2 Molecular composition of exosomes (Sun et al., 2018).

what happens in interactions between two cells but without the presence of a direct link between the cells (Kowal et al., 2016). Second, exosomes can bind to the membranes of target cells, which can then carry "new" surface molecules and possibly obtain new receptors, surface molecules, and, presumably, acquire new adhesion properties (Kowal et al., 2016). Third, exosomes can fuse with target cells and exchange membrane proteins and cytosol between the two cell types. Of course, if any of these mechanisms occur—which remains to be demonstrated, even in vitro—they would have to be highly regulated, like all other modes of intercellular communication (Kowal et al., 2016).

In the context of the interaction between cancer stem cells (CSCs) and nonCSCs, exosomes are considered important information transmitters by transmitting strain-associated substances to nonCSCs, making them regain their strain phenotype. On the one hand, cancer cells can mobilize and alter the phenotypic attributes and functions of stromal cells in the tumor microenvironment by releasing exosomes. On the other hand, these formed cells or CSCs transmit specific molecules to cancer cells via exosomes that are required for tumor growth, metastasis, and drug resistance, to promote tumorigenicity or stemness phenotype of cancer cells (Alenquer & Maria, 2015).

16.2.3 Roles of exosomes in bladder cancer

Within a tumor, cell transmission is an important dynamic process. It is now known that exosomes are an integral part of this process. Different physiological conditions in the microenvironment change the situation of cancer cells, which release more exosomes than healthy cells. Also, their content is different from that of the normal cell, suggesting a particular sorting phenomenon that promotes tumor proliferation (Jeppesen et al., 2019).

In particular, exosomal noncoding RNAs (ncRNAs) play vital roles in the initiation and progression of many cellular processes related to BC, in addition to their involvement in modulating the expression of various key signaling and molecular pathways that play important regulatory roles in BC metastasis (Table 16.1).

16.3 Urinary biomarkers for bladder cancer diagnosis

Konety (2006) determined that the ideal BC biomarker is an objective, noninvasive, easily interpretable marker with high sensitivity and specificity (Konety, 2006). Urinary biomarkers for the detection of BC represent an attractive alternative. Urine is directly in contact with the urothelial bladder cells, thus constituting a valuable source of biomarkers of various natures such as proteins, DNA, metabolites, various types of RNA, and single nucleotide polymorphisms. The presence or changes in the presentation or expression of these molecules are likely to be associated with BC (Leiblich. 2017). It has been reported that urinary EVs are a source of biomarkers for BC diagnosis. Specifically, exosomal ncRNAs have been detected in plasma, serum, urine, and other body fluids. The expression levels of some exosomal ncRNAs are related to the clinical classification and diagnosis of BC and can be considered biomarkers of BC.

According to Elsharkawi et al., tumor-derived exosomes could be a useful biological device for the early detection of BC. Using the ELISA technique, they determined the concentration of these exosomes in urine and serum samples from BC patients and healthy controls. Exosome concentrations in BC patients were higher than in the healthy group in serum and urine samples at different stages of the disease (Elsharkawi et al., 2019).

Exosomal content presents a variety of biomarkers of diagnosis utility. For instance, the level of urinary exosomal CA9 mRNA was significantly higher in BC group in comparison to controls. The area under the ROC curve (AUC) was found to be 0.837 (95% confidence interval [CI]: 0.743–0.859), a sensitivity of 85.18% and a specificity of 83.15% (Wen et al., 2021). In addition, exosomal lncRNA PTENP1 represented a promising new biomarker for the diagnosis of BC with an AUC = 0.743 (95% CI = 0.645–0.840), 65.4% sensitivity, and 84.2% specificity (Zheng et al., 2018).

Exosomal DNA is another valuable source of biomarkers. The relative nature and quantity of DNA species present in exosomes from cell culture supernatants and biological fluids are being actively studied. Different types (single-stranded, double-stranded, mitochondrial) and several types of DNA are present in exosomes (Kalluri & LeBleu, 2016). In fact, urine exosomal DNA analysis revealed somatic driver variants in genes associated with BC (Zhou et al., 2021).

TABLE 16.1 The roles of exosomal noncoding RNAs in bladder cancer.

Exosomal content		Target	Mechanism	References
LncRNAs	LINC01133	Wnt signaling pathway	Limits the viability, proliferation, migration, and invasion of cells.	Yang et al. (2021)
	PTENP1	PTEN	Exosomal PTENP1 regulates PTEN expression via competitive binding to miR-17	Zheng et al. (2018)
	LNMAT2	hnRNPA2B1	Bladder cancer cell-secreted exosome-mediated lymphangiogenesis promoted LN metastasis in BCa in a VEGF-C-independent manner.	Chen et al. (2020)
	LINC00960 and LINC02470.	β-catenin signaling, Notch signaling, and Smad2/3 signaling pathways	Exosome-derived LINC00960 and LINC02470 from high-grade bladder cancer cells promote the malignant behaviors of recipient low-grade bladder cancer cells and induce epithelial-mesenchymal transition (EMT) by upregulating β-catenin signaling, Notch signaling, and Smad2/3 signaling.	Huang et al. (2020)
MicroRNAs	miR-21	PI3K/AKT	Exosomal miR-21 derived from bladder cancer cells inhibited phosphatase and tensin homolog activation of the PI3K/AKT signaling pathway in macrophages and enhanced STAT3 expression to promote M2 phenotypic polarization.	Lin et al. (2020)
	miR-375−3p	Wnt/β-catenin.	Potential suppressor in bladder cancer via the Wnt/β-catenin pathway, inhibiting the expression of FZD8.	Li et al. (2020)
	microRNA-133b	Wnt/β-catenin signaling pathway by targeting EZH2.	Exosomal miR-133b may inhibit tumor growth in vivo. In addition, exosomal miR-133b may contribute to suppressing bladder cancer proliferation by upregulating dual-specificity protein phosphatase 1 (DUSP1).	Xu et al. (2019)
	miR-4792	FOXC1/c-Myc Signaling	Exosomal miR-4792 downregulated FOXC1 and c-Myc.	Wu et al. (2022)
	microRNA-133b	DUSP1	Exosomal miR-133b upregulated dual-specificity protein phosphatase 1 (DUSP1).	Cai et al. (2020)
	miRNA-217	Hippo-YAP pathway	Exosomal miR-217 mimic stimulated YAP and its target proteins including Cyr61, CTGF, and ANKRD1.	Huang et al. (2021)

16.3.1 Exosomes therapy applications for bladder cancers

Several methods are usually applied for the treatment of patients with BC, including tumor surgery, chemotherapy, radiation therapy, stem cell transformation, and radical cystectomy. However, as we note, these methods have many side effects such as reduced bioavailability, nonselectivity, toxicity, rapid clearance, and limited ability to cause metastasis. In addition, researchers are looking for new treatment methods with few side effects and more therapeutic effects.

Nowadays, nanotechnology has tremendously improved the diagnosis and treatment of a wide variety of cancers. Recently, several nanoparticles (NPs), such as polymeric NPs, lipid NPs, and metallic NPs, have been used to facilitate the treatment of BC. Different forms of NPs can improve the solubility of drugs, and multifunctional NPs have interesting results against kidney, bladder, prostate, and bowel cancer. NPs are also used as drug delivery devices to improve the effects and interactions between drugs and the urothelium. In addition, nanotechnology can also be combined with other recent technologies to improve their effectiveness. Exosomes and other EVs constitute additional NPs of natural origin that can be used for cancer therapy.

New therapeutic application of exosome targeting BC has been investigated. As described above, cancer cells communicate their exosomes not only to cells in the microenvironment (fibroblasts, endothelial cells, and immune cells) and to cancer cells themselves but also to cells at distant and premetastatic sites. These exosomes are then transferred to their target cells, and they modify the phenotype of these target cells to their advantage. Deletion of exosome synthesis-related genes, such as Rab27a, Rab27b, Rab35, and nSMase2, can prevent cancer cell-based exosome production, and this approach effectively inhibits cancer metastasis. Another method of exosome targeting therapy is to block exosome uptake by recipient cells (Mathieu et al., 2019).

Moreover, exosomes have been reported to be nanocarriers that can be used in the treatment of many tumors by releasing their cargoes into the targeted site. Exosomes can be used as nanocarriers for antitumor therapeutic agents or siRNAs. The benefits of this method include increased drug efficacy, increased drug bioavailability, in addition to nontoxicity or reduced toxicity. Wang et al., for example, developed a dual-functional exosome-based superparamagnetic NP system that uses exosomes as a targeted drug carrier to treat cancer cells (Wang et al., 2020).

16.4 Conclusions

Concerning their function in cancer propagation and their biological characteristics, exosomes have remarkable potential in cancer therapy. To date, multiple exosome-based cancer treatment strategies have already been investigated and developed, including naturally occurring immune cell exosomes to eliminate cancer cells, activity-inhibiting exosomes derived from cancer cells, and gene and drug delivery exosomes. However, significant challenges remain. First, the distinction between exosomes from different sources is not yet clear.

Second, the number of exosomes to achieve a therapeutic effect may vary significantly from one cancer to another. Third, the evolutionary nature and heterogeneity of the tumor may influence the therapeutic outcome. In addition, the different functions of exosomes derived from different sources are not fully studied.

In particular, the knowledge of how exosomes can be tailored to possess a high degree of selectivity toward specific cancer cells remains unclear. Finally, the storage mode and stability capacity of exosomes remain poorly defined. Because of these challenges, it is essential to systematically characterize exosomes from different cells/tissues to determine the most effective cells for specific cancer therapy. It is also necessary to identify specific surface markers of cancer cells to design exosomes as drug carriers with high specificity for cancer cells. Owing to the difficulty and heterogeneity of the tumor, exosome therapy for cancer may need to be combined with other approaches. Finally, scientific trials of exosome-based cancer therapy are essential to evaluate the efficacy of this application. Although challenges remain, it is clear that exosomes offer new and critical opportunities for cancer treatment.

Acknowledgments

Authors would like to thank the Minister of National Education, Professional Training, Higher Education and Scientific Research and the School of Sciences and Techniques, The University Hassan II of Casablanca. Many thanks to members of Virology, Oncology and Medical Biotechnology team at FSTM-UH2C for all their financial support.

References

Alenquer, Marta, & Maria, João Amorim (2015). Exosome biogenesis, regulation, and function in viral infection. *Viruses*, *7*(9), 5066–5083.

Bebelman, M. P., Smit, M. J., Pegtel, D. M., & Baglio, S. R. (2018). Biogenesis and function of extracellular vesicles in cancer. *Pharmacology & Therapeutics*, *188*, 1–11.

Cai, X., Qu, L., Yang, J., Xu, J., Sun, L., Wei, X., Qu, X., Bai, T., Guo, Z., & Zhu, Y. (2020). Exosome-transmitted microRNA-133b inhibited bladder cancer proliferation by upregulating dual-specificity protein phosphatase 1. *Cancer Medicine*, *9*(16), 6009–6019. Available from https://doi.org/10.1002/cam4.3263.

Chen, C., Luo, Y., He, W., Zhao, Y., Kong, Y., Liu, H., Zhong, G., Li, Y., Li, J., Huang, J., Chen, R., & Lin, T. (2020). Exosomal long noncoding RNA LNMAT2 promotes lymphatic metastasis in bladder cancer. *The Journal of Clinical Investigation*, *130*(1), 404–421. Available from https://doi.org/10.1172/JCI130892.

Crescitelli, R., Lässer, C., Szabó, T. G., Kittel, A., Eldh, M., Dianzani, I., & Lötvall, J. (2013). Distinct RNA profiles in subpopulations of extracellular vesicles: Apoptotic bodies, microvesicles and exosomes. *Journal of Extracellular Vesicles*, *2*(1), 20677.

Elsharkawi, F., Elsabah, M., Shabayek, M., & Khaled, H. (2019). Urine and serum exosomes as novel biomarkers in detection of BC. *Asian Pacific Journal of Cancer Prevention: APJCP*, *20*, 2219–2224.

Huang, C. S., Ho, J. Y., Chiang, J. H., Yu, C. P., & Yu, D. S. (2020). Exosome-derived LINC00960 and LINC02470 promote the epithelial-mesenchymal transition and aggressiveness of bladder cancer cells. *Cells*, *9*(6), 1419. Available from https://doi.org/10.3390/cells9061419.

Huang, Z. M., Wang, H., & Ji, Z. G. (2021). Bladder mesenchymal stromal cell-derived exosomal miRNA-217 modulates bladder cancer cell survival through Hippo-YAP pathway. *Inflammation Research: Official Journal of the European Histamine Research Society*, *70* (9), 959–969. Available from https://doi.org/10.1007/s00011-021-014947.

Javalet, C. (2016). *Rôle des exosomes comme nouvelle voie de communication entre les neurones* (doctoral dissertation). Français: Université Grenoble Alpes.

Jeppesen, D. K., Fenix, A. M., Franklin, J. L., Higginbotham, J. N., Zhang, Q., Zimmerman, L. J., & Coffey, R. J. (2019). Reassessment of exosome composition. *Cell*, *177*(2), 428–445.

Kalluri, R. (2016). The biology and function of exosomes in cancer. *The Journal of Clinical Investigation*, *126*(4), 1208–1215.

Kalluri, R., & LeBleu, V. S. (2016). *Discovery of double-stranded genomic DNA in circulating exosomes. Cold Spring Harbor Symposia on Quantitative Biology* (Vol. 81, pp. 275–280). Cold Spring Harbor Laboratory Press, January.

Kalluri, R., & LeBleu, V. S. (2020). The biology, function, and biomedical applications of exosomes. *Science (New York, N.Y.)*, *367*(6478).

Konety, B. R. (2006). Molecular markers in bladder cancer: A critical appraisal. *Urologic Oncology*, *24*, 326–337.

Kowal, J., Arras, G., Colombo, M., Jouve, M., Morath, J. P., Primdal-Bengtson, B., & Théry, C. (2016). Proteomic comparison defines novel markers to characterize heterogeneous populations of extracellular vesicle subtypes. *Proceedings of the National Academy of Sciences of the United States of America*, *113*(8), E968–E977.

Leiblich, A. (2017). Recent developments in the search for urinary biomarkers in bladder cancer. *Current Urology Reports*, *18*, 100.

Li, Q., Huyan, T., Cai, S., Huang, Q., Zhang, M., Peng, H., Zhang, Y., Liu, N., & Zhang, W. (2020). The role of exosomal miR-375-3p: A potential suppressor in bladder cancer via the Wnt/β-catenin pathway. *FASEB Journal: Official Publication of the Federation of American Societies for Experimental Biology*, *34*(9), 12177–12196. Available from https://doi.org/10.1096/fj.202000347R.

Lin, f, yin, h B., li, x Y., zhu, g M., he, w Y., & gou, x (2020). Bladder cancer cell-secreted exosomal miR-21 activates the PI3K/AKT pathway in macrophages to promote cancer progression. *International Journal of Oncology*, *56*(1), 151–164. Available from https://doi.org/10.3892/ijo.2019.4933.

Mathieu, M., Martin-Jaular, L., Lavieu, G., & Théry, C. (2019). Specificities of secretion and uptake of exosomes and other extracellular vesicles for cell-to-cell communication. *Nature Cell Biology*, *21*(1), 9–17.

McAndrews, K. M., & Kalluri, R. (2019). Mechanisms associated with biogenesis of exosomes in cancer. *Molecular Cancer*, *18*(1), 1–11.

Pitt, J. M., Kroemer, G., & Zitvogel, L. (2016). Extracellular vesicles: Masters of intercellular communication and potential clinical interventions. *The Journal of Clinical Investigation, 126*(4), 1139–1143.

Soung, Y. H., Ford, S., Zhang, V., & Chung, J. (2017). Exosomes in cancer diagnostics. *Cancers, 9*(1), 8.

Sun, Z., Wang, L., Dong, L., & Wang, X. (2018). Emerging role of exosome signalling in maintaining cancer stem cell dynamic equilibrium. *Journal of Cellular and Molecular Medicine, 22*(8), 3719–3728.

Sung, H., Ferlay, J., Siegel, R. L., Laversanne, M., Soerjomataram, I., Jemal, A., & Bray, F. (2021). Global cancer statistics 2020: GLOBOCAN estimates of incidence and mortality worldwide for 36 cancers in 185 countries. *CA: A Cancer Journal for Clinicians, 71*(3), 209–249.

Théry, C., Witwer, K. W., Aikawa, E., Alcaraz, M. J., Anderson, J. D., Andriantsitohaina, R., & Jovanovic-Talisman, T. (2018). Minimal information for studies of extracellular vesicles 2018 (MISEV2018): A position statement of the International Society for Extracellular Vesicles and update of the MISEV2014 guidelines. *Journal of Extracellular Vesicles, 7*(1), 1535750.

Wang, Y., Zhang, Y., Cai, G., & Li, Q. (2020). Exosomes as actively targeted nanocarriers for cancer therapy. *International Journal of Nanomedicine, 15*, 4257.

Wen, J., Yang, T., Mallouk, N., Zhang, Y., Li, H., Lambert, C., & Li, G. (2021). Urinary exosomal CA9 mRNA as a novel liquid biopsy for molecular diagnosis of BC. *International Journal of Nanomedicine, 14*(16), 4805–4811.

Wu, J. H., Sun, K. N., Chen, Z. H., He, Y. J., & Sheng, L. (2022). Exosome-mediated miR-4792 transfer promotes bladder cancer cell proliferation via enhanced FOXC1/c-Myc signaling and warburg effect. *Journal of Oncology, 2022*, 5680353. Available from https://doi.org/10.1155/2022/5680353.

Yang, H., Qu, H., Huang, H., Mu, Z., Mao, M., Xie, Q., Wang, K., & Hu, B. (2021). Exosomes-mediated transfer of long noncoding RNA LINC01133 represses bladder cancer progression via regulating the Wnt signaling pathway. *Cell Biology International, 45*(7), 1510–1522. Available from https://doi.org/10.1002/cbin.11590.

Yáñez-Mó, M., Siljander, P. R. M., Andreu, Z., Bedina Zavec, A., Borràs, F. E., Buzas, E. I., & De Wever, O. (2015). Biological properties of extracellular vesicles and their physiological functions. *Journal of Extracellular Vesicles, 4*(1), 27066.

Zhang, H., Freitas, D., Kim, H. S., Fabijanic, K., Li, Z., Chen, H., & Lyden, D. (2018). Identification of distinct nanoparticles and subsets of extracellular vesicles by asymmetric flow field-flow fractionation. *Nature Cell Biology, 20*(3), 332–343.

Zheng, R., Du, M., Wang, X., Xu, W., Liang, J., Wang, W., Lv, Q., Qin, C., Chu, H., Wang, M., Yuan, L., Qian, J., & Zhang, Z. (2018). Exosome-transmitted long non-coding RNA PTENP1 suppresses bladder cancer progression. *Molecular Cancer, 17*(1), 143. Available from https://doi.org/10.1186/s12943-018-0880-3.

Zhou, X., Kurywchak, P., Wolf-Dennen, K., Che, S. P. Y., Sulakhe, D., D'Souza, M., Xie, B., Maltsev, N., Gilliam, T. C., Wu, C. C., McAndrews, K. M., LeBleu, V. S., McConkey, D. J., Volpert, O. V., Pretzsch, S. M., Czerniak, B. A., Dinney, C. P., & Kalluri, R. (2021). Unique somatic variants in DNA from urine exosomes of individuals with bladder cancer. *Molecular Therapy: Methods & Clinical Development., 22*, 360–376. Available from https://doi.org/10.1016/j.omtm.2021.05.010, PMID: 34514028; PMCID: PMC8408559.

Zöller, Margot (2016). *Exosomes in cancer disease. Cancer Gene Profiling* (pp. 111–149). New York, NY: Humana Press.

Chapter 17

Upper urinary tract urothelial cell carcinoma

Mohammed Mrabti[1,2], Abdelilah Laraqui[3], Alami Mohamed[1], Youssef Ennaji[5] and Moulay Mustapha Ennaji[4]

[1]Urology Department, Mohammed V Military Hospital, Rabat, Morocco, [2]Research and Biosafety Laboratory, Mohammed V Construction Teaching Hospital, Mohammed V University, Rabat, Morocco, [3]Laboratory of Human Pathologies Biology, Faculty of Sciences, and Genomic Center of Human Pathologies, Faculty of Medicine and Pharmacy, Bio-Path Laboratory, Faculty of sciences-Agdal, Mohammed V University, Rabat, Morocco, [4]Group Leader Research team of Virology, Oncology, and Biotechnologies, Head of Laboratory of Virology, Oncology, Biosciences, Environment and New Energies (LVO-BEEN), Faculty of Sciences and Techniques Mohammedia, University Hassan II of Casablanca, Casablanca, Morocco, [5]Team of Virology, Oncology, and Biotechnologies, Laboratory of Virology, Oncology, Biosciences, Environment and New Energies (LVO-BEEN), Faculty of Sciences and Techniques Mohammedia, University Hassan II of Casablanca, Casablanca, Morocco

17.1 Introduction

The urinary excretory tract is internally lined with a distinctive multilayered urothelium, which is often referred to as transitional epithelium, uroepithelium, or paramalpighian epithelium. The upper tract urothelial carcinomas (UTUC) are thus lesions that have developed in the pyelocal cavities and/or the ureter. They are rare tumors representing about 5%−10% of urothelial tumors with an incidence of 1−2 cases per 100,000 inhabitants each year in Western countries (Petros, 2020; Roupret et al., 2018). Although they share common features with bladder tumors, UTUC have a distinct genetic profile and prognosis (Amira et al., 2003; Rouprêt et al., 2004). They pose diagnostic (low-growth pathology), therapeutic (radical or conservative surgery, preservation of renal function), and prognostic problems.

Smoking is the main risk factor for UTUC (Ross et al., 1989), and the clinical picture is dominated by hematuria. In addition to the clinical picture, the diagnosis is made on the basis of medical imaging and pathological examination. The standard treatment of UTUC involves surgery with total nephroureterectomy and removal of a bladder flange as the main procedure.

Immunological Implications and Molecular Diagnostics of Genitourinary Cancer.
DOI: https://doi.org/10.1016/B978-0-323-85496-2.00012-9

17.2 Epidemiology

17.2.1 Frequency

UTUC represent only 5%–10% of UTUC (Raman et al., 2011; Henry & Sèbe, 2008; Vincent et al., 2006). They are five times rarer than kidney tumors and 18 times rarer than bladder tumors.

As stated earlier, their annual incidence is estimated to be 1–2 new cases/100,000 population in Western countries (Petros, 2020; Roupret et al., 2018; Boukoffa & Abdallah, 2012). An increase in incidence is currently observed but the cause is still unknown: increasing toxic factors in the environment, better radiological investigations with early diagnosis, or better therapeutic results of bladder tumors with improved survival (De la Taille et al., 2001).

UTUC are multifocal in 30% of cases, bilateral in 2%–8% of cases, and pyelocal locations are about twice as frequent as urethral locations. The latter are distal in two-third of cases. (Tawfiek & Bagley, 1997). A history of bladder cancer exists in 20%–30% of patients with UTUC. In 8%–13% of cases, there is a bladder tumor synchronous with UTUC (Tawfiek & Bagley, 1997).

17.2.2 Age

The average age of discovery of UTUC is 60–65 years. These tumors are exceptional in children and adolescents (Mazroui & Joual, 2002) with the maximum frequency between the fifth and the seventh decade (El Fhal & Ghadouane, 2010).

17.2.3 Sex

There is a clear male predominance for UTUC with a sex ratio between 3 and 4 (Benslama & El Fassi, 2009).

17.2.4 Risk factors—ethiopathogenesis

Many factors have been incriminated in the occurrence of UTUC. These factors are typically related to the subject's environmental exposure and/or genetic profile. Thus, some factors are specific to UTUC, while others are common to bladder cancers (Colin et al., 2010) The mechanisms of carcinogenesis affect the urothelium as a whole, which would explain its multifocal character.

17.2.4.1 Tobacco

Tobacco exposure appears to be by far the most important risk factor for the occurrence of UTUC (De la Taille et al., 2001). Urothelial carcinogenesis related to tobacco exposure is complex and is related to multiple inhaled toxic substances (aromatic amines including arylamine, benzopyrene, and dimethylbenzanthracene) (Colin et al., 2010).

Aromatic amines are metabolized by the body into N-hydroxyalanine, a truly active carcinogen. Certain genetic alterations described at the tumor level, some of which affect the p53 suppressor gene (transversions of GC to CG and GC to TA), could be specific to tobacco-induced tumors.

17.2.4.2 Occupational origin

Certain occupational exposures are well known to be important risk factors for the development of UTUC and bladder carcinoma.

17.2.4.2.1 Aromatic amines

The relationship between UTUC and the handling of substances containing aromatic amines has been established. The aromatic amines incriminated in this carcinogenesis are most certainly benzidine and β-naphthyllanine, whose absorption in the form of dust or vapor can be via the digestive, respiratory, or transcutaneous route (Mazeman, 1972a, 1972b; Shinka et al., 1995).

17.2.4.2.2 Chlorinated solvents

They are also implicated in urothelial carcinogenesis (Saint et al., 2003). These solvents (trichloroethylene, tetrachloroethylene, etc.) are used in the printing industry, in the manufacture of inks and glues, and in dry cleaning. In case of exposure, the risk of developing UTUC is 1.8 (Pesch et al., 2000).

17.2.4.3 Drug origin

17.2.4.3.1 Abuse of analgesics (phenacetin)

Phenacetin (acetophetidine) or N-(4-ethoxyphenyl) acetamide, an aromatic organic compound used alone or in combination with other analgesics, has been implicated as a high-risk factor for ESV cancer through nephrotoxicity (Holmang & Johansson, 2004).

17.2.4.3.2 Cyclophosphamide and ifosfamide

These are anticancer alkylating agents, which induce urothelial lesions (hyperplasia, dysplasia) through their metabolites (acrolein) and are known to be carcinogenic if taken regularly for at least two years. Although a few cases have been reported, there are no studies specifically looking at the risk of developing a urothelial tumor in the upper urinary tract (McDougal et al., 1981).

17.2.4.4 Heredity

Genetic origin has been incriminated by observations of familial forms of UTUC and chromosomal abnormalities (Lynch et al., 1990; Orphali et al., 1986; Vasen et al., 1999).

One of the reported familial forms of tumors is HNPCC (hereditary nonpolyposis colon cancer) or Lynch syndrome II. This syndrome associates the same family colon tumors with other cancers: hepatobiliary, endometrial, ovarian, small intestine, and upper excretory tract. The mechanism of carcinogenesis is genomic instability due to mutation of genes (MMR: mismatch repair) involved in DNA repair. There are two modes of presentation of HNPCC syndrome, the diagnosis of which is based on well-coded criteria (Amsterdam I and II) (Vasen et al., 1999).

17.2.4.5 Other factors

17.2.4.5.1 Lithiasis

The occurrence of UTUC in lithiasis is rare. A history of lithiasis has been found in 5%–8% of patients with UTUC. Nevertheless, the incidence of tumor remains low (around 1%) (Mazeman, 1972a, 1972b) The mechanism of carcinogenesis is thought to be multifactorial.

17.2.4.5.2 Urinary tract infections

The development of urothelial tumors is thought to be related to the weakening of the urothelium because of chronic urinary tract infection. Bilharzia has been described as a particular parasitic infection with proven carcinogenic potential. The carcinogenic mechanism is thought to be due to the chronic irritation and inflammation induced by *Schistosoma haematobium* eggs.

17.2.4.5.3 Aristolochic acid nephropathy (Balkan endemic nephropathy and Chinese herbal nephropathy)

Following the observation of cases of end-stage renal failure in Belgium between 1992 and 1993 in patients who had used Chinese herbal medicines, a pathogen common to Balkan nephropathies was identified. This is aristolochic acid, a component of some Chinese herbs (*Aristolochia fangchi*) and some Balkan plants (*Aristolochia clematitis*) that is responsible for tubulointerstitial nephropathies that can lead to end-stage renal failure and UTUC (Colin et al., 2010). The common genetic feature that has been described is a mutation in the p53 gene.

17.2.4.5.4 Blackfoot disease

A high incidence of UTUC has also been described in Taiwan (Tan et al., 2008; Yang et al., 2002). In this region, which is endemic for a peripheral vasculitis described as "blackfoot disease," UTUC accounts for 20%–26.6% of UTUC. It is thought to be attributable to chronic intoxication by arsenic in well water (Tan et al., 2008; Chiou et al., 2001).

17.2.4.6 History of bladder tumor: in 20%–30% of patients with upper tract urothelial carcinomas

17.2.4.6.1 Anatomopathology

1. Histological type

   By far, the most common tumors of the UTUC are primary epithelial tumors, which can be nonepithelial. Primary epithelial tumors correspond in 95% of cases to UTUC, also known as transitional cell carcinomas (Dekeyser et al., 2009) and are classified into two varieties: papillary epithelial tumors (90% of UTUC) (De la Taille et al., 2001) and nonpapillary epithelial tumors, which are rarer.

2. The pathological stage

Urothelial tumors can be defined according to their penetration into and beyond the urothelial wall; a distinction is made between superficial and

TABLE 17.1 TNM classification 2017 for upper tract urothelial cell carcinoma (Takahashi et al., 2010).

T-Primary tumor		
TX	Primary tumor cannot be assessed	
T0	No evidence of primary tumor	
	Ta	Noninvasive papillary carcinoma
	Tis	Carcinoma in situ
T1	Tumor invades subepithelial connective tissue	
T2	Tumor invades muscularis	
T3	Renal pelvis: Tumor invades beyond muscularis into peripelvic fat or renal parenchyma (ureter); Tumor invades beyond muscularis into periureteric fat	
T4	Tumor invades adjacent organs or through the kidney into perinepheric fat	
N-Regional lymph nodes		
NX	Regional lymph nodes cannot be assessed	
N0	No regional lymph node metastasis	
N1	Metastasis in a single lymph node 2 cm or less in the greatest dimension	
N2	Metastasis in a single lymph node more than 2 cm, or multiple lymph nodes	
M-Distant metastasis		
M0	No distant metastasis	
M1	Distant metastasis	

TNM, Tumor, node, metastasis (classification).
3. Histological grade

infiltrative tumors. The TNM 2017 tumor infiltration classification is shown in Table 17.1. This allows histopronostic and therapeutic groups to be defined.

Urothelial tumors are also classified according to their histological grade; the current reference of grading urothelial tumors is the WHO 2016 classification. This increases the proportion of high-grade carcinomas compared to the WHO 73 classification, based on the tumor architecture (persistence or not of superficial cells in tumor vegetations, disorganization of cell layers) and cell characteristics (abnormalities in shape, size of nuclei structures, and number of mitoses) and according to whether the tumor is well-, moderately, or poorly differentiated.

17.2.4.7 Clinical

17.2.4.7.1 Circumstances of discovery

1. Hematuria

Hematuria is the most common presenting symptom and is present in 70%–80% of cases (Tawfiek & Bagley, 1997; Hall et al., 1998; Inman et al., 2009; Rouprêt et al., 2004), sometimes evoked in over 80% (Mazeman, 1972a, 1972b; El Fhal & Ghadouane, 2010; Gawley et al., 1989; Djokic et al., 2001). The characteristics are variable: usually total, sometimes terminal (for tumors of the lower ureter or prolapsed into the ureteral orifice or because of associated bladder lesions).

- It is painless and often abundant, causing in some cases a state of hemorrhagic shock or even acute retention of urine by bladder clotting.
- Sometimes it can be minimal and only microscopic.
- It is usually permanent or intermittent with sometimes very long remissions (De la Taille et al., 2001).

2. Pain

The second major symptom is pain, which is present in 20%–30% of cases (De la Taille et al., 2001). It can be explained in three ways:

- Ureteral obstruction: this is the most common mechanism. The pain is usually moderate, reduced to a sensation of tension in the flank, radiating to the iliac fossa, constant or intermittent. It is the clinical consequence of hydronephrosis or ureterohydronephrosis secondary to tumor obstruction of the excretory tract. Nephritic colic is rarer and is linked to the sudden tension of the pyelocalicular cavities (clots, tumor fragments, ureteral spasm on the tumor, intussusception of the ureter on the tumor, lithiasis association);
- a locoregional extension of the tumor to the retroperitoneal cellulo-fatty atmosphere and to the neighboring organs: the resulting pain has a topography that depends on the tumor location. They are diffuse, constant, and severe, sometimes simulating a digestive, gynecological, or rheumatological disorder.

- metastatic spread, particularly in the bone (pelvis, lumbar spine): depending on the site, the pain is constant and often throbbing.

3. Urinary tract infection

   It may be asymptomatic or associated with micturition disorders; sometimes it is a febrile state.

4. Other modes of disclosure
   a. Follow-up after treatment of primary bladder cancer
   b. Unusual forms: pyonephrosis, paraneoplastic syndrome
   c. Incidental findings:

A workup for another pathology in 10%–15% of cases (Rouprêt & Cussenot, 2008), or on pathology specimens.

17.2.4.8 Paraclinical

17.2.4.8.1 Imaging

1. The uroscanner

   In addition, to a more complete assessment of the lesion thanks to reconstructions (multiplanar or even surface), it allows its locoregional and metastatic extension to be evaluated. Thus, more than 89% of upper urinary tract tumors can be detected and almost 100% were detected in the study by Tsili et al. (2007). Although the uroscanner has replaced intra veinous uretrpgraphy (IVU) in the assessment of UTUC, it has the disadvantage of being more radiating, hence the importance of using two phases (first phase without contrast medium and second with injection for the nephrographic and excretory times) with "low-dose" protocols.

   The tumor pattern is variable. In the vegetative forms, the lesion is an intracavitary mass in the renal pelvis, calyces, and ureters, of tissue density (40–50 HU), isodense to the renal parenchyma, sometimes heterogeneous and rarely calcified. After injection, enhancement at the early stage is discrete (60–70 HU) and the tumor always remains hypodense to the parenchyma. In the excretory phase, the appearance is that of an intraluminal lacuna with a parietal implantation base often enlarging the calyx or ureter. In infiltrating forms, the appearance is that of a nonspecific, irregular, more or less circumferential parietal thickening, rapidly stenosing the cavities. In the ureter, diagnosis is often difficult because of the difficulty in locating the tumor lesion (Delomez et al., 2002).

   Uro-CT remains insufficient for the detection of certain urothelial mucosal changes without an exophytic component. It does not allow precise determination of local invasion, which is crucial in the choice of treatment.

2. URO-MRI

It involves the examination of choice in cases where the uroscanner is contraindicated owing to renal insufficiency or allergy to iodinated contrast media. The performance of uro-MRI remains inferior to uro-CT in the detection of urothelial tumors owing to a lower spatial resolution and greater artifacts (Girish et al., 2004). Nevertheless, it provides a better approach to parietal extension and assessment of tumor vascularization. The semiology is comparable to that of IVUS on T2 sequences and to that of CT on T1-weighted sequences with gadolinium injection. Few studies have been published in the context of UTUC. Takahashi et al. (2008, 2010) found that uro-MRI has a sensitivity of 70%–80% and a specificity close to 100%, including for small lesions.

1. Retrograde and antegrade opacification

Uretero-pyelography (UPR) is performed during or after urethrocystoscopy. After urethral catheterization and injection of contrast product, the images taken in the operating theater with image intensifiers are not of sufficient quality to detect small lesions. However, it allows visualization of the tumor and washing for cytological study with a positive diagnosis in 93% of cases (Scolierie et al., 2000).

Also, antegrade pyelography, of exceptional indications in UTUC (risk of perirenal tumor dissemination) is performed during endoscopy after placement of a nephrostomy tube. It should be performed with caution (Delomez et al., 2002). However, these indications have been reduced with the development of CT scanning.

17.2.4.8.2 Endoscopy

1. Urethrocystoscopy

   As part of the assessment, urethrocystoscopy is systematically required. It is used to look for damage to the lower urinary tract (urethra, bladder) and to take biopsies for anatomopathological study.

2. Ureteroscopy

   Diagnostic ureteroscopy can nowadays be performed with flexible fiberscopes, allowing analysis of the entire excretory tract up to the pyelocal cavities, including the lower calyces (Dekeyser et al., 2009). This is a particularly innovative tool for completing the staging workup (Lam & Gupta, 2004). It allows the state of the wall where the tumor is implanted to be assessed, a visual macroscopic diagnosis to be made and a histological sample of the lesion to be taken (Shiraishi et al., 2003) which can be used to determine the grade of tumor. Caution should be exercised when taking deep samples owing to the risk of parietal perforation. The contribution of biopsy to tumor grade is nearly 90% with a false negative rate of around 5% (Boorjian & Munver, 2004, 2005). However, it does not contribute much to establishing the stage of tumor invasion owing to the inadequacy of the material taken (Thalmann et al., 2002). With the miniaturization of devices, complications (perforations, stenosis, stripping) are rare (0.5%–4.6%) and less frequent (Lam & Gupta, 2004).

3. Urine cytology

Used as an adjunct to diagnosis, it also allows for screening and following up. Requiring the skills of a trained anatomocytologist, the positiveness of cytology (presence of abnormal cells desquamated in the urine) does not make it possible to affirm the uniqueness of the lesion because of the lack of information on the precise origin of the abnormal cells. However, its reliability varies according to the sampling method and is related to the grade of the tumors studied with 35%–90%: the higher the grade, the better the cytodiagnosis (Scolierie et al., 2000).

4. Optional examinations

In the case of an infiltrating lesion, a thoracic CT scan completes the assessment of distant extension. The classic metastatic locations are lungs (52%), liver (33%), and bone (26%). In the event of clinical signs suggestive of metastatic lesions, a bone scan or brain scan may be performed.

PET scans (FDG or choline labeled) are not recommended as part of the workup for UTUC.

17.2.4.9 Preoperative prognostic factors

The therapeutic orientation of the patient preoperatively is essential in order not to undertreat a patient requiring radical treatment or inversely (Colin et al., 2014). It is proposed that low and high-risk UTUC be differentiated in order to consider conservative treatment in low-risk tumors (Roupret et al., 2014).

- Low-risk UTUC: low grade on biopsy, low cytological grade, potentially complete conservative treatment, noninfiltrative appearance on imaging, and unifocal disease.

The question of tumor size (≤1 cm, previously retained as the limit for conservative treatment) could be modulated for the pyelic location (96% of pyelic lesions of less than 3 cm are not infiltrating) and the potentially complete nature of endoscopic treatment. The size limit indeed evolves toward a definition of high risk from 2 cm (Seisen et al., 2016).

- High-risk UTUC: presence of hydronephrosis, high grade on biopsy, high cytological grade, potentially incomplete resection of conservative treatment, infiltrative appearance on imaging, and multifocal disease. Continued active smoking and a history of bladder injury are associated with recurrence and impaired specific survival.

Other pejorative prognostic factors are useful even if they have not been directly incorporated into preoperative stratification (Colin et al., 2014): ureteral location, sessile tumor architecture, elevated C-reactive protein, neutrophil/lymphocyte ratio > 3.0, operative time greater than three months, high body mass index, and very low score.

17.2.4.10 Treatment

17.2.4.10.1 Localized upper tract urothelial carcinomas

1. Low-risk upper tract urothelial carcinomas

   Conservative treatment: In the case of a single functional or anatomical kidney, comorbidity or comorbidities preventing radical treatment or when this may lead the patient to dialysis, conservative treatment of necessity may be performed for high-risk UTUC. Overall or specific mortality does not appear to be affected by conservative management in these indications of necessity (Pignot et al., 2014).

   - By endoscopic approach: This approach has the main advantage of preserving a closed system, thus reducing the risk of tumor cells spreading outside the urinary tract (Jabbour & Smith, 2006).

     Ureteroscopy: Retrograd intra renal surgery (RIRS) is preferred to rigid ureteroscopy (endoscopic control of the entire urinary tract intraoperatively). There are risks to be aware of, including underestimation of tumor grade and stage, local recurrence in the urinary tract (6%–71% of cases), and progression in case of local recurrence (15%–21%), which may require secondary total nephroureterectomy (11%–40%). For some authors, this risk can be reduced by performing a "second look" ureteroscopy (within 60 days postoperation) (Villa et al., 2015).

     Percutaneous approach: the development of the RIRS has reduced the use of this approach. It can be used in the case of an inferior calyx lesion that is inaccessible to treatment with the RIRS (Pignot et al., 2014; Roupret et al., 2015).

   - Segmental ureterectomy (US, ultrasound):

     Within the elective indications, the results of conservative treatment by segmental ureterectomy are excellent when surgical margins are negative (Pignot et al., 2014; Roupret et al., 2015).

     *US allows for monobloc removal of the tumor with accurate staging and histological grading. The passage of the UTUC is necessary to obtain healthy surgical margins. Orientation of the surgical specimen is necessary for pathological analysis. Direct contact between urine from the tumor ESV and the surgical field should be avoided. Node dissection can be performed at the same time as the US. As with conservative endoscopic treatment, the risk of homolateral recurrence (30%–60%) must be known. Distal US with reimplantation for lower ureter injury has a better recurrence-free survival rate than segmental resection of the iliac or lumbar ureter (Pignot et al., 2014; Roupret et al., 2015). Open partial surgery of the pyelocal cavities is difficult and has a high rate of local recurrence (Pignot et al., 2014; Roupret et al., 2015).

- Instillation of adjuvant topical agents:

* The feasibility of instilling adjuvant topical agents (Bacille de Calmette et Guerrin (BCG) or mitomycin C) has been reported for curative treatment of carcinoma in situ lesions (Dillman et al., 2008) and as adjuvant therapy after conservative treatment of low-risk papillary lesions (Audenet et al., 2014).

* Instillations in the urinary tract appear to decrease the frequency of local recurrence without improving survival only for carcinom in citu (CIS) lesions (2% of all ESVT).

High-risk upper tract urothelial carcinomas * Radical treatment by total nephroureterectomy:

* Open or laparoscopic NUT involves en bloc removal of the kidney, the entire upper urinary excretory tract, and an ipsilateral periorificial bladder flange (Michel & Smith, 2000)

The open route is currently being implemented in a double track:

- Lumbar for release of the kidney and lumbo-iliac ureter.
- Low (median subumbilical or transverse suprapubic) for removal of the pelvic ureter and the periorificial flange. The choice of route (extra or retroperitoneal and transperitoneal) as well as the timing of the approach differs from one operator to another. The extraperitoneal route is generally the most used. Its morbidity is not negligible, and for this reason many techniques have been developed, including the laparoscopic route. The oncological results of laparoscopy are equivalent with less morbidity (Roupret et al., 2015; Neuzillet et al., 2014).

Certain oncological precautions must be observed in case of laparoscopic dissection:

- No opening of the excretory pathway.
- No morcellation of the tumor.
- Use of an endoscopic bag for the extraction of the surgical part in a single block.
- Removal of the kidney, ureter, and bladder neck en bloc.
- Open surgery is preferred for locally advanced tumors (cT3/T4 and/or cN +).

  * Lymph node dissection:

  Node dissection in combination with NUT allows better stratification, guides therapeutic management (adjuvant chemotherapy), and may improve survival (Neuzillet et al., 2014). However, the anatomical limits remain to be defined and depend on the location of the tumor (Neuzillet et al., 2014).

  * Perioperative treatments:

  o Neoadjuvant/adjuvant treatments:

- UTUC are considered chemosensitive tumors.

Neoadjuvant chemotherapy is the concept with the strongest rationale in UTUC. Indeed, there is a significant risk of not being able to administer chemotherapy after NUT (Audenet et al., 2014), owing to decreased renal function. The available data have shown a favorable impact of chemotherapy both neoadjuvant and in the adjuvant setting.

- Adjuvant radiotherapy may improve local control of the disease, but it does not influence the occurrence of metastases or specific or overall survival. It is not recommended.
- Adjuvant intravesical instillations: The rate of bladder recurrence after NUT is around 40% (Audenet et al., 2014). Early postoperative instillation of intravesical chemotherapy reduces this risk (Roupret et al., 2015; O'Brien et al., 2011; Ito et al., 2013).

17.2.4.10.2 Metastatic disease

Local treatment, either surgery or radiotherapy, has no place in metastatic disease outside the symptomatic palliative setting. Platinum-based chemotherapy is the standard of care; most of the data in the literature are extrapolated from prospective trials of metastatic UTUC.

17.3 Surveillance

Posttreatment surveillance of UTUC is necessary to detect local or distant bladder recurrence (Roupret et al., 2015; Colin et al., 2015). After NUT, the risk of local recurrence is low, whereas the risk of distant recurrence (metastasis) depends directly on prognostic factors. This risk of recurrence changes over time and decreases during follow-up (Ploussard et al., 2015).

Monitoring is based on urine cytology, cystoscopy, and uro-TD at a defined rate.

- After conservative treatment:

In the case of conservative treatment, the homolateral excretory tract requires special monitoring because of the high risk of recurrence. An endoscopic "second look" at six weeks after laser treatment is recommended by some experts.

References

Amira, N., Rivet, J., Soliman, H., Cancel-Tassin, G., Duc, A., Janin, A., et al. (2003). Microsatellite instability in urothelial carcinoma of the upper urinary tract. *Journal of Urology*, *170*, 1151–1154.

Audenet, F., Roupret, M., Houede, N., & Colin, P. (2014). Non-surgical treatment modalities available for the treatment of upper tract urothelial carcinomas: State-of-the-art review for the yearly scientific report of the French National Association of Urology. *Progres en Urologie: Journal de l'Association Francaise d'urologie et de la Societe Francaise d'urologie*, *24*(15), 1030–1040.

Benslama, I, & El Fassi, M J. (2009). *Les tumeurs des voies excrétrices supérieures urinaires (à propos de 4cas)* (thèse Doctorat de Médecine), Fès, n 16.

Boorjian, S., Munver, N. G. C. R., et al. (2004). Abnormal selective cytology results predict recurrence of upper-tract transitional-cell carcinoma treated with ureteroscopic laser ablation. *Journal of Endourology / Endourological Society*, *18*, 912–916.

Boorjian, S., Munver, N. G. C. R., et al. (2005). Impact of delay to nephroureterectomy for patients undergoing ureteroscopic biopsy and laser tumor ablation of upper tract transitional cell carcinoma. *Urology*, *66*, 283–287.

Boukoffa, S, & Abdallah, A. The ureters. Available at: <http://www.facmed-annaba.com/medecine/anatomie/20082009/ureteres.pdf> (Accessed 25.6.2012).

Chiou, H. Y., Chiou, S. T., Hsu, Y. H., et al. (2001). Incidence of transitional cell carcinoma and arsenic in drinking water: A follow-up study of 8,102 residents in an arseniasis-endemic area in northeastern Taiwan. *American Journal of Epidemiology*, *153*(5), 411–418.

Colin, P., Irani, J., Drouin, S. J., Shariat, S. F., & Roupret, M. (2014). Prognostic factors of upper tract urothelial carcinomas and impact on survival: A systematic review for the yearly scientific report of the French National Association of Urology. *Progres en Urologie: Journal de l'Association Francaise d'urologie et de la Societe Francaise d'urologie*, *24*(15), 1000–1010.

Colin, P., Neuzillet, Y., Pignot, G., Roupret, M., Comperat, E., Larre, S., et al. (2015). Follow-up of urothelial carcinoma: Review of the Cancer Committee of the French Association of Urology. *Progres en Urologie: Journal de l'Association Francaise d'urologie et de la Societe Francaise d'urologie*, *25*(10), 616–624.

Colin, P., Koenig, P., Ballereau, C., Phé, V., Berthon, N., et al. (2010). Sporadic upper urinary tract tumours: Identification of the interaction between exposure to environmental carcinogens and the genetic susceptibility. *Progres en Urologie: Journal de l'Association Francaise d'urologie et de la Societe Francaise d'urologie*, *20*, 1–10.

De la Taille, A., Meria, P., & et Mazeman, E. (2001). *Tumeurs de la voie excrétrice supérieure*. Paris: EMC (Editions Scientifiques et Médicales Elsevier SAS), Néphrologie-Urologie,18-098-A-10, 18p.

Dekeyser, E., Eiss, D., Debrito, P., et al. (2009). *Imaging of tumours of the excretory tract*. Paris: EMC(Elsevier Masson SAS), Radiodiagnostic-Urology-Gynecology, 34-117-A-50.

Delomez, J., Claudon, M., Darmaillacq, C., et al. (2002). Imaging of upper urinary tract tumors. *European Journal of Radiology*, *83*, 825–841.

Dillman, J. R., Caoili, E. M., Cohan, R. H., Ellis, J. H., Francis, I. R., & Schipper, M. J. (2008). Detection of upper tract urothelial neoplasms: Sensitivity of axial, coronal reformatted, and curved-planar reformatted image-types utilizing 16-row multi-detector CT urography. *Abdominal Imaging*, *33*(6), 707–716.

Djokic, M., Hadzi-Djokic, J., Dragicevic, D., et al. (2001). Tumors of the upper excretory tract: Results of conservative surgery. *Progress in Urology*, *11*, 1231–1238.

El Fhal, A, & Ghadouane, M. (2010). *Tumeurs de la voie excrétrice supérieure(à propos de 8cas)* (thèse de Doctorat de Médecine), Rabat, n 171.

Gawley, W. F., Mehir, M., Harney, J., et al. (1989). Transitional cell carcinoma of upper urinary tract. *Urology*, *33*(6), 459–461.

Girish, G., Chooi, W. K., Morcos, S. K., et al. (2004). Filling defect artefacts in magnetic resonance urography. *European Radiology*, *14*, 145–150.

Hall, M. C., Womack, S., Sagalowsky, A. I., Carmody, T., Erickstad, M. D., et al. (1998). Prognostic factors, recurrence, and survival in transitional cell carcinoma of the upper urinary tract: A 30 year experience in 252 patients. *Urology*, *52*, 594–601.

Henry, N., & Sèbe, P. (2008). *Anatomy of the kidneys and the upper excretory tract*. Paris: EMC (ElsevierMassonSAS), Nephrology, 18-001-C-10.

Holmang, S., & Johansson, S. L. (2004). Synchronous bilateral ureteral and renal pelvic carcinomas: Incidence, etiology, treatment and outcome. *Cancer*, *101*(4), 741–747.

Inman, B. A., Tran, V.-T., Lacombe, L., et al. (2009). Carcinoma of the upper urinary tract. *American Cancer Society*, *115*, 2853–2862.

Ito, A., Shintaku, I., Satoh, M., Ioritani, N., Aizawa, M., Tochigi, T., et al. (2013). Prospective randomized phase II trial of a single early intravesical instillation of pirarubicin (THP) in the prevention of bladder recurrence after nephroureterectomy for upper urinary tract urothelial carcinoma: The THP Monotherapy Study Group Trial. *Journal of Clinical Oncology: Official Journal of the American Society of Clinical Oncology*, *31*(11), 1422–1427.

Jabbour, M.-E., & Smith, A. D. (2006). Conservative treatment of upper excretory tract tumours. Elsevier Masson SAS, surgical techniques. *Urology*, 41–152.

Lam, J. S., & Gupta, M. (2004). Ureteroscopic management of upper tract transitional cell carcinoma. *The Urologic Clinics of North America*, *31*, 115–128.

Lynch, H. T., Ens, J. A., & Lynch, I. F. (1990). The Lynch's syndrome II and urological malignancies. *The Journal of Urology*, *143*, 24–28.

Mazeman, E. (1972a). Les tumeurs de la voie excrétrice supérieure. *Rapport du congrès de l'AFU. J UROL*, *78*, 1–220.

Mazeman, E. (1972b). Tumeurs des voies excrétrices supérieures, calices, bassinet. *Uretère J Urol Nephrol(Paris)*, *78*(Suppl.9), 1–219.

Mazroui, A, & Joual, A. (2002). *Les tumeurs des voies urinaires excrétrices supérieures(à propos de 16cas)* (thèse Doctorat de Médecine), Casablanca, n°113.

McDougal, W. S., Cramer, S. F., & Miller, R. (1981). Invasive carcinoma of the renal pelvis following cyclophosphamide therapy for nonmalignant disease. *Cancer*, *48*(3), 691–695.

Michel, E., & Smith, A. D. (2000). Primary percutaneous approach to upper urinary tract transitional cell carcinoma. *Urologic clinics of North America*, *27*, 4.

Neuzillet, Y., Colin, P., Phe, V., Shariat, S. F., & Roupret, M. (2014). Surgical treatment of upper tract urothelial carcinomas by nephroureterectomy: State of the art review for the yearly scientific report of the French National Association of Urology. *Progres en Urologie: Journal de l'Association Francaise d'urologie et de la Societe Francaise d'urologie*, *24*(15), 1021–1029.

O'Brien, T., Ray, E., Singh, R., Coker, D., & Beard, R. (2011). British Association of urological surgeons section of O. Prevention of bladder tumours after nephroureterectomy for primary upper urinary tract urothelial carcinoma: A prospective, multicentre, randomised clinical trial of a single postoperative intravesical dose of mitomycin C (the ODMIT-C Trial). *European Urology*, *60*(4), 703–710.

Orphali, S. L., Shols, G. W., Hagewood, J., et al. (1986). Familial transitional-cell carcinoma of renal pelvis and upper ureter. *Urology*, *27*, 394–396.

Pesch, B., Haerting, J., Ranft, U., Klimpel, A., Oelschlägel, B., et al. (2000). Occupational risk factor for urothelial carcinoma: Agent-specific results from a case-control study in Germany. *International Journal of Epidemiology*, *29*(2), 238–247.

Petros, F. G. (2020). Epidemiology, clinical presentation, and evaluation of upper-tract urothelial carcinoma. *Translational Andrology and Urology*, *9*(4), 1794.

Pignot, G., Colin, P., Roupret, M., & Traxer, O. (2014). Conservative management of urothelial carcinomas of the upper tract: Systematic review for the yearly scientific report of the French National Association of Urology. *Progres en Urologie: Journal de l'Association Francaise d'urologie et de la Societe Francaise d'urologie*, *24*(15), 1011–1020.

Ploussard, G., Xylinas, E., Lotan, Y., Novara, G., Margulis, V., Roupret, M., et al. (2015). Conditional survival after radical nephroureterectomy for upper tract carcinoma. *European Urology*, *67*(4), 803–812. Available from https://doi.org/10.1016/j.eururo.2014.08.003.

Raman, J. D., Messer, J., Sielatycki, J. A., et al. (2011). Incidence and survival of patients with carcinoma of the ureter and renal pelvis in the USA, 1973–2005. *BJU International*, *107*, 1059–1064. Available from https://doi.org/10.1111/j.1464-410X.2010.09675.x.

Ross, R. K., Pagani-Hill, A., Landolph, J., Gerkins, V., & Henderson, B. E. (1989). Analgesic, cigarette smoking and other risk factors for cancer of the renal pelvis and ureter. *Cancer Research*, *49*, 104s–1048s.

Roupret, M., Babjuk, M., Comperat, E., et al. (2018). European association of urology guidelines on upper urinary tract urothelial carcinoma: 2017 Update. *European Urology*, *73*, 111–122. Available from https://doi.org/10.1016/j.eururo.2017.07.036.

Roupret, M., Babjuk, M., Comperat, E., Zigeuner, R., Sylvester, R. J., Burger, M., et al. (2015). European Association of Urology guidelines on upper urinary tract urothelial cell carcinoma: 2015 update. *European Urology*, *68*(5), 868–879.

Roupret, M., Colin, P., & Yates, D. R. (2014). A new proposal to risk stratify urothelial carcinomas of the upper urinary tract (UTUCs) in a predefinitive treatment setting: Low-risk vs high-risk UTUCs. *European Urology*, *66*(2), 181–183.

Rouprêt, M., & Cussenot, O. (2008). *Les tumeurs de la voie excrétrice supérieure*. Paris: Edition John Libbey Eurotext.

Rouprêt, M., Catto, J., Coulet, F., Azzouzi, A. R., Amira, N., Karmouni, T., et al. (2004). Microsatellite instability as indicator of MSH2 gene mutation in patients with upper urinary tract transitional cell carcinoma. *Journal of Medical Genetics*, 41–91.

Saint, F., Petit, J., & Doutrelot-Philipon, C. (2003). Occupational bladder tumours: Practical modalities for their recognition as an occupational disease. *Progres en Urologie: Journal de l'Association Francaise d'urologie et de la Societe Francaise d'urologie*, *13*(5Suppl.2), 1215–1224.

Scolieri, M. J., Paik, M. L., Brown, S. L., et al. (2000). Limitations of computed tomography in the preoperative staging of upper tract urothelial carcinoma. *Urology*, *56*, 930–934.

Seisen, T., Peyronnet, B., Dominguez-Escrig, J. L., Bruins, H. M., Yuan, C. Y., Babjuk, M., et al. (2016). Oncologic outcomes of kidney-sparing surgery vs radical nephroureterectomy for upper tract urothelial carcinoma: A systematic review by the EAU Non-muscle Invasive Bladder Cancer Guidelines Panel. *European Urology*, *70*(6), 1052–1068.

Shinka, T., Miyai, M., Sawada, Y., Inagaki, T., & Okawa, T. (1995). Factors affecting the occurrence of urothelial tumors in dye workers exposed to aromatic amines. *International Journal of Urology: Official Journal of the Japanese Urological Association*, *4*, 243–248.

Shiraishi, K., Eguchi, S., Mohri, J., & Kamiryo, Y. (2003). Role of ureteroscopic biopsy in the management of upper urinary tract malignancy. *International Journal of Urology*, *10*, 627–630.

Takahashi, N., Glockner, J. F., Hartman, R. P., et al. (2010). Gadolinium enhanced magnetic resonance urography for upper urinary tract malignancy. *The Journal of Urology*, *183*(4), 1330–1365.

Takahashi, N., Kawashima, A., Glockner, J. F., et al. (2008). Small (<2-cm) upper-tract urothelial carcinoma: Evaluation with gadolinium-enhanced three-dimensional spoiled gradient-recalled echo MR urography. *Radiology*, *247*(2), 451–457.

Tan, L. B., Chen, K. T., & Guo, H. R. (2008). Clinical and epidemiological features of patients with genitourinary tract tumour in a blackfoot disease endemic area of Taiwan. *BJU International*, *102*(1), 48–54.

Tawfiek, E. R., & Bagley, D. H. (1997). Upper tract transitional cell carcinoma. *Urology*, *50*, 321–329.

Thalmann, G. N., Markwalder, R., Walter, B., & Studer, U. E. (2002). Long-term experience with bacillus Calmette-Guerin therapy of upper urinary tract transitional cell carcinoma in patients not eligible for surgery. *The Journal of Urology*, *168*, 1381–1385.

Tsili, A. C., Efremidis, S. C., Kalef-Ezra, J., et al. (2007). Multi-detector row CT urography on 16-row CT scanner in the evaluation of urothelial tumors. *European Radiology*, *17*, 1046–1054.

Vasen, H. F., Watson, P., Mecklin, J. P., et al. (1999). New clinical criteria for hereditary nonpolyposis colorectal cancer(HNPCC, Lynch syndrome)proposed by the International Collaborative group on HNPCC. *Gastroenterology*, *116*, 1453–1456.

Villa, L., Cloutier, J., Letendre, J., Ploumidis, A., Salonia, A., Cornu, J. N., et al. (2015). Early repeated ureteroscopy within 6–8 weeks after a primary endoscopic treatment in patients with upper tract urothelial cell carcinoma: Preliminary findings. *World Journal of Urology*, *34*(9), 1201–1206. Available from https://doi.org/10.1007/s00345-015-1753-7.

Vincent, D., Brémond-Gignac, D., Douard, R., Dupont, S., Latrémouille, C., Sèbe, P., et al. (2006). *Dictionary of anatomy* (1st ed.). Paris: Elsevier-Masson.

Yang, M. H., Chen, K. K., Yen, C. C., et al. (2002). Unusually high incidence of upper urinary tract urothelial carcinoma in Taiwan. *Urology*, *59*(5), 681–687.

Chapter 18

Testicular cancer

Mohammed Mrabti[1,2], Youssef Ennaji[5], Abdelilah Laraqui[3], Alami Mohamed[1] and Moulay Mustapha Ennaji[4]

[1]Urology Department, Mohammed V Military Hospital, Rabat, Morocco, [2]Research and Biosafety Laboratory, Mohammed V Construction Teaching Hospital, Mohammed V University, Rabat, Morocco, [3]Laboratory of Human Pathologies Biology, Faculty of Sciences, and Genomic Center of Human Pathologies, Faculty of Medicine and Pharmacy, Bio-Path Laboratory, Faculty of sciences-Agdal, Mohammed V University, Rabat, Morocco, [4]Group Leader Research team of Virology, Oncology, and Biotechnologies, Head of Laboratory of Virology, Oncology, Biosciences, Environment and New Energies (LVO-BEEN), Faculty of Sciences and Techniques Mohammedia, University Hassan II of Casablanca, Casablanca, Morocco, [5]Team of Virology, Oncology, and Biotechnologies, Laboratory of Virology, Oncology, Biosciences, Environment and New Energies (LVO-BEEN), Faculty of Sciences and Techniques Mohammedia, University Hassan II of Casablanca, Casablanca, Morocco

18.1 Introduction

Testicular germ cell tumors (TGCTs) are generally rare but represent the most common solid tumors among young men. The incidence of TGCT differs among ethnic groups. Its rate is the highest in North European countries, such as Norway and Denmark, and the lowest in African and Asian countries (Ghazarian et al., 2015; Murez, 2020; Williamson et al., 2017).

In 2016 the WHO classification of TGCTs led to a division into two major groups: (1) prepubertal-type tumors, which are not derived from germ cell neoplasia in situ (GCNIS) and (2) postpubertal-type tumors, which are GCNIS derived and occur in young men (seminomatous and nonseminomatous germ cell tumors [NSGCT] – embryonal carcinoma, yolk sac tumor, teratoma, and choriocarcinoma essentially). The term "germ cell neoplasia in situ" is consensually accepted as a new terminology for the precursor lesion. In this new classification, the term "spermatocytic seminoma" is replaced by "spermatocytic tumor," reclassified among nonGCNIS-derived tumors (Williamson et al., 2017).

TGCT diagnosis is based on physical examination, biological tests, and radiological assessment. Total inguinal orchiectomy is the first-line treatment allowing characterization of the histological type, local staging, and identification of risk factors for micrometastases.

Immunological Implications and Molecular Diagnostics of Genitourinary Cancer.
DOI: https://doi.org/10.1016/B978-0-323-85496-2.00030-0

Treatment paradigms continue to be refined for TGCTs as research in these areas continues (Ghazarian et al., 2015; Murez, 2020; Stephenson et al., 2019; Williamson et al., 2017).

18.2 Clinical presentation

Most often the diagnosis is made after local symptoms such as palpation of a hard and asymptomatic scrotal mass, sometimes during a painful episode. There is no affinity with a particular side. Bilateral synchronous involvement is extremely rare, and the tumor is localized in 60%–70% of cases.

In less than 5% of cases, the diagnosis will be evoked prior to regional or general symptoms, respiratory distress, gynecomastia, and Virchow's ganglion (Ghazarian et al., 2015; Murez, 2020; Williamson et al., 2017).

18.3 Investigations

18.3.1 Serum tumor markers

The determination of three serum markers is systematically recommended before and after orchiectomy, for their diagnostic and prognostic values: Alpha-fetoprotein (AFP) is mainly produced by endodermal sinus tumors and embryonic carcinoma. Total human chorionic gonadotropin (hCGt) is routinely secreted by choriocarcinoma but can be found in some embryonic carcinomas and in 10%–20% of seminomas. Lactate dehydrogenases (LDH) are nonspecific and correlate with cell turnover and tumor volume (Mai et al., 2009; Stephenson et al., 2019).

HCG: comes from syncytiotrophoblasts, elevated in:

- all choriocarcinomas
- 50% of embryonal carcinomas
- 5%–10% of pure seminomas

Levels in male: <1 ng/mL (10 mIU/mL)
Half-life: 24 h (of beta subunit – 1 h)
AFP: yolk sac, its presence rules out:

- Pure seminoma
- Pure choriocarcinoma
- Half-life: 5–7 days

LDH: marker of bulk of disease and is used to monitor:

- Advanced seminoma
- Marker-negative NSGCT

18.3.2 Imagery

18.3.2.1 Scrotal doppler

Ultrasound is systematically recommended, which makes it possible to distinguish between intra- and extra-testicular lesions and consider certain benign lesions, with a sensitivity > 95% when associated with clinical examination.

Scrotal MRI can be useful in case of an inconclusive ultrasound, to help determine malignancy with sensitivity, specificity, and accuracy of 100%, 87.5%, and 92.8%, respectively (Loehrer et al., 2008; Mai et al., 2009; Stephenson et al., 2019).

18.4 Abdomino-pelvic and thoracic imaging

Abdomino-pelvic CT is routinely recommended for evaluation of the retroperitoneal lymph node stage.

Abdominal MRI can be performed for lymph node evaluation if there is a contraindication to CT scan with injection or if the patient refuses to be irradiated, and it provides results equivalent to a CT scan. The sensitivity is 70%–80% for a threshold target set at 8–10 mm.

Brain imaging (CT scan or MRI) is recommended in case of neurological symptoms and in subjects at risk: choriocarcinoma, IGCCCG poor prognosis (10% of the brain lesions), extensive pulmonary metastases and primary nonseminomatous anterior mediastinal mass.

18FDG positron emission tomography (PET) is not recommended in the initial staging of germinal cell tumors (GCTs).

Other imaging tests (bone scintigraphy, liver ultrasound, etc.) can be envisaged according to the clinical context (Loehrer et al., 2008; Mai et al., 2009; Nayan et al., 2016; Stephenson et al., 2019).

- Classification: histological (Hiester & Albers, 2021; Loehrer et al., 2008; Mai et al., 2009; Murez, 2020; Nayan et al., 2016).

Germinal cell tumors:

- Seminoma: 35%–40% of total testicular tumors
- NSGCTs: group
  - Yolk sac tumor
  - Teratoma:

(Ecto/endo/meso dermal and ± malignant transformation)

- mature
- immature
- malignant nongerm cell
- embryonal carcinoma
- choriocarcinoma
- mixed germ cell tumor

Nongerminal tumors

- Specialized gonadal stromal tumors:
  - Ledig cell tumors

- Sertoli cell tumors
- Gonadoblastoma
- Carcinoids
- Adrenal rests

Mesenchymal tumors

Staging (Ghazarian et al., 2015; Hiester & Albers, 2021; Mai et al., 2009; Murez, 2020; Nayan et al., 2016) (Tables 18.1 and 18.2)

Treatment (Culine et al., 2008; Garcia-del-Muro et al., 2008; Hiester & Albers, 2021; Loehrer et al., 2008; Lorch, 2018; Murez, 2020; Oldenburg et al., 2013; Stephenson et al., 2019)

TABLE 18.1 AJCC: TNMS staging.

AJCC Staging	
Primary tumor (T)	
pTX	Primary tumor cannot be assessed (if no radical orchiectomy has been performed, TX is used)
pTO	No evidence of primary tumor (e.g., histologic scar in testis)
pTis	Intratubular germ cell neoplasia (carcinoma in situ)
pT1	Tumor limited to the testis and epididymis and no vascular/lymphatic invasion
pT2	Tumor limited to the testis and epididymis with vascular/lymphatic invasion or tumor extending through the tunica albuginea with involvement of tunica vaginalis
pT3	Tumor invades the spermatic cord with or without vascular/lymphatic invasion
pT4	Tumor invades the scrotum with or without vascular/lymphatic invasion
Regional lymph nodes (N)	
Clinical	
NX	Regional lymph nodes cannot be assessed
NO	No regional lymph node metastasis
N1	Lymph node mass 2 cm or less in greatest dimension or multiple lymph node masses, none more than 2 cm in greatest dimension
N2	Lymph node mass, more than 2 cm but not more than 5 cm in greatest dimension, or multiple lymph node masses, any one mass greater than 2 cm but not more than 5 cm in greatest dimension
N3	Lymph node mass more than 5 cm in greatest dimension

TABLE 18.2 TNM + Risk groups according to TM levels (Sx, S0, S1, S2, S3).

Distant metastases (M)			
MO	No evidence of distant metastases		
MI	Nonregional nodal or pulmonary metastases		
M2	Nonpulmonary visceral masses		
Serum tumor markers (S)			
	LDH	hCG (mlU/mL)	AFP (ng/mL)
SO	≤N	≤ N	≤ N
S1	<1.5 × N	< 5000	< 1000
S2	1.5–10 × N	5000–50,000	1000–10,000
S3	>10 × N	> 50,000	>10,000

The care is based on a multimodal approach, which includes:

- Surgery
- Chemotherapy
- Radiotherapy

18.5 Surgical management

High inguinal orchiectomy (radical orchiectomy) is performed to:

- avoid local tissue violation
- get the most proximal lymphatics

Radical orchiectomy reduces the tumor burden and represents a curative treatment by: carcinoma in situ (CIS), spermatocytic seminoma, typical seminoma – if low risk and at stage 1 (smaller tumor, no vascular, and rete testis invasion) with close surveillance.

18.6 Retroperitoneal lymphadenectomy for staging

Seminoma: early stages can respond to RT – highly radiosensitive tumor, late stage – chemotherapy

NSGCT: surgery (RPLND, retroperitoneal lymph node dissection) in early stage; in late stage, chemotherapy is mainstay of Tt – monitor by imaging and tumor markers (TM).

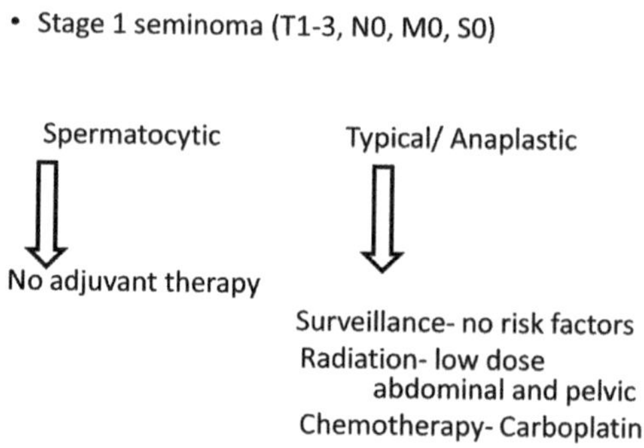

FIGURE 18.1 Treatment of testicular germ cell tumor at stage I.

Postchemotherapy residual LNs:
NSGCT – RPLND,
Seminoma, if <3 cm and no hot spot on PET – can be observed
Treatment of testicular GCT at stage I (Fig. 18.1)
Stage 2a and 2b (T1–3 N1–2, M0)

- Radiation – abdominal and pelvic

(ipsilateral external iliac, bilateral common iliac, the paracaval, para-aortic nodes including the cisterna chyli) – dog leg RT field

- 150 cGy/day, 5 days per week.

Seminoma: Stage IIc and III (N3 / M1–2)
Cisplatin-based chemotherapy:

- A major breakthrough in treatment of testicular tumor
- Three or four cycles depending on response
  - BEP = cisplatin, etoposide, bleomycin
  - VIP = etoposide,cisplatin, ifosfamide
  - VeIP = vinblastine, ifosfamide, and cisplatin

Residual retroperitoneal mass after chemotherapy in seminoma is shown in Fig. 18.2.

The description of anatomical boundaries of right and left template PC-RPLND is shown in Fig. 18.3.

NSGCT – Stage 1 (T1–3, N0, M0, S0–1)
Modified RPLND – node <2 cm – observation
N >2 cm: adjuvant CT – BEPx three cycles.
or
Primary chemotherapy – BEP three cycles
Persistent tumor markers – BEP three cycles
NSGCT – Stage IIa, IIb (T1–3, N1–2, M0, S0–1)

- Diffuse desmoplastic plaque < 3 cm and no hot spot on PET scan : observation
- Discrete mass > 3 cm: surgical resection

Histology

necrosis/ fibrosis → No further Tt

germ cell tumor → CT- VIP : 2-3 cycles

FIGURE 18.2 Residual retroperitoneal mass after chemotherapy in seminoma.

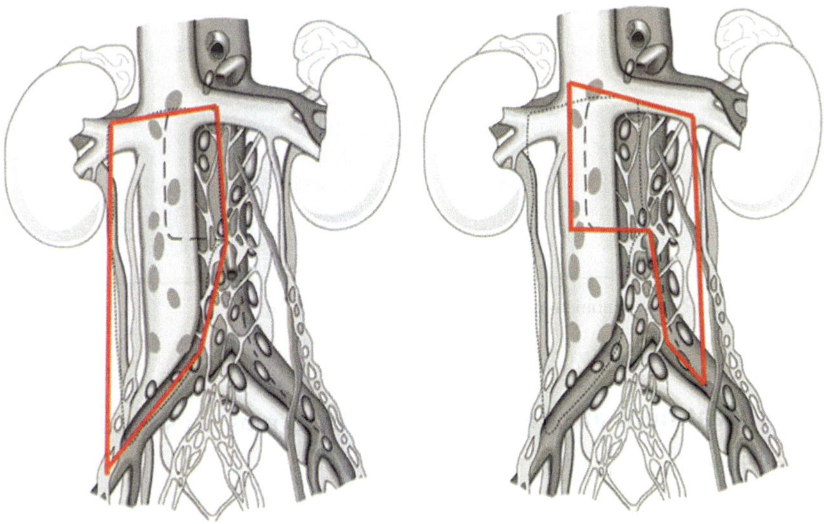

FIGURE 18.3 Graphical description of anatomical boundaries of right and left template PC-RPLND. Template resection of the right side includes the precaval, caval, paracaval, retrocaval, and interaortocaval regions, as well as the region lateral to the common iliac vessels. Template resection of the left side includes pre-, retro-, and para-aortic lymph nodes. The ipsilateral ureter represents the caudal and lateral boundary of resection. In patients without retrocrural or suprahilar lymph nodes, the renal vein is described as the cranial and the crus of the diaphragma as the posterior resection boundary.

- Bilateral nerve sparing RPLND

  Or

- Primary CT – BEP three cycles

  NSGCT- Stage IIc, III (N3/M1–2) (Fig. 18.4)

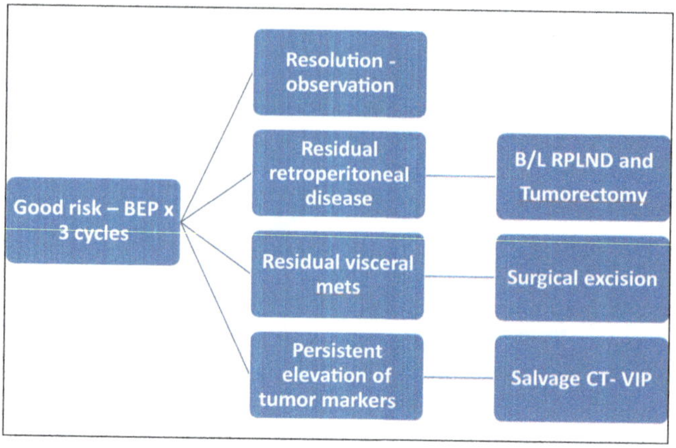

FIGURE 18.4 Nonseminomatous germ cell tumor- Stage IIc, III.

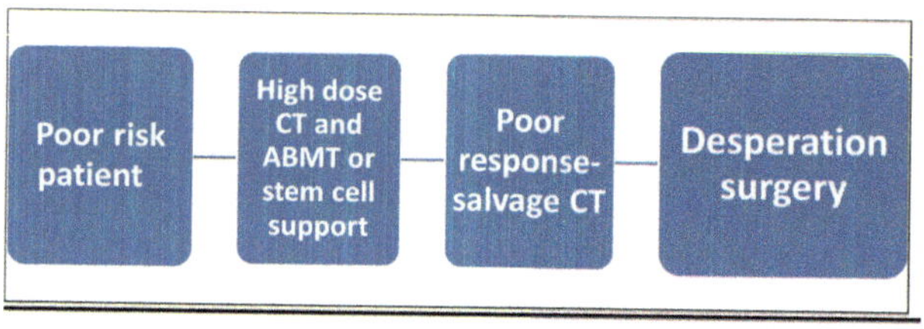

FIGURE 18.5 Nonseminomatous germ cell tumor- Stage IIc, III.

18.7 Treatment after RPLND or residual mass resection

After primary modified RPLND for N0 disease:

- Node < 2 cm → observation
- Node > 2 cm → adjuvant CT (BEP × 3)

After primary B/L nerve sparing RPLND for N1–2

- No further Tt, FU with TM and computed tomography (CT)

Post-chemo residual mass resection:
If residual masse (RM) shows only fibrosis/necrosis → no further Tt
IF RM shows viable tumor cells → further CT required:
If RMS was after first line CT: BEP × 2
If RMS was after second line CT: VEIP × 2 → Increased survival
NSGCT – Stage IIc, III (N3 / M1–2) (Fig. 18.5)
CT refractory testicular tumor

If TM still high after three (low and intermediate risk disease) to four (high-risk disease) cycles → go to second line CT: VIP × four cycles

References

Culine, S., Kramar, A., Theodore, C., et al. (2008). Randomized trial comparing bleomycin/etoposide/cisplatin with alternating cisplatin/cyclophosphamide/doxorubicin and vinblastine/bleomycin regimens of chemotherapy for patients with intermediate- and poor-risk metastatic nonseminomatous germ cell tumors: Genito-Urinary Group of the French Federation of Cancer Centers Trial T93MP. *Journal of Clinical Oncology: Official Journal of the American Society of Clinical Oncology*, *26*, 421–427.

Garcia-del-Muro, X., Maroto, P., Guma, J., et al. (2008). Chemotherapy as an alternative to radiotherapy in the treatment of stage IIA and IIB testicular seminoma: A Spanish Germ Cell Cancer Group Study. *Journal of Clinical Oncology: Official Journal of the American Society of Clinical Oncology*, *26*, 5416–5421.

Ghazarian, A. A., Trabert, B., Devesa, S. S., & McGlynn, K. A. (2015). Recent trends in the incidence of testicular germ cell tumors in the United States. *Andrology*, *3*, 13e8.

Hiester, A., & Albers, P. (2021). Surgical treatment of metastatic germ cell cancer. *Asian Journal of Urology*. Available from https://doi.org/10.1016/j.ajur.2020.05.007.

Loehrer, P. J., Ahlering, T., Buyyounouski, M. K., et al. (2008). Testicular cancer. In R. Pazdur (Ed.), *Cancer Management: A Multidisciplinary Approach* (11th ed., pp. 425–446). Manhasset, NY: CMP Media;.

Lorch, A. (2018). Management of refractory germ cell cancer. *American Society of Clinical Oncology Educational Book*, *38*, 324e9.

Mai, P. L., Friedlander, M., Tucker, K., et al. (2009). The international testicular cancer linkage consortium: A clinicopathologic descriptive analysis of 461 familial malignant testicular germ cell tumor kindred. *Urologic Oncology*, [Epub ahead of print].

Murez, T. (2020). French ccAFU guidelines – update 2020–2022: Testicular germ cell tumors. *Progres en Urologie: Journal de l'Association Francaise d'urologie et de la Societe Francaise d'urologie*, 12S, 30, S280.

Nayan, M., Jewett, M. A., Anson-Cartwright, L., Bedard, P. L., Moore, M., Chung, P., et al. (2016). The association between institution at orchiectomy and outcomes on active surveillance for clinical stage I germ cell tumours. *Canadian Urological Association Journal*, *10*, 204e9.

Oldenburg, J., Fossa, S. D., Nuver, J., Heidenreich, A., Schmoll, H. J., Bokemeyer, C., et al. (2013). Testicular seminoma and non-seminoma: ESMO clinical practice guidelines for diagnosis, treatment and follow-up. *Annals of Oncology: Official Journal of the European Society for Medical Oncology / ESMO*. Available from https://doi.org/10.1093/annonc/mdt304, 24:vi125e32.

Stephenson, A., Eggener, S. E., Bass, E. B., Chelnick, D. M., Daneshmand, S., Feldman, D., et al. (2019). Diagnosis and treatment of early stage testicular cancer: AUA guideline. *The Journal of Urology*, *202*, 272e81.

Williamson, S. R., Delahunt, B., Magi-Galluzzi, C., Algaba, F., Egevad, L., Ulbright, T. M., et al. (2017). The world health organization 2016 classification of testicular germ cell tumours: A review and update from the international society of urological pathology testis consultation panel. *Histopathology*, *70*(3), 335–346.

Chapter 19

A comprehensive survey on spectrum of BRCA1 and BRCA2 pathogenic variants in breast and ovarian cancer

Oubaida ElBiad[1,2], Abdelilah Laraqui[6], Moulay Mustapha Ennaji[5], Bouabid Badaoui[3] and Khalid Ennibi[2,4]

[1]*Laboratory of Research and Biosafety L3, Military Teaching Hospital Mohammed V, Rabat, Morocco,* [2]*Sequencing Unit, Laboratory of Virology, Center for Virology, Infectious and Tropical Diseases, Mohammed V Military Teaching Hospital, Faculty of Medicine and Pharmacy, Mohammed V University, Rabat, Morocco,* [3]*Biodiversity, Ecology and Genome Laboratory, Faculty of Sciences, Mohammed V University, Rabat, Morocco,* [4]*Center for Virology, Infectious and Tropical Diseases, Mohammed V Military Teaching Hospital, Faculty of Medicine and Pharmacy, Mohammed V University, Rabat, Morocco,* [5]*Group Leader Research team of Virology, Oncology, and Biotechnologies, Head of Laboratory of Virology, Oncology, Biosciences, Environment and New Energies (LVO-BEEN), Faculty of Sciences and Techniques Mohammedia, University Hassan II of Casablanca, Casablanca, Morocco,* [6]*Laboratory of Human Pathologies Biology, Faculty of Sciences, and Genomic Center of Human Pathologies, Faculty of Medicine and Pharmacy, Bio-Path Laboratory, Faculty of sciences-Agdal, Mohammed V University, Rabat, Morocco*

19.1 Introduction

In 2021 breast cancer (BC) was reported as the most common cancer worldwide, with an estimated 2.3 million new cases, representing 11.7% of all cancer cases (Sung et al., 2021). It has now overtaken lung cancer as the world's mostly commonly diagnosed cancer. As per the GLOBOCAN Cancer Tomorrow prediction tool, by 2040, incident cases are expected to increase by more than 46%. The increasing global BC burden is mainly observed in low- and middle-income countries, particularly women under the age of 50 years (World Health Organisation, 2018).

Since 2008, worldwide BC incidence and mortality have increased by more than 20% and by 14%, respectively. Age-standardized BC mortality in high-income countries dropped by 40% between the 1980 and 2020.

Immunological Implications and Molecular Diagnostics of Genitourinary Cancer.
DOI: https://doi.org/10.1016/B978-0-323-85496-2.00007-5

Countries that have succeeded in reducing BC mortality have been able to achieve an annual BC mortality reduction of 2%–4% per year. If an annual mortality reduction of 2.5% per year occurs worldwide, 2.5 million BC deaths would be avoided between 2020 and 2040.

BReast CAncer gene (BRCA) 1 and 2 are the most known genes associated with hereditary breast and/or ovarian cancer (HBOC) risk (Mavaddat et al., 2013). Individuals identified as harboring inherited pathogenic variants (PVs) in BRCA1 or BRCA2 are at a significantly elevated lifetime risk of developing BC and OC and face treatment choices ranging from prophylactic surgery to increased surveillance (Domchek & Weber, 2006; Miki et al., 1994; Wooster et al., 1995). PVs in BRCA1 and BRCA2 genes are inherited in an autosomal dominant manner (Haber, 2002), and one in 300–800 persons in the general population are estimated to have a PV in BRCA1 or BRCA2 genes (Garcia & Powell, 2015).

19.2 BRCA1

The gene encoding for BRCA1, cloned in 1994, was first mapped to the long arm of the chromosome 17 (17q21) comprising 24 exons (22 coding exons) that translate into a large protein of 1863 amino acids with a molecular weight of 220 kDa and an mRNA that is 7.8 kb in length (Brzovic et al., 1998).

BRCA1 is comprised of different biding domains (Fig. 19.1). At its N-terminal region, BRCA1 contains a series of eight repeats of the Cys3-His-Cys4 motif called the really interesting new gene (RING), which is a zinc-finger motif domain, a catalytic domain involved in protein ubiquitination and protein–protein interaction. In fact, the RING domain of BRCA1 is

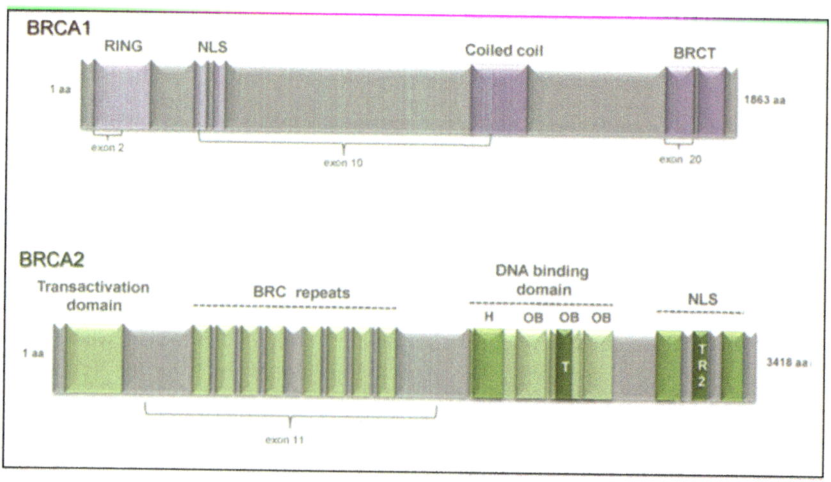

FIGURE 19.1 BRCA1 and BRCA2 functional domains. *Modified from source Gorodetska I, Kozeretska I, Dubrovska A. BRCA genes: The role in genome stability, cancer stemness and therapy resistance. Journal of Cancer. 2019;10(9):2109–2127. doi: 10.7150/jca.30410.*

essential for interaction with BARD1 protein (BRCA1-associated RING domain protein 1), forming an E3 ubiquitin ligase complex. In addition, this domain contains two nuclear export sequence (NES) motifs (Savage & Harkin, 2015).

The central part of BRCA1 contains two nuclear localization signals (NLS), located at the largest exons 11 and 13 (representing 65% of BRCA1 sequence), allowing the protein to return to the nucleus. The central part contains binding sites for several proteins including retinoblastoma protein (RB), cMyc, Rad50, and Rad51. It also has a coiled-coil domain, which interacts directly with the N-terminal part of PALB2 following DNA damage (Gorodetska et al., 2019).

The C-terminal part of BRCA1 has polypeptide motifs called BRCA1 C-terminal domains (BRCT) repeated in tandem. This BRCT domain mediates phosphoprotein interactions between BRCA1 and proteins phosphorylated by ATM and ATR, two kinases activated by DNA damage. The tandem of two BRCT domains appears to be involved in other manners such as protein--protein interactions with CtIP, ABRAXAS, and BRIP1 proteins, as well as mediating DNA binding and nonphosphoprotein interactions (Clark et al., 2012; Gorodetska et al., 2019).

19.3 BRCA2

Mary-Claire King and her group found that families with a high incidence of male BC did not to carry BRCA1 mutations, leading to the search for other BRCAs. A year later after cloning BRCA1, BRCA2 was mapped to the long arm of the chromosome 13 (13q12) as the second BC susceptibility gene. Comprising 27 exons, BRCA2 gene encodes a 11,386 bp mRNA transcript, which translates into a large nuclear protein of 3418 amino acids with a high molecular weight of 384 kDa. Although BRCA1 and BRCA2 share functional similarities, it is important to note that there is no homology between them (Narod & Foulkes, 2004; Wooster et al., 1995).

The large size of BRCA2 protein can accommodate interactions with numerous protein partners via its functional domains (Fig. 19.1). The N-terminal part of the BRCA2 protein contains a transcriptional activation domain (TAD) that recruits PALB2 (Xia et al., 2006). BRCA2 exon 11 encodes eight conserved motifs termed BRC repeats. Each of these repeats is composed of about 30 residues and mediate binding and regulation of RAD51 on resected DNA substrates (Chatterjee et al., 2016; Bork et al., 1996; Chen et al., 1998). A DNA-binding domain (DBD) composed of five parts is located at the carboxyl terminus, an α-helical domain (HD), 3 oligonucleotide-binding domains (OB1, OB2, and OB3), which bind the single-stranded DNA (ssDNA), and a tower domain (TD), which facilitates the binding of BRCA2 to double-stranded DNA (dsDNA) (Gorodetska et al., 2019). Two more NLS have been identified in the C-terminal region of BRCA2 (Esashi et al., 2005).

19.4 BRCA-associated breast and ovarian cancer

BRCA1-associated BCs frequently show a poorly differentiated infiltrating ductal histotype, high proliferative activity (ki-67), a high Nottingham grade and display medullary morphology, and a triple-negative and/or a basal-like immunophenotype (Massihnia et al., 2016). These tumors are associated with higher mortality and morbidity and therefore involve only the use of conventional chemotherapy as therapeutic option. Instead, BRCA2-associated BCs have a molecular profiling that resembles the luminal A or B tumor subtypes (Larsen et al., 2013; Waddell et al., 2010), as well as a slight increase in the incidence of the lobular histotype compared to sporadic forms (Dossus & Benusiglio, 2015; Lakhani et al., 1998). In contrast, BCs in BRCA2-PVs carriers are similar to sporadic luminal-type tumors that are positive for hormone receptors and lack expression of human epidermal growth factor receptor 2.

In OC, the prevalence of BRCA1/2 PVs is high (17%–20%), especially in patients with serous tumors (Alsop et al., 2012) and increases up to 23%–25% in the high-grade serous histotype (Rust et al., 2018), regardless of the age of diagnosis and family history. For this reason, and according to current guidelines, the BRCA test is performed in all non-mucinous and non-borderline ovarian epithelial carcinomas, fallopian tube carcinomas, and primary peritoneal carcinomas. on the other hand, individuals and family members possibly carriers of BRCA PV will be referred to dedicated high-risk follow-up programs and specific risk reduction strategies.

Furthermore, nowadays, genetic testing result has substantial clinical implications for patient care (Incorvaia et al., 2020). In addition to preventive pathways for early diagnosis and cancer risk reduction developed for individuals at high-risk and their relatives, BRCA testing has become a predictive biomarker of therapy response (Gori et al., 2019).

19.5 BRCA1 and BRCA2 genes mutations in breast and/or ovarian cancer

BRCA1 gene PVs cause BC in women with a possibility of 60%–80% and also cause increased risk of OC development in women. Germline mutations in BRCA2 gene are seen in approximately 35% of families with early-onset BC in women and also lead to an increased risk of OC development in women and BC in men (Gazalla Ayub et al., 2014).

Current investigations have reported several differences and significant heterogeneity in the incidence and geographic distribution of PVs in BRCA genes (Manchanda & Gaba, 2018; Rebbeck et al., 2018). In North Africa, BRCA PV frequency varies widely from $\approx 1\%$ (Morocco) in sporadic BC (Laraqui et al., 2012) to 37.5% (Tunisia) in HBOC (Troudi et al., 2007). The spectrum and prevalence of BRCA PVs vary mainly because of population-specific recurrent/founder variants. A few studies have reported a founder effect of such recurrent or unique variants through haplotype analysis. Prevalence studies of BRCA gene variants suggest that these genetic alterations can explain a high-frequency BC in some populations than others and may contribute to differences in cancer risk between populations and racial/ethnic minorities (Ferla et al., 2007; Figlioli et al., 2021; Rebbeck et al., 2018). Accurate identification of the population-specific variant spectrum is therefore the first step toward incorporating appropriate BRCA genetic testing into clinical practice in certain populations and racial/ethnic groups (Rashid et al., 2019).

19.6 BRCA1 and BRCA2 recurrent/founder variants in North Africa

BRCA1 founder variants explain around 36.4% (47/129) of BC and outnumber BRCA2 founder variants by a ratio of ≈3:1. Clear founder effects have been reported in Morocco (BRCA1 c.5309G > T) and Tunisia (BRCA1 c.211dupA). Furthermore, the BRCA1 c.798_799detTT was identified in 14% (18/129) of BRCA1 carriers in North African populations. It was initially thought to be specific to Algeria (19.23%, 5/26) (Cherbal et al., 2010; Uhrhammer et al., 2008) but was eventually found to be prevalent in Tunisia (7.4%, 4/54) (Fourati et al., 2014; Troudi et al., 2007; Troudi et al., 2008) and Morocco (18.4%, 9/49) (Bakkach et al., 2020; El Ansari et al., 2020; Jouali et al., 2020; Laraqui et al., 2012; Mansouri et al., 2020; Tazzite et al., 2012). Haplotype analysis of some families carrying these PV revealed the presence of a common allele (Uhrhammer et al., 2008). The BRCA1 c.798_799detTT frameshift variant is cited twice in the Breast Cancer Information Core (BIC) database, without any ethnic origin indicated. Interestingly, the c.798_799delTT and c.5309G > T variants in BRCA1 have been identified in sporadic BC patients in North Africa, and hence, their presence in patients without a history of BC and/or OC cannot be attributed to the de novo mutational event. To our knowledge, the BRCA1 c.798_799delTT variant has been identified in Spain (John et al., 2007), in southern Italy (Russo et al., 2007; Ten years of BRCA testing in calabrian population & Request PDF, 2022), and in France (Muller et al., 2004). This restricted geographical distribution to close Mediterranean countries could be ascribed to geographical proximity and migration flow history.

The c.1310_1313delAAGA variant in BRCA2 represents another common PV in North African populations whose founder effect through haplotype analysis is required for confirmation in this region. According to the BIC database, the BRCA2 c.1310_1313delAAGA PV was found in different European patients and was recorded several times in the French Universal Mutation database-BRCA2 (UMD-BRCA2) and classified as founder variant (Caputo et al., 2012). The c.1310_1313delAAGA PV, located in coding exon

9 of the BRCA2 gene, results from a deletion of four nucleotides at nucleotide positions 1310–1313. This deletion causes a frameshift, which changes a Lysine to an Isoleucine at codon 437, and creates a premature stop codon at position 22 of the new reading frame. In addition, it is important to highlight that one of the three Ashkenazi Jewish founder variants (i.e., BRCA1 c.5266dup) is frequently observed in Tunisian BRCA1 carriers (20.4%, 11/54) (ElBiad et al., 2022).

The BRCA1 c.5266dup has been mainly observed in Italy in some families from the Northeastern coast of Sicily (Incorvaia et al., 2020). BRCA1 c.5266dup was reported as a founder variant in several European populations as well with a low proportion of individuals who self-identify as Jewish (Janavičius, 2010). Previous studies have indicated that the mutation was introduced into the Ashkenazi Jewish genetic pool approximately 400–500 years ago in Poland, but the mutation originated from a single common European ancestor long before it became an Ashkenazi Jewish founder mutation (Hamel et al., 2011). The BRCA1 c.5266dupC variant is the second most frequently reported PV in the BIC database.

19.7 BRCA1 and BRCA2 recurrent/founder variants worldwide

Because of common ancestral haplotypes, several founder variants have been identified in various areas and races. For example, the well-known founder variants are c.68_69delAG, c.5266dupC in BRCA1, and c.5946_5946delT in BRCA2 in the Ashkenazi Jewish population (Struewing et al., 1995; Struewing et al., 1997). The c.824_825ins10, c.1713_1717delAGAAT, c.5177_5180del4, c.4357 + 1G > A variants in BRCA1 and c.4471_4474delCTGA variant in BRCA2 have been identified as a potential Afro-American founder variant (Olopade et al., 2003; Pal et al., 2004; Pal et al., 2015). A high frequency of founder c.771_775del5 BRCA2 PV was identified in Iceland (Thorlacius et al., 1997). The founder BRCA2 c.771_775del5 variant was reported to cause the familial clustering of both female and male BC cases (Johannesdottir et al., 1996; Thorlacius et al., 1997). The c.2685_2686del variant in BRCA1 and c.9672dup variant in BRCA2 have been reported as founder mutations for the Dutch population (Leegte et al., 2005). A French-Canadian founder status is evident for c.4327C > T in BRCA1 and c.8537_8538delAG in BRCA2 (Tonin et al., 1998). The founder effect of c.68_69delAG, c.181T > G, c.676delT, c.1687 C > T, c.3700_3704delGTAAA, c.3756_3759delGTCT, c.4035delA, c.5251C > T, c.5266dupC in BRCA1 and c.658_659delGT, c.3847_3848delGT, c.5946delT, c.7913_7917delTTCCT in BRCA2 is characteristic of Central European population (Janavičius, 2010).

In BRCA1 gene, three large genomic deletions (deletion of exon 20, exon 24, and exons 23 and 24) and the c.5212G > A PV have been characterized as population-specific founder variants by haplotype analysis in the

Greek population (Fostira et al., 2020). The c.1140dupG and c.4136_4137delCT variants in BRCA1 were identified as novel putative founder variants in Middle Eastern patients (Bu et al., 2016). In addition to c.2641G > T, c.68_69delAG, c.5266dupC, and c.1374delC recurrent variants in BRCA1, haplotype analysis confirmed the founder status of c.5771_5774del and c.7934del variants in BRCA2 and revealed an additional founder variant in BRCA2, c.582G > A, in South African families (Reeves et al., 2004). In Latin America, clear founder effects have been reported in Mexico (BRCA1 del exons 9–12), Brazil (BRCA1 c.5266dupC and BRCA2 c.156_157insAlu), and Colombia (BRCA1 c.3331_3334delCAAG, BRCA1 c.5123C > A, and BRCA2 c.2808_2811delACAA) (Ossa & Torres, 2016).

In the Middle Eastern population, nine PVs were recurrent in epithelial OC, and founder mutation analysis revealed only two mutations (BRCA1 c.4136_4137delCT and BRCA1 c.1140dupG) sharing the same haplotypes, thus representing founder mutations (Siraj et al., 2019). Studying the founder effect of these variants can provide a comprehensive analysis of a population's evolution and its migration pathways.

Besides recurrent/founder variants, two BRCA1 PVs (c.211dupA and c.5309G > T) identified in North Africa were not reported previously. The c.211dupA and c.5309G > T variants in the BRCA1 gene were found as unique to the Tunisian and Moroccan populations, respectively (Fourati et al., 2014; Mighri et al., 2020; Riahi et al., 2015; Troudi et al., 2007; Troudi et al., 2008).

19.8 BRCA1- and BRCA2-specific variants in North Africa and Worldwide

A specific variant in BRCA genes has been found with high prevalence in restricted populations as a consequence of a founder effect. The specific founder variant of c.303T > G and c.2641G > T in BRCA1 gene were reported in the Yoruba population from Nigeria (Zhang et al., 2009) and in the Afrikaner population from South Africa (Reeves et al., 2004), respectively. Geographical clustering of c.3481_3491del11 and c.5128G > T variants in BRCA1 in the Alsace–Lorraine region at the north-east and in the north-east of France, respectively, suggests a founder effect (Muller et al., 2004; Ramus & Gayther, 2009).

In the southwest of the Netherland, the founder effect of c.4186–1643_4357 + 2020del3835 variant in BRCA1 gene and c.5351dupA variant in BRCA2 gene were prevalent in Catholic (West Brabant clustering) and Protestant (South Beveland clustering) families, respectively, reflecting religious endogamy (Verhoog et al., 2001). The c.4964_4982del19 variant in BRCA1 gene has been identified as a founder variant in a geographically and historically homogeneous population from Calabria, a south Italian region (Baudi et al., 2001). Significant regional founder effect has been demonstrated for c.3228_3229delAG, c.3285delA, c.1380dupA, and c.5062_5064del3 variants in BRCA1 gene in Tuscany in central Italy (Papi et al., 2009). The c.5062_5064delGTT variant in BRCA1 gene and c.8537_8538delAG variant in BRCA2 gene have been described as founder variants in Middle Sardinia and in South and Middle Sardinia, respectively (Malacrida et al., 2008). Figlioli et al. showed that the BRCA1 c.190T > C is a founder variant in BC families from Bergamo province in the Northern Italian region (Figlioli et al., 2021). The c.3048_3052dupTGAGA variant is the western Swedish BRCA1 founder variant (Einbeigi et al., 2001). The BRCA1 c.131G PV was considered a specific founder variant in the Lebanese population (Geredeli et al., 2019). In Saudi Arabia, six PVs were reported to be unique and founder PVs in Saudis with OC; four in BRCA1 gene (c.711_712insTGAA, c.1140dupG, c.5054C > T, c.5530delC) and two in BRCA2 gene (c.2667delT and c.5760_5770del11) genes (Alhuqail et al., 2018).

Identification of specific and recurrent/founder variants that could be included in a low-cost PV panel, used as a first line screening approach, would be useful in the North African region. Advance of a screening panel for specific/recurrent and founder PVs offers a simple, rapid, and affordable routine molecular diagnostic method for the clinical management of BC and/ or OC patients and their unaffected family members (Kwong et al., 2018). The PV panel can also include other recurrent worldwide PVs such as BRCA1c.1016dupA, which has also been reported in other countries (Italy, Germany, and French Canada). However, allelotyping results indicated an independent origin of this PV. This would justify the inclusion of the BRCA1c.1016dupA into targeted variant screening panels in any population, regardless of ethnic origin (Caputo et al., 2012).

References

Alhuqail, A. J., Alzahrani, A., Almubarak, H., et al. (2018). High prevalence of deleterious BRCA1 and BRCA2 germline mutations in arab breast and ovarian cancer patients. *Breast Cancer Research and Treatment*, *168*(3), 695–702. Available from https://doi.org/10.1007/S10549-017-4635-4.

Alsop, K., Fereday, S., Meldrum, C., et al. (2012). BRCA mutation frequency and patterns of treatment response in BRCA mutation-positive women with ovarian cancer: A report from the Australian ovarian cancer study group. *Journal of Clinical Oncology: Official Journal of the American Society of Clinical Oncology*, *30*(21), 2654–2663. Available from https://doi.org/10.1200/JCO.2011.39.8545.

Bakkach, J., Mansouri, M., Derkaoui, T., et al. (2020). Contribution of BRCA1 and BRCA2 germline mutations to early onset breast cancer: A series from north of Morocco. *BMC Cancer*, *20*(1). Available from https://doi.org/10.1186/s12885-020-07352-9.

Baudi, F., Quaresima, B., Grandinetti, C., et al. (2001). Evidence of a founder mutation of BRCA1 in a highly homogeneous population from southern Italy with breast/ovarian cancer. *Human Mutation*, *18*(2), 163–164. Available from https://doi.org/10.1002/HUMU.1167.

Bork, P., Blomberg, N., & Nilges, M. (1996). Internal repeats in the BRCA2 protein sequence. *Nature Genetics*, *13*(1), 22–23. Available from https://doi.org/10.1038/NG0596-22.

Brzovic, P. S., Meza, J., King, M. C., & Klevit, R. E. (1998). The cancer-predisposing mutation C61G disrupts homodimer formation in the NH2-terminal BRCA1 RING finger domain. *The Journal of Biological Chemistry*, *273*(14), 7795–7799. Available from https://doi.org/10.1074/JBC.273.14.7795.

Bu, R., Siraj, A. K., Al-Obaisi, K. A. S., et al. (2016). Identification of novel BRCA founder mutations in middle eastern breast cancer patients using capture and Sanger sequencing analysis. *International Journal of Cancer. Journal International du Cancer*, *139*(5), 1091–1097. Available from https://doi.org/10.1002/IJC.30143.

Caputo, S., Benboudjema, L., Sinilnikova, O., et al. (2012). Description and analysis of genetic variants in French hereditary breast and ovarian cancer families recorded in the UMD-BRCA1/BRCA2 databases. *Nucleic Acids Research*, *40*(Database issue), D992. Available from https://doi.org/10.1093/NAR/GKR1160.

Chatterjee, G., Jimenez-Sainz, J., Presti, T., Nguyen, T., & Jensen, R. B. (2016). Distinct binding of BRCA2 BRC repeats to RAD51 generates differential DNA damage sensitivity. *Nucleic Acids Research*, *44*(11), 5256. Available from https://doi.org/10.1093/NAR/GKW242.

Chen, P. L., Chen, C. F., Chen, Y., Xiao, J., Sharp, Z. D., & Lee, W. H. (1998). The BRC repeats in BRCA2 are critical for RAD51 binding and resistance to methyl methanesulfonate treatment. *Proceedings of the National Academy of Sciences of the United States of America*, *95*(9), 5287–5292. Available from https://doi.org/10.1073/PNAS.95.9.5287.

Cherbal, F., Bakour, R., Adane, S., Boualga, K., Benais-Pont, G., & Maillet, P. (2010). BRCA1 and BRCA2 germline mutations screening in Algerian breast/ovarian cancer families. *Disease Markers*, *28*(6), 377–384. Available from https://doi.org/10.3233/DMA-2010-0718.

Clark, S. L., Rodriguez, A. M., Snyder, R. R., Hankins, G. D. V., & Boehning, D. (2012). Structure-function of the tumor suppressor BRCA1. *Computational and Structural Biotechnology Journal*, *1*(1)e201204005. Available from https://doi.org/10.5936/CSBJ.201204005.

Domchek, S. M., & Weber, B. L. (2006). Clinical management of BRCA1 and BRCA2 mutation carriers. *Oncogene*, *25*(43), 5825–5831. Available from https://doi.org/10.1038/SJ.ONC.1209881.

Dossus, L., & Benusiglio, P. R. (2015). Lobular breast cancer: Incidence and genetic and non-genetic risk factors. *Breast Cancer Research: BCR*, *17*(1). Available from https://doi.org/10.1186/S13058-015-0546-7.

Einbeigi, Z., Bergman, A., Kindblom, L. G., et al. (2001). A founder mutation of the BRCA1 gene in Western Sweden associated with a high incidence of breast and ovarian cancer. *European Journal of Cancer*, *37*(15), 1904–1909. Available from https://doi.org/10.1016/S0959-8049(01)00223-4.

El Ansari, F. Z., Jouali, F., Marchoudi, N., et al. (2020). Screening of BRCA1/2 genes mutations and copy number variations in patients with high risk for hereditary breast and ovarian cancer syndrome (HBOC). *BMC Cancer*, *20*(1), 1–11. Available from https://doi.org/10.1186/s12885-020-07250-0.

ElBiad, O., Laraqui, A., El Boukhrissi, F., et al. (2022). Prevalence of specific and recurrent/founder pathogenic variants in BRCA genes in breast and ovarian cancer in North Africa. *BMC Cancer*, *22*(1), 1–19. Available from https://doi.org/10.1186/S12885-022-09181-4, *2022 221*.

Esashi, F., Christ, N., Cannon, J., et al. (2005). CDK-dependent phosphorylation of BRCA2 as a regulatory mechanism for recombinational repair. *Nature*, *434*(7033), 598–604. Available from https://doi.org/10.1038/NATURE03404.

Ferla, R., Calò, V., Cascio, S., et al. (2007). Founder mutations in BRCA1 and BRCA2 genes. *Annals of Oncology, The Official Journal of the European Society for Medical Oncology, 18* (Suppl 6). Available from https://doi.org/10.1093/ANNONC/MDM234. (SUPPL. 6).

Figlioli, G., De Nicolo, A., Catucci, I., et al. (2021). Analysis of Italian BRCA1/2 pathogenic variants identifies a private spectrum in the population from the Bergamo Province in Northern Italy. *Cancers (Basel).*, *13*(3), 1–11. Available from https://doi.org/10.3390/CANCERS13030532.

Fostira, F., Kostantopoulou, I., Apostolou, P., et al. (2020). One in three highly selected Greek patients with breast cancer carries a loss-of-function variant in a cancer susceptibility gene. *Journal of Medical Genetics*, *57*(1), 53–61. Available from https://doi.org/10.1136/JMEDGENET-2019-106189.

Fourati, A., Louchez, M. M., Fournier, J., et al. (2014). Screening for common mutations in BRCA1 and BRCA2 genes: Interest in genetic testing of Tunisian families with breast and/or ovarian cancer. *Bulletin du Cancer*, *101*(11), E36–E40. Available from https://doi.org/10.1684/bdc.2014.2049.

Garcia, C., & Powell, C. B. (2015). A comprehensive approach to the identification and management of the BRCA patient. *Obstetrical & Gynecological Survey*, *70*(2), 131–143. Available from https://doi.org/10.1097/OGX.0000000000000156.

Gazalla Ayub, S., Rasool, S., Ayub, T., Khan, S. N., Wani, K. A., & Andrabi, K. I. (2014). Mutational analysis of the BRCA2 gene in breast carcinoma patients of Kashmiri descent. *Molecular Medicine Reports*, *9*(2), 749–753. Available from https://doi.org/10.3892/MMR.2013.1862.

Geredeli, C., Yasar, N., & Sakin, A. (2019). Germline mutations in BRCA1 and BRCA2 in breast cancer patients with high genetic risk in Turkish population. *International Journal of Breast Cancer*, *2019*. Available from https://doi.org/10.1155/2019/9645147.

Gori, S., Barberis, M., Bella, M. A., et al. (2019). Recommendations for the implementation of BRCA testing in ovarian cancer patients and their relatives. *Critical Reviews in Oncology/Hematology*, *140*, 67–72. Available from https://doi.org/10.1016/J.CRITREVONC.2019.05.012.

Gorodetska, I., Kozeretska, I., & Dubrovska, A. (2019). BRCA genes: The role in genome stability, cancer stemness and therapy resistance. *Journal of Cancer*, *10*(9), 2109–2127. Available from https://doi.org/10.7150/jca.30410.

Haber, D. (2002). Prophylactic oophorectomy to reduce the risk of ovarian and breast cancer in carriers of BRCA mutations. *The New England Journal of Medicine*, *346*(21), 1660–1662. Available from https://doi.org/10.1056/NEJMED020044.

Hamel, N., Feng, B. J., Foretova, L., et al. (2011). On the origin and diffusion of BRCA1 c.5266dupC (5382insC) in European populations. *European Journal of Human Genetics: EJHG*, *19*(3), 300. Available from https://doi.org/10.1038/EJHG.2010.203.

Incorvaia, L., Fanale, D., Badalamenti, G., et al. (2020). Hereditary breast and ovarian cancer in families from Southern Italy (Sicily)-prevalence and geographic distribution of pathogenic variants in BRCA1/2 Genes. *Cancers (Basel).*, *12*(5). Available from https://doi.org/10.3390/CANCERS12051158.

Janavičius, R. (2010). Founder BRCA1/2 mutations in the Europe: Implications for hereditary breast-ovarian cancer prevention and control. *EPMA Journal*, *1*(3), 397. Available from https://doi.org/10.1007/S13167-010-0037-Y.

Johannesdottir, G., Gudmundsson, J., Bergthorsson, J. T., et al. (1996). Advances in Brief 14. Landspilalinn. /Ill Reykjavik, Â¡celami; Institute of Oncology. University Hospital. S-221 85 Luna. Sweden. *Cancer Research*, *56*, 3663–3665, Accessed February 28, 2022. Available from http://aacrjournals.org/cancerres/article-pdf/56/16/3663/2461047/cr0560163663.pdf.

John, E. M., Miron, A., Gong, G., et al. (2007). Prevalence of pathogenic BRCA1 mutation carriers in 5 US racial/ethnic groups. *JAMA: The Journal of the American Medical Association, 298*(24), 2869–2876. Available from https://doi.org/10.1001/JAMA.298.24.2869.

Jouali, F., Zahra, F., Ansari, E., et al. (2020). EGFR, BRCA1, BRCA2 and TP53 genetic profile in Moroccan triple negative breast cancer cases. *International Journal of Molecular Epidemiology and Genetics, 11*(1), 16, Accessed February 28, 2022. /pmc/articles/PMC7373717/.

Kwong, A., Shin, V. Y., Ma, E., et al. (2018). Screening for founder and recurrent BRCA mutations in Hong Kong and US Chinese populations. *Hong Kong Medical Journal*, 24, Acccessed February 28, 2022. Available from http://www.hkmj.org.

Lakhani, S. R., Jacquemier, J., Sloane, J. P., et al. (1998). Multifactorial analysis of differences between sporadic breast cancers and cancers involving BRCA1 and BRCA2 mutations. *Journal of the National Cancer Institute, 90*(15), 1138–1145. Available from https://doi.org/10.1093/JNCI/90.15.1138.

Laraqui, A., Uhrhammer, N., Lahlou-Amine, I., et al. (2012). Mutation screening of the BRCA1 gene in early onset and familial breast/ovarian cancer in Moroccan population. *International Journal of Medical Sciences, 10*(1), 60–67. Available from https://doi.org/10.7150/ijms.5014.

Larsen, M. J., Kruse, T. A., Tan, Q., et al. (2013). Classifications within molecular subtypes enables identification of BRCA1/BRCA2 mutation carriers by RNA tumor profiling. *PLoS One, 8*(5). Available from https://doi.org/10.1371/JOURNAL.PONE.0064268.

Leegte, B., van der Hout, A. H., Deffenbaugh, A. M., et al. (2005). Phenotypic expression of double heterozygosity for BRCA1 and BRCA2 germline mutations. *Journal of Medical Genetics, 42*(3), e20. Available from https://doi.org/10.1136/JMG.2004.027243.

Malacrida, S., Agata, S., Callegaro, M., et al. (2008). BRCA1 p.Val1688del is a deleterious mutation that recurs in breast and ovarian cancer families from Northeast Italy. *Journal of Clinical Oncology: Official Journal of the American Society of Clinical Oncology, 26*(1), 26–31. Available from https://doi.org/10.1200/JCO.2007.13.2118.

Manchanda, R., & Gaba, F. (2018). Population based testing for primary prevention: A systematic review. *Cancers (Basel)., 10*(11). Available from https://doi.org/10.3390/CANCERS10110424.

Mansouri, M., Derkaoui, T., Bakkach, J., et al. (2020). Screening of BRCA1 and BRCA2 germline mutations in unselected triple-negative breast cancer patients: A series from north of Morocco. *Precision Medical Sciences, 9*(1), 43–48. Available from https://doi.org/10.1002/prm2.12009.

Massihnia, D., Galvano, A., Fanale, D., et al. (2016). Triple negative breast cancer: Shedding light onto the role of pi3k/akt/mtor pathway. *Oncotarget., 7*(37), 60712. Available from https://doi.org/10.18632/ONCOTARGET.10858.

Mavaddat, N., Peock, S., Frost, D., et al. (2013). Cancer risks for BRCA1 and BRCA2 mutation carriers: Results from prospective analysis of EMBRACE. *Journal of the National Cancer Institute, 105*(11), 812–822. Available from https://doi.org/10.1093/JNCI/DJT095.

Mighri, N., Hamdi, Y., Boujemaa, M., et al. (2020). Identification of novel BRCA1 and RAD50 mutations associated with breast cancer predisposition in Tunisian patients. *Frontiers in Genetics, 11*(November). Available from https://doi.org/10.3389/fgene.2020.552971.

Miki, Y., Swensen, J., Shattuck-Eidens, D., et al. (1994). A strong candidate for the breast and ovarian cancer susceptibility gene BRCA1. *Science, 266*(5182), 66–71. Available from https://doi.org/10.1126/science.7545954.

Muller, D., Bonaiti-Pellié, C., Abecassis, J., Stoppa-Lyonnet, D., & Fricker, J. P. (2004). BRCA1 testing in breast and/or ovarian cancer families from northeastern France identifies two common mutations with a founder effect. *Familial Cancer, 3*(1), 15–20. Available from https://doi.org/10.1023/B:FAME.0000026819.44213.DF.

Narod, S. A., & Foulkes, W. D. (2004). BRCA1 and BRCA2: 1994 and beyond. *Nature Reviews. Cancer, 4*(9), 665–676. Available from https://doi.org/10.1038/NRC1431.

Olopade, O. I., Fackenthal, J. D., Dunston, G., Tainsky, M. A., Collins, F., & Whiffield-Broome, C. (2003). Breast cancer genetics in African Americans. *Cancer, 97*(1 SUPPL.), 236–245. Available from https://doi.org/10.1002/cncr.11019.

Ossa, C. A., & Torres, D. (2016). Founder and recurrent mutations in BRCA1 and BRCA2 genes in Latin American countries: State of the art and literature review. *The Oncologist, 21*(7), 832. Available from https://doi.org/10.1634/THEONCOLOGIST.2015-0416.

Pal, T., Bonner, D., Cragun, D., et al. (2015). A high frequency of BRCA mutations in young black women with breast cancer residing in Florida. *Cancer, 121*(23), 4173–4180. Available from https://doi.org/10.1002/CNCR.29645.

Pal, T., Permuth-Wey, J., Holtje, T., & Sutphen, R. (2004). BRCA1 and BRCA2 mutations in a study of African American breast cancer patients. *Cancer Epidemiology, Biomarkers & Prevention, 13*(11), 1794–1803, Accessed February 28, 2022. Available from http://aacr-journals.org/cebp/article-pdf/13/11/1794/1748644/1794-1799.pdf.

Papi, L., Putignano, A. L., Congregati, C., et al. (2009). Founder mutations account for the majority of BRCA1-attributable hereditary breast/ovarian cancer cases in a population from Tuscany, Central Italy. *Breast Cancer Research and Treatment, 117*(3), 497–504. Available from https://doi.org/10.1007/S10549-008-0190-3.

Ramus, S. J., & Gayther, S. A. (2009). The Contribution of BRCA1 and BRCA2 to Ovarian Cancer. *Molecular Oncology, 3*(2), 138. Available from https://doi.org/10.1016/J.MOLONC.2009.02.001.

Rashid, M. U., Muhammad, N., Naeemi, H., et al. (2019). Spectrum and prevalence of BRCA1/2 germline mutations in Pakistani breast cancer patients: Results from a large comprehensive study. *Hereditary Cancer in Clinical Practice, 17*(1). Available from https://doi.org/10.1186/s13053-019-0125-5.

Rebbeck, T. R., Friebel, T. M., Friedman, E., et al. (2018). Mutational spectrum in a worldwide study of 29,700 families with BRCA1 or BRCA2 mutations. *Human Mutation, 39*(5), 593. Available from https://doi.org/10.1002/HUMU.23406.

Reeves, M. D., Yawitch, T. M., Van Der Merwe, N. C., Van Den Berg, H. J., Dreyer, G., & Van Rensburg, E. J. (2004). BRCA1 mutations in South African breast and/or ovarian cancer families: Evidence of a novel founder mutation in Afrikaner families. *International Journal of Cancer. Journal International du Cancer, 110*(5), 677–682. Available from https://doi.org/10.1002/IJC.20186.

Riahi, A., Kharrat, M., Ghourabi, M. E., et al. (2015). Mutation spectrum and prevalence of BRCA1 and BRCA2 genes in patients with familial and early-onset breast/ovarian cancer from Tunisia. *Clinical Genetics, 87*(2), 155–160. Available from https://doi.org/10.1111/cge.12337.

Russo, A., Calò, V., Agnese, V., et al. (2007). BRCA1 genetic testing in 106 breast and ovarian cancer families from Southern Italy (Sicily): A mutation analyses. *Breast Cancer Research and Treatment, 105*(3), 267–276. Available from https://doi.org/10.1007/S10549-006-9456-9.

Rust, K., Spiliopoulou, P., Tang, C. Y., et al. (2018). Routine germline BRCA1 and BRCA2 testing in patients with ovarian carcinoma: Analysis of the Scottish real-life experience. *BJOG: An International Journal of Obstetrics and Gynaecology, 125*(11), 1451–1458. Available from https://doi.org/10.1111/1471-0528.15171.

Savage, K. I., & Harkin, D. P. (2015). BRCA1, a "complex" protein involved in the maintenance of genomic stability. *The FEBS Journal, 282*(4), 630–646. Available from https://doi.org/10.1111/FEBS.13150.

Siraj, A. K., Bu, R., Iqbal, K., et al. (2019). Prevalence, spectrum, and founder effect of BRCA1 and BRCA2 mutations in epithelial ovarian cancer from the Middle East. *Human Mutation, 40*(6), 729–733. Available from https://doi.org/10.1002/HUMU.23736.

Struewing, J. P., Abeliovich, D., Peretz, T., et al. (1995). The carrier frequency of the BRCA1 185delAG mutation is approximately 1 percent in Ashkenazi Jewish individuals. *Nature Genetics, 11*(2), 198–200. Available from https://doi.org/10.1038/NG1095-198.

Struewing, J. P., Hartge, P., Wacholder, S., et al. (1997). The risk of cancer associated with specific mutations of BRCA1 and BRCA2 among Ashkenazi Jews. *The New England Journal of Medicine, 336*(20), 1401–1408. Available from https://doi.org/10.1056/NEJM199705153362001.

Sung, H., Ferlay, J., Siegel, R. L., et al. (2021). Global cancer statistics 2020: GLOBOCAN estimates of incidence and mortality worldwide for 36 cancers in 185 countries. *CA: A Cancer Journal for Clinicians, 71*(3), 209–249. Available from https://doi.org/10.3322/CAAC.21660.

Tazzite, A., Jouhadi, H., Nadifi, S., et al. (2012). BRCA1 and BRCA2 germline mutations in Moroccan breast/ovarian cancer families: Novel mutations and unclassified variants. *Gynecologic Oncology, 125*(3), 687–692. Available from https://doi.org/10.1016/j.ygyno.2012.03.007.

Ten years of BRCA testing in calabrian population | Request PDF. Accessed February 28, 2022. <https://www.researchgate.net/publication/285914506_Ten_years_of_BRCA_testing_in_calabrian_population>.

Thorlacius, S., Sigurdsson, S., Bjarnadottir, H., et al. (1997). Study of a single BRCA2 mutation with high carrier frequency in a small population. *American Journal of Human Genetics, 60*(5), 1079, Accessed February 28, 2022. /pmc/articles/PMC1712443/?report = abstract.

Tonin, P. N., Mes-Masson, A. M., Futreal, P. A., et al. (1998). Founder BRCA1 and BRCA2 mutations in French Canadian breast and ovarian cancer families. *American Journal of Human Genetics, 63*(5), 1341. Available from https://doi.org/10.1086/302099.

Troudi, W., Uhrhammer, N., Romdhane, K. B., et al. (2008). Complete mutation screening and haplotype characterization of BRCA1 gene in Tunisian patients with familial breast cancer. *Cancer Biomarkers., 4*(1), 11–18. Available from https://doi.org/10.3233/CBM-2008-4102.

Troudi, W., Uhrhammer, N., Sibille, C., et al. (2007). Contribution of the BRCA1 and BRCA2 mutations to breast cancer in Tunisia. *Journal of Human Genetics, 52*(11), 915–920. Available from https://doi.org/10.1007/s10038-007-0195-5.

Uhrhammer, N., Abdelouahab, A., Lafarge, L., Feille, V., Dib, A. B., & Bignon, Y. J. (2008). BRCA1 mutations in Algerian breast cancer patients: High frequency in young, sporadic cases. *International Journal of Medical Sciences, 5*(4), 197–202. Available from https://doi.org/10.7150/ijms.5.197.

Verhoog, L. C., Van Den Ouweland, A. M. W., Berns, E., et al. (2001). Large regional differences in the frequency of distinct BRCA1/BRCA2 mutations in 517 Dutch breast and/or ovarian cancer families. *European Journal of Cancer, 37*(16), 2082–2090. Available from https://doi.org/10.1016/S0959-8049(01)00244-1.

Waddell, N., Arnold, J., Cocciardi, S., et al. (2010). Subtypes of familial breast tumours revealed by expression and copy number profiling. *Breast Cancer Research and Treatment, 123*(3), 661–677. Available from https://doi.org/10.1007/S10549-009-0653-1.

Wooster, R., Bignell, G., Lancaster, J., et al. (1995). Identification of the breast cancer susceptibility gene BRCA2. *Nature, 378*(6559), 789–792. Available from https://doi.org/10.1038/378789A0.

World Health Organisation. (2018). Latest global cancer data : Cancer burden rises to 18. 1 million new cases and 9. 6 million cancer deaths in 2018 latest global cancer data: Cancer burden rises to 18. 1 million new cases and 9. 6 million cancer deaths in 2018. *International Agency for Research on Cancer* (September), 13–15.

Xia, B., Sheng, Q., Nakanishi, K., et al. (2006). Control of BRCA2 cellular and clinical functions by a nuclear partner, PALB2. *Molecular Cell*, *22*(6), 719–729. Available from https://doi.org/10.1016/J.MOLCEL.2006.05.022.

Zhang, B., Fackenthal, J. D., Niu, Q., et al. (2009). Evidence for an ancient BRCA1 mutation in breast cancer patients of Yoruban ancestry. *Familial Cancer*, *8*(1), 15–22. Available from https://doi.org/10.1007/S10689-008-9205-9.

Chapter 20

Molecular and epidemiological characterization of bladder tumors

Ikram Tiabi[3], Anouar Tadlaoui Kaoutar[3], Youssef Ennaji[3], Soukayna Alaoui Sosse[3], Mohammed Nabil Benchekroun[3], Mohammed Mrabti[3], Abdelilah Laraqui[2] and Moulay Mustapha Ennaji[1]

[1]Group Leader Research team of Virology, Oncology, and Biotechnologies, Head of Laboratory of Virology, Oncology, Biosciences, Environment and New Energies (LVO-BEEN), Faculty of Sciences and Techniques Mohammedia, University Hassan II of Casablanca, Casablanca, Morocco, [2]Laboratory of Human Pathologies Biology, Faculty of Sciences, and Genomic Center of Human Pathologies, Faculty of Medicine and Pharmacy, Bio-Path Laboratory, Faculty of sciences-Agdal, Mohammed V University, Rabat, Morocco, [3]Team of Virology, Oncology, and Biotechnologies, Laboratory of Virology, Oncology, Biosciences, Environment and New Energies (LVO-BEEN), Faculty of Sciences and Techniques Mohammedia, University Hassan II of Casablanca, Casablanca, Morocco

20.1 Introduction

Bladder cancer is the ninth most common cancer worldwide (Mahdavifar et al., 2016), representing a global incidence of 10.1% in men and 2.5% in women, This frequency varies with geographic distribution and the country of origin.

This cancer is the second most common genitourinary cancer after prostate cancer (Ploeg et al., 2009) (Fig. 20.3). In 2012 429,800 new cases were diagnosed worldwide with 165,100 deaths and a sex ratio of 3:1 (Torre et al., 2012).

In recent years, its incidence has been higher in developed countries and in some African countries, with an increase in morbidity in North African and Middle Eastern countries (Mahdavifar et al., 2016; Malats & Real, 2015).

In Tunisia, bladder cancer occupies the first place with respect to urological cancer cases among men and the second place for all malignant cancers (Cancer Registry of Northern Tunisia, 1999–2003).

In Morocco, bladder cancer constituted 3.1% of the cases observed within the period 2008–12. Furthermore, 85.3% of bladder cancer cases were

Immunological Implications and Molecular Diagnostics of Genitourinary Cancer.
DOI: https://doi.org/10.1016/B978-0-323-85496-2.00026-9

among men, compared to 14.7% in women (Registry of Cancer in the Greater Casablanca 2008–12).

During the 5 years under review, 752 cases of bladder cancer were identified, corresponding to 3.7 per 100,000 population (1.1 per 100,000 women and 6.5 per 100,000 men). The normalization on the world population has resulted in a rate of 4.7 per 100,000 (1.3 per 100,000 for women and 8.6 per 100,000 for men) (Registry of Cancer of the Greater Casablanca 2008–12).

20.2 Anatomy of the urinary system

The urinary system corresponds to the set of organs that allow the production of urine and its evacuation from the body. It includes the two kidneys and the urinary tract, with anatomical differences between men and women (Kiemeney et al., 2008, 2010) (Fig. 20.1).

20.2.1 Kidneys

The nephron is the structural and functional unit of the kidney; it ensures the formation of urine. A nephron is composed of a glomerulus and a renal tube (Rafnar et al., 2009). An adult human kidney has about 1 million nephrons. The number of nephrons, determined at birth, is highly variable. It depends

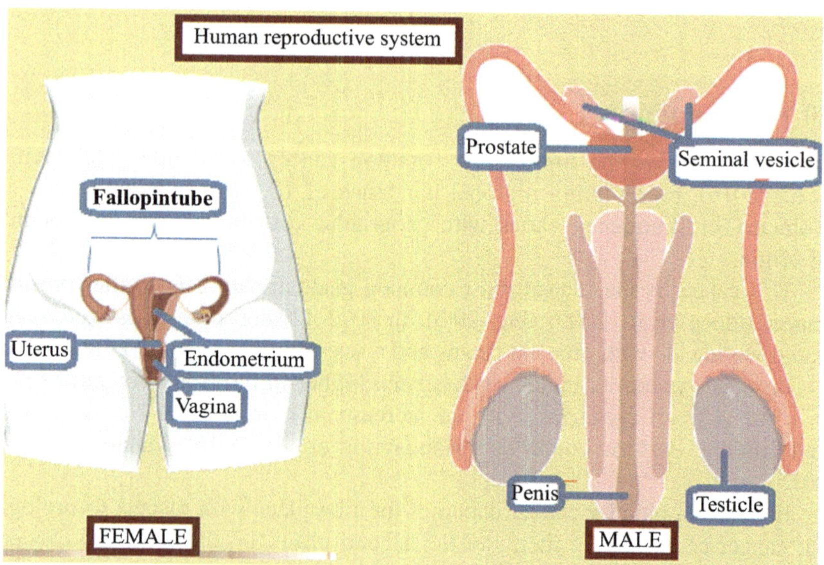

FIGURE 20.1 **Diagram illustrating the anatomy of the urogenital system in men and the location of the bladder in both sexes.**

on several factors including gestational age, intrauterine growth retardation, growth, and the nutritional status of the mother.

20.2.2 Urinary tract

They are composed of all the pipes through which urine passes between the kidneys and the external environment. When the urine leaves the kidney, it flows into a long channel called the ureter (Wu et al., 2009), which is about 25 cm in size and has a diameter between 3 and 5 mm. The urinary tract consists of two ureters, each of which connects a kidney to the bladder where the urine is collected (Rafnar et al., 2009).

20.2.3 Bladder

The bladder is a reservoir that collects urine, fed through the ureters and evacuated through the urethra. It is entirely located in the pelvic cavity when empty, behind the pubic symphysis, and protrudes 3 cm into the abdomen when full (Fig. 20.2).

From the outside, the bladder is composed of three faces: superior, anteroinferior, and posteroinferior (also known as the base). There are three edges: two lateral edges and one posterior edge placed at the union of the superior and posteroinferior faces. There are two lateral angles and an anterior angle called the apex of the bladder (Sylvester et al., 2006).

From the inside, three orifices can be distinguished: the urethral orifice (bladder neck), anterior and medial, and the two narrow and elliptical ureteral orifices. These three points define a triangular area: Lieutaud's bladder trigone (see Fig. 20.2).

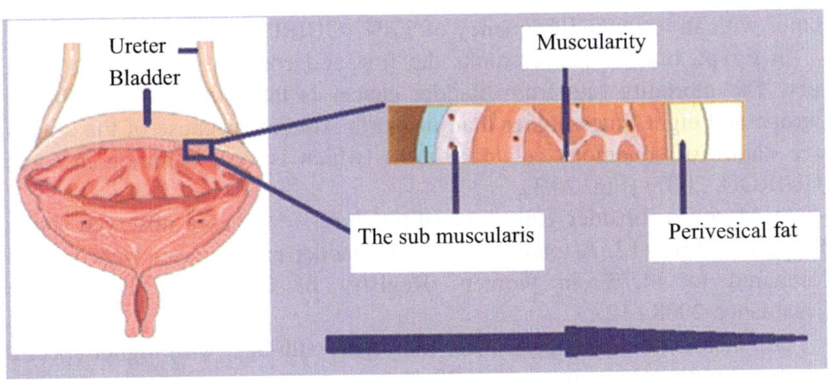

FIGURE 20.2 Diagram showing the different layers of the bladder wall.

20.3 Bladder cancer

Bladder cancer is a tumor that develops at the base of the bladder wall. It represents a multifactorial pathology that can be benign or evolve very quickly to a malignant tumor (Figueroa et al., 2015). It is considered one of the most common malignant cancers worldwide and is the most common cancer of the urinary excretory tract and the second most common cancer of the genitourinary tract after prostate cancer (Egger et al., 1997).

20.3.1 Epidemiology

Bladder tumors constitute 3%–4% of all types of cancer and are the second most common urologic tumor worldwide, next in frequency to prostate cancer in men (Stenzl et al., 2011).

There is a large geographical difference in the incidence rate of bladder cancer worldwide with the highest incidence in Eastern Europe, North Africa, the Middle East, and North America. The lowest incidence rate is found in Asia and underdeveloped regions of Africa (Louis et al., 2012).

In the European community, bladder cancer is the fourth leading cause of cancer in men. It is estimated to account for 4.1% of cancer deaths in men and 1.8% in women in Europe (Ferlay et al., 2008).

The development of transitional cell carcinoma constitutes over 90% of bladder cancers in Western countries, in contrast to North African countries, where the frequency of squamous cell carcinoma is greater (Stenzl et al., 2011).

In France, about 12,000 new bladder cancer cases were diagnosed in 2012 (fifth most frequent cancer) with 4772 deaths (fifth rank), of which 75% were in men. The average age of occurrence is 65 years. Its frequency is increased by about 1% per year, but its mortality rate remains constant among men and women (Rébillard et al., 2010).

In Burkina Faso, bladder tumors are the seventh most common malignant tumor with an estimated frequency of 3.8% (GUIROU, 2007).

In Egypt, bladder cancer ranks the first and constitutes 28% of all cancers. The mortality rate from bladder cancer is three times higher than in Europe and eight times higher than in North America because of the aggressive nature of squamous cell carcinoma, which is very common in Egypt (GUIROU, 2007) (Fig. 20.3).

In Morocco, bladder cancer constituted 3.1% of cases observed within the period 2008–12. A total of 85.3% of bladder cancer cases were in men, compared to 14.7% in women (Registry of Cancer in The Greater Casablanca 2008–12).

The incidence of bladder cancer increased with age, with higher specific rates in men than in women. (Fig. 20.4).

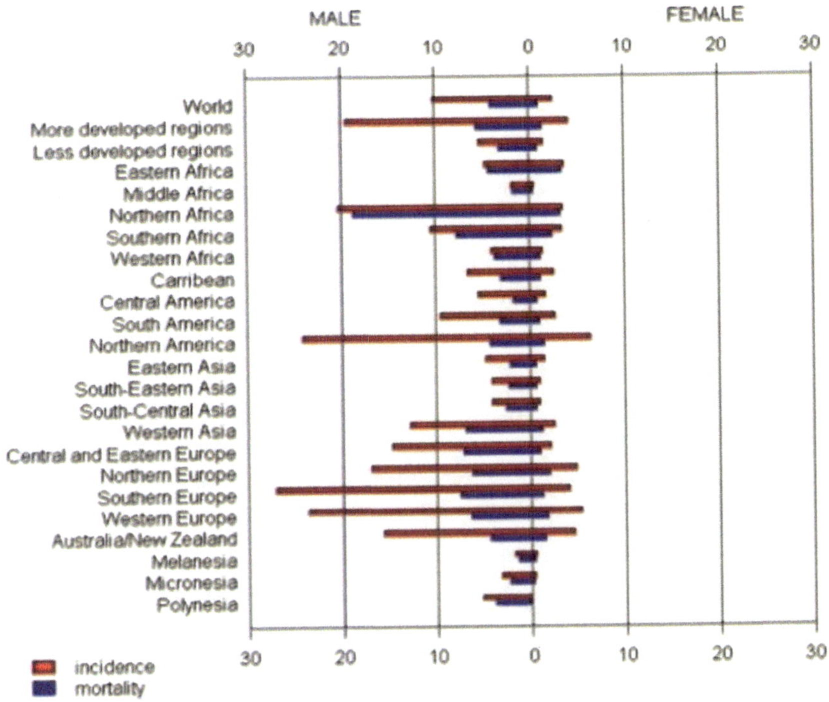

FIGURE 20.3 **Worldwide incidence of bladder cancer in both sexes (Ploeg et al., 2009).**

20.3.2 Risk factors for bladder cancer

A number of environmental factors have a carcinogenic role. However, the site of responsibility of one of these factors is generally difficult to establish on a daily basis, and some genetic factors are also involved, in addition to certain environmental factors (Coulange & Cs, 2003).

1. Tobacco is considered the most frequent risk factor. It is implicated in one in two cases in men and one in three cases in women (Coulange & Cs, 2003). The relative risk varies from two to five. Forty-three of the 3500 chemical compounds in tobacco are classified as carcinogens. It is directly implicated in 30%–40% of bladder tumors (Desgrandchamps, 1995).
2. Diabetes may be involved in bladder cancer through the risk of increased urinary tract infections.
3. Some professional uses are regarded as carcinogenic, for example, hydrocarbons, chlorinated water, aromatic amines, aluminum. Occupations at risk are found in the dyeing, rubber, tar, and metallurgy industries. Aromatic amines and their derivatives are considered an occupational risk factor for bladder cancer (Table 20.1).

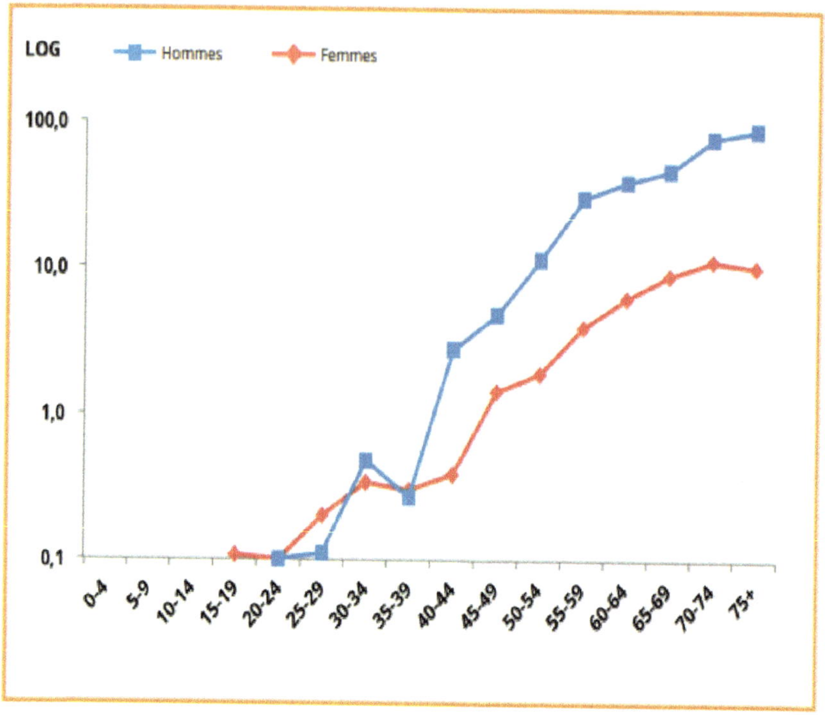

FIGURE 20.4 Gender-specific incidence rates of bladder cancer (Greater Casablanca Cancer Registry 2008–12).

Table 20.1 summarizes the different risk factors for bladder cancer known to date. (Coulange & Cs, 2003): Table 20.1 (Amaral et al., 2010; Coulange & Cs, 2003; Desgrandchamps, 1995; Egger et al., 1997; Ferlay et al., 2008; Figueroa et al., 2015; Goebell & Knowles, 2010; Guirou, 2007; Hamosh, 2016; Kavoussi et al., 2012; Kiemeney et al., 2008, 2010; Mahdavifar et al., 2016; Malats & Real, 2015; Morales & Pang, 1986; Neuzillet et al., 2012; Perret et al., 2013; Pfister et al., 2010; Ploeg et al., 2009; Rafnar et al., 2009; Rébillard et al., 2010; Stamatiou et al., 2009; Stenzl et al., 2011; Sylvester et al., 2006; Torre et al., 2012; Wu et al., 2009; Zhu et al., 2004).

20.3.3 The diagnosis

In case of a suspected tumor, it is currently recommended to perform several paraclinical examinations, enumerated as follows (Pfister et al., 2010):

1. urinary cytology, which allows the detection of tumor cells in the urine. Its particularities will be described later.

TABLE 20.1 The different risk factors for bladder cancer known to date (Coulange & Cs, 2003).

Agent involved	Carcinogenic effect	Mechanism of carcinogenesis	Involved agent documented
Practical exposures: aromatic amine industry Dye industry Rubber industry	Potantialization	Exposures to aromatic amines and other chemical carcinogens diesel and low hydration	Yes
Painting Leather industry aluminum industry machine operators	----------	---------	-----------
Drink intake	Potantialization	--------	-----------
Chlorite and arsenic water	----------	Direct carcinogenic action	Yes
Drugs: phenacetin cycloptiosphamide phanabarbita	Potantialization Prevenlion	-------- -------- --------	Yes Yes Yes
Idulcorents	Potantialization	Not known	Inadéquat

2. Ultrasound via the suprapubic route (sensitivity of detection of a bladder tumor).
3. particularly for polypoid tumors > 5 mm (Stamatiou et al., 2009).
4. venous endoscopy, which allows the number, size, topography and in particular the appearance of the lesions to be determined.
5. uroscanner to exclude an associated upper urinary tract lesion.

20.4 Six-molecular characterization of bladder tumors

The uncontrolled proliferation of urothelial cells seen in bladder cancer is usually the consequence of a combination of several factors: genetic, including chromosomal aberrations (deletions/duplications) and genetic alterations (point mutations), and epigenetic. Knowing that NMIT and TVIM are marked by different molecular modifications, it is essential in the molecular events that condition the mechanism of tumor progression to determine biological markers that can be used to establish not only prognostic markers but also diagnostic criteria and new targets for therapeutic action (Goebell & Knowles, 2010).

20.4.1 Point mutations

In this context, a large number of polymorphisms have been linked to bladder cancer. Among the oldest polymorphisms identified, we can mention mutations in the FGFR, P53, Rb1 genes, in particular FGFR3 genes of the EGFR family and genes of the RAS family. It has been established that 80% of Ta G1/G2 tumors are known to have mutations in RAS family genes (mainly HRAS and KRAS) and FGFR3 genes, exclusive of each other (65% for FGFR3 and 15% for RAS) (Goebell & Knowles, 2010).

20.4.1.1 RAS family genes

In tumor cells, mutations in the HRAS gene lead to a permanent activation of the HRAS protein, which causes a chain of phosphorylations leading to an increase in the rate of cell proliferation (Hamosh, 2016). Zhu et al. (2004) showed that mutations in the HRAS gene are present in 30%–40% of urothelial carcinomas.

20.4.1.2 The FGFR3 gene

FGFR3 activation is done by ligand binding, and it can also be constitutively active after mutation in some cancers. Approximately 70% of stage Ta (Ta –Non-invasive papillary carcinoma) bladder tumors have activator mutations in the FGFR3 gene compared to a frequency of 10%–20% in invasive tumors (Neuzillet et al., 2012). Fig. 20.5 shows the mutation frequencies of the FGFR3 and TP53 genes involved in the developmental pathways of urothelial tumors.

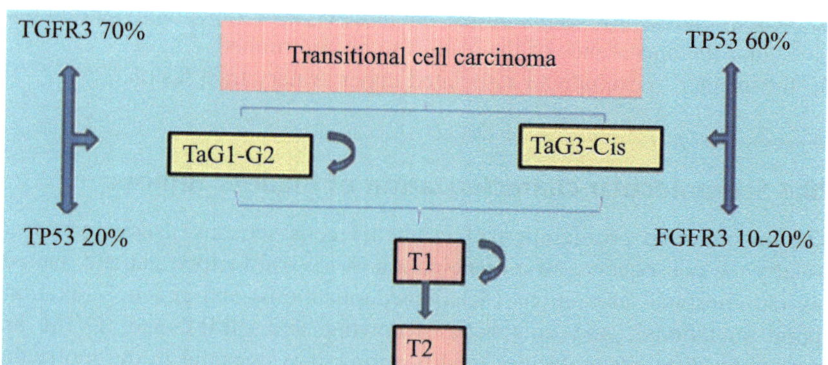

FIGURE 20.5 Frequencies of FGFR3 and TP53 gene mutations in the two pathways of bladder tumor progression (Neuzillet et al., 2012).

20.4.1.3 The p53 gene

This is a tumor suppressor gene that encodes a nuclear phosphoprotein of 393 amino acids and a molecular weight of 53 kilodaltons (kDa). This protein is a transcription factor that binds specifically to the regulatory domains of the genes it controls. It controls gene expression and is involved in the regulation of the cell cycle, differentiation, apoptosis, and maintenance of genome integrity (Amaral et al., 2010). Humans have only one functional p53 gene located on the short arm of chromosome 17.

The p53 protein is therefore stabilized and activated in response to various molecular stresses, including DNA damage, hypoxia, viral infections, and oncogene activation. It is modified in many posttranslational ways, which allow it to activate its functionality as a transcription factor (Amaral et al., 2010).

20.5 Chromosomal aberrations

TCGA also identified 2529 structural aberrations and over 1000 gene fusions including translocations that promote cancer development and proliferation. Thus the HER2 gene (involved in cell growth) was associated with translocations in several bladder tumors with different partners such as DIP2B, a gene involved in DNA methylation (Morales & Pang, 1986).

20.5.1 Epigenetic aberrations

Epigenetic modifications, including changes in DNA methylation, histone modification, and chromatin modification and remodeling have also been reported in bladder tumors. Thus 34% of tumors possess CpG islands, which contain hypermethylated tumor suppressor genes, inducing repression of these genes (Perret et al., 2013). A very large number of somatic mutations in chromatin remodeling genes have also been observed in urothelial carcinomas.

20.6 Conclusion

Bladder cancer is a major public health problem. On the effect site, it is the second source of mortality in men after lung cancer. And despite the many therapeutic approaches developed to fight this cancer, the frequency of recurrence is still high; the progression of the disease to a more aggressive stage is possible and often concludes with the death of the patient due to the reduced effectiveness of these treatments.

Acknowledgments

Authors would like to thank the Minister of National Education, Professional Training, Higher Education and Scientific Research and express gratitude to members of Virology, Oncology and Medical Biotechnology team at FSTM-Hassan II University of Casablanca, for all their efforts to support us during all stages of this research.

References

Amaral, J., Xavier, J., & Steer, C. J. (2010). The role of p53 in apoptosis. *Urologic Oncology, 9* (45), 409–428.

Coulange, C., & Cs (2003). Cancer De La Vessie.

Desgrandchamps, F. (1995). Epidémiologie Des Tumeurs Epithéliales De Vessie. Encyclopédie Médico-Chirurgicale.

Egger, M., Smith, G. D., Schneider, M., & Minder, C. (1997). Bias in meta-analysis detected by a simple, graphical test. *BMJ (Clinical Research ed.), 315*(7109), 629–634. Available from https://doi.org/10.1136/bmj.315.7109.629.

Ferlay, J., Randi, G., Bosetti, C., Levi, F., Negri, E., Boyle, P., & La Vecchia, C. (2008). Declining mortality from bladder cancer in Europe. *BJU International, 101*(1), 11–19. Available from https://doi.org/10.1111/j.1464-410X.2007.07239.x.

Figueroa, J. D., Koutros, S., & S, J. (2015). Modification of occupational exposures on bladder cancer risk by common genetic polymorphisms. *Journal of the National CancerInsti-Tute, 107.*

Goebell, P. J., & Knowles, M. A. (2010). Bladder cancer or bladder cancers? Genetically distinct malignant conditions of the urothelium. *Urologic Oncology: Seminars and Original Investigations, 28*(4), 409–428. Available from https://doi.org/10.1016/j.urolonc.2010.04.003.

Guirou. (2007). Prise En Charge Des Tumeurs Vésicales Dans Le Service D'urologie Du Chu Du Point G A Propos De 86 Cas.

Hamosh, A. (2016). Bladder cancer. Phenotype-Gene Relationships.

Kavoussi, L. R., Novick, A. C., Partin, A. W., & PETERS, C. A. (2012). Campbell-Walsh urology.

Kiemeney, L. A., Sulem, P., Besenbacher, S., Vermeulen, S. H., Sigurdsson, A., Thorleifsson, G., Gudbjartsson, D. F., Stacey, S. N., Gudmundsson, J., Zanon, C., Kostic, J., Masson, G., Bjarnason, H., Palsson, S. T., Skarphedinsson, O. B., Gudjonsson, S. A., Witjes, J. A., Grotenhuis, A. J., Verhaegh, G. W., & Stefansson, K. (2010). A sequence variant at 4p16.3 confers susceptibility to urinary bladder cancer. *Nature Genetics, 42*(5), 415–419. Available from https://doi.org/10.1038/ng.558.

Kiemeney, L. A., Thorlacius, S., Sulem, P., Geller, F., Aben, K. K. H., Stacey, S. N., Gudmundsson, J., Jakobsdottir, M., Bergthorsson, J. T., Sigurdsson, A., Blondal, T., Witjes, J. A., Vermeulen, S. H., Hulsbergen-Van De Kaa, C. A., Swinkels, D. W., Ploeg, M., Cornel, E. B., Vergunst, H., Thorgeirsson, T. E., & Stefansson, K. (2008). Sequence variant on 8q24 confers susceptibility to urinary bladder cancer. *Nature Genetics, 40*(11), 1307–1312. Available from https://doi.org/10.1038/ng.229.

Louis, E., Mary, J. Y., Vernier–Massouille, G., Grimaud, J. C., Bouhnik, Y., Laharie, D., & Groupe D'etudes Thérapeutiques Des Affections Inflammatoires, Digestives. (2012). Maintenance of remission among patients with Crohn's disease on antimetabolite therapy after infliximab therapy is stopped. *Gastroenterology, 142*(1), 63–70.

Mahdavifar, N., Ghoncheh, M., Pakzad, R., Momenimovahed, Z., & Salehiniya, H. (2016). Epidemiology, incidence and mortality of bladder cancer and their relationship with the development index in the world. *Asian Pacific Journal of Cancer Prevention, 17*(1), 381–386. Available from https://doi.org/10.7314/APJCP.2016.17.1.381.

Malats, N., & Real, F. X. (2015). Epidemiology of bladder cancer. *Hematology/Oncology Clinics of North America, 29*(2), 177–189. Available from https://doi.org/10.1016/j.hoc.2014.10.001.

Morales, A., & Pang, A. S. D. (1986). Prophylaxis and therapy of an experimental bladder cancer with biological response modifiers. *Journal of Urology, 135*(1), 191–193. Available from https://doi.org/10.1016/S0022-5347(17)45560-1.

Neuzillet, Y., Paoletti, X., Ouerhani, S., Mongiat-Artus, P., Soliman, H., de The, H., Sibony, M., Denoux, Y., Molinie, V., Herault, A., Lepage, M. L., Maille, P., Renou, A., Vordos, D., Abbou, C. C., Bakkar, A., Asselain, B., Kourda, N., El Gaaied, A., ... Radvanyi, F. (2012). A meta-analysis of the relationship between FGFR3 and TP53 mutations in bladder cancer. *PLoS One, 7*(12). Available from https://doi.org/10.1371/journal.pone.0048993.

Perret, R., Sierro, S. R., Botelho, N. K., Corgnac, S., Donda, A., & Romero, P. (2013). Adjuvants that improve the ratio of antigen-specific effector to regulatory T cells enhance tumor immunity. *Cancer Research, 73*(22), 6597–6608. Available from https://doi.org/10.1158/0008-5472.CAN-13-0875.

Pfister, C., Roupret, M., & Wallerand, H. (2010). Oncology commitee of the french association of urology recommendations onco-urology: Urothelial tumors. *Progres en Urologie: Journal de l'Association Francaise d'urologie et de la Societe Francaise d'urologie, 4*, 255–274.

Ploeg, M., Aben, K. K. H., & Kiemeney, L. A. (2009). The present and future burden of urinary bladder cancer in the world. *World Journal of Urology, 27*(3), 289–293. Available from https://doi.org/10.1007/s00345-009-0383-3.

Rafnar, T., Sulem, P., Stacey, S. N., Geller, F., Gudmundsson, J., Sigurdsson, A., Jakobsdottir, M., Helgadottir, H., Thorlacius, S., Aben, K. K. H., Blöndal, T., Thorgeirsson, T. E., Thorleifsson, G., Kristjansson, K., Thorisdottir, K., Ragnarsson, R., Sigurgeirsson, B., Skuladottir, H., Gudbjartsson, T., & Stefansson, K. (2009). Sequence variants at the TERT-CLPTM1L locus associate with many cancer types. *Nature Genetics, 41*(2), 221–227. Available from https://doi.org/10.1038/ng.296.

Rébillard, X., Grosclaude, P., Lebret, T., Patard, J.-J., Pfister, C., Richaud, P., Rigaud, J., Salomon, L., & Soulié, M. (2010). Projection de l'incidence et de la mortalité par cancer urologique en France en 2010. *Progrès En Urologie*, S211–S214. Available from https://doi.org/10.1016/s1166-7087(10)70041-5.

Stamatiou, K., Papadoliopoulos, I., Dahanis, S., Zafiropoulos, G., & Polizois, K. (2009). The accuracy of ultrasonography in the diagnosis of superficial bladder tumors in patients presenting with hematuria. *Annals of Saudi Medicine, 29*(2), 134–137. Available from https://doi.org/10.4103/0256-4947.51802.

Stenzl, A, Witfies, J. A., Cowan, N. (2011). Guideline on bladder cancer muscle invasive and metastatic. European Association of urologie.

Sylvester, R. J., Van Der Meijden, A. P. M., Oosterlinck, W., Witjes, J. A., Bouffioux, C., Denis, L., Newling, D. W. W., & Kurth, K. (2006). Predicting recurrence and progression in individual patients with stage Ta T1 bladder cancer using EORTC risk tables: A combined analysis of 2596 patients from seven EORTC trials. *European Urology, 49*(3), 466–477. Available from https://doi.org/10.1016/j.eururo.2005.12.031.

Torre, L. A., Bray, F., Siegel, F., Ferly, R. L., Lortet-Tieulent, J., & Jemal. (2012). Global cancer statistics. *CA: A Cancer Journal for Clinicians, 65*, 87–108.

Wu, X., Ye, Y., Kiemeney, L. A., Sulem, P., Rafnar, T., Matullo, G., Seminara, D., Yoshida, T., Saeki, N., Andrew, A. S., Dinney, C. P., Czerniak, B., Zhang, Z. F., Kiltie, A. E., Bishop, D. T., Vineis, P., Porru, S., Buntinx, F., Kellen, E., & Gu, J. (2009). Genetic variation in the prostate stem cell antigen gene PSCA confers susceptibility to urinary bladder cancer. *Nature Genetics*, *41*(9), 991–995. Available from https://doi.org/10.1038/ng.421.

Zhu, D., Xing, D., Shen, X., & Liu, J. (2004). A method to quantitatively detect H-ras point mutation based on electrochemiluminescence. *Biochemical and Biophysical Research Communications*, *324*(2), 964–969. Available from https://doi.org/10.1016/j.bbrc.2004.09.121.

Chapter 21

Impact of signaling in the development pathway of genitourinary cancers

Ikram Tiabi[2], Kaoutar Anouar Tadlaoui[2], Youssef Ennaji[2], Soukayna Alaoui Sosse[2], Yassine Kasmi[2], Imane Saif[2], Mohammed Nabil Benchekroun[1] and Moulay Mustapha Ennaji[1]

[1]Group Leader Research team of Virology, Oncology, and Biotechnologies, Head of Laboratory of Virology, Oncology, Biosciences, Environment and New Energies (LVO-BEEN), Faculty of Sciences and Techniques Mohammedia, University Hassan II of Casablanca, Casablanca, Morocco, [2]Team of Virology, Oncology, and Biotechnologies, Laboratory of Virology, Oncology, Biosciences, Environment and New Energies (LVO-BEEN), Faculty of Sciences and Techniques Mohammedia, University Hassan II of Casablanca, Casablanca, Morocco

21.1 Introduction

Cellular signaling refers to all the communication channels established between cells. This signaling leads in the cell that receives a message from another cell, to the realization of different actions, direct or indirect, including the transcription of genes allowing the execution of the received orders. The signals exchanged mainly concern reproduction and differentiation, adhesion and motility, survival and death. Thanks to multiple genetic or epigenetic mechanisms, the cancer cell can take advantage of this signaling, divert it from its purpose, and use the same to multiply, migrate, and survive (Robert, 2010a,b,c).

The signaling provided by growth factors is certainly the best known, in particular because of its role in oncogenesis (Centenera et al., 2008).

Indeed, this signalling opens multiple pathways; the latter is entirely devoted to growth factors and their receptors; the main signaling pathways that are activated downstream of the interaction of a growth factor and a receptor. Growth factors and their receptors are divided into different categories because of the mode of activation of the latter. The most important category is that of receptors with tyrosine kinase activity (RTK); a second class is that of receptors that activate a cytoplasmic tyrosine kinase, and a last class is that of receptors with serine/threonine kinase activity (Spiegel et al., 1998).

Immunological Implications and Molecular Diagnostics of Genitourinary Cancer.
DOI: https://doi.org/10.1016/B978-0-323-85496-2.00010-5

21.2 General principles of cell signaling

Cellular communication is a fundamental element in the life of multicellular organisms. Cells are required to exchange the information necessary to carry out their actions. However, this communication is already present in single-celled organisms, such as yeast, which must also exchange data, only to find sexual partners. The basis of cellular communication is therefore universal. Signaling molecules are transmitted by one cell, recognized by another, which then sets up a transduction pathway for the signal received, which leads to an effector system that takes the signal into account. The diversity of the transduction systems of this information is extremely important, both at the level of signal transmission and at the level of effector activation. However, it is certainly possible to discover global patterns, that is, common structures of information, if one makes an effort to look for them (Robert, 2010a,b,c).

21.3 Impact of androgen receptor alterations on signaling pathways related to cell differentiation and prostate cancer progression

21.3.1 Androgen receptor

21.3.1.1 Genomic signaling pathway of the androgen receptor

Androgens are male sex hormones that belong to the steroid hormone family. They are important in the development and maintenance of male characteristics of reproductive tissues (maintenance of secondary sexual characteristics and development and maintenance of fertility) (Handelsman, 2010).

The most important circulating androgen in mammals is testosterone. The vast majority of testosterone is synthesized in the testes by the Leydig cells from cholesterol. It is also formed in smaller proportions by androstenedione and dehydroepiandrosterone (DHEA), which is secreted by the adrenal glands. Testosterone biosynthesis involves a series of enzymatic reactions (Yin & Hu, 2014).

In the absence of ligand, the androgen receptor (AR) is located in the cytoplasm, where it is complexed to chaperone proteins such as HSP70 and HSP90, as well as to heat shock proteins and proteins.

Together these proteins maintain the receptor in a conformationally favorable state for ligand binding. Binding of dihydrotestosterone (DHT) results in a conformational change of the ligand-binding domain (LBD), which promotes dissociation of the receptor from its chaperone proteins.

The receptor then presumably homodimerizes through LBD and is phosphorylated at serine residues, including serine S81 (Koryakina et al., 2014).

In addition, and following ligand binding, unmasking of the Nuclear localization signals (NLS) ensues, along with transfer of the receptor into the nucleus of the organism (Bennett et al., 2010; Li & Al-Azzawi, 2009).

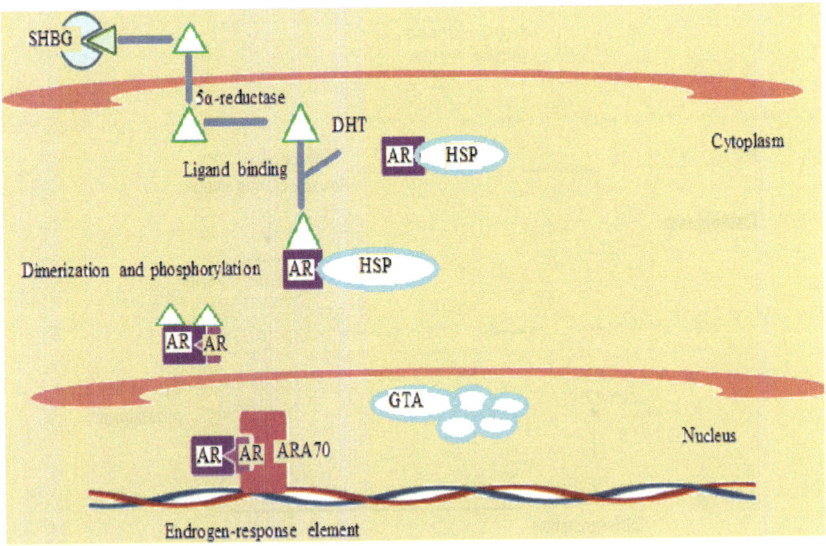

FIGURE 21.1 Genomic signaling pathway of the androgen receptor.

Once in the nucleus, each AR binds to a half-site of the existing AREs in the DNA and then dimerization occurs through the D-boxes present in the second zinc of the DNA-binding domain (DBD) (Fig. 21.1) (Centenera et al., 2008).

21.4 Oncogenic alterations

21.4.1 Sphingosine kinase 1/sphingosine 1-phosphate

21.4.1.1 The sphingosine kinase 1/sphingosine 1-phosphate signaling pathway

Sphingolipids are very complex lipids, isolated and mentioned in 1884 by JLW Thudichum. They are constituents of biological membranes and are formed from a common sphingoid base, sphinganine, which is a long carbon chain alcohol resulting from the condensation of a palmitic fatty acid (C16) and a serine. Sphingosine is the most abundant derivative of sphingolipids. It is found in 90% of sphingolipids in animals, while phytosphingosine (4-hydroxysphinganine) is the largest form in plants (Spiegel et al., 1998).

The production of sphingolipid compounds can be performed de novo through the condensation of a fatty acid (palmitic acid) and a serine, followed by the degradation of membrane sphingomyelins as a result of glycosphingolipid degradation. Sphingolipids are irreversibly degraded to phosphoethanolamine and hexadecenal. For a long time, sphingolipids were perceived as simple constituents of the plasma membrane and could be employed as plasma

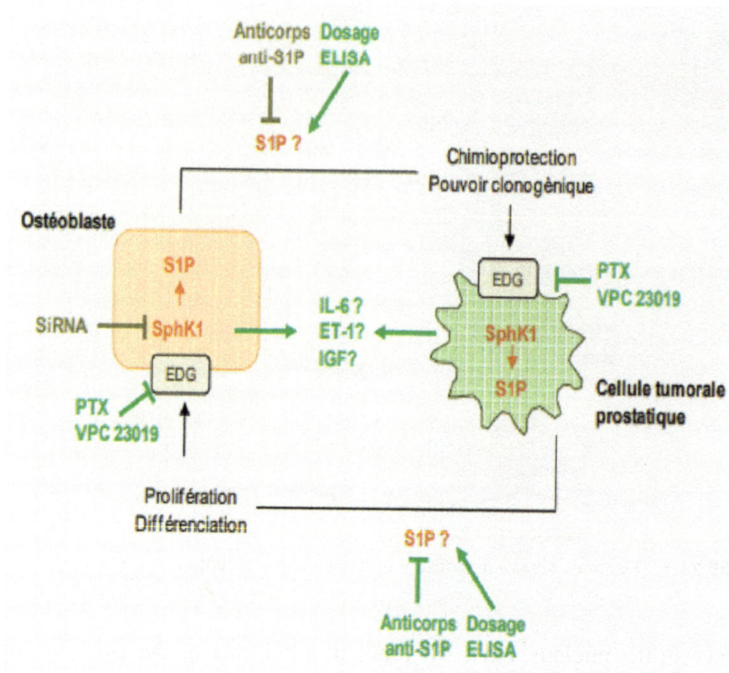

FIGURE 21.2 The paracrine dialog between osteoblast and prostate cell (Martin, 2009).

membrane that can be used as substrate for β-oxidation and glycolysis. However, studies in the last two decades have shown that they cause major biological effects in a number of biological processes (Xia et al., 2000).

Ceramide, sphingosine, and sphingosine 1-phosphate are identified as mediators involved in the regulation of proliferation, apoptosis/survival, cell migration, senescence, and inflammatory phenomena (Cuvillier et al., 1996).

An interaction has been reported to occur between the osteoblast and the prostate cells (Martin, 2009). There is a paracrine communication from the tumor cell to the osteoblast (proliferation and differentiation), and reciprocally, the osteoblast is also able to modulate the chemosensitivity and clonogenic capacity of the prostate tumor cells (Fig. 21.2).

21.5 Oncogenic alterations

21.5.1 Bone metastases of prostate cancer

Metastases are a frequent consequence of certain cancers. They result from the penetration of a tissue or an organ by tumor cells after their diffusion from the starting site. They constitute about 98% of malignant bone tumors. Bone is the preferred site for metastasis in the three most common human cancers, namely, lung, breast, and prostate. Bone metastases develop in

TABLE 21.1 Incidence of bone metastases in postmortem examinations of various cancers. (Coleman & Rubens, 1987).

Primary tumour	Incidence of bone metastases (%)
Breast	73
Prostate	68
Thyroid	42
Kidney	35
Lung	36
Tractus gastro-intestinal	5

15%–30% of people with lung carcinoma and in over 70% of advanced breast and prostate cancers (Table 21.1). It has been reported that 350,000 people die from the consequences of bone metastases each year in the United States (Coleman & Rubens, 1987; Mundy, 2002).

21.6 Growth factor signaling pathway

There are a few hundred growth factors that can activate an RTK and a few dozen receptors that can recognize them. These are grouped into families of corresponding homologous proteins.

The growth factors of the epidermal growth factor (EGF) family act with the receptors of the EGF family and interfere with those receptors (Robert, 2010a,b,c).

The terms "epidermal" or "fibroblastic" growth factors are more related to the circumstances of their discovery than to a specificity of the target tissue. Epithelial tissues can express epidermal growth factor receptors, whereas nonepithelial tissues can express fibroblastic growth factor receptors. (Beenken & Mohammadi, 2009).

Table 21.2 enumerates some of the major families of growth factors and their receptors. There are nearly 60 RTKs divided into about 20 families, and the number of growth factors that correspond to them is much larger. The associated growth factors are much more important. All RTKs have a single transmembrane domain, a homologous intracellular part that ensures the catalytic activity, and another extracellular part that completely varies from one family to another (Harris et al., 2003).

Among the best known signaling systems are the growth factor model and RTK activity (Fig. 21.3). A molecular protein, emitted by a cell, identifies a receptor located in the membrane of another cell. A conformational modification leads to the dimerization of the receptor, its autophosphorylation, and the activation of a signal transduction system that involves, according to different pathways, a cascade of kinases generally leading to the activation of

TABLE 21.2 The main families of growth factor receptors (Beenken & Mohammadi, 2009).

Families	Receptors	Ligands
EGF receptors	EGFR ERBB2 ERBB3 ERBB	EGF TGFα HBEGF Epigene (EPGN) Epirgulin (EREG) Betacellulin (BTC) Amphiregulin (AREG) Neuregulins 1 to 4 (NRG1-4)
FGF receptors	FGFR1 FGFR2 FGFR3 FGFR4	FGF1 to FGF10 FGF15 to FGF23
VEGF receptors	FLT1 (VEGFR1) KDR (VEGFR2) FLT4 (VEGFR3)	VEGFA to VEGFD
PDGF receptors and related receptors	PDGFRα PDGFRβ KIT FLT3 CSF1R	PDGFA to PDGFD SCF/KITLG FLT3LG CSF1
Insulin receptors	INSR IGF1R [IGF2R] INSRR	Insulin IGF1 IGF2
Angiopoietin receptors	TIE1 TEK (TIE2)	ANGPT1–4

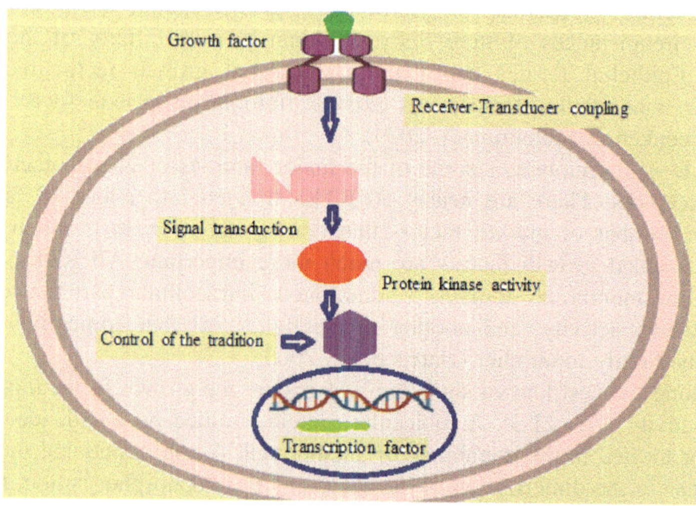

FIGURE 21.3 The receptor model with tyrosine kinase activity. The signal (growth factor).

transcription factors, and sometimes to the activation of those stimulating translation (Suteau et al., 2020).

The signal (growth factor) is identified at the membrane by an RTK. The receptor is split in two after a conformational change related to ligand binding and is susceptible to autophosphorylation on tyrosine residues. Following a series of events that promote coupling between the activated receptor and transducers, a series of kinases organized in a cascade leads to the activation of transcription factors and/or translation factors that allow the cell to present the proteins necessary to take up the message received (Robert, 2010a,b,c).

21.7 Oncogenic alterations

Mutations or overexpression of growth factors may have an essential role in oncogenesis, but the essential role of molecular alterations of growth factors in oncogenesis has been rarely established. Germline inactivating mutations in growth factors are indeed responsible for various cancers. On the other hand, germline growth factor inactivating mutations are the cause of several hereditary diseases, including dwarfism. At the level of growth factor receptors, many alterations are observed in cancers, and it is at this level that the greatest number of proto-oncogenes are observed. We will indicate the main alterations as we present the families of receptors, without being exhaustive (Ciardiello & Tortora, 2008).

21.7.1 Phosphatidylinositol-3-kinase

21.7.1.1 Phosphatidylinositol-3-kinase signaling pathway

Phosphoinositide 3-kinases (PI3Ks) are part of a conserved family of lipid kinases that phosphorylate proteins in the body and 30-hydroxyl group of phosphoinositides. The most commonly characterized product of this reaction is phosphatidylinositol-3,4,5-trisphosphate, or PIP3, an essential second messenger that recruits AKT to activate growth, proliferation, and survival mechanisms (Cantley, 2002). PIP3 is negatively controlled by dephosphorylation by the tumor suppressor phosphatase and tensin homolog (PTEN). PIP3 production is a feature of PI3K subclass I, which can be subdivided into class IA and class IB. To date, only class IA PI3Ks have been implicated in human cancer. In human cancer, common genetic alterations in these enzymes and their pathways have been found. These enzymes and their effectors have made the PI3K pathway one of the most frequently dysregulated pathways in cancer. Currently, a significant effort is being made to develop pan- and isoform-specific PI3K inhibitors for the treatment of cancer (Barault et al., 2008).

Interactions of p85 through its SH2 domain on a phosphorylated tyrosine receptor, an adaptor receptor, or an anchor protein, underlie the recruitment

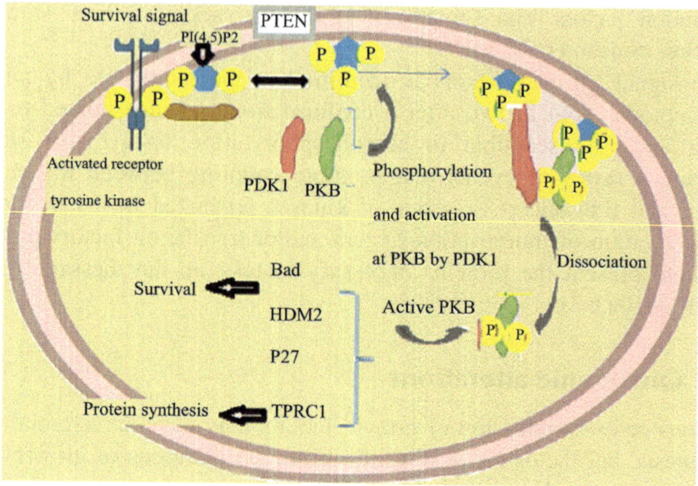

FIGURE 21.4 PI3K/AKT signaling pathway.

of p110 to the membrane where it meets its of its substrates. The most classical pathway activated downstream of PI3K is the AKT pathway (Yuzawa et al., 2007). The generation site of PIP3 leads to the recruitment of PH domain signaling proteins such as PDK1, mTORc1, and AKT. The serine/threonine kinases PDK1 and mTORc1 phosphorylate AKT at its serine 473 and threonine 308 (Yuzawa et al., 2007), resulting in full activation of the serine/threonine kinase AKT. The PI3K/AKT pathway has a major role in cell survival and metabolism (Mol et al., 2003).

The binding of a growth factor to its RTK leads to its activation through autophosphorylation by triggering a PI-3-Kinase (PI3K). The latter transmits to the membranes PIP2 and PIP3, and the reversible reaction is carried out by the phosphatase PTEN. The creation of PIP3 by PI3K leads to the recruitment of the pleckstrin domain proteins AKT/PKB and PDK1 to the membrane. PDK1 is phosphorylated and in turn phosphorylates AKT/PKB (Fig. 21.4), resulting in its activation. AKT/PKB dissociates from the membrane and stimulates its cytosolic and nuclear targets via phosphorylation. These targets then lead to an amplification of protein synthesis and survival signals that allow cell growth (adapted from Alberts et al., 2002).

21.8 Oncogenic alterations

The PI3K pathway is unique in that all major components of this pathway have been identified as mutated or amplified in a large number of cancers. Therefore, a very large number of tumor types are likely to benefit from the

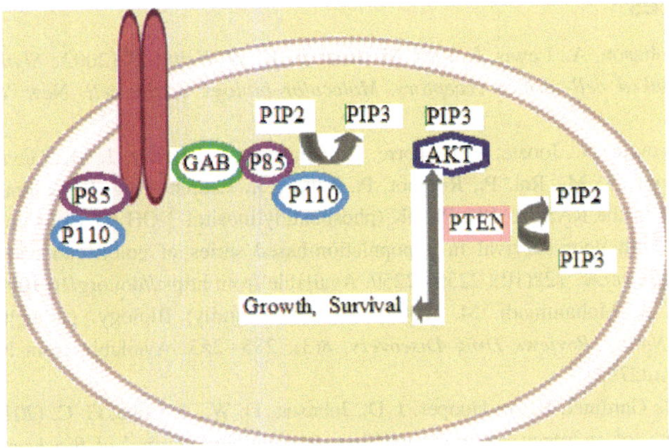

FIGURE 21.5 The PI3K signaling axis.

development of PI3K inhibitors. The mechanism of PI3K signaling in cancer begins with the engagement of growth factors by RTKs (Fig. 21.5). PI3K is then attracted to receptors anchored in the plasma membrane. It is then activated and phosphorylates PIP2 to produce PIP3. Through its pleckstrin (PH) homology domain, the nodal kinase AKT (also known as PKB) links to PIP3, where it is activated by two phosphorylation events and triggers a complex cascade of signals that control growth, proliferation, survival, and motility, and counteracts this process by dephosphorylating PIP3 to prevent AKT activation. Unlike any other major signaling pathway in the cell, each member of this signaling axis is frequently altered in cancer (Yuan & Cantley, 2008).

21.9 Conclusion

Over the past two decades, the development of targeted therapies has led to a substantial increase in the management and cure of cancers. The knowledge of the processes of carcinogenesis mechanisms has revealed the key role of molecular modifications leading to the activation of oncogenes such as the disease genes Ras, EGFR, KIT, and HER2 in the development, multiplication, and survival of tumors. This has led to the development of therapeutic strategies to prevent these oncogenes, using, for example, new chemical molecules or antibodies that have shown their effectiveness in the treatment of certain cancers such as breast cancer, bronchial cancer, or chronic myeloma.

21.10 Acknowledgments

Authors would like to thank the Ministry of National Education, Professional Training, Higher Education and Scientific Research and express gratitude to the members of Virology, Oncology and Medical Biotechnology team at FSTM-Hassan II University of Casablanca, for all their efforts and support during all work stages of this research.

References

Alberts, B., Johnson, A., Lewis, J., Raff, M., Roberts, K., & Walter, P. (2002). *Signaling through enzyme-linked cell-surface receptors. Molecular biology of the cell.* New York: Garland Science.

Barault, L., Veyrie, N., Jooste, V., Lecorre, D., Chapusot, C., Ferraz, J. M., Lièvre, A., Cortet, M., Bouvier, A. M., Rat, P., Roignot, P., Faivre, J., Laurent-Puig, P., & Piard, F. (2008). Mutations in the RAS-MAPK, PI(3)K (phosphatidylinositol-3-OH kinase) signaling network correlate with poor survival in a population-based series of colon cancers. *International Journal of Cancer*, *122*(10), 2255–2259. Available from https://doi.org/10.1002/ijc.23388.

Beenken, A., & Mohammadi, M. (2009). The FGF family: Biology, pathophysiology and therapy. *Nature Reviews Drug Discovery*, *8*(3), 235–253. Available from https://doi.org/10.1038/nrd2792.

Bennett, N. C., Gardiner, R. A., Hooper, J. D., Johnson, D. W., & Gobe, G. C. (2010). Molecular cell biology of androgen receptor signalling. *International Journal of Biochemistry and Cell Biology*, *42*(6), 813–827. Available from https://doi.org/10.1016/j.biocel.2009.11.013.

Cantley, L. C. (2002). The phosphoinositide 3-kinase pathway. *Science*, *296*(5573), 1655–1657. Available from https://doi.org/10.1126/science.296.5573.1655.

Centenera, M. M., Harris, J. M., Tilley, W. D., & Butler, L. M. (2008). The contribution of different androgen receptor domains to receptor dimerization and signaling. *Molecular Endocrinology*, *22*(11), 2373–2382. Available from https://doi.org/10.1210/me.2008-0017.

Ciardiello, F., & Tortora, G. (2008). EGFR antagonists in cancer treatment. *New England Journal of Medicine*, 1160–1174. Available from https://doi.org/10.1056/nejmra0707704.

Coleman, R. E., & Rubens, R. D. (1987). The clinical course of bone metastases from breast cancer. *British Journal of Cancer*, *55*(1), 61–66. Available from https://doi.org/10.1038/bjc.1987.13.

Cuvillier, O., Pirianov, G., Kleuser, B., Vanek, P. G., Cosot, O. A., Gutkind, J. S., & Spiegel, S. (1996). Suppression of ceramide-mediated programmed cell death by sphingosine- 1-phosphate. *Nature*, *381*(6585), 800–803. Available from https://doi.org/10.1038/381800a0.

Handelsman, D. J. (2010). *Androgen physiology, pharmacology, and abuse* (pp. 2469–2498). Elsevier BV. Available from https://doi.org/10.1016/b978-1-4160-5583-9.00137-4.

Harris, R. C., Chung, E., & Coffey, R. J. (2003). EGF receptor ligands. *Experimental Cell Research*, *284*(1), 2–13. Available from https://doi.org/10.1016/S0014-4827(02)00105-2.

Koryakina, Y., Ta, H. Q., & Gioeli, D. (2014). Androgen receptor phosphorylation: Biological context and bifunctional consequences. *Endocrine-Related Cancer*, *21*(4), T131–T145.

Li, J., & Al-Azzawi, F. (2009). Mechanism of androgen receptor action. *Maturitas*, *63*(2), 142–148. Available from https://doi.org/10.1016/j.maturitas.2009.03.008.

Martin, C. (2009). *Rôle de la signalisation sphingosine kinase-1 sphingosine 1-phosphate dans les interactions stroma-cellules épithéliales au sein des métastases osseuses du cancer de la prostate* (Doctoral dissertation).

Mol, C. D., Lim, K. B., Sridhar, V., Zou, H., Chien, E. Y. T., Sang, B. C., Nowakowski, J., Kassel, D. B., Cronin, C. N., & McRee, D. E. (2003). Structure of a c-Kit product complex reveals the basis for kinase transactivation. *Journal of Biological Chemistry*, *278*(34), 31461–31464. Available from https://doi.org/10.1074/jbc.C300186200.

Mundy, G. R. (2002). Metastasis to bone: Causes, consequences and therapeutic opportunities. *Nature Reviews Cancer*, *2*(8), 584–593. Available from https://doi.org/10.1038/nrc867.

Robert, J. (2010a). *Introduction Principes généraux de la signalisation cellulaire. Signalisation cellulaire et cancer. Oncologie pratique* (pp. 15–19). Paris: Springer.

Robert, J. (2010b). *Les facteurs de croissance et les récepteurs à activité tyrosine kinase. Signalisation cellulaire et cancer. Oncologie pratique* (pp. 21–43). Paris: Springer.

Robert, J. (2010c). Signalisation cellulaire et cancer. *Bulletin du Cancer*, *97*(11), 1215–1222. Available from https://doi.org/10.1684/bdc.2010.1199.

Spiegel, S., Cuvillier, O., Edsall, L., Kohama, T., Menzeleev, R., Olivera, A., Thomas, D., Tu, Z., Van Brooklyn, J., & Wang, F. (1998). Roles of sphingosine-1-phosphate in cell growth, differentiation, and death. *Biochemistry (Moscow)*, *63*(1), 69–73.

Suteau, V., Seegers, V., Munier, M., Rousselet, M. C., Hamy, A., Rodien, P., & Briet, C. (2020). Les récepteurs couplés aux protéines G comme potentielles cibles dans le cancer thyroïdien réfractaire. *Annales d'Endocrinologie*, 145. Available from https://doi.org/10.1016/j.ando.2020.07.054.

Xia, P., Gamble, J. R., Wang, L., Pitson, S. M., Moretti, P. A. B., Wattenberg, B. W., D'Andrea, R. J., & Vadas, M. A. (2000). An oncogenic role of sphingosine kinase. *Current Biology*, *10*(23), 1527–1530. Available from https://doi.org/10.1016/S0960-9822(00)00834-4.

Yin, L., & Hu, Q. (2014). CYP17 inhibitors—abiraterone, C17, 20-lyase inhibitors and multi-targeting agents. *Nature Reviews Urology*, *11*(1).

Yuan, T. L., & Cantley, L. C. (2008). PI3K pathway alterations in cancer: Variations on a theme. *Oncogene*, *27*(41), 5497–5510. Available from https://doi.org/10.1038/onc.2008.245.

Yuzawa, S., Opatowsky, Y., Zhang, Z., Mandiyan, V., Lax, I., & Schlessinger, J. (2007). Structural basis for activation of the receptor tyrosine kinase KIT by stem cell factor. *Cell*, *130*(2), 323–334. Available from https://doi.org/10.1016/j.cell.2007.05.055.

Chapter 22

Prostate cancer: genetic changes and viral-mediated immune regulation

Soukayna Alaoui Sosse[5], Berjas Abumsimir[5,6], Ihsane Ali Mahasneh[2,3], Mohammed Mrabti[3], Abdelilah Laraqui[4] and Moulay Mustapha Ennaji[1]

[1]Group Leader Research team of Virology, Oncology, and Biotechnologies, Head of Laboratory of Virology, Oncology, Biosciences, Environment and New Energies (LVO-BEEN), Faculty of Sciences and Techniques Mohammedia, University Hassan II of Casablanca, Casablanca, Morocco, [2]Department of Biotechnology, Faculty of Science, Univeristy of Sharjah, Sharjah, United Arab Emirates, [3]Research and Biosafety Laboratory, Mohammed V Military Teaching Hospital, Laboratory of Human Pathologies Biology, Faculty of Sciences, and Genomic Center of Human Pathologies, Faculty of Medicine and Pharmacy, Mohammed V University, Rabat, Morocco, [4]Laboratory of Human Pathologies Biology, Faculty of Sciences, and Genomic Center of Human Pathologies, Faculty of Medicine and Pharmacy, Bio-Path Laboratory, Faculty of sciences-Agdal, Mohammed V University, Rabat, Morocco, [5]Team of Virology, Oncology, and Biotechnologies, Laboratory of Virology, Oncology, Biosciences, Environment and New Energies (LVO-BEEN), Faculty of Sciences and Techniques Mohammedia, University Hassan II of Casablanca, Casablanca, Morocco, [6]Pharmacological and Diagnostic Research Centre (PDRC), Department of Medical Laboratory Sciences, Faculty of Allied Medical Sciences, Al-Ahliyya Amman University (AAU), Amman, Jordan

22.1 Introduction

Prostate cancer (PCa) is a public health problem mostly reported in developed countries. It is the fifth most common cause of male tumors of all ages in the world and the second most common cause of cancer death in men. Its annual incidence is constantly increasing: a man born in 1940 had a 0.7% risk of developing prostate cancer, while a man born in 1910 had a risk of only 2.7%. Thus this cancer is characterized in Moroccan regions by a diagnosis most often late, at a locally advanced or metastatic stage. This delay in diagnosis is linked, among other things, to the lack of screening, the low awareness of the medical population regarding this pathology, and the difficulties of access to healthcare.

The pathogenesis of PCa involves both hereditary and environmental factors. The molecular events involved in the development or progression of PCa are still unclear. A recent body of literature highlights the role of viral infections in the

Immunological Implications and Molecular Diagnostics of Genitourinary Cancer.
DOI: https://doi.org/10.1016/B978-0-323-85496-2.00020-8

initiation or progression of PCa. In this regard, it has been reported that certain viruses interact with host proteins and cause changes in genetic, immunological, and inflammatory events that lead to the initiation or progression of PCa

In this chapter, we focus specifically on the possible viral etiology of PCa and the evidence for viral-mediated genetic changes and associated immune dysregulation.

22.2 Epidemiology of prostate cancer

According to the statistics reported by the International Agency for Research on Cancer, nearly 680,000 PCas were diagnosed worldwide in 2002. It is the second most common cancer among men. The incidence rate standardized to the world population is 25.3/100,000. The US and Northern Europe have the highest incidence rate. In the United States, more than 230,000 new cases of PCa were diagnosed in 2004 (Crawford, 2003).

A US study suggested that a 50-year-old man had a 42% risk of developing histological CaP, a 9.5% risk of developing clinical PCa and a 2.9% risk of dying from it (Scher & Zelefsky, 2000). With an aging population, the number of PCa instances in the US is expected to increase fourfold by 2030 (Crawford, 2003). In the European Union, about 2.3 million new cases of cancer were diagnosed in 2006 and more than 1.1 million deaths from cancer were recorded. In Africa, there have been a few studies that report 4.5/100,000 in Senegal against 11.5/1000,00 in Liberia. The Kingdom of Morocco has 30,000 new cases of cancer per year according to the Directorate of Epidemiology and Disease Control. According to a study conducted between 1986 and 1987 by the National Institute of Oncology of Rabat, PCa accounted for 2.4% of cancers in men. In 1990 PCa accounted for 1.3% of male genital cancers collected by the oncology center of the CHU IBN ROCHD in Casablanca (Acharki, 1993). An anatomopathological study carried out between 1990 and 1995 at the national level reported 249 cases of PCa out of 1609 patients tested, that is, a frequency of 15.5% (Benaissa et al., 1996). According to a study conducted between 1992 and 2002 in the region of Marrakech-Tensift-Al Haouz, on a total of 1370 urological cancer patients, PCa was the most common urological cancer with a percentage of 58.10% followed by bladder cancer (32.91%).

In men, PCa is the most frequent type of cancer. It is the third-leading cause of cancer death, accounting for over 10% of all cancer deaths. Asia has the lowest rate of PCa (Fig. 22.1).

In the US, 3% of men alive today may die from PCa. Around three decades ago, mortality increased in the US by 3.1% per year between 1987 and 1991 and then decreased by 1.9% per year until 1995.

The number of deaths decreased from 37,400 in 1999 to 31,900 in 2000 and a 25% decrease has been observed since the early 1990s due to more common use of prostate-specific antigen (PSA) test. In France, mortality was estimated at 10,104 cases in 2000 fourth only to bronchopulmonary, colorectal, and breast cancers (and second only to bronchopulmonary cancer in men; Fig. 22.2).

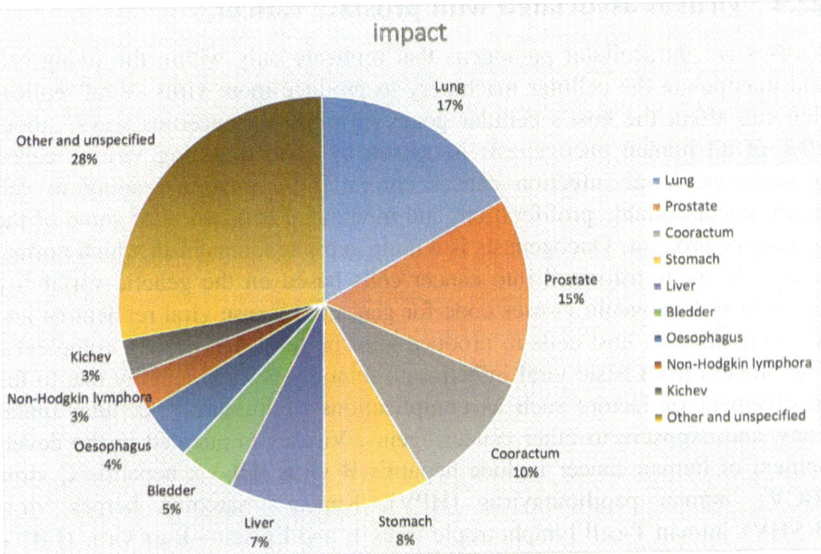

FIGURE 22.1 Diagram of the incidence of different cancers in the world. Little epidemiological data are available on the incidence of PCa in Asia, where screening is rarely used.

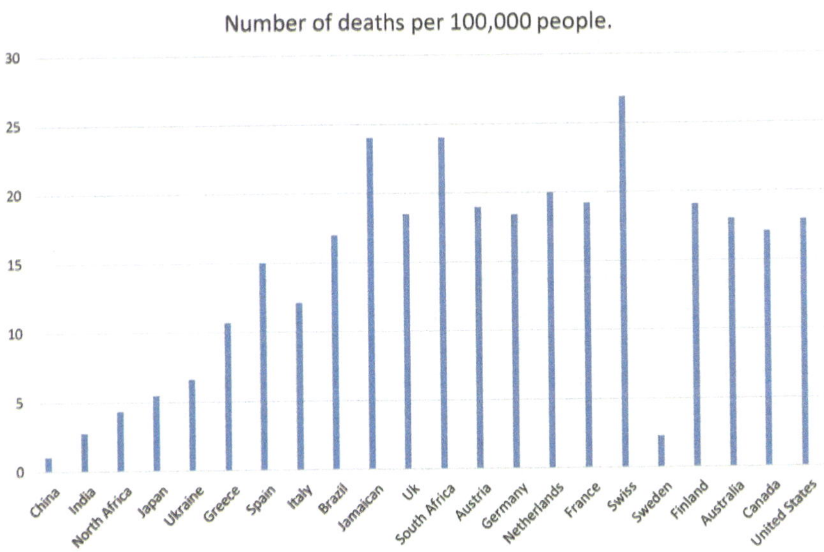

FIGURE 22.2 Mortality of PCa by country (age standardized; statistics year 2000). Mortality varies by country but with less variation than that for incidence.

22.3 Viruses associated with prostate cancer

Viruses are intracellular pathogens that replicate only within the living cell and manipulate the cellular machinery to produce more virus. Viral replication can affect the host's cellular genes in multiple cancerous ways. About 20% of all human oncogenesis is caused by cancer-causing viruses called oncoviruses. Viral infection causes chronic inflammation leading to cell death, uncontrollable proliferation, and modulated expression of some of the regulatory proteins. Oncogenesis is a multistep phenomenon in which normal host cells are transformed into cancer cells based on the genetic variability of the host. Oncogenic viruses code for genes that cause viral replication and transformation of host cells to produce viral proteins and protein complexes. The process from basic viral infection to tumorigenesis is lengthy due to the involvement of factors such as complications of immunity, cellular mutations, and exposure to other cancer agents. Viruses implicated in the development of human cancer include hepatitis B virus (HBV), hepatitis C virus (HCV), human papillomavirus (HPV), Kaposi's sarcoma herpes virus (KSHV), human T-cell lymphotropic virus 1, and Epstein–Barr virus (EBV)

22.3.1 Human papillomavirus

HPV infection is an established etiologic factor for cervical, uterine, vulvar, vaginal, penile, and anal cancers. Given its anatomical proximity to anogenital and urinary sites, the prostate has been extensively investigated for HPV infection. Studies reported in the literature, primarily in Western populations, have varied considerably in terms of study design and methodology. As a result, findings are also inconsistent, with only a few studies showing statistically significant differences in HPV infection between PCa patients and controls (Hrbacek et al., 2013). More recently, studies in Mediterranean and Asian populations have suggested an association between HPV, particularly the high-risk subtypes 16 and 18, and PCa (Atashafrooz & Rokhbakhsh-Zamin, 2016; Whitaker et al., 2013). The strength of the association varies by geographic distribution (Yang et al., 2015). In addition, studies have found significant positive associations of PCa with sexual activity and sexually transmitted diseases (Chung et al., 2013; Spence et al., 2014), including HPV, further suggesting that an infectious etiology being involved in prostate carcinogenesis. HPV warrants a more rigorous investigation, particularly to reconcile the diversity of findings reported within the same populations (Ghasemian et al., 2013; Yow et al., 2014).

22.3.2 Herperviruses

Herpesviruses can be transmitted both sexually and nonsexually and are highly prevalent in some populations (Pagano, 2007). Herpesviruses, such as

EBV and HHV-8, have been associated with human malignancies (Sunil et al., 2010). In PCa, CMV, HSV-1, HSV-2, HHV-8, and EBV infections have been studied (Hrbacek et al., 2013). A recent study in men from Tobago, a region with one of the highest PCa incidence and mortality rates, showed that HHV-8 establishes a latent prostate infection associated with macrophage infiltration and inflammation (Henning et al., 2016). However, a metaanalysis to explore the association between infections caused by several sexually transmitted pathogens, including HSV-1, HSV-2, HHV-8, and CMV, found no significant association with an increased risk of PCa (Caini et al., 2014).

22.3.3 BK

BK virus is ubiquitous and infects approximately 90% of the world's population, most often in childhood. It persists in the body in a latent state in the urinary tract and is susceptible to reactivation during cellular immune deficiency; it is then responsible for hemorrhagic cystitis and nephropathy, which can lead to graft loss in kidney transplant recipients. The genome of polyomaviruses encodes two early proteins, the T antigen (AgT) and the t antigen (Agt), whose oncogenic power is exerted through interactions with cellular antioncogenic proteins, mainly p53 and pRB. BK virus has transforming potential in vitro and in vivo in a mouse model, alone or in combination with other oncogenes. The potential role of BK virus in human cancers has been discussed for a long time but remains controversial.

PCa is one of the leading causes of death in men in Western countries. The p53 protein, a major antioncogene, is implicated in the progression of PCa by losing its ability to bind to the cell's DNA and regulate its division cycle

22.3.4 XMRV

The first molecular studies of XMRV (Xenotropic Murine Leukemia virus-related Virus) chromosomal integration sites have been completed in two PCa cases homozygous for R462Q. The data confirm that XMRV replicated well in epithelial tissue in addition to stromal cells, and that viral DNA integrated in the vicinity of genes encoding important transcription factors, similar to what has already been widely described with murine leukemia viruses (MLVs) (Dong et al., 2007).

These remarkable observations highlight once again that retroviruses circulate within populations, especially since they can replicate at a high level like HIV-1. The presence of XMRV raises many questions, starting with its origin, variability, mode of transmission, incidence in the general population, as well as the molecular determinants of the virus (Corbin et al., 1994) and of the host responsible for pathologies such as PCa.

22.4 Carcinogenesis of the prostate: interaction between host genetics and viral infection

PCa is one of the most common malignancies in men and the second leading cause of cancer death in men worldwide (Rawla, 2019). The different types of epithelial tumors of the prostate are acinar adenocarcinoma, intraductal carcinoma, ductal adenocarcinoma, urothelial carcinoma, squamous neoplasms, adenosquamous carcinoma, and squamous cell carcinoma. Acinar adenocarcinoma is the most common of these tumors (Montironi et al., 2017). Several factors, such as age, race, diet, and family history of PCa are involved in the development and progression of PCa. In addition to these factors, PCa can be initiated or progressed by viral infections, but the exact cause of PCa is unknown (Gann, 2002). As stated previously, many viruses are known to interact with host proteins and cause changes in genetic, immunological, and inflammatory events that lead to tumor initiation or progression (Martinez-Fierro et al., 2010). Viral products, for example, the large T antigen of polyomaviruses, or the E6/E7 proteins of HPV, can transform prostate cells and interfere with interferon (IFN) signaling pathways (Zheng, 2010). Host genetics add an additional layer of complexity to the molecular pathways involved in PCa initiation or progression, where polymorphisms in certain genes may promote viral progression or poor control of viral infections, potentially allowing the virus to exert its cytopathic effects or transform normal prostate cells.

The prostate serves as a possible target for HPV infection for anatomical reasons; HPV E5, E6, and E7 oncoproteins are essential for viral replication and play a critical carcinogenic role through different mechanisms (Duensing & Münger, 2002; Hemmat & Baghi, 2018). The capabilities of the E6 and E7 oncoproteins of high-risk HPVs are related to the targeting of tumor suppressor signaling pathways via a number of mechanisms such as the induction of p53 and pRB degradation via E6 and E7, respectively (Duensing & Münger, 2002). Polymorphism (proline or arginine) at position 72 of the p53 gene is known to modulate E6-mediated degradation of p53 protein, where p53 with arginine at position 72 is more sensitive to E6-mediated proteasomal degradation compared to proline at the same position. Studies both supporting and opposing this observation have been published for cervical cancer; however, only one study on PCa supports the observation that proline at position 72 is associated with a reduced risk of PCa (Leiros et al., 2005). In addition to HPV, simian virus 40 (SV40) is also known to induce epithelial tumor transformation of prostate cells in transgenic models, although the direct role of SV40 infection and PCa development has not been proven in clinical studies (Deeb et al., 2007). SV40 large-T and small-T antigens have been extensively studied because of their role in tumorigenesis. The main function of large-T antigen is to bind and target p53 and Rb proteins for degradation, which promotes cell replication and transformation [36]. The small-T antigen itself does not cause transformation but provides the necessary mitogenic signals that facilitate cell transformation (Kasper & Smith, 2004). The small-T antigen, for example, interacts with and inhibits PP21, a serine-threonine protein phosphatase. The inhibition of PP2A constitutively activates the Wnt pathway, which promotes cell proliferation. In addition, the inhibition of PP2A induces changes in the actin cytoskeleton and tight junctions, leading to a loss of cell polarity and promoting tumor invasiveness (Kasper & Smith, 2004) (Fig. 22.3).

The complex interplay between host genetics, host immunity, and viral infection can initiate and promote PCa. Key viral factors, for example, lead to inhibition of cell cycle proteins such as p53 and RB by SV40 and HPV, inhibition of antigen receptor signaling by HHV-8, and vice versa, activation of Wnt by SV40 and activation of VEGF, Janus kinase / STAT3, and NF-κ B by HHV-8, which ultimately promote uncontrolled androgen-independent cell growth as well as angiogenesis, etc. Viruses are also involved in chronic inflammation that can directly lead to PCa. The host factor includes variations in cancer susceptibility genes, such as the R462Q variation in the RNASEL gene, which altered interferon activity, resulting in poor viral control. Similarly, antibody titer to the viral protein (large T-antigen of BK virus) increased IL-10 levels that promoted differentiation of immunosuppressive M2 macrophages. PCa cells also upregulate testosterone levels, which suppress Th1 diffraction, resulting in decreased clearance of viral particles and cancer cells due to the compromised cytotoxic T-cell response (Abidi et al., 2018).

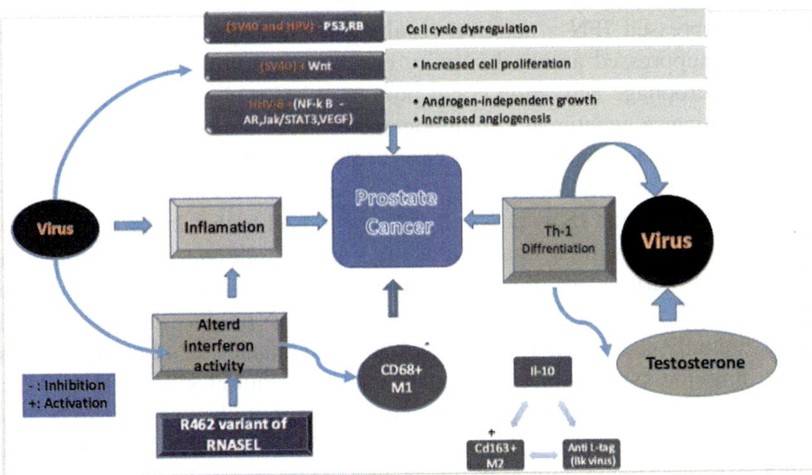

FIGURE 22.3 **The interaction between host genetics, host immunity, and viral infection that can lead to the progression of PCa (Abidi et al., 2018).**

22.5 Viral-mediated immune deregulation

Tumor cells establish an inflammatory terrain, the tumor microenvironment to support tumor growth (Lin & Zhang, 2017). The two pillars of this microenvironment are cancer associated fibroblasts (CAFs) and tumor associated macrophages (TAMs), (Porta et al., 2011). CAFs and TAMs help tumor cells maintain an environment that is conducive to their growth (structural and metabolic environment) and protective of the immune system (inflammatory and immunosuppressive environment). The site of inflammation has been shown to be a precursor to prostate intraepithelial neoplasia. Since viruses play an important role in the etiology of PCa, their role in promoting a proinflammatory microenvironment, that is, inflammatory pathways that contribute to the development of PCa, cannot be compromised. Many inflammation genes have SNPs (single-nucleotide polymorphism), some of which are associated with increased risk of PCa.

22.5.1 RNASEL (Ribonuclease L)

This gene involved in innate immunity has unexpectedly emerged as a candidate gene for PCa susceptibility. It is located at 1q25 and is a component of the innate immune system required for its antiviral and antiproliferative roles (Hassel et al., 1993; Silverman, 2003). Inactivating mutations (E265X and M1I) in RNASEL identify two familial CaP types: E265X present in individuals of European ancestry and M1I in individuals of African ancestry (Carpten et al., 2002; Smith et al., 1996). It is possible that hosts with a susceptible genetic background, such as the presence of the R462Q variant of the RNASEL/HPC gene, have decreased CD68 + M1 macrophage activation due to suppressed IFN-γ activity, resulting in widespread dissemination of PCa. The suppressed antiviral activity of IFN coupled with decreased CD68 + M1 macrophage activation could promote viral replication in the prostate milieu and cause genetic and immunogenic changes that lead to PCa progression. Likewise, increased antibody titer to the large-T antigen (L-Tag) of the BK polyoma virus has been shown to be associated with increased IL-10 versus IFN-γ expression (Sais et al., 2012). It is possible that large-T antigen of SV40 also causes similar changes. These reports highlight the possible contribution of viruses in promoting impaired macrophage differentiation. Macrophages, in general, have also been shown to produce arginase, which can potentially induce anergy in lymphocytes. Changes in other cells of the innate immune system have also been reported. Natural killer cell dysfunction has also been demonstrated. This could be due to the presence of TGF-β in the PCa tumor milieu. The increase in absolute neutrophil count was found to be associated with high tumor grade (Strasner & Karin, 2015).

22.5.2 Toll-like receptors

As key players in innate immunity, Toll-like receptors (TLRs) recognize Pathogen Associated Molecular Patterns (PAMP) molecular motifs (Janeway & Medzhitov, 2002). In humans, 11 TLRs have been identified. Their function is the recognition of pathogens and the activation of the cell that carries them.

The activation of TLRs is initiated by their binding to PAMP or DAMP ligand molecules.

One of the most studied TLRs is TLR4. This receptor recognizes Gram-negative bacterial products, including lipopolysaccharide (Poltorak et al., 1998) and the heat shock protein HSP60 (heat shock protein 60) (Ohashi et al., 2000). In the Swedish CAPS study, an SNP in the 3'UTR region of TLR4 (11381 G/C) was found to be associated with PCa risk. Carriers of the GC and CC genotypes had respectively 26% and 39% increased risk of PCa (before age 65) compared to men with the wild-type GG genotype. A North American study reported that eight TLR4 SNPs were associated with a lower risk of PCa.

22.5.2.1 Macrophage inhibitory cytokine 1

The cytokine macrophage inhibitory cytokine 1 (MIC-1) encodes a protein that carries characteristics close to the growth factor β (TGF-β) superfamily. MIC-1 plays a vital role in inflammation by regulating macrophage activity. The Swedish CAPS study shows that the nonsynonymous H6D variant is associated with a lower risk of sporadic PCa (OR = 0.80, 95% CI = 0.66–0.97) and familial PCa (OR = 0.61, 95% CI = 0.42–0.89) (Lindmark et al., 2004).

22.5.2.2 Interleukin-1 receptor antagonist

Interleukin-1 receptor antagonist (IL-1RN) is a member of the interleukin-1 family. It is a receptor antagonist, secreted by various cell types, including immune cells, epithelial cells, and adipocytes. It is an inhibitor of the proinflammatory effect of IL1α and IL1β (Dinarello, 1994). Among the evaluated SNPs of IL-1RN, one had a higher frequency (38.7%) in PCa patients compared with controls (33.5%; $P = .009$; Lindmark et al., 2005).

Furthermore, a link between the innate and adaptive immune system is also compromised due to the decreased number of dendritic cells (DCs) in PCa tissue (Troy et al., 1998). However, functional DCs are present in the periphery of the tumor, which could be an incentive to develop immunotherapy for PCa.

Aberrant function of the adaptive immune system has been reported in PCa. B-cell function appears to be compromised in PCa by testosterone, as increased testosterone levels correlate with a decreased antibody response to vaccination (Furman et al., 2014). Testosterone has also been postulated to maintain T-cell tolerance to virus and tumor antigen by inhibiting Th1 differentiation, which is a critical step in viral clearance, and T-cell response to tumor antigen (Fig. 22.2). CD4 + Th1 cells were found to be biased toward differentiation into regulatory T cells (T-reg) or Th17 (Strasner & Karin, 2015). The number of Th17 cells was found to be directly proportional to the Gleason score (Stefanos, et al., 2008). Altered Th1 differentiation of CD^{4+} T cells has been shown to be mediated by inhibition of IL-12-induced Stat4 phosphorylation by testosterone (Kissick et al., 2014). Androgens also negatively alter IFN-γ signaling as well as Th17 differentiation (Kissick et al., 2014). Furthermore, androgen deprivation therapy in humans has been reported to enhance CD4 + T cell differentiation and promote T-cell infiltration into the PCa microenvironment [53]. In mouse models, castration has been shown to enhance CD8 + T cell response (Kissick et al., 2014). Interestingly, the presence of BK polyoma has been shown to be associated with increased expression of CD4 + CD25 + FoxP + cells, which in turn produce the immunosuppressive cytokines IL-10 and TGF-β (Sais et al., 2012).

22.5.3 Other genes linked to inflammation

A few other inflammation genes are thought to be related to PCa. For example, certain variant alleles of IL-10 and IL8 are associated with PCa (McCarron et al., 2002). Serum levels of IL-1, IL-18, IL-6, and MIC-1/GDF-15 are correlated with PCa risk and cancer prognosis. While the role of IL-6 in PCa is well documented, studies on serum IL-18 or its diagnostic utility are still limited. In a cohort of 149 patients, serum IL-18 was shown to be significantly higher in locally advanced PCa than in benign prostatic hyperplasia (BPH) and control patients (Dwivedi et al., 2011). The expression of IL-18 BP (Interleukin-18 binding protein) transporter protein is increased in patients with large-volume PCa. Moreover, high serum IL-18 BP level was correlated with Gleason score (Fujita et al., 2011). Clinical evidence suggests that serum levels of MIC-1, in combination with PSA, may improve the specificity of PCa detection (Bauskin et al., 2006; Selander et al., 2007). Using an experimental rat model, where chronic inflammation was induced by a chemical compound (carrageenan), an association was identified between overexpression of inflammasome proteins (IL1b, CASP1 and NLRP1) and prostate damage, suggesting that activation of the inflammasome complex may produce an inflammatory state similar to BPH in humans (Chen et al., 2013; Kashyap et al., 2015).

Finally, serum IL-6 levels (one of the best markers of chronic inflammation) are elevated in patients with untreated metastatic or castration-resistant PCa and are negatively correlated with tumor survival and response to chemotherapy (Nguyen et al., 2014). IL-6 (via signaling pathways involving signal transducers and activators of transcription, Janus kinase, mitogen-

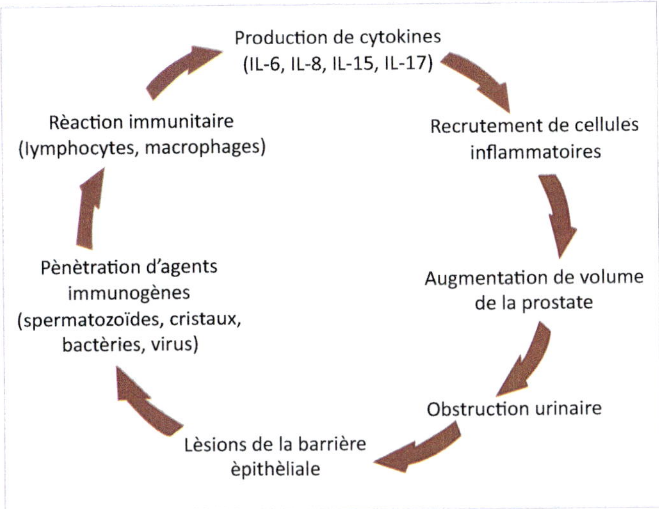

FIGURE 22.4 **Causes and consequences of chronic prostate inflammation (Robert et al., 2010).**

activated protein kinases, extracellular signal-regulated kinases, phosphoinositide 3-kinase) is capable of promoting PCa cell proliferation and inhibiting apoptosis in vitro and in vivo (Shankar et al., 2015) (Fig. 22.4).

22.6 Conclusion

PCa is the second leading cause of cancer and the fifth leading cause of cancer death worldwide. Carcinogenesis is associated with multiple factors such as age, diet, heredity and environment. However, the mechanisms determining the initiation of PCa remain poorly understood. In this chapter we observed a complex interaction between host genetics, host immunity and viral infection which leads to the initiation or the promotion of prostate cancer. These data support the need to develop antiviral and immunomodulatory therapeutic agents for the treatment of PCa, indeed, immune therapy has been shown to increase the overall survival of patients diagnosed with PCa (Maia & Hansen, 2017).

Acknowledgment

Authors would like to thank the Ministry of National Education, Professional Training, Higher Education and Scientific Research and express gratitude to members of Virology, Oncology and Medical Biotechnology team at FSTM-Hassan II University of Casablanca, for all their efforts to support us during all stages of this research.

References

Abidi, S. H., Bilwani, F., Ghias, K., & Abbas, F. (2018). Viral etiology of prostate cancer: Genetic alterations and immune response. A literature review. *International Journal of Surgery*, *52*, 136–140. Available from https://doi.org/10.1016/j.ijsu.2018.02.050.

Acharki, A. (1993). Répartition des cancers: Expérience du service d'oncologie du CHU Ibn Rochd de Casablanca (19275 cas).

Atashafrooz, F., & Rokhbakhsh-Zamin, F. (2016). Frequency and type distribution of human papilloma virus in patients with prostate cancer, Kerman, southeast of Iran. *Asian Pacific Journal of Cancer Prevention*, *17*(8), 3951–3956. Available from http://www.apocpcontrol.org/paper_file/issue_abs/Volume17_No8/3951-3956%205.28%20Fatemeh%20Atashafrooz.pdf.

Bauskin, A. R., Brown, D. A., Kuffner, T., Johnen, H., Lou, X. W., Hunter, M., & Breit, S. N. (2006). Role of macrophage inhibitory cytokine-1 in tumorigenesis and diagnosis of cancer. *Cancer Research*, *66*(10), 4983–4986. Available from https://doi.org/10.1158/0008-5472.CAN-05-4067.

Benaissa, M., Babin, P., Quellard, N., Pezennec, L., Cenatiempo, Y., & Fauchère, J. L. (1996). Changes in Helicobacter pylori ultrastructure and antigens during conversion from the bacillary to the coccoid form. *Infection and immunity*, *64*(6), 2331–2335.

Caini, S., Gandini, S., Dudas, M., Bremer, V., Severi, E., & Gherasim, A. (2014). Sexually transmitted infections and prostate cancer risk: A systematic review and *meta*-analysis. *Cancer Epidemiology*, *38*(4), 329–338. Available from https://doi.org/10.1016/j.canep.2014.06.002.

Carpten, J., Nupponen, N., Isaacs, S., Sood, R., Robbins, C., Xu, J., Faruque, M., Moses, T., Ewing, C., Gillanders, E., Hu, P., Bujnovszky, P., Makalowska, I., Baffoe-Bonnie, A., Faith, D., Smith, J., Stephan, D., Wiley, K., Brownstein, M., … Trent, J. (2002). Germline mutations in the ribonuclease L gene in families showing linkage with HPC1. *Nature Genetics*, *30*(2), 181–184. Available from https://doi.org/10.1038/ng823.

Chen, C. S., Chang, P. J., Lin, W. Y., Huang, Y. C., & Ho, D. R. (2013). Evidences of the inflammasome pathway in chronic prostatitis and chronic pelvic pain syndrome in an animal model. *The Prostate*, *73*(4), 391–397. Available from https://doi.org/10.1002/pros.22580.

Chung, S. D., Lin, Y. K., Huang, C. C., & Lin, H. C. (2013). Increased risk of prostate cancer following sexually transmitted infection in an Asian population. *Epidemiology and Infection*, *141*(12), 2663–2670. Available from https://doi.org/10.1017/S0950268813000459.

Corbin, A., Prats, A. C., Darlix, J. L., & Sitbon, M. (1994). A nonstructural gag-encoded glycoprotein precursor is necessary for efficient spreading and pathogenesis of murine leukemia viruses. *Journal of Virology*, *68*(6), 3857–3867. Available from https://doi.org/10.1128/jvi.68.6.3857-3867.1994.

Crawford, E. D. (2003). Epidemiology of prostate cancer. *Urology*, *62*(6), 3–12. Available from https://doi.org/10.1016/j.urology.2003.10.013.

de Sanjosé, S., Bruni, L., & Alemany, L. (2014). HPV in genital cancers (at the exception of cervical cancer) and anal cancers. *La Presse Médicale*, e423–e428. Available from https://doi.org/10.1016/j.lpm.2014.10.001.

De Stefano, V., Za, T., Rossi, E., Vannucchi, A. M., Ruggeri, M., Elli, E., … Barbui, T. (2008). Recurrent thrombosis in patients with polycythemia vera and essential thrombocythemia: incidence, risk factors, and effect of treatments. *haematologica*, *93*(3), 372–380.

Deeb, K. K., Michalowska, A. M., Yoon, C. Y., Krummey, S. M., Hoenerhoff, M. J., Kavanaugh, C., Li, M. C., Demayo, F. J., Linnoila, I., Deng, C. X., Lee, E. Y. H. P., Medina, D., Shih, J. H., & Green, J. E. (2007). Identification of an integrated SV40 T/t-antigen cancer signature in aggressive human breast, prostate, and lung carcinomas with poor prognosis. *Cancer Research*, *67*(17), 8065–8080. Available from https://doi.org/10.1158/0008-5472.CAN-07-1515.

Dinarello, C. A. (1994). The interleukin-1 family: 10 years of discovery. *FASEB Journal*, *8*(15), 1314–1325.

Dong, B., Kim, S., Hong, S., Gupta, J. D., Malathi, K., Klein, E. A., Ganem, D., DeRisi, J. L., Chow, S. A., & Silverman, R. H. (2007). An infectious retrovirus susceptible to an IFN antiviral pathway from human prostate tumors. *Proceedings of the National Academy of Sciences of the United States of America*, *104*(5), 1655–1660. Available from https://doi.org/10.1073/pnas.0610291104.

Duensing, S., & Münger, K. (2002). The human papillomavirus type 16 E6 and E7 oncoproteins independently induce numerical and structural chromosome instability. *Cancer Research*, *62* (23), 7075–7082.

Dwivedi, S., Goel, A., Natu, S. M., Mandhani, A., Khattri, S., & Pant, K. K. (2011). Diagnostic and prognostic significance of prostate specific antigen and serum interleukin 18 and 10 in patients with locally advanced prostate cancer: A prospective study. *Asian Pacific Journal of Cancer Prevention*, *12*(7), 1843–1848. Available from http://www.apocp.org/cancer_-download/Volume12_No7/1843-1848%20c%206.27%20Shailendra%20Dwivedi.pdf.

Ferlay, J., Autier, P., Boniol, M., Heanue, M., Colombet, M., & Boyle, P. (2007). Estimates of the cancer incidence and mortality in Europe in 2006. *Annals of Oncology*, *18*(3), 581–592. Available from https://doi.org/10.1093/annonc/mdl498.

Fujita, K., Ewing, C. M., Isaacs, W. B., & Pavlovich, C. P. (2011). Immunomodulatory IL-18 binding protein is produced by prostate cancer cells and its levels in urine and serum correlate with tumor status. *International Journal of Cancer*, *129*(2), 424–432. Available from https://doi.org/10.1002/ijc.25705.

Furman, D., Hejblum, B. P., Simon, N., Jojic, V., Dekker, C. L., Thiebaut, R., Tibshirani, R. J., & Davis, M. M. (2014). Systems analysis of sex differences reveals an immunosuppressive role for testosterone in the response to influenza vaccination. *Proceedings of the National Academy of Sciences of the United States of America*, *111*(2), 869–874. Available from https://doi.org/10.1073/pnas.1321060111.

Gann, P. H. (2002). Risk factors for prostate cancer. *Reviews in Urology*, *4*.

Ghasemian, E., Monavari, S. H. R., Irajian, G. R., Nodoshan, M. R. J., Roudsari, R. V., & Yahyapour, Y. (2013). Evaluation of human papillomavirus infections in prostatic disease: A cross-sectional study in Iran. *Asian Pacific Journal of Cancer Prevention*, *14*(5), 3305–3308. Available from https://doi.org/10.7314/APJCP.2013.14.5.3305.

Häggman, M. J., Macoska, J. A., Wojno, K. J., & Oesterling, J. E. (1997). The relationship between prostatic intraepithelial neoplasia and prostate cancer: Critical issues. *Journal of Urology*, *158*(1), 12–22. Available from https://doi.org/10.1097/00005392-199707000-00004.

Hassel, B. A., Zhou, A., Sotomayor, C., Maran, A., & Silverman, R. H. (1993). A dominant negative mutant of 2-5A-dependent RNase suppresses antiproliferative and antiviral effects of interferon. *EMBO Journal*, *12*(8), 3297–3304. Available from https://doi.org/10.1002/j.1460-2075.1993.tb05999.x.

Hemmat, N., & Baghi, H. B. (2018). Human papillomavirus E5 protein, the undercover culprit of tumorigenesis. *Infectious Agents and Cancer*, *13*(1). Available from https://doi.org/10.1186/s13027-018-0208-3.

Henning, J. D., Bunker, C. H., Patrick, A. L., & Jenkins, F. J. (2016). Human herpesvirus 8 establishes a latent infection in prostates of Tobago men resulting in increased macrophage infiltration. *The Prostate*, *76*(8), 735–743. Available from https://doi.org/10.1002/pros.23163.

Hrbacek, J., Urban, M., Hamsikova, E., Tachezy, R., & Heracek, J. (2013). Thirty years of research on infection and prostate cancer: No conclusive evidence for a link. A systematic review. *Urologic Oncology: Seminars and Original Investigations*, *31*(7), 951–965. Available from https://doi.org/10.1016/j.urolonc.2012.01.013.

Janeway, C. A., & Medzhitov, R. (2002). Innate immune recognition. *Annual Review of Immunology*, *20*, 197–216. Available from https://doi.org/10.1146/annurev.immunol.20.083001.084359.

Kashyap, M., Pore, S., Wang, Z., Gingrich, J., Yoshimura, N., & Tyagi, P. (2015). Inflammasomes are important mediators of prostatic inflammation associated with BPH. *Journal of Inflammation (United Kingdom)*, *12*(1). Available from https://doi.org/10.1186/s12950-015-0082-3.

Kasper, S., & Smith, J. A. (2004). Genetically modified mice and their use in developing therapeutic strategies for prostate cancer. *Journal of Urology*, *172*(1), 12–19. Available from https://doi.org/10.1097/01.ju.0000132122.93436.aa, Lippincott Williams and Wilkins.

Kissick, H. T., Sanda, M. G., Dunn, L. K., Pellegrini, K. L., On, S. T., Noel, J. K., & Arredouani, M. S. (2014). Androgens alter T-cell immunity by inhibiting T-helper 1 differentiation. *Proceedings of the National Academy of Sciences of the United States of America*, *111*(27), 9887–9892. Available from https://doi.org/10.1073/pnas.1402468111.

Leiros, G. J., Galliano, S. R., Sember, M. E., Kahn, T., Schwarz, E., & Eiguchi, K. (2005). Detection of human papillomavirus DNA and p53 codon 72 polymorphism in prostate carcinomas of patients from Argentina. *BMC Urology*, *5*. Available from https://doi.org/10.1186/1471-2490-5-15.

Lin, C., & Zhang, J. (2017). Inflammasomes in inflammation-induced cancer. *Frontiers in Immunology*, *8*. Available from https://doi.org/10.3389/fimmu.2017.00271.

Lindmark, F., Zheng, S. L., Wiklund, F., Bälter, K. A., Sun, J., Chang, B., Hedelin, M., Clark, J., Johansson, J. E., Meyers, D. A., Adami, H. O., Isaacs, W., Grönberg, H., & Xu, J. (2005). Interleukin-1 receptor antagonist haplotype associated with prostate cancer risk. *British Journal of Cancer*, *93*(4), 493–497. Available from https://doi.org/10.1038/sj.bjc.6602729.

Lindmark, F., Zheng, S. L., Wiklund, F., Bensen, J., Bälter, K. A., Chang, B., Hedelin, M., Clark, J., Stattin, P., Meyers, D. A., Adami, H. O., Isaacs, W., Grönberg, H., & Xu, J. (2004). H6D polymorphism in macrophage-inhibitory cytokine-1 gene associated with prostate cancer. *Journal of the National Cancer Institute*, *96*(16), 1248–1254. Available from https://doi.org/10.1093/jnci/djh227.

Lumme, S., Tenkanen, L., Langseth, H., Gislefoss, R., Hakama, M., Stattin, P., Hallmans, G., Adlercreutz, H., Saikku, P., Stenman, U. H., Tuohimaa, P., Luostarinen, T., & Dillner, J. (2016). Longitudinal biobanks-based study on the joint effects of infections, nutrition and hormones on risk of prostate cancer. *Acta Oncologica*, *55*(7), 839–845. Available from https://doi.org/10.3109/0284186X.2016.1139178.

Maia, M. C., & Hansen, A. R. (2017). A comprehensive review of immunotherapies in prostate cancer. *Critical Reviews in Oncology/Hematology*, *113*, 292–303. Available from https://doi.org/10.1016/j.critrevonc.2017.02.026.

Martinez-Fierro, M. L., Leach, R. J., Gomez-Guerra, L. S., Garza-Guajardo, R., Johnson-Pais, T., Beuten, J., Morales-Rodriguez, I. B., Hernandez-Ordoñez, M. A., Calderon-Cardenas, G., Ortiz-Lopez, R., Rivas-Estilla, A. M., Ancer-Rodriguez, J., & Rojas-Martinez, A. (2010). Identification of viral infections in the prostate and evaluation of their association with cancer. *BMC Cancer*, *10*. Available from https://doi.org/10.1186/1471-2407-10-326.

McCarron, S. L., Edwards, S., Evans, P. R., Gibbs, R., Dearnaley, D. P., Dowe, A., Southgate, C., Easton, D. F., Eeles, R. A., & Howell, W. M. (2002). Influence of cytokine gene polymorphisms on the development of prostate cancer. *Cancer Research*, *62*(12), 3369–3372.

Montironi, R., Gasparrini, S., Cimadamore, A., Mazzucchelli, R., Massari, F., Cheng, L., Lopez-Beltran, A., Briganti, A., & Scarpelli, M. (2017). Morphologic variants of epithelial and neuroendocrine tumors of the prostate. The pathologist's point of view. *European Urology, Supplements*, *16*(12), 223–231. Available from https://doi.org/10.1016/j.eursup.2017.08.010.

Mygatt, J. G., Singhal, A., Sukumar, G., Dalgard, C. L., & Kaleeba, J. A. R. (2013). Oncogenic herpesvirus HHV-8 promotes androgen- independent prostate cancer growth. *Cancer Research*, *73* (18), 5695–5708. Available from https://doi.org/10.1158/0008-5472.CAN-12-4196.

Nguyen, D. P., Li, J., & Tewari, A. K. (2014). Inflammation and prostate cancer: The role of interleukin 6 (IL-6). *BJU International*, *113*(6), 986–992. Available from https://doi.org/10.1111/bju.12452.

Ohashi, K., Burkart, V., Flohé, S., & Kolb, H. (2000). Cutting edge: heat shock protein 60 is a putative endogenous ligand of the toll-like receptor-4 complex. *The Journal of Immunology*, *164*(2), 558–561.

Pagano, J. S. (2007). Is Epstein-Barr virus transmitted sexually? *Journal of Infectious Diseases*, *195*(4), 469–470. Available from https://doi.org/10.1086/510861.

Poltorak, A., He, X., Smirnova, I., Liu, M. Y., Huffel, C. V., Du, X., ... Beutler, B. (1998). Defective LPS signaling in C3H/HeJ and C57BL/10ScCr mice: mutations in Tlr4 gene. *Science*, *282*(5396), 2085–2088.

Porta, C., Riboldi, E., & Sica, A. (2011). Mechanisms linking pathogens-associated inflammation and cancer. *Cancer Letters*, *305*(2), 250–262. Available from https://doi.org/10.1016/j.canlet.2010.10.012.

Rajarubendra, N., Lawrentschuk, N., Bolton, D. M., Klotz, L., & Davis, I. D. (2011). Prostate cancer immunology – an update for urologists. *BJU International*, *107*(7), 1046–1051. Available from https://doi.org/10.1111/j.1464-410X.2010.09820.x.

Rawla, P. (2019). Epidemiology of prostate cancer. *World Journal of Oncology*, 63–89. Available from https://doi.org/10.14740/wjon1191.

Robert, G., Salagierski, M., Schalken, J. A., & de La Taille, A. (2010). Inflammation et hyperplasie bénigne de la prostate: Cause ou conséquence? *Progrès En Urologie*, 402–407. Available from https://doi.org/10.1016/j.purol.2010.03.007.

Sais, G., Wyler, S., Hudolin, T., Banzola, I., Mengus, C., Bubendorf, L., Wild, P. J., Hirsch, H. H., Sulser, T., Spagnoli, G. C., & Provenzano, M. (2012). Differential patterns of large tumor antigen-specific immune responsiveness in patients with BK polyomavirus-positive prostate cancer or benign prostatic hyperplasia. *Journal of Virology*, *86*(16), 8461–8471. Available from https://doi.org/10.1128/JVI.00005-12.

Scher, I. J., & Zelefsky, M. J. (2000). Prostate cancer. In: *Clinical oncology*.

Selander, K. S., Brown, D. A., Sequeiros, G. B., Hunter, M., Desmond, R., Parpala, T., Risteli, J., Breit, S. N., & Jukkola-Vuorinen, A. (2007). Serum macrophage inhibitory cytokine-1 concentrations correlate with the presence of prostate cancer bone metastases. *Cancer Epidemiology Biomarkers and Prevention*, *16*(3), 532–537. Available from https://doi.org/10.1158/1055-9965.EPI-06-0841.

Sfanos, K. S., Bruno, T. C., Maris, C. H., Xu, L., Thoburn, C. J., Demarzo, A. M., Meeker, A. K., Isaacs, W. B., & Drake, C. G. (2008). Phenotypic analysis of prostate-infiltrating lymphocytes reveals T H17 and Treg skewing. *Clinical Cancer Research*, *14*(11), 3254–3261. Available from https://doi.org/10.1158/1078-0432.CCR-07-5164.

Shankar, E., Bhaskaran, N., MacLennan, G. T., Liu, G., Daneshgari, F., & Gupta, S. (2015). Inflammatory signaling involved in high-fat diet induced prostate diseases. *Journal of Urology Research*, *2*.

Silverman, R. H. (2003). Implications for RNase L in prostate cancer biology. *Biochemistry*, *42* (7), 1805–1812. Available from https://doi.org/10.1021/bi027147i.

Smith, J. R., Freije, D., Carpten, J. D., Grönberg, H., Xu, J., Isaacs, S. D., Brownstein, M. J., Bova, G. S., Guo, H., Bujnovszky, P., Nusskern, D. R., Damber, J. E., Bergh, A., Emanuelsson, M., Kallioniemi, O. P., Walker-Daniels, J., Bailey-Wilson, J. E., Beaty, T. H., Meyers, D. A., ... Isaacs, W. B. (1996). Major susceptibility locus for prostate cancer on chromosome 1 suggested by a genome-wide search. *Science (New York, N.Y.)*, *274*(5291), 1371–1374. Available from https://doi.org/10.1126/science.274.5291.1371.

Spence, A. R., Rousseau, M. C., & Parent, M. É. (2014). Sexual partners, sexually transmitted infections, and prostate cancer risk. *Cancer Epidemiology*, *38*(6), 700–707. Available from https://doi.org/10.1016/j.canep.2014.09.005.

Strasner, A., & Karin, M. (2015). Immune infiltration and prostate cancer. *Frontiers in Oncology*, *5*(MAY). Available from https://doi.org/10.3389/fonc.2015.00128.

Sunil, M., Reid, E., & Lechowicz, M. J. (2010). Update on HHV-8-associated malignancies. *Current Infectious Disease Reports*, *12*(2), 147–154. Available from https://doi.org/10.1007/s11908-010-0092-5.

Troy, A., Davidson, P., Atkinson, C., & Hart, D. (1998). Phenotypic characterisation of the dendritic cell infiltrate in prostate cancer. *Journal of Urology*, *160*(1), 214–219. Available from https://doi.org/10.1016/S0022-5347(01)63093-3.

Whitaker, N. J., Glenn, W. K., Sahrudin, A., Orde, M. M., Delprado, W., & Lawson, J. S. (2013). Human papillomavirus and Epstein Barr virus in prostate cancer: Koilocytes indicate potential oncogenic influences of human papillomavirus in prostate cancer. *The Prostate*, *73* (3), 236–241. Available from https://doi.org/10.1002/pros.22562.

Yang, L., Xie, S., Feng, X., Chen, Y., Zheng, T., Dai, M., Ke Zhou, C., Hu, Z., Li, N., & Hang, D. (2015). Worldwide prevalence of human papillomavirus and relative risk of prostate cancer: A meta-analysis. *Scientific Reports*, *5*. Available from https://doi.org/10.1038/srep14667.

Yow, M. A., Tabrizi, S. N., Severi, G., Bolton, D. M., Pedersen, J., Longano, A., Garland, S. M., Southey, M. C., & Giles, G. G. (2014). Detection of infectious organisms in archival prostate cancer tissues. *BMC Cancer*, *14*(1). Available from https://doi.org/10.1186/1471-2407-14-579.

Zheng, Z. M. (2010). Viral oncogenes, noncoding RNAs, and RNA splicing in human tumor viruses. *International Journal of Biological Sciences*, *6*(7), 730–755. Available from https://doi.org/10.7150/ijbs.6.730.

Chapter 23

Dramatic impact of partial loss of PTEN function on tumorigenesis and progression of prostate cancer

Moussa Koita[6], Soukayna Alaoui Sosse[4], Berjas Abumsimir[6,7], Ihsane Ali Mahasneh[2], Mohammed Mrabti[3,4], Abdelilah Laraqui[5] and Moulay Mustapha Ennaji[1]

[1]Group Leader Research team of Virology, Oncology, and Biotechnologies, Head of Laboratory of Virology, Oncology, Biosciences, Environment and New Energies (LVO-BEEN), Faculty of Sciences and Techniques Mohammedia, University Hassan II of Casablanca, Casablanca, Morocco, [2]Faculty of Science, Department of Biotechnology, University of Sharjah, Sharjah, UAE, [3]Research and Biosafety Laboratory, Mohammed V Military Teaching Hospital, Rabat, Morocco, [4]Laboratory of Human Pathologies Biology, Faculty of Sciences, and Genomic Center of Human Pathologies, Faculty of Medicine and Pharmacy, Mohammed V University, Rabat, Morocco, [5]Research and Biosafety Laboratory, Mohammed V Military Teaching Hospital, Laboratory of Human Pathologies Biology, Faculty of Sciences, and Genomic Center of Human Pathologies, Faculty of Medicine and Pharmacy, Mohammed V University, Rabat, Morocco, [6]Team of Virology, Oncology, and Biotechnologies, Laboratory of Virology, Oncology, Biosciences, Environment and New Energies (LVO-BEEN), Faculty of Sciences and Techniques Mohammedia, University Hassan II of Casablanca, Casablanca, Morocco, [7]Pharmacological and Diagnostic Research Centre (PDRC), Department of Medical Laboratory Sciences, Faculty of Allied Medical Sciences, Al-Ahliyya Amman University (AAU), Amman, Jordan

23.1 Introduction

Prostate cancer is the second most frequently detected male cancer in the world, with over 1 million new cases recorded worldwide annually (Bray et al., 2018). Although most men do not die from this disease, prostate cancer is one of the leading causes of cancer-related deaths in men, with more than 350,000 deaths per year worldwide (Bray et al., 2018). The leading cause of death by prostate cancer is the emergence of incurable, metastatic, and effective treatments to castration and current treatments, such as androgen deprivation therapy and reward, demand for new therapeutic strategies.

Immunological Implications and Molecular Diagnostics of Genitourinary Cancer.
DOI: https://doi.org/10.1016/B978-0-323-85496-2.00015-4

Tumorigenesis is a genetic/epigenetic process triggered by the activation of oncogenes and inactivation of tumor suppressor genes. Phosphatase and tensin homolog deleted on chromosome 10 (PTEN) is one of the most frequently inactive tumor suppressor genes in human cancers, due to genetic alterations or transcriptional/posttranscriptional inhibition; moreover, even a partial loss of its function (haploinsufficiency) can lead to neoplastic transformation (Milella et al., 2015). Loss of the tumor suppressor PTEN is observed in patients with treated prostate cancer. Although the frequency of PTEN loss in prostate cancer patients varies among studies, largely due to differences in the methodological approaches used, recent studies involving large cohorts of prostate cancer patients have indicated that PTEN is lost in approximately 15%–20% of primary prostate cancers (Jamaspishvili et al., 2018; Lotan et al., 2017). A higher frequency of PTEN loss is observed in more aggressive stages of disease, including castration prostate cancer and metastatic disease, with PTEN loss in 40%–60% of these cases (Jamaspishvili et al., 2018; Lotan et al., 2011). The most common cause of PTEN loss of function in prostate cancer is homozygous genomic deletion of PTEN. However, several mechanisms have also been reported, including inactivation of somatic mutations (primarily truncated nonsense or frameshift mutations), deletion of PTEN-targeting microRNAs (miRNAs), and inactivation of posttranslational modifications (e.g., phosphorylation and ubiquitylation). Rare epiphytic silencing via PTEN promoter methylation has also been observed in prostate cancer patients.

Therefore, we will refer to genetic mutations and loss of the protein as "PTEN loss" and discuss its impacts on tumorigenesis and progression of prostate cancer.

23.1.1 Gross Anatomical Features

The normal adult gland is about the size of a walnut and resembles a cone measur- ing approximately 4 cm (transverse) 3 cm (vertical) and 2 cm (anteroposterior) and weighs approximately 20 grams in adults. The gland comprises of glandular and stromal elements, tightly fused within a capsule. The prostate is positioned subperitoneally below the pelvic diaphragm. It lies posterior to the symphysis pubis, anterior to the rectum and inferior to the urinary bladder surrounding its neck. Being pyramidal in shape, it has a base superiorly, a neck inferiorly along with anterior, posterior and two inferolateral surfaces. The anterior surface lies behind the pubic arch (see Fig. 23.1).

The prostate is divided into three zones:

- **The peripheral zone**: This is the area closest to the rectum, palpable during a digital rectal exam. It is the largest zone of the prostate, and three-fourth of malignant tumors occur in this zone (Fig. 23.2).

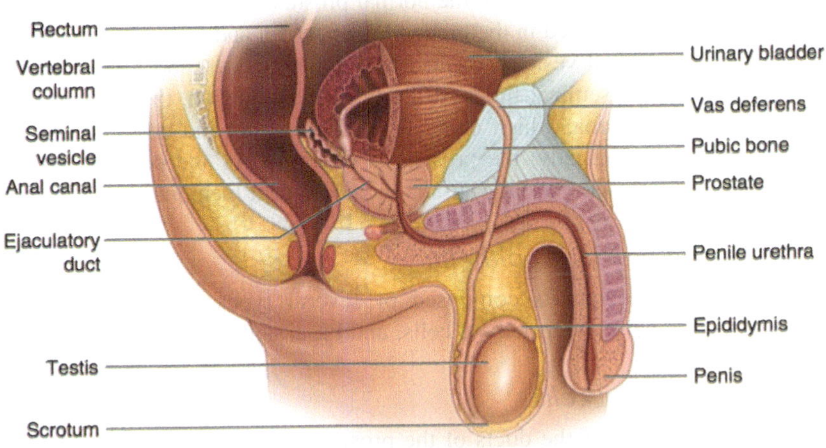

FIGURE 23.1 Side view of the prostate of the prostate.

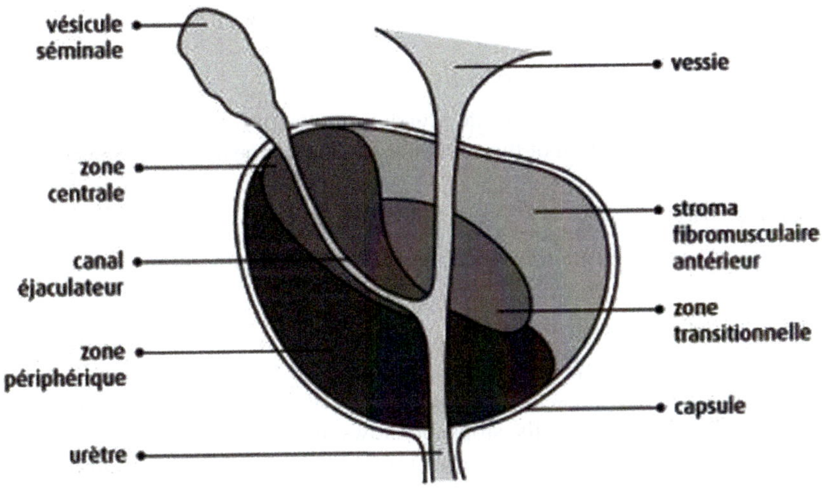

FIGURE 23.2 Zones of the prostate.

- **The transitional zone**: This is the zone that surrounds the beginning of the urethra. Until the age of 40 years, it represents only 5% of the prostate, but with aging, it grows to become the largest part of the prostate. This is called prostate adenoma or benign prostatic hyperplasia, which affects almost all men over the age of 70 years. Prostate tumors located in this zone are difficult to palpate on a rectal exam but can be detected by a biopsy.
- **The central zone**: This represents 20% of the prostate and surrounds the ejaculatory ducts.

The function and histology of the normal prostate are described as follows. The prostate is involved in the production of semen and in particular of prostatic fluid. The seminal vesicles, located behind the bladder, above the prostate, produce most of the seminal fluid. At the time of ejaculation, the seminal fluid mixes with spermatozoa, which come from the testicles and pass through the vas deferens. Histologically, the prostate is composed of the prostatic epithelium, separated from the prostatic stroma by a basement membrane.

23.1.1.1 The prostatic epithelium

The prostate epithelium is composed of several types of cells: epithelial cells, endocrine cells, intermediate cells, and basal cells.

23.1.1.2 Epithelial cells

They line the lumen of the ducts of the prostate gland, express the androgen receptor, and secrete the elements that make up the seminal fluid of the semen. These are a protein called prostate-specific antigen (PSA) and the enzyme is called prostatic acid phosphatase. Their volume and function are greatly affected by castration.

23.1.1.3 Neuroendocrine cells

Intraglandular, they are part of the secretory epithelium and have a role in the growth and differentiation of the epithelium via autocrine and paracrine control.

23.1.1.4 Basal cells

They have a reserve role to regenerate the prostatic epithelium.

23.1.1.5 The prostatic stroma

It contains the extracellular matrix, fibroblasts, capillaries, lymphatic endothelial cells, smooth muscle cells, neuroendocrine cells, and axons. The contraction of the muscle cells stops or slows the urine stream and controls ejaculation. This stroma acts as a vector for growth factors and intercellular communication through paracrine pathways. It is thus involved in differentiation, growth, and proliferation (Fig. 23.3).

23.2 Epidemiology

The (Fig 23.4) show the most commonly diagnosed cancers and leading causes of cancer death, respectively,for men at the national level. The maps reveal substantial global diversity in leading cancer types, particularly for incidence in men (8 different cancer types) and for mortality in both men (8 types). In men, prostate cancer is the most frequently diagnosed cancer in 112 countries, followed by lung cancer in 36 countries, and colorectal cancer and liver cancer each in 11 countries (Fig 23.4), (Sung et al.,2020). The highest incidence and mortality rates globally

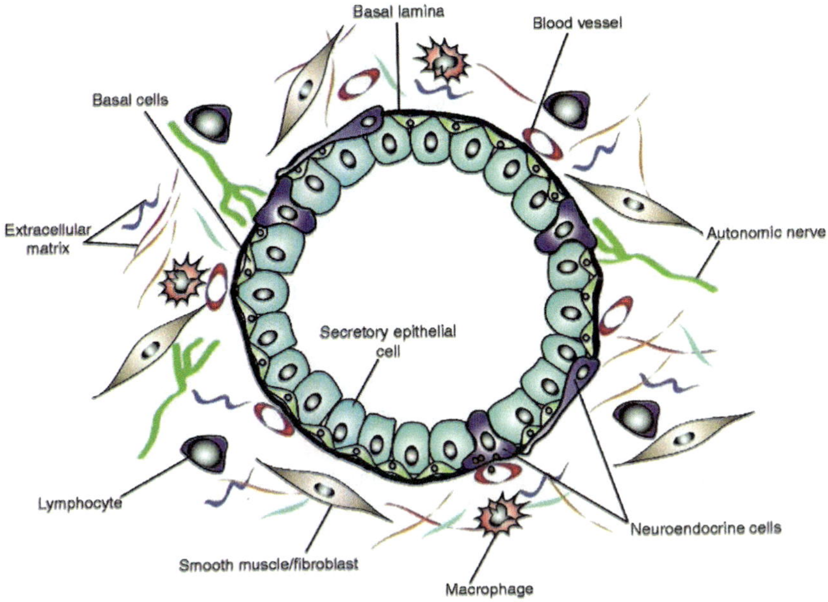

FIGURE 23.3 Cell composition of the normal prostate.

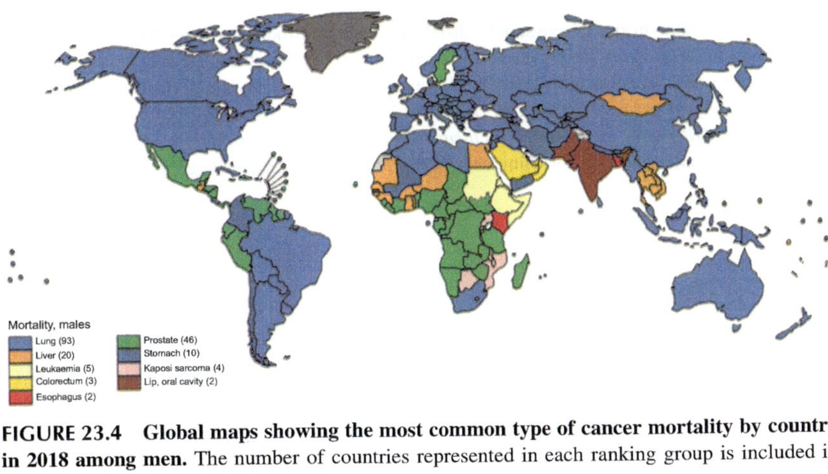

FIGURE 23.4 **Global maps showing the most common type of cancer mortality by country in 2018 among men.** The number of countries represented in each ranking group is included in the legend. *From GLOBOCAN (2018).*

are seen in Guadeloupe and Barbados (Fig 23.5), respectively. Although incidence rates are high in Australia/ New Zealand, Northern and Western Europe (eg, Norway, Sweden, Ireland), and North America (particularly in the United States), mortality rates do not follow those of in- cidence, with mortality rates elevated in the Sub-Saharan Africa regions (eg, Benin, South Africa, Zambia, and Zimbabwe) as well as the Caribbean (Barbados, Jamaica, and Haiti) (Fig 23.6).

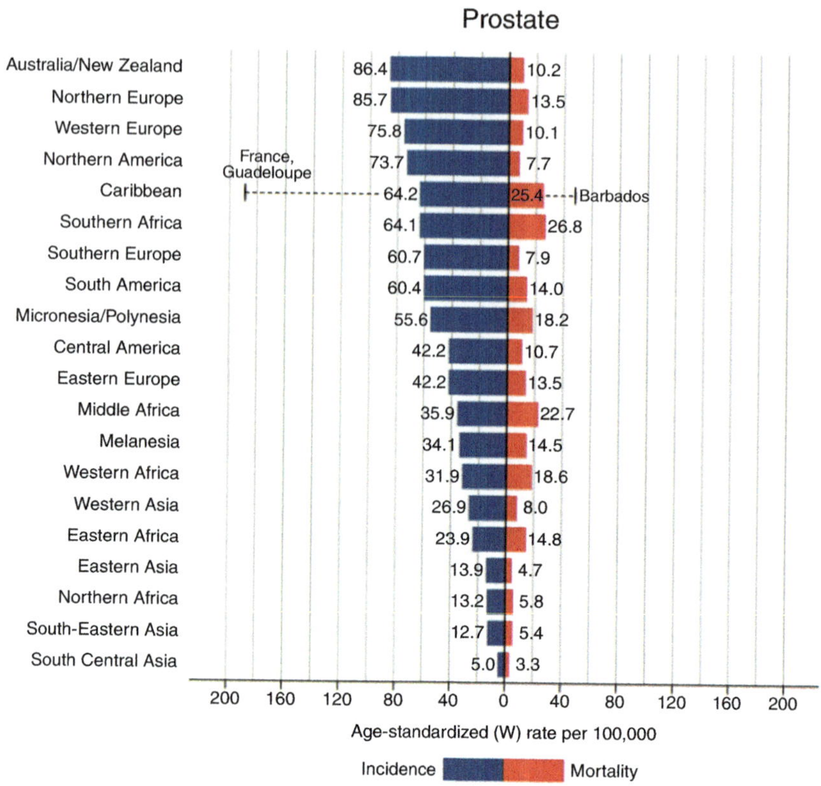

FIGURE 23.5 Bar graph of age-standardized incidence and mortality rates by region for prostate cancers in 2018. Rates are presented in descending order of the global age-standardized rate (W), and the highest national age-standardized rates for incidence and mortality are overlaid. *From Bray, F., Ferlay, J., Soerjomataram, I., Siegel, R. L., Torre, L. A. & Jemal, A. (2018). Global cancer statistics 2018: GLOBOCAN estimates of incidence and mortality worldwide for 36 cancers in 185 countries.* CA Cancer Journal for Clinicians, *68(6), 394–424. https://doi.org/10.3322/caac.21492.*

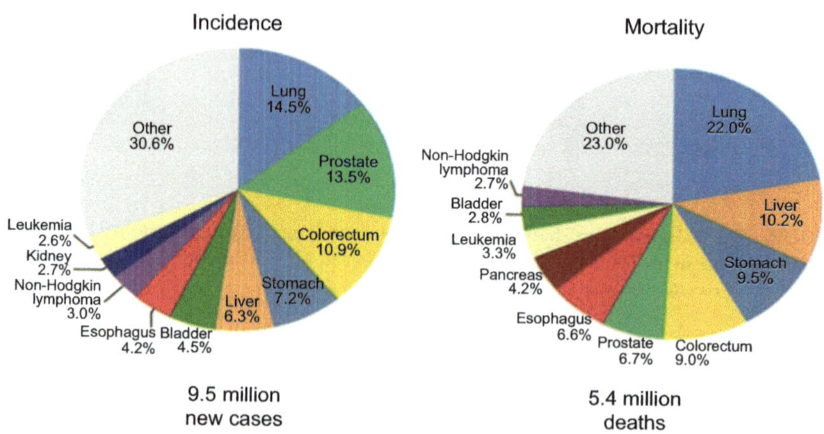

FIGURE 23.6 Pie charts show the distribution of cases and deaths for the 10 most common cancers in 2018 for men. The area of the pie chart reflects the proportion of total cases or deaths; nonmelanoma skin cancers are included in the "other" category. *From GLOBOCAN (2018).*

23.3 The PI3K/Akt signaling pathway

Activation of intracellular class I PI3Ks is driven by a variety of cell surface receptors that promote cell growth and proliferation, including many growth factor-activated members of receptor tyrosine kinases, cytokine receptors, some integrins, and a subset of G protein-coupled receptors, including several chemokine receptors (Vanhaesebroeck et al., 2012). These activated receptors directly or indirectly recruit and activate class I PI3K, which in turn phosphorylate a small fraction of plasma membrane phosphatidylinositol-4,5-bisphosphate (PIP2) to generate phosphatidylinositol-3,4,5-trisphosphate (PIP3), a membrane-associated lipid that acts as a second messenger driving downstream signaling (Fig. 23.7).

Fig. 23.7 Overview of the class I PI3 kinase signalling cascade. The binding of diverse ligands to their cognate cell surface receptors activates PI3K. The relevant ligand/ receptor pairs include many growth factors and cytokines, as well as chemokines and neurotransmitters and their receptors. The diagram uses a receptor tyrosine kinase as an example, although many

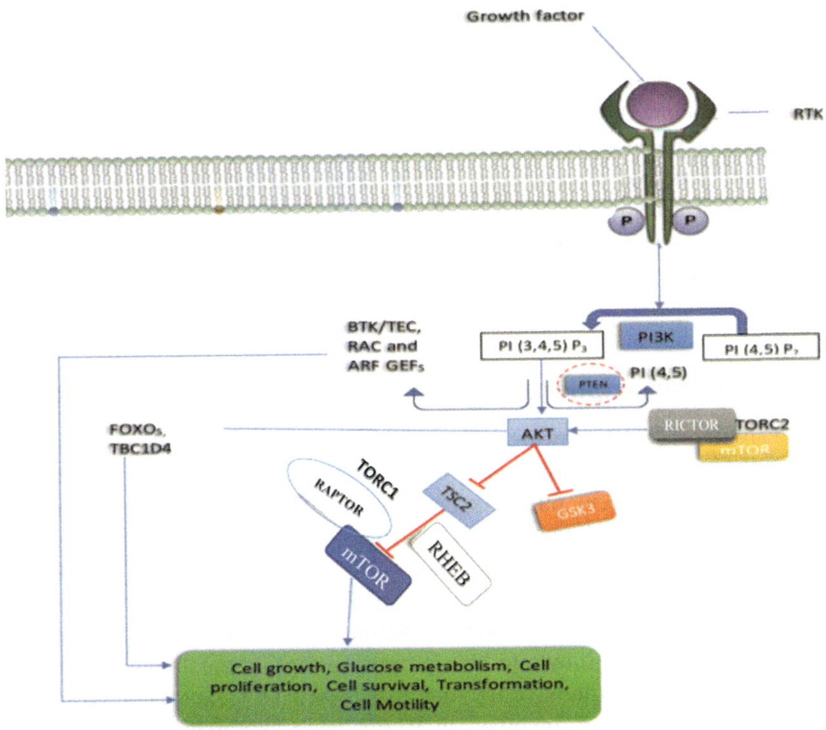

FIGURE 23.7 **The PI3K/Akt signaling pathwa**. Overview of the PI3 class I kinase signaling cascade.

G-protein coupled receptors and integrins also activate PI3K. Activated PI 3-kinase phosphorylates the membrane phos- phoinositide PI(4,5)P2 converting a small fraction of this lipid to PI(3,4,5)P3 which then continues the signalling cascade by regulating a large group of PIP3-binding proteins including AKT. AKT influences cellular behaviour by phosphorylating its substrates including FOXO transcription factors, TSC1 and TSC2, TBC1D4 and GSK3. PTEN acts as an antagonist to PI3K de-phosphorylating PIP3 and converting it back to PIP2.

23.4 Changes in PTEN activity in health and disease

Given the biological importance of its functions and the profound pathological effects that arise as a consequence of subtle disruptions on its expression and activity, it is unsurprising that PTEN levels are tightly regulated through multiple physiological mechanisms (Brito et al., 2015; Lee et al., 2018). These mechanisms of PTEN regulation act at transcriptional, post-transcrip-tional and post-translational levels. Significantly, these physiological mechanisms appear to be subverted in some cancers to suppress PTEN expression and activity. In particular, strong evidence has established the role of promoter methylation and miRNAs suppressing PTEN ex- pression in certain tumour types and these effects are discussed in more detail below (Fig. 23.7). Moreover, PTEN regulation by the transcriptional product of its pseudogene (PTENP1) has gained great interest recently, thus adding a further degree of complexity to the already intricate regulation of PTEN expression (Haddadi et al., 2018). Notably, PTENP1 contains similar 3'UTR miRNA binding sites to PTEN, and has been proposed to act as a miRNA sponge with significance in a number of cancers (Tay, et al., 2011) (Fig. 23.8).

23.5 Posttranscriptional regulation of PTEN by noncoding RNAs

An example of PTEN downregulation is miRNA124, which plays an important role in ovarian cancer development as well as cisplatin resistance. A plethora of different miRNAs have been linked to PTEN regulation in human cancers, including miR19a in leukemia, miR22 in prostate cancer, and miR26a in high-grade glioma. Interestingly, the contribution of miRNAs to tumorigenesis through the regulation of PTEN levels tends to be dependent on the type of cancer. Direct inhibition of miRNA function to increase PTEN expression has shown to be a promising tool in oncology. In addition, miRNA regulation could have indirect effects on PTEN expression by targeting transcription factors involved in PTEN gene expression. However, the broader biological effects of most of the newly discovered miRNAs are still unknown. Further studies are needed to gain knowledge about their functions and thus discover their therapeutic potential.

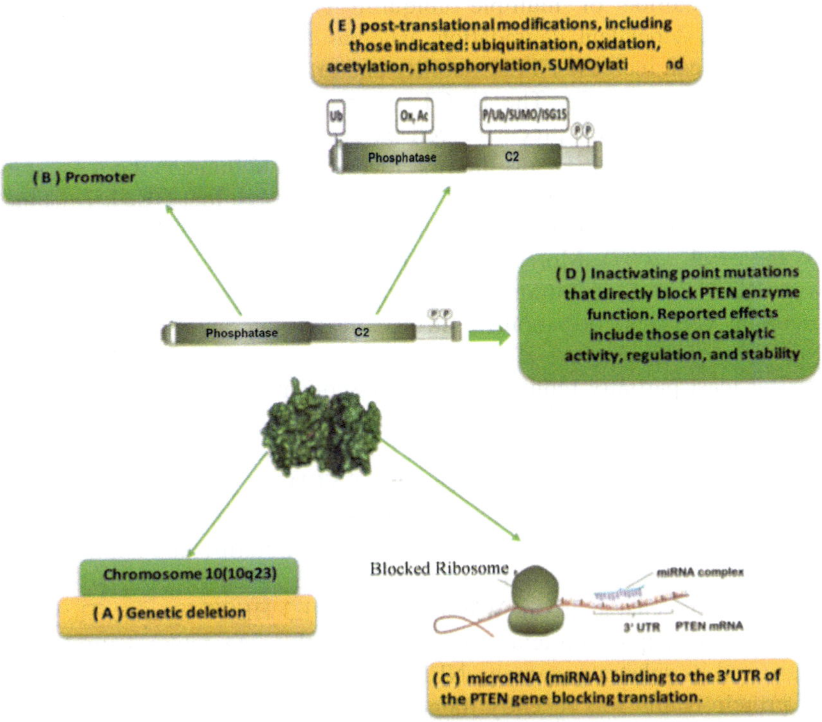

FIGURE 23.8 Changes in PTEN activity in health and disease PTEN regulatory mechanisms act at the transcriptional, posttranscriptional and posttranslational levels: (A) genetic deletion and mutation; (B) promoter hypermethylation; (C) microRNA (miRNA) binding to the 3′ UTR of the PTEN gene blocking translation; (D) inactivating point mutations that directly block PTEN enzyme function. Reported effects include those on catalytic activity, regulation, and stability of the protein; (E) posttranslational modifications, including those indicated: ubiqutination, oxidation, acetylation, phosphorylation, SUMOylation, and ISGylation. *From Verrastro, I., Tveen-Jensen, K., Woscholski, R., Spickett, C. M. & Pitt, A. R. (2016). Reversible oxidation of PTEN alters its interactions with signaling and regulatory proteins. Free Radical Biology and Medicine, 90, 24–34. https://doi.org/10.1016/j.freeradbiomed.2015.11.0046.*

23.6 Posttranslational modification: phosphorylation

These C-terminal phosphorylation events promote the maintenance of a closed but more stable conformation in which the C-tail binds to the C2 and phosphatase domains, blocking the active site perhaps by acting as a pseudosubstrate (Masson et al., 2016; Vazquez et al. 2000). In agreement with this, Thr366 appears to undergo slow auto dephosphorylation (Tibarewal et al., 2012).

23.7 Posttranslational modification: ubiquitination

Ubiquitination of PTEN by E3 Ubiquitin (Ub) ligases affects its catalytic activity as well as its stability and subcellular localization. It has been shown that the addition of multiple ubiquitin chains can target PTEN for proteasome-dependent degradation, whereas the addition of a single ubiquitin unit can increase PTEN stability and promote its nuclear localization (Trotman et al., 2007). The HECT (homologous to E6AP C terminus) domain protein neural precursor cell expressed, developmentally downregulated 4–1 (NEDD4–1) was the first identified and remains the most studied Ub ligase of PTEN. Wang and colleagues showed that NEDD4–1 binds to PTEN, catalyzing its polyubiquitination and inducing PTEN degradation (Wang et al., 2007). Moreover, NEDD4–1 levels are inversely correlated with PTEN levels in tumor biopsies, while overexpression of NEDD4–1 promotes cell transformation in vitro, indicating an oncogenic function of NEDD4–1. However, the effects of NEDD4–1 on PTEN should be considered at least partially redundant, as a subsequent analysis in two different strains of NEDD4–1-deficient mice found no apparent change in the regulation of PTEN levels and its subcellular distribution (Fouladkou et al., 2008). Other studies on the mechanisms of NEDD4–1-mediated PTEN ubiquitination have involved several adapters and ubiquitin ligase-activating proteins. For example, it has been proposed that Ndfip1 and Ndfip2 act as potent activators of several E3 ubiquitin ligases, including NEDD4–1, by binding to the characteristic WW domains of E3 HECT ligases. They also function as adaptor proteins by promoting the interaction between the ligase and its substrate, namely, NEDD4–1 and PTEN. Similarly, the adaptor protein Numb was recently found to be a binding partner of NEDD4–1 and plays an active role in modulating PTEN ubiquitination (Shao et al., 2017). PTEN has multiple ubiquitination sites, and it seems likely that several Ub-ligases are involved in the mono- and polyubiquitination of PTEN, possibly with some redundancy between related ligases (Gupta et al., 2016; Wang, et al., 2007). WWP2, a member of the NEDD4 family of proteins, has been reported to tag PTEN for degradation through a ubiquitination-dependent pathway (Maddika, et al., 2011). Interestingly, in vitro ubiquitin transferase assays revealed that purified WWP2 appears to be more active than NEDD4–1 in ubiquitinating unphosphorylated PTEN, suggesting that the two enzymes may exhibit distinct ubiquitination preferences for PTEN depending on the phosphorylation profile of the phosphatase (Chen, et al., 2016). In addition, the RING X-linked inhibitor of apoptosis protein domain E3 ligase and the C-terminus chaperone-assisted E3 ligase of Hsc70-interacting protein have both been reported to induce ubiquitination and regulate PTEN proteasome turnover (Van Themsche et al., 2009).

In contrast to the growing number of E3 ubiquitin ligases that have been linked to PTEN to date, the regulation of PTEN deubiquitination remains poorly understood. C-terminal ubiquitin hydrolase 13 (USP13) was found to reverse PTEN ubiquitination, leading to its stabilization in breast cancer cells. Other deubiquitinating enzymes that have been associated with PTEN include outer domain-containing protein 3 (OTUD3) and herpes virus-associated ubiquitin-specific protease 7 (HAUSP, also known as USP7).

23.8 Other ubiquitin-like modifications: SUMOylation and ISGylation

More recently, PTEN has been reported as one of the first validated substrates of ISGylation in cancer biology. As with ubiquitin, ISG15 conjugation to protein substrates requires a cascade that includes an E1 activator protein (UBE1L), an E2 conjugator protein (UBCH8), and an E3-ligase, typically HERC5. Although the E3-ligase(s) involved in the final step of ISG15 conjugation of PTEN remain unidentified, the functional consequences of ISGylation of PTEN are linked to its destabilization in in vitro studies, suggesting that ISG15 conjugation may control PTEN protein levels. Conversely, the deubiquitinating enzyme ubiquitin specific peptidase 18 (USP18) has been reported to reverse PTEN ISGylation. Furthermore, immunostaining of USP18 and PTEN was positively correlated in human lung cancer samples, suggesting the role of USP18 as a potential therapeutic target in cancer (Mustachio et al., 2017).

23.8.1 Posttranslational modification: oxidation

Like other members of the PTP family, PTEN contains a reactive nucleophilic cysteine catalytic site that is susceptible to oxidation. Indeed, several studies have shown that the catalytic activity of PTEN is subject to physiological regulation by reactive oxygen species (ROS). Reversible oxidation of the Cys124 site by ROS can promote the formation of a disulfide bond with Cys71, which in turn suppresses the phosphatase activity of PTEN (Lee et al., 2002). In addition, it has been shown that endogenic ROS generated in stimulated cells promote transient oxidation and thus inactivation of a fraction of the PTEN protein pool, and this correlates with ROS-dependent activation of downstream Akt signaling (Kwon et al., 2004; Leslie et al., 2003). Reversible oxidation of PTEN appears to be regulated by thioredoxin-interacting protein (Txnip), which acts as a negative regulator of thioredoxin- and NADPH-dependent disulfide bond reduction in proteins. Studies in a total Txnip knockout mouse model showed accumulation of oxidized PTEN and increased Akt signaling in oxidized tissues (Hui et al., 2008). Similarly, peroxidase peroxiredoxin 1 (Prdx1) and more recently apoptosis-inducing factor have been reported to protect PTEN from H_2O_2-mediated oxidation through direct interaction, thereby promoting the tumor suppressor functions of PTEN (Cao et al., 2009; Shen et al., 2015). Interestingly, analysis of the PTEN interactome using in vitro affinity capture showed that the redox status of PTEN can also alter its protein–protein interactions, suggesting that

ROS may also play a role in regulating the phosphatase-independent functions of PTEN (Verrastro et al., 2016).

23.8.2 Posttranslational modification: acetylation

The activity of the lipid phosphatase PTEN is subject to modulation by acetylation. Okumura and colleagues provided the first evidence for PTEN acetylation by reporting that the histone acetyltransferase PCAF (p300/CBP-associated factor) acetylates PTEN at Lys125 and Lys128, both located in the catalytic pocket. Acetylation at these residues inhibits the lipid phosphatase activity of PTEN and thus prevents PTEN from negatively regulating the Akt signaling pathway. Intriguingly, PTEN acetylation by PCAF appears to occur only in the presence of growth factors, indicating that PCAF may be a regulator of PTEN in response to mitogenic stimulation (Okumura et al., 2006).

Similarly, the histone acetyltransferase CBP targets PTEN on Lys402, which is located in its extreme C-terminal PDZ (PSD-95/Discs large/ZO-1 homologous) binding sequence. Acetylation of Lys402 does not directly affect the catalytic activity of PTEN but instead enhances its interaction with certain PDZ proteins, including MAGI-2. Sirtuin deacetylase 1 (SIRT1) has been shown to be responsible for PTEN deacetylation in this context (Ikenoue et al., 2008). In SIRT1 knockout cells, PTEN was hyperacetylated and excluded from the nucleus, which correlates with increased Akt activity, suggesting that acetylation may be involved in modulating PTEN subcellular localization and activity.

23.9 PTEN loss in prostate cancer

A recent study identified six genes in a minimally deleted region on 10q23 in prostate cancer datasets that were lost along with PTEN. Two particularly intriguing genes are KLLN (a target of p53, which encodes the protein killin) and multiple inositol-polyphosphate phosphatase 1 (MINPP1), a histidine phosphatase involved in inositol-3-phosphate metabolism. Another study also reported that genes lost in the 10q23 region, including the cell surface death receptor FAS and 3′-phosphoadenosine 5′-phosphosulfate synthase 2 (PAPSS2), as well as PTEN were involved in the biochemical recurrence of PSA (Ibeawuchi et al., 2015). FAS and PTEN may cooperate to induce programmed cell death, and PAPSS2 may have a role in androgen synthesis. PAPSS2 has been shown to be weakly expressed in prostate tumors (Ibeawuchi et al., 2015). In a number of cases, PTEN status according to FISH and IHC has been reported for prostate tumors, and in many cases, there is good agreement between the techniques. However, PTEN function is known to be regulated at transcriptional, posttranscriptional, and translational levels, and the question remains to what extent dysregulation of these processes might contribute to prostate cancer development. A preliminary comparison of the frequency of PTEN loss using sequencing, CGH, FISH, or IHC showed that IHC consistently showed higher frequencies of PTEN loss than FISH or other genetic assessments, which is consistent with the hypothesis that PTEN may be regulated at this level in prostate cancer.

The question of what mechanisms might be involved is therefore relevant. There is relatively little evidence for the role of promoter methylation in prostate cancer (Krohn et al., 2012), compared to other tumors. Conversely, there is increasing evidence that suppression of PTEN levels by miRNAs plays a role in prostate cancer progression (Irshad et al., 2013). Nevertheless, a number of miRNAs have been implicated in PTEN regulation in prostate cancer, including mir4534 (Nip et al., 2016), mir153, and mir410–3p, and a number of miRNA levels are altered in tumor tissues compared to nontumor human prostate samples (e.g., Poliseno et al., 2010).

23.9.1 Tumor PTEN affects immune infiltration

Extensive evidence suggests a central role of tumor PTEN status in modulating immune tumor microenvironment (TME) infiltrate and cancer cell/TME interactions in different tumor histotypes (Fig. 23.9).

23.9.2 Various genetic aberrations in the PI3K-AKT-mTOR pathway in prostate cancer

Furthermore, genomic and transcriptomic profiling revealed that genetic alterations and deregulation of gene expression of PI3K pathway components

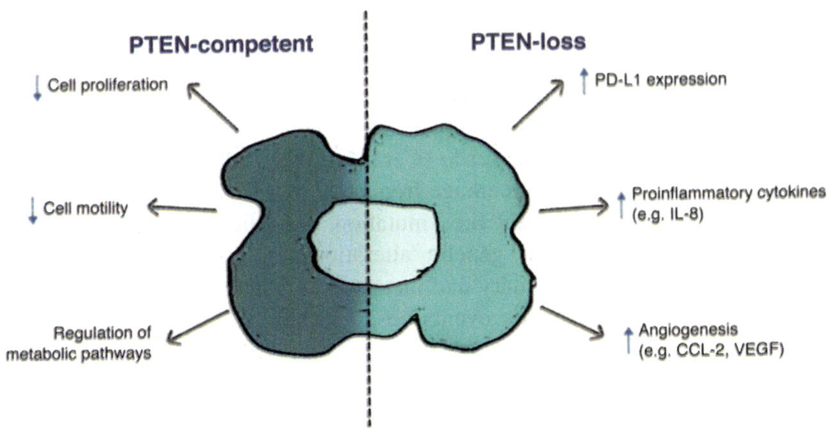

FIGURE 23.9 Schematic illustration of PTEN function in tumor cells. The status of PTEN in cancer cells affects both the biological characteristics of cancer cell survival and the composition of the tumor microenvironment (TME), depending on the expression of specific ligands (i.e., PD-L1) and soluble factors (i.e., IL-8, CCL-2, VEGF).

TABLE 23.1 Frequency of common genetic alterations in the PI3K-AKT-mTOR pathway genes in prostate cancer.

Common types of genetic alterations in PI3K-AKT-mTOR pathway genes	Frequency in prostate cancer (%)
PTEN deletion/mutation	16.4–32
DEPTOR amplification	5.1–21.4
SGR mutation/amplification	5.6–20.5 (SGK3)
	0.2–2.7 (SGK1)
FOXO deletion	0.0–15.2 (FOXO1)
	4.5–13.4 (FOXO3)
MAP3K7	5.9–14.8
RRAGD deletion	6.5–14.4
SESN1 mutation/deletion	5.4–13.6
PIK3CA mutation/amplification	5.5–11.5
PIK3C2B mutation/amplification	1.4–11.5
PDPK1 amplification	0–8.1

are common in prostate cancer patients and are present in 42% of primary prostate cancer samples and 100% of metastatic prostate cancer samples. Deregulation of the PI3K-AKT-mTOR pathway reflects a variety of genetic alterations, primarily loss of PTEN function. To improve our understanding of the frequency and diversity of genetic aberrations in the PI3K-AKT-mTOR pathway in prostate cancer, we used the cBioPortal platform to study three publicly available prostate cancer genomic datasets with primary and/or metastatic patient samples for a panel of 68 genes that encode key components/effectors of the PI3K cascade (Cerami et al., 2012; Gao et al., 2013). OncoPrints displaying the percentage frequency of each type of genetic aberration assessed in each dataset (i.e., mutation, amplification, and deep deletion of a gene) show that genetic alterations in the PI3K-AKT-mTOR pathway are common in primary and metastatic prostate cancer and illustrate that the wide range of genetic events observed tend to coexist (summarized in Table 23.1).

23.10 Conclusion

Loss of PTEN, which negatively regulates the PI3K-AKT-mTOR pathway, is strongly linked to advanced prostate cancer progression and poor clinical outcome. As a result, several therapeutic approaches are being explored to combat PTEN-deficient tumors. These include classical inhibition of the PI3K-AKT-mTOR signaling network, as well as novel approaches that restore PTEN function or target PTEN regulation of chromosome stability, DNA damage repair and TME. Although targeting PTEN-deficient prostate cancer remains a clinical challenge, emerging advances in precision medicine indicate that PTEN loss provides a valuable biomarker for stratifying prostate cancer patients for treatment, which may improve the overall outcome.

Acknowledgment

Authors would like to thank the Ministry of National Education, Professional Training, Higher Education and Scientific Research and express gratitude to the members of Virology, Oncology and Medical Biotechnology team at FSTM-Hassan II University of Casablanca, for all their efforts to support us during all the stages of this research

References

Bray, F., Ferlay, J., Soerjomataram, I., Siegel, R. L., Torre, L. A., & Jemal, A. (2018). Global cancer statistics 2018: GLOBOCAN estimates of incidence and mortality worldwide for 36 cancers in 185 countries. *CA Cancer Journal for Clinicians*, *68*(6), 394–424. Available from https://doi.org/10.3322/caac.21492.

Brito, M. B., Goulielmaki, E., & Papakonstanti, E. A. (2015). Focus on PTEN regulation. *Frontiers in Oncology*, 5. Available from https://doi.org/10.3389/fonc.2015.00166.

Cao, J., Schulte, J., Knight, A., Leslie, N. R., Zagozdzon, A., Bronson, R., Manevich, Y., Beeson, C., & Neumann, C. A. (2009). Prdx1 inhibits tumorigenesis via regulating PTEN/AKT activity. *EMBO Journal*, *28*(10), 1505–1517. Available from https://doi.org/10.1038/emboj.2009.101.

Cerami, E., Gao, J., Dogrusoz, U., Gross, B. E., Sumer, S. O., Aksoy, B. A., Jacobsen, A., Byrne, C. J., Heuer, M. L., Larsson, E., Antipin, Y., Reva, B., Goldberg, A. P., Sander, C., & Schultz, N. (2012). The cBio Cancer Genomics Portal: An open platform for exploring multidimensional cancer genomics data. *Cancer Discovery*, *2*(5), 401–404. Available from https://doi.org/10.1158/2159-8290.CD-12-0095.

Chen, Z., Thomas, S. N., Bolduc, D. M., Jiang, X., Zhang, X., Wolberger, C., & Cole, P. A. (2016). Enzymatic Analysis of PTEN Ubiquitylation by WWP2 and NEDD4-1 E3 Ligases. *Biochemistry*, *55*(26), 3658–3666. Available from https://doi.org/10.1021/acs.biochem.6b00448.

Fouladkou, F., Landry, T., Kawabe, H., Neeb, A., Lu, C., Brose, N., Stambolic, V., & Rotin, D. (2008). The ubiquitin ligase Nedd4-1 is dispensable for the regulation of PTEN stability and localization. *Proceedings of the National Academy of Sciences of the United States of America*, *105*(25), 8585–8590. Available from https://doi.org/10.1073/pnas.0803233105.

Gao, J., Aksoy, B. A., Dogrusoz, U., Dresdner, G., Gross, B., Sumer, S. O., Sun, Y., Jacobsen, A., Sinha, R., Larsson, E., Cerami, E., Sander, C., & Schultz, N. (2013). Integrative analysis of complex cancer genomics and clinical profiles using the cBioPortal. *Science Signaling*, *6* (269), pl1. Available from https://doi.org/10.1126/scisignal.2004088.

González-Santamaría, J., Campagna, M., Ortega-Molina, A., Marcos-Villar, L., De La Cruz-Herrera, C. F., González, D., Gallego, P., Lopitz-Otsoa, F., Esteban, M., Rodríguez, M. S., Serrano, M., & Rivas, C. (2012). Regulation of the tumor suppressor PTEN by SUMO. *Cell Death and Disease*, *3*(9), e393. Available from https://doi.org/10.1038/cddis.2012.135.

Gupta, A., Maccario, H., Kriplani, N., & Leslie, N. R. (2016). *In cell and in vitro assays to measure PTEN ubiquitination. Methods in Molecular Biology* (Vol. 1388, pp. 155–165). Humana Press Inc. Available from https://doi.org/10.1007/978-1-4939-3299-3_11.

Haddadi, N., Lin, Y., Travis, G., Simpson, A. M., McGowan, E. M., & Nassif, N. T. (2018). PTEN/PTENP1: "Regulating the regulator of RTK-dependent PI3K/Akt signalling," new targets for cancer therapy. *Molecular Cancer*, *17*(1). Available from https://doi.org/10.1186/s12943-018-0803-3.

Hui, S. T. Y., Andres, A. M., Miller, A. K., Spann, N. J., Potter, D. W., Post, N. M., Chen, A. Z., Sachithanantham, S., Jung, D. Y., Kim, J. K., & Davis, R. A. (2008). Txnip balances metabolic and growth signaling via PTEN disulfide reduction. *Proceedings of the National Academy of Sciences of the United States of America*, *105*(10), 3921–3926. Available from https://doi.org/10.1073/pnas.0800293105.

Ibeawuchi, C., Schmidt, H., Voss, R., Titze, U., Abbas, M., Neumann, J., Eltze, E., Hoogland, A. M., Jenster, G., Brandt, B., & Semjonow, A. (2015). Exploring prostate cancer genome reveals simultaneous losses of PTEN, FAS and PAPSS2 in patients with PSA recurrence after radical prostatectomy. *International Journal of Molecular Sciences*, *16*(2), 3856–3869. Available from https://doi.org/10.3390/ijms16023856.

Ikenoue, T., Inoki, K., Zhao, B., & Guan, K. L. (2008). PTEN acetylation modulates its interaction with PDZ domain. *Cancer Research*, *68*(17), 6908–6912. Available from https://doi.org/10.1158/0008-5472.CAN-08-1107.

Irshad, S., Bansal, M., Castillo-Martin, M., Zheng, T., Aytes, A., Wenske, S., Le Magnen, C., Guarnieri, P., Sumazin, P., Benson, M. C., Shen, M. M., Califano, A., & Abate-Shen, C. (2013). A molecular signature predictive of indolent prostate cancer. *Science Translational Medicine*, *5*(202). Available from https://doi.org/10.1126/scitranslmed.3006408, 202ra122–202ra122.

Jamaspishvili, T., Berman, D. M., Ross, A. E., Scher, H. I., De Marzo, A. M., Squire, J. A., & Lotan, T. L. (2018). Clinical implications of PTEN loss in prostate cancer. *Nature Reviews Urology*, *15*(4), 222–234. Available from https://doi.org/10.1038/nrurol.2018.9.

Krohn, A., Diedler, T., Burkhardt, L., Mayer, P. S., De Silva, C., Meyer-Kornblum, M., Kötschau, D., Tennstedt, P., Huang, J., Gerhäuser, C., Mader, M., Kurtz, S., Sirma, H., Saad, F., Steuber, T., Graefen, M., Plass, C., Sauter, G., Simon, R., & Schlomm, T. (2012). Genomic deletion of PTEN is associated with tumor progression and early PSA recurrence in ERG fusion-positive and fusion-negative prostate cancer. *American Journal of Pathology*, *181*(2), 401–412. Available from https://doi.org/10.1016/j.ajpath.2012.04.026.

Kwon, J., Lee, S. R., Yang, K. S., Ahn, Y., Kim, Y. J., Stadtman, E. R., & Rhee, S. G. (2004). Reversible oxidation and inactivation of the tumor suppressor PTEN in cells stimulated with peptide growth factors. *Proceedings of the National Academy of Sciences of the United States of America*, *101*(47), 16419–16424. Available from https://doi.org/10.1073/pnas.0407396101.

Lee, S. R., Yang, K. S., Kwon, J., Lee, C., Jeong, W., & Rhee, S. G. (2002). Reversible inactivation of the tumor suppressor PTEN by H2O2. *Journal of Biological Chemistry*, *277*(23), 20336–20342. Available from https://doi.org/10.1074/jbc.M111899200.

Lee, Y. R., Chen, M., & Pandolfi, P. P. (2018). The functions and regulation of the PTEN tumour suppressor: New modes and prospects. *Nature Reviews. Molecular Cell Biology, 19* (9), 547–562. Available from https://doi.org/10.1038/s41580-018-0015-0.

Leslie, N. R., Bennett, D., Lindsay, Y. E., Stewart, H., Gray, A., & Downes, C. P. (2003). Redox regulation of PI 3-kinase signalling via inactivation of PTEN. *EMBO Journal, 22* (20), 5501–5510. Available from https://doi.org/10.1093/emboj/cdg513.

Lotan, T. L., Gurel, B., Sutcliffe, S., Esopi, D., Liu, W., Xu, J., Hicks, J. L., Park, B. H., Humphreys, E., Partin, A. W., Han, M., Netto, G. J., Isaacs, W. B., & De Marzo, A. M. (2011). PTEN protein loss by immunostaining: Analytic validation and prognostic indicator for a high risk surgical cohort of prostate cancer patients. *Clinical Cancer Research, 17*(20), 6563–6573. Available from https://doi.org/10.1158/1078-0432.CCR-11-1244.

Lotan, T. L., Heumann, A., Rico, S. D., Hicks, J., Lecksell, K., Koop, C., Sauter, G., Schlomm, T., & Simon, R. (2017). PTEN loss detection in prostate cancer: Comparison of PTEN immunohistochemistry and PTEN FISH in a large retrospective prostatectomy cohort. *Oncotarget, 8*(39), 65566–65576. Available from https://doi.org/10.18632/oncotarget.19217.

Maddika, S., Kavela, S., Rani, N., Palicharla, V. R., Pokorny, J. L., Sarkaria, J. N., & Chen, J. (2011). WWP2 is an E3 ubiquitin ligase for PTEN. *Nature Cell Biology, 13*(6), 728–733. Available from https://doi.org/10.1038/ncb2240.

Masson, G. R., Perisic, O., Burke, J. E., & Williams, R. L. (2016). The intrinsically disordered tails of PTEN and PTEN-L have distinct roles in regulating substrate specificity and membrane activity. *Biochemical Journal, 473*(2), 135–144. Available from https://doi.org/10.1042/BJ20150931.

Meng, F., Henson, R., Wehbe–Janek, H., Ghoshal, K., Jacob, S. T., & Patel, T. (2007). MicroRNA-21 regulates expression of the PTEN tumor suppressor gene in human hepatocellular cancer. *Gastroenterology*, 647–658. Available from https://doi.org/10.1053/j.gastro.2007.05.022.

Milella, M., Falcone, I., Conciatori, F., Incani, C., Inzerilli, N., Nuzzo, C. M., Vaccaro, V., Vari, S., Cognetti, F., et al. (2015). Multiple functions in human malignant tumors. *Frontiers in Oncology*, 5.

Mustachio, L. M., Kawakami, M., Lu, Y., Rodriguez-Canales, J., Mino, B., Behrens, C., Wistuba, I., Bota-Rabassedas, N., Yu, J., Jack Lee, J., Roszik, J., Zheng, L., Liu, X., Freemantle, S. J., & Dmitrovsky, E. (2017). The ISG15-specific protease USP18 regulates stability of PTEN. *Oncotarget, 8*(1), 3–14. Available from https://doi.org/10.18632/oncotarget.13914.

Nip, H., Dar, A. A., Saini, S., Colden, M., Varahram, S., Chowdhary, H., Yamamura, S., Mitsui, Y., Tanaka, Y., Kato, T., Hashimoto, Y., Shiina, M., Kulkarni, P., Dasgupta, P., Imai-Sumida, M., Tabatabai, Z. L., Greene, K., Deng, G., Dahiya, R., & Majid, S. (2016). Oncogenic microRNA-4534 regulates PTEN pathway in prostate cancer. *Oncotarget, 7*(42), 68371–68384. Available from https://doi.org/10.18632/oncotarget.12031.

Okumura, K., Mendoza, M., Bachoo, R. M., DePinho, R. A., Cavenee, W. K., & Furnari, F. B. (2006). PCAF modulates PTEN activity. *Journal of Biological Chemistry, 281*(36), 26562–26568. Available from https://doi.org/10.1074/jbc.M605391200.

Poliseno, L., Salmena, L., Riccardi, L., Fornari, A., Song, M. S., Hobbs, R. M., Sportoletti, P., Varmeh, S., Egia, A., Fedele, G., Rameh, L., Loda, M., & Pandolfi, P. P. (2010). Identification of the miR-106b˜25 microRNA cluster as a proto-oncogenic PTEN- targeting intron that cooperates with its host gene MCM7 in transformation. *Science Signaling, 3*. Available from https://doi.org/10.1126/scisignal.2000594ra29.

Sekuklu, S. D., Donoghue, M. T. A., & Spillane, C. (2009). miR-21 as a key regulator of oncogenic processes. *Biochemical Society Transactions*, *37*(4), 918–925. Available from https://doi.org/10.1042/BST0370918.

Shao, C., Li, Z., Ahmad, N., & Liu, X. (2017). Regulation of PTEN degradation and NEDD4–1 E3 ligase activity by Numb. *Cell Cycle (Georgetown, Tex.)*, *16*(10), 957–967. Available from https://doi.org/10.1080/15384101.2017.1310351.

Shen, S. M., Guo, M., Xiong, Z., Yu, Y., Zhao, X. Y., Zhang, F. F., & Chen, G. Q. (2015). AIF inhibits tumor metastasis by protecting PTEN from oxidation. *EMBO Reports*, *16*(11), 1563–1580. Available from https://doi.org/10.15252/embr.201540536.

Song, M. S., Salmena, L., Carracedo, A., Egia, A., Lo-Coco, F., Teruya-Feldstein, J., & Pandolfi, P. P. (2008). The deubiquitinylation and localization of PTEN are regulated by a HAUSP-PML network. *Nature*, *455*(7214), 813–817. Available from https://doi.org/10.1038/nature07290.

Sung, H., Ferlay, J., Siegel, R. L., Laversanne, M., Soerjomataram, I., Jemal, A., & Bray, F. (2021). Global cancer statistics 2020: GLOBOCAN estimates of incidence and mortality worldwide for 36 cancers in 185 countries. *CA: a cancer journal for clinicians*, *71*(3), 209–249.

Tay, Y., Kats, L., Salmena, L., Weiss, D., Tan, S. M., Ala, U., Karreth, F., Poliseno, L., Provero, P., Di Cunto, F., Lieberman, J., Rigoutsos, I., & Pandolfi, P. P. (2011). Coding-independent regulation of the tumor suppressor PTEN by competing endogenous mRNAs. *Cell*, *147*(2), 344–357. Available from https://doi.org/10.1016/j.cell.2011.09.029.

Tibarewal, P., Zilidis, G., Spinelli, L., Schurch, N., Maccario, H., Gray, A., Perera, N. M., Davidson, L., Barton, G. J., & Leslie, N. R. (2012). PTEN protein phosphatase activity correlates with control of gene expression and invasion, a tumor-suppressing phenotype, but not with AKT activity. *Science Signaling*, *5*(213). Available from https://doi.org/10.1126/scisignal.2002138.

Trotman, L. C., Wang, X., Alimonti, A., Chen, Z., Teruya-Feldstein, J., Yang, H., Pavletich, N. P., Carver, B. S., Cordon-Cardo, C., Erdjument-Bromage, H., Tempst, P., Chi, S. G., Kim, H. J., Misteli, T., Jiang, X., & Pandolfi, P. P. (2007). Ubiquitination regulates PTEN nuclear import and tumor suppression. *Cell*, *128*(1), 141–156. Available from https://doi.org/10.1016/j.cell.2006.11.040.

Van Themsche, C., Leblanc, V., Parent, S., & Asselin, E. (2009). X-linked inhibitor of apoptosis protein (XIAP) regulates PTEN ubiquitination, content, and compartmentalization. *Journal of Biological Chemistry*, *284*(31), 20462–20466. Available from https://doi.org/10.1074/jbc.C109.009522.

Vanhaesebroeck, B., Stephens, L., & Hawkins, P. (2012). PI3K signalling: The path to discovery and understanding. *Nature Reviews. Molecular Cell Biology*, *13*(3), 195–203. Available from https://doi.org/10.1038/nrm3290.

Vazquez, F., Ramaswamy, S., Nakamura, N., & Sellers, W. R. (2000). Phosphorylation of the PTEN tail regulates protein stability and function. *Molecular and Cellular Biology*, *20*(14), 5010–5018. Available from https://doi.org/10.1128/MCB.20.14.5010-5018.2000.

Verrastro, I., Tveen-Jensen, K., Woscholski, R., Spickett, C. M., & Pitt, A. R. (2016). Reversible oxidation of phosphatase and tensin homolog (PTEN) alters its interactions with signaling and regulatory proteins. *Free Radical Biology and Medicine*, *90*, 24–34. Available from https://doi.org/10.1016/j.freeradbiomed.2015.11.004.

Wang, X., Trotman, L. C., Koppie, T., Alimonti, A., Chen, Z., Gao, Z., Wang, J., Erdjument-Bromage, H., Tempst, P., Cordon-Cardo, C., Pandolfi, P. P., & Jiang, X. (2007). NEDD4-1 is a proto-oncogenic ubiquitin ligase for PTEN. *Cell*, *128*(1), 129–139. Available from https://doi.org/10.1016/j.cell.2006.11.039.

Chapter 24

Association between glucose consumption and cancer development: prostate cancer and bladder cancer

Mouad Najih[2], Youssef Ennaji[2], Ikram Tiabi[2] and Moulay Mustapha Ennaji[1]

[1]Group Leader Research team of Virology, Oncology, and Biotechnologies, Head of Laboratory of Virology, Oncology, Biosciences, Environment and New Energies (LVO-BEEN), Faculty of Sciences and Techniques Mohammedia, University Hassan II of Casablanca, Casablanca, Morocco, [2]Team of Virology, Oncology, and Biotechnologies, Laboratory of Virology, Oncology, Biosciences, Environment and New Energies (LVO-BEEN), Faculty of Sciences and Techniques Mohammedia, University Hassan II of Casablanca, Casablanca, Morocco

24.1 Introduction

Genitourinary cancers are classified as the most common malignant diseases in men. They form a specialized field focusing on cancers in relation with urinary system and the male reproductive system. These include prostate cancer, kidney cancer, bladder cancer, testicular cancer, and cancers of the penis. In this chapter, we will talk about the two most common genitourinary cancers in the world (Guo et al., 2021).

Prostate cancer is the second most frequent cancer and the fifth leading cause of death among men. In 2018 approximately 1.3 million new cases of prostate cancer and 359,000 associated deaths were reported worldwide. It is also the most diagnosed cancer among men in over one-half of the countries of the world. Fortunately, prostate cancer mortality rates have declined in many countries, and this is due to early diagnosis through screening in addition to improved treatment, which results in an extended life expectancy for some men with this metastatic disease (Bray et al., 2018).

Bladder cancer is the 10th most frequent cancer in worldwide. In 2018 approximately 549,000 new cases of bladder cancer and 200,000 associated deaths were reported worldwide. Bladder cancer is more common in men,

Immunological Implications and Molecular Diagnostics of Genitourinary Cancer.
DOI: https://doi.org/10.1016/B978-0-323-85496-2.00002-6

with respective incidence and mortality four times higher in men than in women (Bray et al., 2018).

Bladder cancer is a disease that consists of two parts, 70% of patients have superficial tumors, which are often recurrent but harmless, and 30% have muscle-invasive cancer, which is associated with a high risk of death from distant metastases.

In cancer cells, metabolism is reprogrammed to aerobic glycolysis, which contributes to the aggressive phenotype.

Otto Warburg was the first to discover that tumor cells, unlike their normal counterparts, use glycolysis instead of mitochondrial oxidative phosphorylation for glucose metabolism, even in the presence of oxygen (Warburg effect; Shaw, 2006).

24.2 Glycose metabolism

24.2.1 General scheme of dietary carbohydrate assimilation

In the intestine, glucose is found in carbohydrates, amino acids in proteins, and chylomicrons in lipids (Tortora & Derrickson, 2007). Glucose then passes through the circulation to the liver cells or hepatocytes, where it is stored. It can also be used directly by the cells of the body that require energy. In particular, glucose is degraded in the cytosol and then in the mitochondria into CO_2, H_2O, and adenosine triphosphate (ATP; Schiaffino & Reggiani, 2011).

In the intestinal lumen, glucose, fructose, and galactose are found and all three reach the liver via the blood where they get degraded. If too much sugar is consumed, the liver will be saturated, forcing the body to store it as fat in the adipose tissue. Later, when the body needs them again, the liver will be able to produce glucose from noncarbohydrate substances, which is called gluconeogenesis (Tortora & Derrickson, 2007).

Blood glucose uptake by skeletal muscle occurs by a facilitated diffusion process and requires glucose transporters (GLUT) in the sarcolemma and T-tubules. Blood glucose is also taken up by skeletal muscles, requiring the presence of GLUT in the sarcolemma and T-tubules (Birk & Wojtaszewski, 2006). Twelve GLUTs (GLUT1–GLUT12) as well as the proton/myoinositol cotransporter (HMIT) have been identified. GLUTs are proteins with 12 transmembrane domains. Their tissue expression is specific to each GLUT, as is their affinity for various saccharides. GLUTs are divided into three classes. This classification is based primarily on the amino acid sequence and glucose affinity of the different GLUTs (Cantó et al., 2006).

Class I includes GLUT1–4; class II includes GLUT5, GLUT7, GLUT9, and GLUT11. Class III includes all other GLUTs as well as HMIT [4, 5]. The different types of GLUTs are shown in Table 24.1. For skeletal muscle tissue, GLUT1 and GLUT4 are the most widely studied GLUTs to date (Carling, 2004).

TABLE 24.1 Metabolic alteration in prostate cancer (Elia et al., 2016).

	Prostate			Breast		Liver
	Normal cells	**Cancer cells**	**Metastatic cells**	**Triple negative**	**Estrogen positive**	**Cancer cells**
Ox Phos	Inactive	Active	Inactive	Inactive	Active	Inactive
Krebs cycle	Inactive	Active	Inactive	Inactive	Active	Inactive
Glucose	Consumed	Consumed	Consumed	Consumed	–	Consumed
Lactate	–	Consumed	Accumulated	Secreted	Imported	Secreted
Citrate	Secreted	Consumed	–	–	Consumed	–

24.2.2 Carbohydrate catabolism

Carbohydrate catabolism refers to the breakdown of glucose molecules into more energetic molecules (Cantó et al., 2006).

24.2.3 Glycolysis (or Embden–Meyerhof pathway)

The glycolysis reaction, which takes place in the cytoplasm, is explained in detail in Fig. 24.1. The glucose site can follow the pentose phosphate replacement pathway, glucose-6- phosphate, to re-enter glycolysis as fructose-6-phosphate or glyceraldehyde-3-phosphate (Kuettner et al., 2010; Kuser et al., 2000). Neoglucogenesis uses reversible reactions catalyzed by numerous glycolysis enzymes, as well as specific enzymes for nonreversible reactions: phosphoenolpyruvate carboxykinase and fructose-1,6-bisphosphatase. In glycolysis, reactions in the opposite direction are catalyzed by pyruvate kinase and phosphofructokinase (Fig. 24.1).

The other steps in glycolysis are all catalyzed by enzymes that can perform the reaction in both directions. In *Saccharomyces cerevisiae*, however, a number of steps are catalyzed by multiple enzymes, all of which are specialized in glycolysis or gluconeogenesis. For example, the reaction that converts 2-phosphoglycerate to phosphoenolpyruvate is catalyzed by enolase-catalyzed enolpyruvate, encoded by the ENO1 and ENO2 genes. ENO2 is expressed primarily in the presence of glucose, whereas ENO1 is expressed under conditions of gluconeogenesis. In *S. cerevisiae*, some gene-encoding enzymes have homologs following complete duplication and paralogs following complete genome duplication. This is the case for HXK1 and HXK2, TDH2 and TDH3, ENO1 and ENO2, and PYK1 and PYK2. Glucose phosphorylation is carried out mainly by hexokinase, which is responsible for the phosphorylation of different types of hexoses (glucose, fructose, mannose, etc.) and also by a glucokinase that is specialized in glucose phosphorylation and whose catalytic role is less high (Verho et al., 2002).

24.3 Regulation of glucose metabolism in cancer cells

Glucose is the primary fuel source in all types of cells. In noncancer cells, glucose is mainly metabolized via oxidative phosphorylation, but in malignant cells, the uncontrolled proliferation needs adjustments in metabolism to provide for their increased energy demands (Afonso et al., 2020). Warburg first reported his observation that cancer cells prefer glycolysis over oxidative phosphorylation to generate ATP, which means that cancer cells have a higher metabolism because of uptake of more glucose as compared to normal cells (Warburg et al., 1924; Najafov & Alessi, 2010). To facilitate the uptake of glucose, tumor cells overexpress on their surface GLUT proteins named GLUTs (Tekade & Sun, 2017).

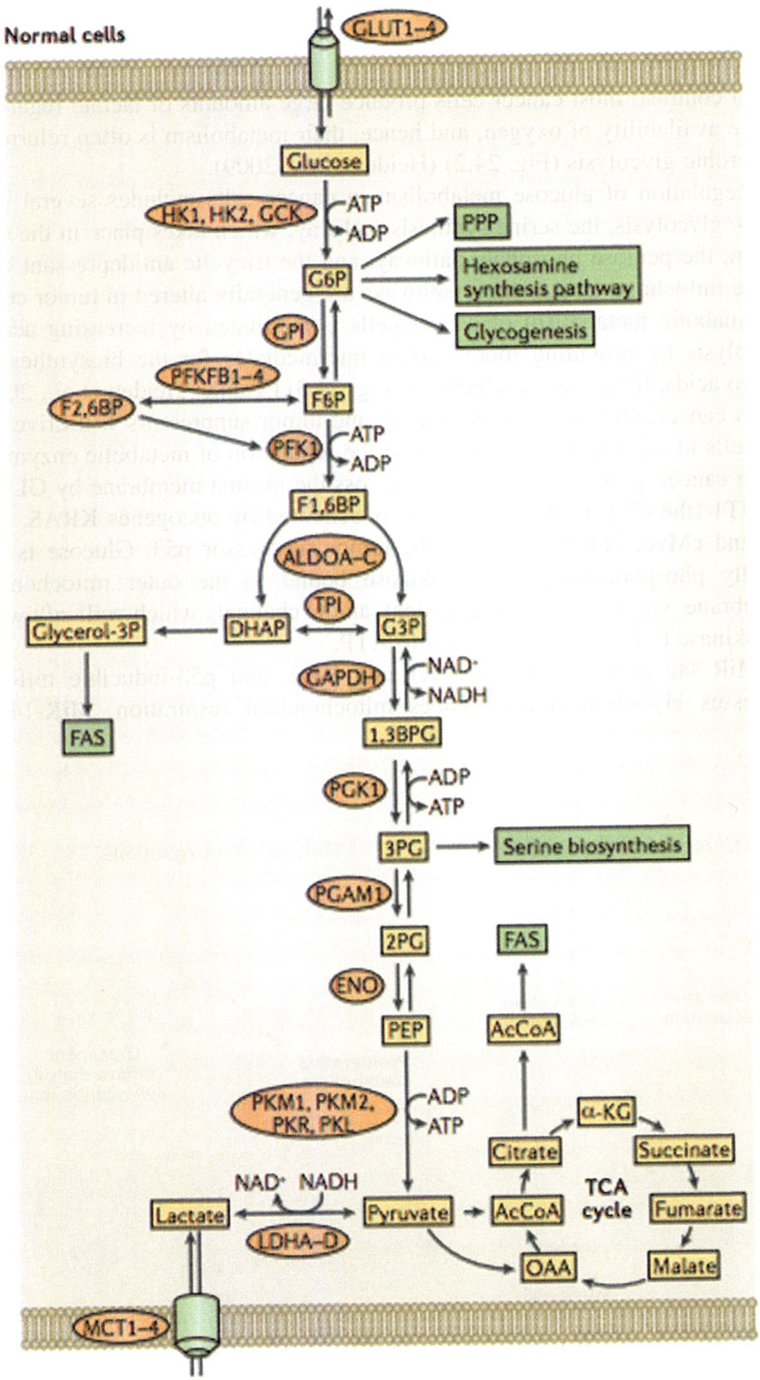

FIGURE 24.1 Regulation of glucose metabolism in normal cells (Hay, 2016).

In the presence of oxygen, normal cells use oxidative phosphorylation to produce energy. It is only under anaerobic conditions that differentiated cells produce large amounts of lactate.

In contrast, most cancer cells produce large amounts of lactate regardless of the availability of oxygen, and hence, their metabolism is often referred to as aerobic glycolysis (Fig. 24.2) (Heiden et al., 2009).

Regulation of glucose metabolism in cancer cells includes several pathways: glycolysis, the serine synthesis pathway, which takes place in the cytoplasm, the pentose phosphate pathway, and the tricyclic antidepressant cycle in the mitochondria. All these pathways are generally altered in tumor cells.

Anabolic metabolism of cancer cells is facilitated by increasing aerobic glycolysis by providing more carbon intermediates for the biosynthesis of amino acids, lipids, and nucleotides (Fig. 24.3) (Vander Heiden et al., 2012).

In cancer, alterations of oncogenes and tumor suppressors will drive cancer cells to aerobic glycolysis through the regulation of metabolic enzymes.

In cancer, glucose is transported across the plasma membrane by GLUTs, GLUT1 (the GLUT 1). This protein is activated by oncogenes KRAS, HIF-1a, and cMyc, but inhibited by the tumor suppressor p53. Glucose is then rapidly phosphorylated by hexokinase bound to the outer mitochondrial membrane via the voltage-dependent anion channel, which will allow the hexokinase to have a direct access to ATP.

MiR-34a acts directly on HK1 and HK2, and p53-inducible miR-34a represses glycolysis and enhances mitochondrial respiration. MiR-143 is

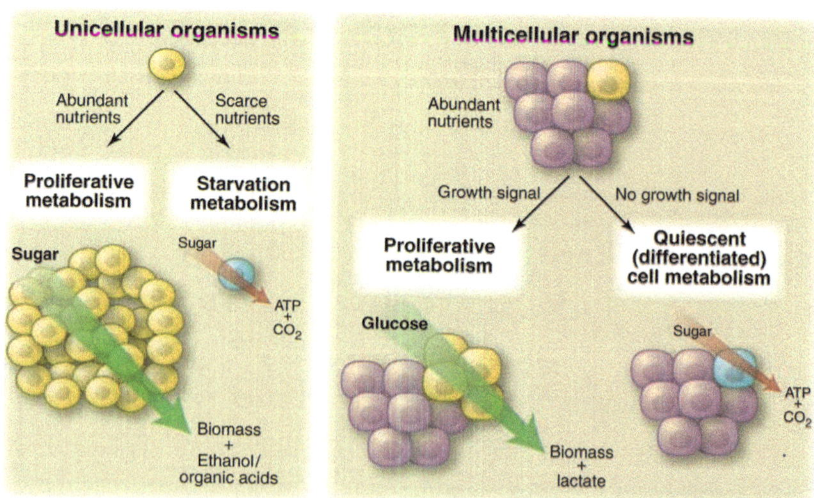

FIGURE 24.2 Schematic representation of the differences between oxidative phosphorylation, anaerobic glycolysis, and aerobic glycolysis (Warburg effect; Heiden et al., 2009).

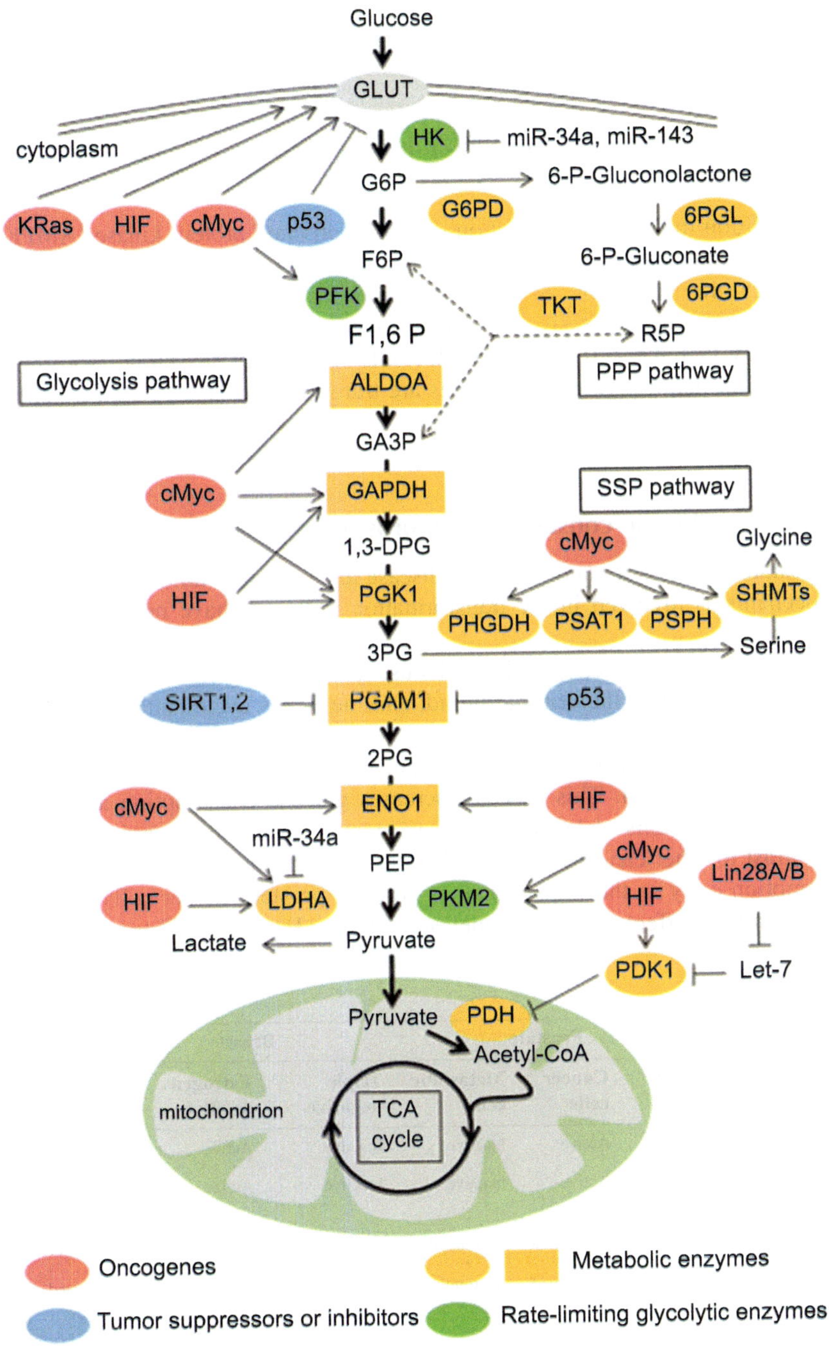

FIGURE 24.3 Regulation of glucose metabolism in cancer cells (Li & Zhang, 2016).

another microarray that regulates HK2 expression in cancer cells (Li & Zhang, 2016).

24.3.1 Activation of hypoxia-inducible factor drives increased glycolysis

In addition to the acute activation of AMP-activated protein kinase (AMPK), hypoxia-inducible factor controls the adaptation of cells to low oxygen levels through the activation of a transcription factor complex. Regarding the angiogenic targets, early studies of hypoxia-responsive element studies revealed that the cell surface GLUT GLUT1 and at least one isoform of almost all major glycolysis enzymes are transcriptionally increased by HIF-1 after hypoxia (Shaw, 2006).

24.3.2 Glucose consumption in prostate cancer

Prostate cancer is a major cause of disease and mortality among men, but the mechanisms involved in the transformation processes have not been clearly elucidated.

In normal prostate, epithelial cells use glucose to synthesize citrate that is secreted as part of the seminal liquid, and the Krebs cycle and the OXPHOS are inhibited.

In prostate cancer, cells corrupt cancer associated fibroblasts to activate the Warburg effect. This process increases glucose consumption and generates large amounts of lactate, which is secreted in the microenvironment. In contrast to other cancer cell types that develop a higher level of glucose consumption early in the transformation process, prostate cancer cells switch to the Warburg effect only in the metastatic stage (Fig. 24.4) (Cutruzzolà et al., 2017).

	Prostate			Breast		Liver
	Normal cells	**Cancer cells**	**Metastatic cells**	**Triple negative**	**Estrogen positive**	**Cancer cells**
Ox Phos	Inactive	Active	Inactive	Inactive	Active	Inactive
Krebs cycle	Inactive	Active	Inactive	Inactive	Active	Inactive
Glucose	Consumed	Consumed	Consumed	Consumed	–	Consumed
Lactate	–	Consumed	Accumulat.	Secreted	Imported	Secreted
Citrate	Secreted	Consumed	–	–	Consumed	–

FIGURE 24.4 Metabolic alteration in prostate cancer (Elia et al., 2016).

24.3.3 Metabolic mechanisms in prostate cancer

24.3.3.1 PGC-1α and glucose metabolism

PGC-1α is also associated with the regulation of glucose metabolism. In particular, in skeletal muscle, this induction of PGC-1α allows the activation of the expression of the GLUT GLUT4 through the activation of the transporter MEF2C (Michael et al., 2001), which allows an increase in glucose uptake in these cells (Michael et al., 2001).

This increase in intracellular glucose concentration is associated with a decrease in glycolysis and an increase in glycogen storage (Wende et al., 2005). Indeed, the induction of PGC-1α leads to the expression of PDK4, via ERRα. This enzyme prevents glucose oxidation by inhibition of PDH and thus promotes glycogen synthesis (Safdar et al., 2011).

24.3.3.2 PGC-1α in prostate cancer

The PGC-1α process in CaP appears to be similar to that in melanoma subpopulations with a difference in PGC-1α expression: a subpopulation overexpressing PGC1α is proliferative but minimally invasive, and a subpopulation underexpressing PGC-1α is highly aggressive.

Studies have indeed revealed that PGC-1α stimulates tumor growth of a subpopulation of androgen-dependent prostate cancer cells through activation of the androgen receptor and thus its host genes (Shiota et al., 2010). It is well estab lished that the androgen-dependent relationship is found in primary prostate tumors that are naïve to any treatment. As a result, in primary prostate tumor, PGC-1α interferes with and activates androgen receptors to alter metabolism, increasing mitochondrial biogenesis and glucose and fatty acid oxidation, which enables CaP cell growth and survival (Shiota et al., 2010). In androgen-dependent CaP cells, the inhibition of PGC-1α causes cell cycle arrest in G1 phase and thus suppresses their growth (Shiota et al., 2010). Subsequently, in these cells, the signaling pathway induces PGC-1α expression in response to androgens, signaling pathway in response to androgens via AMPK (Tennakoon et al., 2014). This increase maintains PGC-1α expression and enhances its influence on tumor metabolism (Tennakoon et al., 2014).

24.3.4 Androgens reprogram prostate cancer cell metabolism

Androgens are key regulators of several metabolic pathways, including aerobic glycolysis and mitochondrial respiration. Indeed, after prolonged treatment with the synthetic androgen R1881, we observed an increase of about 400% in glucose uptake (Fig. 24.5A) as well as a significant increase in lactate production (Fig. 24.5B) in LNCaP-treated cells compared with controls. These results lead toward androgens being a driving force that increases glucose utilization, which is consistent with the reported regulation of glycolytic genes such as hexokinases by the androgen receptor (Audet-Walsh et al., 2017).

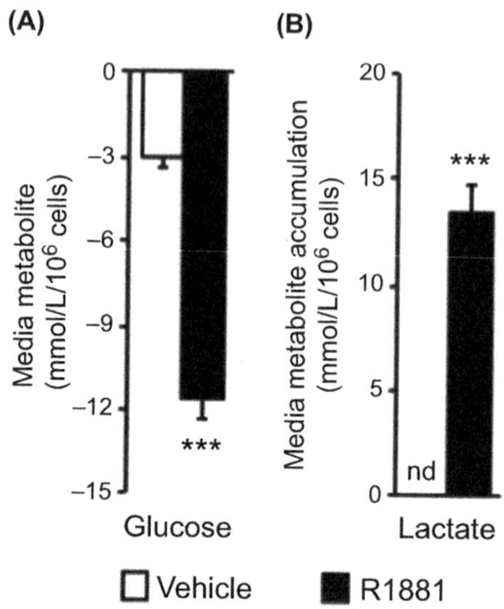

FIGURE 24.5 Androgens induce a metabolic reprogramming in prostate cancer cells. (A) represents glucose consumption and, (B) represents the lactate secretion in extracellular media of LNCaP cells following treatment with R1881 (Audet-Walsh et al., 2017).

24.3.5 Glucose consumption in bladder cancer

Bladder cancer is the second most common urological malignancy, urothelial tumors fall into two major groups superficial and invasive cancer associated with a high risk of death from distant metastases.

All tumor cells, including urothelial cancer cells, depend on glycolysis metabolism (Warburg effect) as the main source of energy to support their growth and uncontrolled proliferation. Therefore overexpression of the glucose receptors GLUT1 and GLUT3 is responsible for the high glycolytic flux (Massari et al., 2016).

To calculate the concentration of glucose in different bladder cancer cell line, a fluorescent glucose analog that accumulates inside tested cells (2-NBDG) is used. Fluorescent imaging of bladder cells showed that 2-NBDG was efficiently accumulated in all tested bladder cancer cells and was low in nontransformed urothelial cells (Fig. 24.6A). This observation was confirmed by a quantitative analysis of accumulated 2-NBDG in cell lysates using a fluorescence plate reader, and a significant difference in glucose consumption (2-NBDG accumulation) was observed in bladder cancer cells compared with nontransformed cells (Fig. 24.6B). The consumption of glucose by bladder cancer cells was higher than normal urothelial cells when cells were incubated for 24 h in 10 mM concentration of glucose (Fig. 24.6C; Whyard et al., 2016).

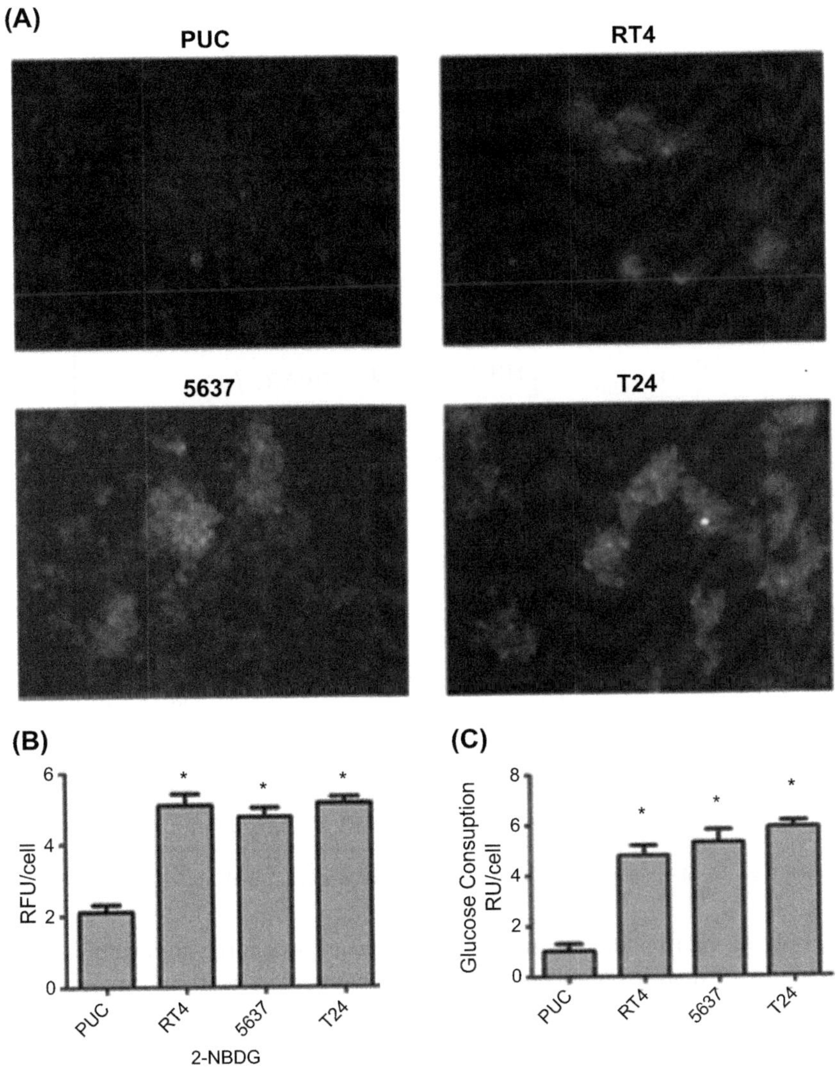

FIGURE 24.6 Glucose consumption by bladder epithelial cells. (A) Images of bladder cells incubated with 50 mM 2-NBDG for 60 min. (B) The level of 2-NBDG absorbed (fluorescence measurement in cell lysates). (C) The level of glucose consumed by bladder epithelial cells. Significantly different results are indicated by (asterisk) compared with untransformed urothelial cells (Whyard et al., 2016).

24.3.6 Metabolic mechanisms in bladder cancer

Increased glucose uptake by GLUT1 results in increased glycolysis, leading to excess glucose, which is ultimately converted to excess pyruvate. Pyruvate is either converted to lactate by lactate dehydrogenase in the

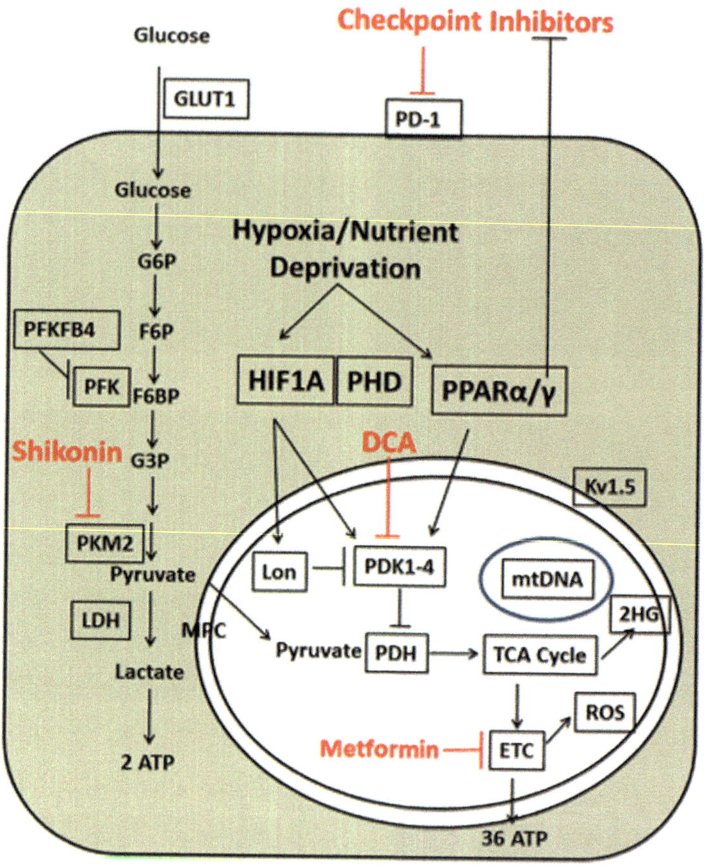

FIGURE 24.7 Metabolic changes in bladder cancer (Woolbright, et al., 2018).

cytoplasm, or it enters the mitochondria by mitochondrial pyruvate carrier. Le pyruvate dans les mitochondries est normalement métabolisé par la prolyl hydroxylases, mais cette interaction est largement bloquée par l'expression de pyruvate dehydrogenase kinase 1–4, qui est régulée à la hausse dans les cancers par les peroxisome proliferator activated receptor, and hypoxia-inducible factor 1A (Fig. 24.7) (Woolbright et al., 2018).

24.4 Conclusion

Cancer cell metabolism is altered that pushes the cells to consume more glucose compared with normal tissue, which contributes to the initiation and progression of tumors. This gives us the opportunity to use the united aspect in all cancer cells to develop this hypothesis.

Therapies that target various aspects of cell metabolism are currently being developed and are primarily focused on glucose metabolism.

Acknowlegment

Authors would like to thank the Ministry of National Education, Professional Training, Higher Education and Scientific Research and express gratitude to members of Virology, Oncology and Medical Biotechnology team at FSTM-Hassan II University of Casablanca, for all their efforts to support us during all stages of this research.

References

Afonso, J., Santos, L. L., Longatto-Filho, A., & Baltazar, F. (2020). Competitive glucose metabolism as a target to boost bladder cancer immunotherapy. *Nature Reviews Urology*, *17*(2), 77–106. Available from https://doi.org/10.1038/s41585-019-0263-6.

Audet-Walsh, É., Yee, T., McGuirk, S., Vernier, M., Ouellet, C., St-Pierre, J., & Giguère, V. (2017). Androgen-dependent repression of ERRγ reprograms metabolism in prostate cancer. *Cancer Research*, *77*(2), 378–389. Available from https://doi.org/10.1158/0008-5472.CAN-16-1204.

Birk, J. B., & Wojtaszewski, J. F. P. (2006). Predominant α2/β2/γ3 AMPK activation during exercise in human skeletal muscle. *The Journal of Physiology*, *577*(3), 1021–1032. Available from https://doi.org/10.1113/jphysiol.2006.120972.

Bray, F., Ferlay, J., Soerjomataram, I., Siegel, R. L., Torre, L. A., & Jemal, A. (2018). Global cancer statistics 2018: GLOBOCAN estimates of incidence and mortality worldwide for 36 cancers in 185 countries. *CA Cancer Journal for Clinicians*, *68*(6), 394–424. Available from https://doi.org/10.3322/caac.21492.

Cantó, C., Chibalin, A. V., Barnes, B. R., Glund, S., Suárez, E., Ryder, J. W., Palacín, M., Zierath, J. R., Zorzano, A., & Gumà, A. (2006). Neuregulins mediate calcium-induced glucose transport during muscle contraction. *Journal of Biological Chemistry*, *281*(31), 21690–21697. Available from https://doi.org/10.1074/jbc.M600475200.

Carling, D. (2004). The AMP-activated protein kinase cascade – a unifying system for energy control. *Trends in Biochemical Sciences*, *29*(1), 18–24. Available from https://doi.org/10.1016/j.tibs.2003.11.005.

Cutruzzolà, F., Giardina, G., Marani, M., Macone, A., Paiardini, A., Rinaldo, S., & Paone, A. (2017). Glucose metabolism in the progression of prostate cancer. *Frontiers in Physiology*, *8*, 97. Available from https://doi.org/10.3389/fphys.2017.00097.

Elia, I., Schmieder, R., Christen, S., & Fendt, S. M. (2016). *Organ-specific cancer metabolism and its potential for therapy. Handbook of Experimental Pharmacology* (Vol. 233, pp. 321–353). Springer New York LLC. Available from https://doi.org/10.1007/164_2015_10.

Guo, C. C., Shen, S. S., & Ro, J. Y. (2021). Pathogenesis and diagnosis of genitourinary cancer. *Cancers*, *13*(2), 1–3. Available from https://doi.org/10.3390/cancers13020347.

Hay, N. (2016). Reprogramming glucose metabolism in cancer: Can it be exploited for cancer therapy? *Nature Reviews Cancer*, *16*(10), 635–649. Available from https://doi.org/10.1038/nrc.2016.77.

Heiden, M. G. V., Cantley, L. C., & Thompson, C. B. (2009). Understanding the warburg effect: The metabolic requirements of cell proliferation. *Science (New York, N.Y.)*, *324*(5930), 1029–1033. Available from https://doi.org/10.1126/science.1160809.

Kuettner, E. B., Kettner, K., Keim, A., Svergun, D. I., Volke, D., Singer, D., Hoffmann, R., Müller, E. C., Otto, A., Kriegel, T. M., & Sträter, N. (2010). Crystal structure of hexokinase KlHxk1 of kluyveromyces lactis: A molecular basis for understanding the control of yeast hexokinase functions via covalent modification and oligomerization. *Journal of Biological Chemistry*, *285*(52), 41019–41033. Available from https://doi.org/10.1074/jbc.M110.185850.

Kuser, P. R., Krauchenco, S., Antunes, O. A. C., & Polikarpov, I. (2000). The high resolution crystal structure of yeast hexokinase PII with the correct primary sequence provides new insights into its mechanism of action. *Journal of Biological Chemistry*, *275*(27), 20814–20821. Available from https://doi.org/10.1074/jbc.M910412199.

Li, Z., & Zhang, H. (2016). Reprogramming of glucose, fatty acid and amino acid metabolism for cancer progression. *Cellular and Molecular Life Sciences*, *73*(2), 377–392. Available from https://doi.org/10.1007/s00018-015-2070-4.

Massari, F., Ciccarese, C., Santoni, M., Iacovelli, R., Mazzucchelli, R., Piva, F., Scarpelli, M., Berardi, R., Tortora, G., Lopez-Beltran, A., Cheng, L., & Montironi, R. (2016). Metabolic phenotype of bladder cancer. *Cancer Treatment Reviews*, *45*, 46–57. Available from https://doi.org/10.1016/j.ctrv.2016.03.005.

Michael, L. F., Wu, Z., Cheatham, R. B., Puigserver, P., Adelmant, G., Lehman, J. J., Kelly, D. P., & Spiegelman, B. M. (2001). Restoration of insulin-sensitive glucose transporter (GLUT4) gene expression in muscle cells by the transcriptional coactivator PGC-1. *Proceedings of the National Academy of Sciences of the United States of America*, *98*(7), 3820–3825. Available from https://doi.org/10.1073/pnas.061035098.

Najafov, A., & Alessi, D. R. (2010). Uncoupling the Warburg effect from cancer. *Proceedings of the National Academy of Sciences of the United States of America*, *107*(45), 19135–19136. Available from https://doi.org/10.1073/pnas.1014047107.

Safdar, A., Little, J. P., Stokl, A. J., Hettinga, B. P., Akhtar, M., & Tarnopolsky, M. A. (2011). Exercise increases mitochondrial PGC-1α content and promotes nuclear-mitochondrial cross-talk to coordinate mitochondrial biogenesis. *Journal of Biological Chemistry*, *286*(12), 10605–10617. Available from https://doi.org/10.1074/jbc.M110.211466.

Schiaffino, S., & Reggiani, C. (2011). Fiber types in Mammalian skeletal muscles. *Physiological Reviews*, *91*(4), 1447–1531. Available from https://doi.org/10.1152/physrev.00031.2010.

Shaw, R. J. (2006). Glucose metabolism and cancer. *Current Opinion in Cell Biology*, *18*(6), 598–608. Available from https://doi.org/10.1016/j.ceb.2006.10.005.

Shiota, M., Yokomizo, A., Tada, Y., Inokuchi, J., Tatsugami, K., Kuroiwa, K., Uchiumi, T., Fujimoto, N., Seki, N., & Naito, S. (2010). Peroxisome proliferator-activated receptor γ coactivator-1α interacts with the androgen receptor (AR) and promotes prostate cancer cell growth by activating the AR. *Molecular Endocrinology*, *24*(1), 114–127. Available from https://doi.org/10.1210/me.2009-0302.

Tekade, R. K., & Sun, X. (2017). The Warburg effect and glucose-derived cancer theranostics. *Drug Discovery Today*, *22*(11), 1637–1653. Available from https://doi.org/10.1016/j.drudis.2017.08.003.

Tennakoon, J. B., Shi, Y., Han, J. J., Tsouko, E., White, M. A., Burns, A. R., Zhang, A., Xia, X., Ilkayeva, O. R., Xin, L., Ittmann, M. M., Rick, F. G., Schally, A. V., & Frigo, D. E. (2014). Androgens regulate prostate cancer cell growth via an AMPK-PGC-1α-mediated metabolic switch. *Oncogene*, *33*(45), 5251–5261. Available from https://doi.org/10.1038/onc.2013.463.

Tortora, G. J., & Derrickson, B. (2007). *Principes d'Anatomie et de Physiologie* (2e Édition (ed.)). Canada: Éditions du Renouveau Pédagogique INC.

Vander Heiden, M. G., Lunt, S. Y., Dayton, T. L., Fiske, B. P., Israelsen, W. J., Mattaini, K. R., Vokes, N. I., Stephanopoulos, G., Cantley, L. C., Metallo, C. M., & Locasale, J. W. (2012). Metabolic pathway alterations that support cell proliferation. *Cold Spring Harbor Symposia on Quantitative Biology*, *76*, 325–334. Available from https://doi.org/10.1101/sqb.2012.76.010900.

Verho, R., Richard, P., Jonson, P. H., Sundqvist, L., Londesborough, J., & Penttilä, M. (2002). Identification of the first fungal NADP-GAPDH from kluyveromyces lactis. *Biochemistry*, *41*(46), 13833–13838. Available from https://doi.org/10.1021/bi0265325.

Warburg, O., Posener, K., & Negelein, E. (1924). Über den stoffwechsel der carcinomzelle. *Naturwissenschaften*, *12*(50), 1131–1137.

Wende, A. R., Huss, J. M., Schaeffer, P. J., Giguère, V., & Kelly, D. P. (2005). PGC-1α coactivates PDK4 gene expression via the orphan nuclear receptor ERRα: A mechanism for transcriptional control of muscle glucose metabolism. *Molecular and Cellular Biology*, *25*(24), 10684–10694. Available from https://doi.org/10.1128/MCB.25.24.10684-10694.2005.

Whyard, T., Waltzer, W. C., Waltzer, D., & Romanov, V. (2016). Metabolic alterations in bladder cancer: Applications for cancer imaging. *Experimental Cell Research*, *341*(1), 77–83. Available from https://doi.org/10.1016/j.yexcr.2016.01.005.

Woolbright, B. L., Ayres, M., & Taylor, J. A. (2018). Metabolic changes in bladder cancer. *Urologic Oncology: Seminars and Original Investigations*, *36*(7), 327–337. Available from https://doi.org/10.1016/j.urolonc.2018.04.010.

Chapter 25

Oncogenic human viruses associated with prostate cancer: molecular epidemiology of Human Papillomavirus and Epstein–Barr virus

Dorine Florence Luthera Ngombe Mouabata[2,3], Christy Parfait Nganga[2], Patrina Joseph Iloukou Mayakia[2,3], Donatien Moukassa[2] and Moulay Mustapha Ennaji[1]

[1]Group Leader Research team of Virology, Oncology, and Biotechnologies, Head of Laboratory of Virology, Oncology, Biosciences, Environment and New Energies (LVO-BEEN), Faculty of Sciences and Techniques Mohammedia, University Hassan II of Casablanca, Casablanca, Morocco, [2]Faculty of Health Sciences, University Marien Ngouabi, Brazzaville, Republic of Congo, [3]Team of Virology, Oncology, and Biotechnologies, Laboratory of Virology, Oncology, Biosciences, Environment and New Energies (LVO-BEEN), Faculty of Sciences and Techniques Mohammedia, University Hassan II of Casablanca, Casablanca, Morocco

25.1 Introduction

Prostate cancer (PCa) is one of the major causes of morbidity and mortality in men around the world and constitutes a line of research for pathologists, urologists, and uro-oncologists. It is the second most common cancer and the eighth leading cause of cancer death in men. Although the lifetime risk of developing a PCa is about 1 in 6 ($\sim$16%), (David Crawford et al., 2014; Howlader et al., 2012) the risk of dying from the disease is only about 2%. The discrepancy between the incidence and lethality of PCa has led to an in-depth review of the management of patients with PCa. The main known risk factors in PCa include increased age, ethnicity, and family history of the disease. PCa is both a biologically and clinically heterogeneous disease that develops amid various genetic and epigenetic changes (Barbieri et al., 2013; Berger et al., 2011). It develops in a minority of people who are persistently infected and only after many years of chronic infection (Schiller & Lowy, 2014). Viral involvement as essential factor or cofactor in the carcinogenesis of PCa worldwide has aroused scientific

Immunological Implications and Molecular Diagnostics of Genitourinary Cancer.
DOI: https://doi.org/10.1016/B978-0-323-85496-2.00021-X

interest for decades. Oncoviruses generally maintain chronic infections in which there is little or no production of viral particles by mechanisms of viral persistence and/or latency. These mechanisms are biologically compatible with the carcinogenic process, as they prevent cell death while keeping the infectious agent hidden from the immune system. Oncogenic viruses are necessary but not sufficient for the development of all types of malignant tumors.

Currently, around 15% of cancer cases worldwide and around 20% of cases in developing countries are associated with infectious agents (zur Hausen, 2009), and 12% of all cancers can be caused by oncoviruses (Bouvard et al., 2009), the vast majority of which (> 85%) occur in developing countries and regions (Grinstein et al., 2002; Lin et al., 2011). Human oncogenic viruses are made up of both RNA and DNA viruses and include several different taxonomic groups. Human oncogenic RNA viruses include Hepatite C virus (HCV) and Human T cell leukomia (HTLV), and human oncogenic DNA viruses include Hepatite B virus (HBV), Human Papillomavirus (HPV), Epstein–Barr virus (EBV), and Kaposi's sarcoma-associated herpesvirus (KSHV). A number of viruses associated with PCa have been identified and can interact with host proteins causing genetic, immunological, and inflammatory changes, which in turn lead to the initiation or progression of PCa as detected through indications based on the analysis of prostatic secretions of men with and without PCa, among which we have the HPV and herpes viruses including cytomegalovirus (Cohen et al., 2007; Hagensee et al., 2011; Khalili et al., 2003a, 2003b; Liu et al., 2005).

The oncogenic potential of high-risk human papillomavirus (HR-HPV) and EBV is well established. In addition, there is recent experimental evidence that has demonstrated that HPV and EBV may increase the oncogenicity of HPV-positive cervical cancer cell cultures (Hagensee et al., 2011), suggesting that the same is true for the epithelial cells of the prostate. HPV and EBV gene sequences have been identified in a very high proportion of samples in benign and malignant prostate tissue. These sequences were localized in the nuclei of epithelial cells of the prostate. These observations confirm the frequent identification in many studies of HR-HPV in PCa and the identification in three studies of EBV in PCa (Bergh et al., 2007; Grinstein et al., 2002; Sfanos et al., 2008).

25.1.1 History, taxonomy, and classification of human papillomavirus and Epstein–Barr virus

EBV is the first human oncogenic virus discovered (Mui et al., 2017). In 1961 following a conference by Denis Burkitt in London, Michael Anthony Epstein decided to search for this infectious agent on biopsies of tumors from this lymphoma by cultivating B cells, which would later take their names (Epstein & Barr, 1964). After three years of unsuccessful research, M. A. Epstein and Yvonne M. Barr established in vitro cell lines derived from Burkitt tumors, formerly called EBV HHV-4, one of eight known human herpes viruses belonging to the family Herpesviridae and to the subfamily *Gammaherpesvirinae* and to the genus *Lymphocryptovirus*. It is known to be a contributing factor in 1%–2% of all cancers (Fitzsimmons & Kelly, 2017). The EBV genome consists of a double-stranded DNA of approximately 172 kb linear, wrapped around a protein structure, composed of 162 capsomers, the icosahedral capsid covering the nucleoid is surrounded by an asymmetric fibrillar assembly called integument and an envelope derived from nuclear membranes and plasma carrying viral glycoproteins.

The European rabbit papillomavirus was the first to be described by Shope in 1933. The viral particles were visualized by electron microscopy in 1950 (Strauss et al., 1949). In 1984 Harald zur Hausen, with Lutz Gissman, first discovered HVP16 and then HVP18 responsible for around 70% of cervical cancers. For discovering that HPV can cause cancer in humans, zur Hausen won a Nobel Prize in 2008 (zur Hausen, 2009). Long classified in the same family of *Papovaviridae* as polyomaviruses, papillomaviruses (PV) form since 2002 a full family called: *Papillomaviridae*. In humans, PVs are called the "human papillomavirus." HPV contains a double-stranded DNA genome circular of about 8000 base pairs (bp) contained in an icosahedral symmetry, nonenveloped capsule formed of 72 capsomers arranged in a penta- or hexavalent manner (Andersson et al., 2008; Buck et al., 2008; Pereira et al., 2009). The viral genome is divided into three regions: the early region (E) containing E1, E2, E4, E5, E6, and E7, which are associated with viral replication, and the late region, which encodes the major (L1) and minor capsid (L2). This L1 gene is used as a basis for the classification of PV and the noncoding region also called the long control region. The oncogenic potential of HPV is determined by the oncogenes E6 and E7, which interact and inhibit the activities of critical components of cell cycle regulatory systems, in particular E6 with p53 and E7 with Rb. A total of 100 members of this family have been described, and among them, more than a dozen (types 16, 18, 31, 33, 35, 45, 51, 52, 56, 58, 59, 62, 66, and 68) have been classified as high risk owing to their epidemiological association with cancers (Zur Hausen, 2008) (19).

25.2 Molecular epidemiology of human papillomavirus and Epstein–Barr virus associated with prostate cancer worldwide

The number and percentage of human cancers linked to persistent unidentified viral infections is increasing (19). This may be true in the case of PCa. Although the prostate is an opening for several viral infections, some of which have oncogenic potential, a few studies have focused on the relationship between PCa and viral infection. Further data must be gathered to clarify the role of HPV and EBV in PCa carcinogenesis as well as their coinfection (Fatemipour et al., 2021).

25.2.1 Epidemiology of prostate cancer worldwide

PCa is the second most common cancer in men with 1,414,259 (14.1%) new cases diagnosed in the world, and in 2020 it is placed in 3rd position after lung and breast cancer for both sexes according to statistics from the International Agency for Research on Cancer. However in terms of mortality, PCa ranks eighth with an estimate of 375,304 deaths in 2020. According to the World Health Organization (WHO), recent data show a higher incidence of PCa in Europe and America in men with 500,827 and 454,096 new cases, respectively, and lower in Africa, while it is in Asia that the highest death rate has been recorded with 120,593 deaths. In Africa, the incidence of PCa is heterogeneous and varies considerably between regions; and it ranks first in terms of incidence in males. PCa is one of the main causes of death in men in many African countries representing 93,173 (29.7%) new cases (Globocan Africa 2020). A more refined analysis of the distribution of PCa by region in 2021 shows that the highest incidence is in East and West Africa with an estimate of 26,392 and 23,622 new cases, respectively.

25.2.2 Human papillomavirus and prostate cancer

Among the viruses responsible for human cancers, HPV occupies a preponderant place, being responsible for about 30% of all cancers linked to infectious agents. HPV is estimated to be responsible for 610,000 cancer cases and 250,000 deaths each year. According to the WHO, 85% of these deaths occur in developing countries. However, HPV is not just a public health problem in developing countries since it infects approximately 6.2 million people in the United States. HR-HPV infection is the most common infection in young, sexually active individuals. Indeed, it is estimated that around 75%–80% of sexually active people will be infected during their lifetime. HPV is the established etiological factor in cancers of the cervix, vulva, vagina, penis, and anus (de Sanjosé et al., 2014). Given its anatomical proximity to the anogenital and urinary sites, the prostate has been extensively studied for HPV infection. Although the link between HPV and cervical cancer is clearly established, the link of HPV to PCa is still questionable and hotly debated by researchers.

Studies in Mediterranean and Asian populations have suggested a link between HPV, particularly high-risk subtypes 16 and 18, and PCa (Atashafrooz & Rokhbakhsh-Zamin, 2016a, 2016b; Singh et al., 2015; Whitaker et al., 2013). The strength of the association varies according to geographic distribution. In addition, studies have found positive associations of PCa with sexual activity and sexually transmitted diseases, including HPV, suggesting that an infectious etiology may be involved in prostate carcinogenesis. HPV justifies a more rigorous investigation, in particular to reconcile the diversity of the results reported within the same populations

(Ghasemian et al., 2013; Tolstov et al., 2014a, 2014b). Several recent meta-analysis studies have shown that HPV infection is associated with an increased risk in the occurrence of PCa, which indicates a potential link between HPV and PCa. Another metaanalysis with an overall systematic review, using data from 24 studies involving 5546 cases of PCa, found a significant positive association between HPV infection and risk of PCa. Genotype 16 was found more frequently in patients with PCa, which significantly increased the risk of cancer (Moghoofei et al., 2019). Abdolmaleki et al. explored the role of HPV in PCa and found no association; only 3 of 133 samples analyzed in total were positive, HR-HPV-18 was positive in 2 (3.4%) of 58 cases and 1 (1.3%) of 75 controls (Abdolmaleki et al., 2018). In 2018 Martha I Dávila Rodriguez detected the HR-HPV in PCa, in a case-control study using normal and benign prostate tissue as a control, which showed the presence of HPV in 13 of 87 samples (62 with primary PCa and 25 with benign prostatic hyperplasia [BPH]), with a statistically significant high frequency in prostatic adenocarcinoma (19.4%) than patients with BPH (4%). The HPV genotype detected was HPV-11 considered to be low risk, and it had a higher prevalence (46.1%); HR-HPV 51, 52, and 66 were detected in six patients with PCa, while HPV-18 was detected in one patient with BPH. The result of another study on the Mexican population also showed that HR-HPV was detected in 37/189 (19.6%) PCa samples compared to 16/167 of the BPH samples. HPV 52 and 58 were the most frequently detected genotypes in the study population (Medel-Flores et al., 2018). This causal inference for HPV in male cancer is corroborated by (1) evidence that HPV infection can be quite common in the male population, up to 20% in a recent study of young Italian men by Mazzoli et al. (2008), (2) epidemiological studies demonstrating a clear protective effect of circumcision in men and women, and (3) a series of epidemiological studies demonstrating an association between infection by HPV and PCa.

25.2.3 Epstein–Barr virus

EBV is an ubiquitous human herpesvirus infecting over 90% of the world's adult population with oncogenic activity (Tsao et al., 2015). It is known to be a contributing factor in 1% to 2% of all cancers (Fitzsimmons and Kelly, 2017). It is involved in the development of a large number of lymphoid and epithelial cancers, including Hodgkin's and nonHodgkin's lymphomas, Burkitt's lymphoma, carcinoma of the nasopharynx, and posttransplant lymphoproliferative disorder (Shah & Young, 2009). It has been proposed that various epithelial carcinomas such as those of breast, kidney, colon, lung, stomach, and prostate could also be included in the list of EBV-related neoplasms (Shah and Young, 2009). A few attempts have been made to investigate the possible association of EBV with PCa (Bergh et al., 2007; Grinstein et al., 2002; Sfanos et al., 2008; Smelov et al., 2016; Whitaker et al., 2013).

Although EBV has a high distribution in the global population with known oncogenic potential, few studies have explored the possible association of EBV with PCa. Grinstein et al. confirmed the presence of EBV in 7 (37%) of the 18 adenocarcinomas of the prostate in American patients (Grinstein et al., 2002). Another study also identified EBV in 16 of 200 (8%) normal, benign, and malignant prostate tissues in American men (Sfanos et al., 2008). A result concerning the development of PCa by EBV was obtained by Bergh et al, who demonstrated the presence of EBV infection in 31 out of 352 (9.4%) benign, malignant, and normal prostate tissues in Sweden (Bergh et al., 2007). In 2019 Malekshahi et al. conducted a case-control study to identify the presence of the BK virus and EBV genome in BPH and PCa prostate samples in Iran. EBV was only detected in one PCa tissue sample among the 121 prostate tissues examined. These results provide further evidence against a causal role of EBV in the development of PCa (Malekshahi et al., 2020). In a study conducted in Australia, EBV was identified in equal proportion (40%, 4/10 cases) in malignant and normal prostate tissues (Whitaker et al., 2013).

25.2.4 Epidemiology of human papillomavirus and Epstein–Barr virus coinfection

HPV and EBV are human DNA oncogenic viruses. The International Agency for Research on Cancer has included both EBV and HPV as viruses causing neoplastic disease (Perera et al., 2010). Viral infections are estimated to contribute to 15%–20% of all human cancers such as PCa, breast cancer, and brain cancer (Alibek et al., 2013). EBV and HPV are believed to be linked to 38% of all cancers associated with viruses (Mesri et al., 2014). Numerous studies have shown that HPV infection is linked to NPC as an etiological factor (Giannoudis et al., 1995; Punwaney et al., 1999; Rassekh et al., 1998; Singhi et al., 2012) and that EBV is also present in cervical cancer uterus (Prayitno, 2006; Sasagawa et al., 2000) and PCa (Whitaker et al., 2013). In addition, experimental evidence has confirmed that HPV and EBV work together to promote the proliferation of cultured cervical cells (Ammatuna et al., 2000), suggesting that the same holds true for prostate epithelial cells. These observations are consistent with those of studies on HR-HPV and on EBV in PCa (Grinstein et al., 2002; Sfanos et al., 2008). In a study, the HPV type 18 and EBV gene (EBNA-1) sequences were identified in a high and approximately equal proportion of malignant, benign, and normal prostate samples. The sequences were localized in the nuclei of prostate epithelial cells. EBV only was identified in 4/10 (40%) of malignant samples, 2/10 (20%) of benign, and 4/10 (40%) of normal fixed archival prostates. HPV alone was identified in 7/10 (70%) smart samples, 7/10 (70%) benign, and 1/10 (10%) of normal samples; these differences were found to be statistically significant. The frequency of EBV and HPV coinfection was significantly higher in PCa 22/40 (55%) as compared to benign 6/40 (15%) and normal samples from the prostate 12/40 (30%). The study by Whitaker et al. helped understand the association between HPV and EBV and the potential oncogenic influences of each other (Whitaker et al., 2013). The identification of EBV and HPV in fresh samples was confirmed by sequencing the PCR product of selected samples of DNA extracts from the fresh frozen samples. Variations were observed in the sequences, which indicated the possibility of no contamination. Only HPV type 18 has been identified. The frequency of infections with these viruses can vary by geographic region.

25.3 Implications and associations of human papillomavirus and Epstein–Barr virus prostate cancer

The inflammation is suggested by the presence of inflammatory cells in the prostate in patients with BPH and PCa, and it is associated with carcinogenesis and the progression of PCa. Infections, especially sexually transmitted infections and those that affect the urogenital tractus, are possible causes of intraprostatic inflammation. It is therefore plausible that in men with preexisting prostatic inflammation, an HR-HPV infection, often localized to the prostate, may contribute to the development of chronic and regenerative inflammation, which is a risk factor for PCa (Farkona et al., 2016). HPV oncogenesis has been proven in several cancers, but its role in PCa is complex and differs from cervical cancer associated with HPV. Its oncogenicity is due to persistent infection with the expression of two early proteins, E6 and E7, inhibiting the protein suppressors of cell tumors such as Rb and p53. Currently, it is clear that the oncoproteins of HPV contribute not only to the initiation of cancer but also to its promotion and progression. Although each oncoprotein (E5, E6, and E7) has a unique action on carcinogens, they act as a driver of cancer progression. HPV infections can directly trigger prostate oncogenesis and influence oncogenesis indirectly via APOBEC enzymes. HPVs may collaborate with other pathogens in prostate oncogenesis (Farkona et al., 2016). Recent studies have shown that HPVs can have oncogenic mechanisms in addition to the influences of HPV E6 and E7 oncoproteins. These include the APOBEC3B proteins, which are a source of genome-wide mutations and may lead to an increased risk of several cancers, including PCa (Ohba et al., 2014). The mechanisms of APOBEC-related mutation processes remained unknown, until recent observations by Ohba et al. and Vieira et al., who have independently demonstrated that HPV infections cause overexpression of the APOBEC3B protein (Ohba et al., 2014; Vieira et al., 2014). An additional mechanism for oncogenesis associated with HPV has been investigated by Kundu et al. (2008). They demonstrated that components present in HPV and other pathogens can influence Toll-like receptor pathways contribute to the malignant transformation of the benign prostate epithelium.

Primary EBV infection, which often occurs early in childhood, is frequently asymptomatic. The targets of this virus are multiple. B lymphocytes and epithelial cells are conventional targets. For viral infections associated with carcinogenesis, EBV has been well studied; it has been reported to infect over 90% of the adult population but is only rarely associated with oncogenesis (Malekshahi et al., 2020). The reason why EBV exerts its oncogenic influences in a particular patient is unknown but is likely associated with cofactors. The frequency of this viral infection may vary depending on the geographic regions. EBV can manipulate the cellular microenvironment through the exosomal transfer of viral and cellular factors. Important signaling functions of exosomes are altered by LMP-1 in infected B cells. In cancers associated with EBV, these virus-modified exosomes can influence tumor growth in neighboring cells, inhibit immune function, or stimulate angiogenesis (Meckes, 2015). Few attempts have been made to investigate the possible association of EBV with PCa, but a few studies have demonstrated the presence of EBV in PCa.

25.3.1 Coinfection of human papillomavirus and Epstein–Barr virus

EBV and HPV are the causative agents of multiple malignant tumors; they infect and spread in epitheliums. The latent gene EBV is differently expressed in these malignant tumors (Raab-Traub, 2012; Suzuki, 2012). The productive phases of both viruses are linked to stratified epithelia, highlighting the possibility that these viruses can affect the life cycle of EBV and HPV. These oncogene viruses induce cancer by various mechanisms that do not include the viral episome or the lytic replication; for example, the immune system can have both roles – deleterious and protective – with increasing immunosuppression in cancers associated with human viruses and with the activation of response to DNA damages (Mesri et al., 2014; Nikitin et al., 2010). Recently, a family of proteins that includes the catalytic polypeptide 3 (APOBEC3) of the mARN editing enzymė of lipoprotein apo B has been developed. It is characterized with its ability to provide innate immunity against various exogenous pathogens, including viral infection (Cullen, 2006; Harris & Dudley, 2015). The cytidine deaminases of the APOBEC3 family all have specificness for single-stranded DNA, which can be exposed during the double-stranded DNA replication or transcription. Human genes APOBEC3A (hA3A, hA3B and hA3H) are expressed in the keratinocytes and skin; all induce hypermutation in the DNA of HPV-16 upon stimulation by the interféron beta in the benign and precancerous lesions during natural viral infection (Kukimoto et al., 2015; Vartanian et al., 2008; Wang et al., 2014). Interestingly, APOBEC3 is able to edit both EBV and HPV by inducing cytidine–uracil mutations in viral DNA (Suspène et al., 2011) and that it increases the chances of integration of viral DNA into the host by inducing mutations and instability of the genome after viral infection.

In a study regarding the double expression of EBV, the protein membrane latent-1 (LPM-1) and human HPV-16 E6 on mouse primary embryonic fibroblasts (MEF) via NF-signaling Kb, a conspicuous difference was found in the induction of the components of the DNA damage response (DDR) versus viral gene expression. All viral expressions in this study damaged the DNA, but only the coexpression of LMP-1 and E6 suppressed DDR and induced a transformation. Their results indicated that in addition to the activation of NF Kb signaling by expression of LMP-1 in primary MEFs, inhibition of a tumor suppressor gene, like p53 or RB, is necessary for transformation, and transformation is associated with removal of DDR. However, in addition to the expression of LMP-1, this study suggests that an additional oncogenic factor such as HPV-16 E6 or EBNA-1, may be strongly associated at the oncogenic transformation in coinfected cells by EBV and HPV. We have demonstrated these synergistic mechanisms using the coexpression of HPV and EBV genes in primary MEFs, but molecular mechanisms remain to be clarified (Shimabuku et al., 2014a, 2014b).

In a recent study regarding EBV/HPV coinfection in PCa, the HPV/EBV coinfection was present in 14.9% of PCa samples, and high-risk strains (HPV-16 and 18) were responsible for 50% and 30% of the 10 PCa samples coinfected with HPV/EBV, respectively. The maximum percentage of integration of the HPV genome was found in the PCa group coinfected with HPV/EBV (8/10, 80%). CD44 as a cell membrane receptor with multifunctional potential was highly expressed in many cancers such as PCa, which explains the cell–cell adhesion and the metastasis and tumor invasion. In this study, the mean CD44 expression level was significantly higher in the EBV-positive samples than in EBV-negative samples, and there was a positive correlation between LMP-1 and LPM-2 expression level and CD44 expression level. The existence of HPV and EBV is likely to be the cause of these changes, and the viral infection plays an important role in contributing to the resistance of anoïkis and development of PCa. Although there was no significant association between HPV/EBV coinfection and PCa, the expression pattern of certain cellular factors involved in tumor progression and metastasis was different between PCa infected with the virus and between HPV/EBV PCa samples coinfected with mono EBV or mono HPV infection. These differences may mean that the simultaneous presence of these viruses altered the pattern of expression of cellular factors compared to mono-infection (Nahand et al., 2021).

25.4 Conclusion

PCa is the most commonly diagnosed among men in most Western countries. Its incidence varies between countries and between different ethnic groups.

The prostate gland in men represents a complex organ where many viral infections with oncogenic DNA viruses such as HPV and EBV occur, implicating the potential role of these viruses in the progression of PCa. Since HPV has been identified in some studies of PCa, it is known to be highly oncogenic in cervical glandular epithelial cells, and there is no obvious reason why it should not be oncogenic in the prostate. Further studies are required to elucidate whether EBV and HPV coinfection plays a role in the development of malignant prostate tumors. Moreover, the control of the detailed mechanisms of this viral coinfection will represent potential targets for the development of new antiviral therapies.

References

Abdolmaleki, K., Ramezanzadeh., & Roshani, D. (2018). No association between human papillomavirus and prostate cancer. *International Journal of Cancer Management, 30.*

Alibek, K., Kakpenova, A., & Baiken, Y. (2013). Role of infectious agents in the carcinogenesis of brain and head and neck cancers. *Infectious Agents and Cancer, 8*(1), 1–9. Available from https://doi.org/10.1186/1750-9378-8-7.

Ammatuna, P., Giovannelli, L., Giambelluca, D., Mancuso, S., Rubino, E., Colletti, P., Mazzola, G., Belfiore, P., & Lima, R. (2000). Presence of human papillomavirus and Epstein-Barr virus in the cervix of women infected with the human immunodeficiency virus. *Journal of Medical Virology, 62*(4), 410–415. Available from https://doi.org/10.1002/1096-9071(200012)62:4 < 410::AID-JMV3 > 3.0.CO;2-J.

Andersson, K., Waterboer, T., Kirnbauer, R., Slupetzky, K., Iftner, T., De Villiers, E. M., Forslund, O., Pawlita, M., & Dillner, J. (2008). Seroreactivity to cutaneous human papillomaviruses among patients with nonmelanoma skin cancer or benign skin lesions. *Cancer Epidemiology Biomarkers and Prevention, 17*(1), 189–195. Available from https://doi.org/10.1158/1055-9965.EPI-07-0405.

Atashafrooz, F., & Rokhbakhsh-Zamin, F. (2016a). Frequency and type distribution of human papilloma virus in patients with prostate Cancer, Kerman, southeast of Iran. *Asian Pacific Journal of Cancer Prevention, 17*(8), 3953–3958.

Atashafrooz, F., & Rokhbakhsh-Zamin, F. (2016b). Frequency and type distribution of human papilloma virus in patients with prostate cancer, Kerman, southeast of Iran. *Asian Pacific Journal of Cancer Prevention, 17*(8), 3951–3956. Available from http://www.apocpcontrol.org/paper_file/issue_abs/Volume17_No8/3951-3956%205.28%20Fatemeh%20Atashafrooz.pdf.

Barbieri, C. E., Bangma, C. H., Bjartell, A., Catto, J. W. F., Culig, Z., Grönberg, H., Luo, J., Visakorpi, T., & Rubin, M. A. (2013). The mutational landscape of prostate cancer. *European Urology, 64*(4), 567–576. Available from https://doi.org/10.1016/j.eururo.2013.05.029.

Berger, M. F., Lawrence, M. S., Demichelis, F., Drier, Y., Cibulskis, K., Sivachenko, A. Y., Sboner, A., Esgueva, R., Pflueger, D., Sougnez, C., Onofrio, R., Carter, S. L., Park, K., Habegger, L., Ambrogio, L., Fennell, T., Parkin, M., Saksena, G., Voet, D., & Garraway, L. A. (2011). The genomic complexity of primary human prostate cancer. *Nature, 470*(7333), 214–220. Available from https://doi.org/10.1038/nature09744.

Bergh, J., Marklund, I., Gustavsson, C., Wiklund, F., Grönberg, H., Allard, A., Alexeyev, O., & Elgh, F. (2007). No link between viral findings in the prostate and subsequent cancer development. *British Journal of Cancer*, *96*(1), 137–139. Available from https://doi.org/10.1038/sj.bjc.6603480.

Bouvard, V., Baan, R., Straif, K., Grosse, Y., Secretan, B., El Ghissassi, F., Benbrahim-Tallaa, L., Guha, N., Freeman, C., Galichet, L., & Cogliano, V. (2009). A review of human carcinogens–Part B: Biological agents. *The Lancet Oncology*, *10*(4), 321–322. Available from https://doi.org/10.1016/s1470-2045(09)70096-8.

Buck, C. B., Cheng, N., Thompson, C. D., Lowy, D. R., Steven, A. C., Schiller, J. T., & Trus, B. L. (2008). Arrangement of L2 within the papillomavirus capsid. *Journal of Virology*, *82* (11), 5190–5197. Available from https://doi.org/10.1128/JVI.02726-07.

Cohen, S. B., Graham, M. E., Lovrecz, G. O., Bache, N., Robinson, P. J., & Reddel, R. R. (2007). Protein composition of catalytically active human telomerase from immortal cells. *Science (New York, N.Y.)*, *315*(5820), 1850–1853. Available from https://doi.org/10.1126/science.1138596.

Cullen, B. R. (2006). Role and mechanism of action of the APOBEC3 family of antiretroviral resistance factors. *Journal of Virology*, *80*(3), 1067–1076. Available from https://doi.org/10.1128/JVI.80.3.1067-1076.2006.

David Crawford, E., Ventii, K., & Shore, N. D. (2014). New biomarkers in prostate cancer. *Oncology (United States)*, *28*(2). Available from http://www.cancernetwork.com/printpdf/196735.

de Sanjosé, S., Bruni, L., & Alemany, L. (2014). HPV in genital cancers (at the exception of cervical cancer) and anal cancers. *La Presse Médicale*, *43*(12), e423–e428. Available from https://doi.org/10.1016/j.lpm.2014.10.001.

Epstein, M. A., & Barr, Y. M. (1964). Cultivation in vitro of human lymphoblasts from Burkitt's malignant lymphoma. *The Lancet*, *283*(7327), 252–253. Available from https://doi.org/10.1016/S0140-6736(64)92354-2.

Farkona, S., Diamandis, E. P., & Blasutig, I. M. (2016). Cancer immunotherapy: The beginning of the end of cancer? *BMC Medicine*, *14*(1), 1–18. Available from https://doi.org/10.1186/s12916-016-0623-5.

Fatemipour, M., Nahand, J. S., Fard Azar, M. E., Baghi, H. B., Taghizadieh, M., Sorayyayi, S., Hussen, B. M., Mirzaei, H., Moghoofei, M., & Bokharaei-Salim, F. (2021). Human papillomavirus and prostate cancer: The role of viral expressed proteins in the inhibition of anoikis and induction of metastasis. *Microbial Pathogenesis*, 152. Available from https://doi.org/10.1016/j.micpath.2020.104576.

Fitzsimmons, L., & Kelly, G. L. (2017). EBV and apoptosis: The viral master regulator of cell fate? *Viruses*, *9*(11), 339. Available from https://doi.org/10.3390/v9110339.

Ghasemian, E., Monavari, S. H. R., Irajian, G. R., Nodoshan, M. R. J., Roudsari, R. V., & Yahyapour, Y. (2013). Evaluation of human papillomavirus infections in prostatic disease: A cross-sectional study in Iran. *Asian Pacific Journal of Cancer Prevention*, *14*(5), 3305–3308. Available from https://doi.org/10.7314/APJCP.2013.14.5.3305.

Giannoudis, A., Ergazaki, M., Segas, J., Giotakis, J., Adamopoulos, G., Gorgoulis, V., & Spandidos, D. A. (1995). Detection of Epstein-Barr virus and human papillomavirus in nasopharyngeal carcinoma by the polymerase chain reaction technique. *Cancer Letters*, *89*(2), 177–181. Available from https://doi.org/10.1016/0304-3835(94)03667-8.

Grinstein, S., Preciado, M. V., Gattuso, P., Chabay, P. A., Warren, W. H., de Matteo, E., & Gould, V. E. (2002). Demonstration of Epstein-Barr virus in carcinomas of various sites. *Cancer Research*, *62*(17), 4876–4878.

Hagensee, M.E., Clark, R., Cameron, J.E., D'Angelo, A. (2011).Epstein Barr virus interacts with human papilloma virus to decrease apoptosis in vitro and increase cervical dysplasia in vivo.

In: *International Centre Genetic Engineering Biotechnology DNA Tumour virus Meeting proceedings*.

Harris, R. S., & Dudley, J. P. (2015). APOBECs and virus restriction. *Virology*, *479–480*, 131–145. Available from https://doi.org/10.1016/j.virol.2015.03.012.

Howlader, N., Noone, A. M., Krapcho, M., Garshell, J., Neyman, N., Altekruse, S. F., Kosary, C. L., Yu, M., Ruhl, J., Tatalovich, Z., Cho, H., Mariotto, A., Lewis, D. R., Chen, H. S., Feuer, E. J., Cronin, K. A., editors. SEER Cancer Statistics Review, 1975–2010. National Cancer Institute; Bethesda, MD: http://seer.cancer.gov/csr/1975_2010/, based on November 2012 SEER data submission, posted to the SEER web site, April 2013.

Humans IWG on the E of CR to. IARC Monographs on the Evaluation of Carcinogenic Risks to Humans. A Review of Human Carcinogens. (2011a). *Biological agents. Volume 100 B. A review of human carcinogens*.

Humans IWG on the E of CR to. IARC Monographs on the Evaluation of Carcinogenic Risks to Humans. A Review of Human Carcinogens. (2011b). *Biological agents. Volume 100 B. A review of human carcinogens*.

Khalili, K., Del Valle, L., Wang, J. Y., Darbinian, N., Lassak, A., Safak, M., et al. (2003a). T-antigen of human polyomavirus JC cooperates withIGF-IR signaling system in cerebellar tumors. *Anticancer Research*, *23*, 2035–2042.

Khalili, K., Del Valle, L., Wang, J. Y., Darbinian, N., Lassak, A., Safak, M., & Reiss, K. (2003b). T-antigen of human polyomavirus JC cooperates with IGF-IR signaling system in cerebellar tumors of the childhood-medulloblastomas. *Anticancer Research*, *23*(Issue 3 A), 2035–2041.

Kukimoto, I., Mori, S., Aoyama, S., Wakae, K., Muramatsu, M., & Kondo, K. (2015). Hypermutation in the E2 gene of human papillomavirus type 16 in cervical intraepithelial neoplasia. *Journal of Medical Virology*, *87*(10), 1754–1760. Available from https://doi.org/10.1002/jmv.24215.

Kundu, S. D., Lee, C., Billips, B. K., Habermacher, G. M., Zhang, Q., Liu, V., Wong, L. Y., Klumpp, D. J., & Thumbikat, P. (2008). The toll-like receptor pathway: A novel mechanism of infection-induced carcinogenesis of prostate epithelial cells. *The Prostate*, *68*(2), 223–229. Available from https://doi.org/10.1002/pros.20710

Lin, Y., Mao, Q., Zheng, X., Yang, K., Chen, H., Zhou, C., & Xie, L. (2011). Human papillomavirus 16 or 18 infection and prostate cancer risk: A *meta*-analysis. *Irish Journal of Medical Science*, *180*(2), 497–503. Available from https://doi.org/10.1007/s11845-011-0692-6.

Liu, B., Hong, S., Tang, Z., Yu, H., & Giam, C.-Z. (2005). HTLV-I Tax directly binds the Cdc20-associated anaphase-promoting complex and activates it ahead of schedule. *Proceedings of the National Academy of Sciences*, *102*(1), 63–68. Available from https://doi.org/10.1073/pnas.0406424101.

Malekshahi, S. S., Yavarian, J., Salehi, R., Babaei, F., Ahmadi, S. A., Ghavami, N., Naseri, M., Hosseini, M., Mokhtari-Azad, T., & Shafiei-Jandaghi, N. Z. (2020). Epstein-Barr and BK virus in cancerous and noncancerous prostate tissue. *Future Virology*, *15*(1), 13–17. Available from https://doi.org/10.2217/fvl-2019-0140.

Mazzoli, S., Cai, T., Mondaini, N., & Bartoletti, R. (2008). HPV vaccination program: Women's health under male protection. *European Urology Supplements*, *7*(3), 156. Available from https://doi.org/10.1016/s1569-9056(08)60338-3.

Meckes, D. G. (2015). Exosomal communication goes viral. *Journal of Virology*, *89*(10), 5200–5203. Available from https://doi.org/10.1128/JVI.02470-14.

Medel-Flores, O., Valenzuela-Rodríguez, V. A., Ocadiz-Delgado, R., Castro-Muñoz, L. J., Hernández-Leyva, S., Lara-Hernández, G., Silva-Escobedo, J. G., Vidal, P. G., & Sánchez-

Monroy, V. (2018). Association between HPV infection and prostate cancer in a Mexican population. *Genetics and Molecular Biology*, *41*(4), 781–789. Available from https://doi.org/10.1590/1678-4685-gmb-2017-0331.

Mesri, E. A., Feitelson, M. A., & Munger, K. (2014). Human viral oncogenesis: A cancer hallmarks analysis. *Cell Host and Microbe*, *15*(3), 266–282. Available from https://doi.org/10.1016/j.chom.2014.02.011.

Moghoofei, M., Keshavarz, M., Ghorbani, S., Babaei, F., Nahand, J. S., Tavakoli, A., Mortazavi, H. S., Marjani, A., Mostafaei, S., & Monavari, S. H. (2019). Association between human papillomavirus infection and prostate cancer: A global systematic review and meta-analysis. *Asia-Pacific Journal of Clinical Oncology*, *15*(5), e59–e67. Available from https://doi.org/10.1111/ajco.13124.

Mui, U. N., Haley, C. T., & Tyring, S. K. (2017). Viral oncology: Molecular biology and pathogenesis. *Journal of Clinical Medicine*, *6*(12), 111. Available from https://doi.org/10.3390/jcm6120111.

Nahand, J. S., Khanaliha, K., Mirzaei, H., Moghoofei, M., Baghi, H. B., Esghaei, M., et al. (2021). Rôle possible de la co-infection HPV/EBV dans la résistance et le développement d'Anoikis dans le cancer de la prostate. *BMC Cancer*, *21*, 926. Available from https://doi.org/10.1186/s12885-021-08658-y.

Nikitin, P. A., Yan, C. M., Forte, E., Bocedi, A., Tourigny, J. P., White, R. E., Allday, M. J., Patel, A., Dave, S. S., Kim, W., Hu, K., Guo, J., Tainter, D., Rusyn, E., & Luftig, M. A. (2010). An ATM/Chk2-mediated DNA damage-responsive signaling pathway suppresses Epstein-Barr virus transformation of primary human B cells. *Cell Host and Microbe*, *8*(6), 510–522. Available from https://doi.org/10.1016/j.chom.2010.11.004.

Ohba, K., Ichiyama, K., Yajima, M., Gemma, N., Nikaido, M., Wu, Q., Chong, P. P., Mori, S., Yamamoto, R., Wong, J. E. L., & Yamamoto, N. (2014). In vivo and in vitro studies suggest a possible involvement of HPV infection in the early stage of breast carcinogenesis via APOBEC3B induction. *PLoS One*, *9*(5), e97787. Available from https://doi.org/10.1371/journal.pone.0097787.

Pereira, R., Hitzeroth, I. I., & Rybicki, E. P. (2009). Insights into the role and function of L2, the minor capsid protein of papillomaviruses. *Archives of Virology*, *154*(2), 187–197. Available from https://doi.org/10.1007/s00705-009-0310-3.

Perera, R. A. P. M., Samaranayake, L. P., & Tsang, C. S. P. (2010). Shedding dynamics of Epstein-Barr virus: A type 1 carcinogen. *Archives of Oral Biology*, *55*(9), 639–647. Available from https://doi.org/10.1016/j.archoralbio.2010.06.009.

Prayitno, A. (2006). Cervical cancer with human papilloma virus and Epstein Barr virus positive. *Journal of Carcinogenesis*, *5*, 13. Available from https://doi.org/10.1186/1477-3163-5-13.

Punwaney, R., Brandwein, M. S., Zhang, D. Y., Urken, M. L., Cheng, R., Park, C. S., Li, H. B., & Li, X. (1999). Human papillomavirus may be common within nasopharyngeal carcinoma of Caucasian Americans: Investigation of Epstein-Barr virus and human papillomavirus in eastern and western nasopharyngeal carcinoma using ligation-dependent polymerase chain reaction. *Head and Neck*, *21*(1), 21–29. Available from https://doi.org/10.1002/(SICI)1097-0347(199901)21:1 < 21::AID-HED3 > 3.0.CO;2-Z.

Raab-Traub, N. (2012). Novel mechanisms of EBV-induced oncogenesis. *Current Opinion in Virology*, *2*(4), 453–458. Available from https://doi.org/10.1016/j.coviro.2012.07.001.

Rassekh, C. H., Rady, P. L., Arany, I., Tyring, S. K., Knudsen, S., Calhoun, K. H., Seikaly, H., & Bailey, B. J. (1998). Combined Epstein-Barr virus and human papillomavirus infection in nasopharyngeal carcinoma. *The Laryngoscope*, *108*(3), 362–367. Available from https://doi.org/10.1097/00005537-199803000-00010.

Sasagawa, T., Shimakage, M., Nakamura, M., Sakaike, J., Ishikawa, H., & Inoue, M. (2000). Epstein-Barr virus (EBV) genes expression in cervical intraepithelial neoplasia and invasive cervical cancer: A comparative study with human papillomavirus (HPV) infection. *Human Pathology*, *31*(3), 318–326. Available from https://doi.org/10.1016/S0046-8177(00)80245-2.

Schiller, J. T., & Lowy, D. R. (2014). Virus infection and human cancer: An overview. *Recent Results in Cancer Research*, *193*, 1–10. Available from https://doi.org/10.1007/978-3-642-38965-8_1.

Sfanos, K. S., Sauvageot, J., Fedor, H. L., Dick, J. D., De Marzo, A. M., & Isaacs, W. B. (2008). A molecular analysis of prokaryotic and viral DNA sequences in prostate tissue from patients with prostate cancer indicates the presence of multiple and diverse microorganisms. *The Prostate*, *68*(3), 306–320. Available from https://doi.org/10.1002/pros.20680.

Shah, K. M., & Young, L. S. (2009). Epstein-Barr virus and carcinogenesis: Beyond Burkitt's lymphoma. *Clinical Microbiology and Infection*, *15*(11), 982–988. Available from https://doi.org/10.1111/j.1469-0691.2009.03033.x.

Shimabuku, T., Tamanaha, A., Kitamura, B., Tanabe, Y., Tawata, N., Ikehara, F., et al. (2014a). *Dual expression of Epstein-Barr virus, latent membrane protein-1 and human papillomavirus-16 E6 transform*. 15.

Shimabuku, T., Tamanaha, A., Kitamura, B., Tanabe, Y., Tawata, N., Ikehara, F., Arakaki, K., & Kinjo, T. (2014b). Dual expression of Epstein-Barr virus, latent membrane protein-1 and human papillomavirus-16 E6 transform primary mouse embryonic fibroblasts through NF-κB signaling. *International Journal of Clinical and Experimental Pathology*, *7*(5), 1920–1934. Available from http://www.ijcep.com/files/ijciep0000270.pdf.

Singh, N., Hussain, S., Kakkar, N., Singh, S. K., Sobti, R. C., & Bharadwaj, M. (2015). Implication of high risk Human papillomavirus HR-HPV infection in prostate cancer in Indian population—A pioneering case-control analysis. *Scientific Reports*, *5*(1), 1–4. Available from https://doi.org/10.1038/srep07822.

Singhi, A. D., Califano, J., & Westra, W. H. (2012). High-risk human papillomavirus in nasopharyngeal carcinoma. *Head and Neck*, *34*(2), 213–218. Available from https://doi.org/10.1002/hed.21714.

Smelov, B., Mühr, A., Eklund , Komyakov, G., et al. (2016). Detection of DNA viruses in prostate cancer. *Scientific Reports*, *28*.

Strauss, M. J., Shaw, E. W., Bunting, H., & Melnick, J. L. (1949). "Crystalline" virus-like particles from skin papillomas characterized by intranuclear inclusion bodies. *Proceedings of the Society for Experimental Biology and Medicine*, *72*(1), 46–50. Available from https://doi.org/10.3181/00379727-72-17328.

Suspène, R., Aynaud, M. M., Koch, S., Pasdeloup, D., Labetoulle, M., Gaertner, B., Vartanian, J. P., Meyerhans, A., & Wain-Hobson, S. (2011). Genetic editing of herpes simplex virus 1 and epstein-barr herpesvirus genomes by Human APOBEC3 cytidine deaminases in culture and in vivo. *Journal of Virology*, *85*(15), 7594–7602. Available from https://doi.org/10.1128/JVI.00290-11.

Suzuki, R. (2012). NK/T-cell lymphomas: Pathobiology, prognosis and treatment paradigm. *Current Oncology Reports*, *14*(5), 395–402. Available from https://doi.org/10.1007/s11912-012-0245-9.

Tolstov, Y., Hadaschik, B., Pahernik, S., Hohenfellner, M., & Duensing, S. (2014a). *Human papillomaviruses in urological malignancies: A critical assessment. Urologic Oncology: Seminars and Original Investigations*. Elsevier, 46-e19.

Tolstov, Y., Hadaschik, B., Pahernik, S., Hohenfellner, M., & Duensing, S. (2014b). Human papillomaviruses in urological malignancies: A critical assessment. *Urologic Oncology:*

Seminars and Original Investigations, *32*(1), 46. Available from https://doi.org/10.1016/j.urolonc.2013.06.012, e27.

Tsao, S. W., Tsang, C. M., To, K. F., & Lo, K. W. (2015). The role of Epstein-Barr virus in epithelial malignancies. *Journal of Pathology*, *235*(2), 323–333. Available from https://doi.org/10.1002/path.4448.

Vartanian, J. P., Guétard, D., Henry, M., & Wain-Hobson, S. (2008). Evidence for editing of human papillomavirus DNA by APOBEC3 in benign and precancerous lesions. *Science (New York, N.Y.)*, *320*(5873), 230–233. Available from https://doi.org/10.1126/science.1153201.

Vieira, V. C., Leonard, B., White, E. A., Starrett, G. J., Temiz, N. A., Lorenz, L. D., Lee, D., Soares, M. A., Lambert, P. F., Howley, P. M., & Harris, R. S. (2014). Human papillomavirus E6 triggers upregulation of the antiviral and cancer genomic DNA deaminase APOBEC3B. *mBio*, *5*(6). Available from https://doi.org/10.1128/mBio.02234-14.

Wang, Z., Wakae, K., Kitamura, K., Aoyama, S., Liu, G., Koura, M., Monjurul, A. M., Kukimoto, I., & Muramatsu, M. (2014). APOBEC3 deaminases induce hypermutation in human papillomavirus 16 DNA upon beta interferon stimulation. *Journal of Virology*, *88*(2), 1308–1317. Available from https://doi.org/10.1128/JVI.03091-13.

Whitaker, N. J., Glenn, W. K., Sahrudin, A., Orde, M. M., Delprado, W., & Lawson, J. S. (2013). Human papillomavirus and Epstein Barr virus in prostate cancer: Koilocytes indicate potential oncogenic influences of human papillomavirus in prostate cancer. *The Prostate*, *73*(3), 236–241. Available from https://doi.org/10.1002/pros.22562.

Zur Hausen, H. (2008). Papillomaviruses-to vaccination and beyond. *Biochemistry (Moscow)*, *73*(5), 498–503. Available from https://doi.org/10.1134/S0006297908050027.

zur Hausen, H. (2009). Papillomaviruses in the causation of human cancers – A brief historical account. *Virology*, *384*(2), 260–265. Available from https://doi.org/10.1016/j.virol.2008.11.046.

Chapter 26

Genitourinary cancers immune biomarkers: a comprehensive overview

Lamyae El Khalki[1,2,3,*], Hassan Ait Mouse[1,*], Abdeslam Jaafari[1,*], Moulay Mustapha Ennaji[4,*] and Abdelmajid Zyad[1,*]

[1]Team of Experimental Oncology and Natural Substances; Cellular & Molecular Immunopharmacology, Faculty of Sciences and Technology, University of Sultan Moulay Slimane, Beni Mellal, Morocco, [2]Department of Microbiology, Immunology, and Inflammation, Temple University, Philadelphia, PA, United States, [3]Center for Inflammation and Lung Research, Temple University, Philadelphia, PA, United States, [4]Group Leader Research team of Virology, Oncology, and Biotechnologies, Head of Laboratory of Virology, Oncology, Biosciences, Environment and New Energies (LVO-BEEN), Faculty of Sciences and Techniques Mohammedia, University Hassan II of Casablanca, Casablanca, Morocco

26.1 Introduction

A link between cancer and immune system was proposed two decades ago when scientists reported that tumors could grow in chronic inflammation sites (Balkwill & Mantovani, 2001). This observation eventually led to a hypothesis that both inflammatory and immune cells can – using different cellular and molecular mediators – play an important role in the promotion of tumor development and its elimination (Fridman et al., 2012). The ability of the immune system to recognize and eliminate transformed cells early is called tumor immunosurveillance. Immunoediting refers to a process that can describe how pro- and antitumorigenic responses of the immune system can, through selecting for less immunogenic clones, alter the clinical evolution of a tumor (Dunn et al., 2002).

Given the high morbidity and mortality associated with genitourinary cancers, improving early diagnosis and medical treatment is an important issue for achieving better clinical outcomes. Most cancer types are highly complicated process and exhibit heterogeneity among patients. As proteins directly control the characteristics of cells, they make a powerful tool for

* These authors contributed equally.

Immunological Implications and Molecular Diagnostics of Genitourinary Cancer.
DOI: https://doi.org/10.1016/B978-0-323-85496-2.00009-9

cancer research, through profiling the functional proteins and monitoring their expression changes according to cancer progression and development. Therefore cancer studies focus on discovering biomarkers that can serve for cancer diagnosis, treatment, and other clinical applications (Chen et al., 2019).

26.2 Immune response in urogenital cancers

Certain key immune cells play an important role in the physiopathology of urogenital cancers. In bladder cancer, it seems that the adaptive immune system has an antitumor effect, while the innate immune system promotes a pro-tumor effect. As progenitors of granulocytes, macrophages, dendritic cells (DCs), and myeloid-derived suppressor cells (MDSCs) are involved in tumorigenesis and metastasis process by promoting tumor cell survival and angiogenesis (Zhu et al., 2012). Neutrophils can have an anticancer effect by targeting cancerous cells. On the other hand, they can also promote tumor development by stimulating excessive inflammation, releasing growth factors, and secreting matrix-degrading enzymes (Suttmann et al., 2006). Concerning tumor-associated macrophages, it has been shown that they promote angiogenesis in bladder carcinomas (Van Der Horst et al., 2012). In fact, it has been reported that, in invasive bladder cancer, the number of tissue-infiltrated macrophages is significantly increased compared to superficial cancers. In this environment, macrophages promote tumor angiogenesis by releasing angiogenic factors to reverse the hypoxia. However, in doing so, they contribute to tumor growth and invasion (Solinas et al., 2009). Chen et al. reported that IL-6 may promote more malignant cancer phenotypes, and elevated serum levels of IL-6 in bladder, ovarian, and prostate cancers, is linked to poor prognosis and increased metastasis. In fact, IL-6 levels are increased in both the urine and serum of patients with urothelial bladder carcinoma and in muscle-invasive bladder cancer compared to controls (Chen et al., 2013). Furthermore, some studies, in vivo and in vitro, have shown that inhibition of IL-6 release inhibited development of bladder cancer (Chen et al., 2013). Tumor necrosis factor-α (TNF-α) promotes bladder cancer by stimulating the secretion of two enzymes involved in tumor development (thymidine phosphorylase) and tumor invasion (matrix metalloprotease-9) (Chen et al., 2013).

Regarding kidney cancer, it has been shown that T lymphocyte-DC cross talk, dysfunctional neutrophils migration, immune cell metabolism, DC maturation, and abnormal expression of cytokines and chemokines have been highlighted in renal cell carcinoma and stroma cells (Murphy et al., 2015). Concerning testicular cancer, a clear link between immune system response (immune cells and cytokine profiles) and testicular germ cell tumors has been reported using prognostic biomarkers. The microenvironnement of testicular tumors is characterized by the presence of B cells, DCs, and increased level of IL-6 (Chovanec et al., 2019).

Over the past years, some cancer prostate-associated molecules have been reported including, inter alia, prostate specific antigen (PSA), poly A polymerase (PAP), prostate-specific membrane antigen, prostate stem cell antigen. Unfortunately, the majority of antigens are nonimmunogenic owing to the fact that they are self-proteins, and also, soluble antigens, like PSA and PAP, are mainly tolerant. On the other hand, many prostate-associated-derived peptides, which can activate cytotoxic T lymphocytes (CTL), have been identified, and consequently, they could be used to kill tumor cells by peptide-specific CTL (Van Parijs & Abbas, 1998). Thus in attempt to break the tolerance to such antigens, cancer vaccines generating CTL and/or antibodies from B cells are being developed (Bou-Dargham et al., 2020).

26.3 Immunotherapy of urogenital cancers

In the last few years, immunotherapy has secured a prominent place as anticancer treatment. It is typically used as a complement to conventional methods such as surgery, chemotherapy, and radiotherapy. However, in some cancers, immunotherapy could be used as first-line treatment (Jagodinsky et al., 2020). Coley toxin is a bacterial preparation, which was used in the first clinical application of immunotherapy against cancer in the 1890s. In the 1990s, IL-2 was used to treat metastatic renal and melanoma (Atkins et al., 1999). Nowadays, immune checkpoint inhibitors, T-cell transfer therapy, monoclonal antibodies, treatment vaccines, and immune system modulators are different types of therapy aiming to stimulate the immune system against cancer (Bladder et al., 2020).

26.3.1 Checkpoint's inhibitors

The immune system uses proteins called "checkpoints" that need to be turned on (or off) to start an immune response against cancer or infection. Over the last years, checkpoint inhibitors (anti-PD1 and anti-PD-L1) are increasingly used to treat some solid tumors (Pierantoni et al., 2019). It has been reported that high levels of PD-L1 are associated with advanced and aggressive bladder tumors with poor survival outcomes (Nakanishi et al., 2007; Inman et al., 2007), which explain the benefit of this therapy against high tumor mutational burden, such as bladder cancer. Their mechanism of action is related to a greater T cell-mediated antitumor immune response (Samstein et al., 2019). Molecular features of bladder cancer, as genetically heterogenous disease, considerably influence the efficacy of the immune checkpoint inhibitors Table 26.1.

26.3.1.1 Anti-PD-1/ anti-PD-L1

In kidney cancer, several types of immunotherapies, such as immune checkpoint inhibitors, can be used especially in combined therapy: (Pembrolizumab + axitinib) or (nivolumab + cabozantinib) as the first treatment in advanced

TABLE 26.1 Approved checkpoint inhibitors used in bladder cancer treatment (Wołącewicz et al., 2020; Lopez-Beltran et al., 2021).

Compound	Trade name	Company	Target	Line of therapy	Characteristics
Atezolizumab	Tecentriq	Genentech	PDL-1	First	ORR: 23% (9% cRR) mPFS: 2.7 mo mOS: 15.9 mo
Avelumab	Bavencio	Merck	PDL-1	First	mOS: 21.4 vs. 14.3 mo (A vs. BSC, all pts) ($p = 0.001$) mOS: NE vs. 17.1 mo (A vs. BSC, PD-L1 $\geq$ 5% TC +) ($p < 0.001$)
Durvalumab	Imfinzi	AstraZeneca	PDL-1	First	mOS: 14.4 vs. 12.1 mo (D vs. chemo, PD-L1 +) ($p = 0.30$) mOS: 15.1 vs. 12.1 (D + T vs. chemo, all pts) ($p = 0.075$)
Nivolumab	Opdivo	Bristol-Meyers Squibb	PD-1	First	ORR: 19.6% (52/265). Paterns of responses unrelated to PD-L1 status
Pembrolizumab	Keytruda	Merck	PD-1	Second	mOS: 10.3 vs. 7.4 (P vs chemo, all pts) ($p = 0.002$) mOS: 8.0 vs. 5.2 (P vs chemo, PD-L1 status CPS $\geq$ 10%) ($p = 0.005$)
Ipilimumab	Yervoy	Bristol-Meyers Squibb	CTL-4	Second	–

N, number of patients; *NMIBC*, nonmuscle invasive bladder cancer; *BCG*, bacillus Calmette–Guerin; *cRR*, complete response rate; *MIBC*, muscle-invasive bladder cancer; *pCR*, pathologic complete remission; *pts*, patients; *PD-L1*, programmed cell-death ligand 1; *mMIBC*, metastatic muscle-invasive bladder cancer; *c-DDP unfit*, cisplatin-ineligible; *I*, first-line; *ORR*, objective response rate; *mPFS*, median progression-free survival; *mo*, months; *mOS*, median overall survival; *chemo.*, chemotherapy; *BSC*, best supportive care; *NE*, not estimable; *TXT*, docetaxel; *PTX*, paclitaxel; *II*, second-line; *CPS*, combined positive score.

kidney cancer, (nivolumab + ipilimumab) [Cytotoxic T lymphocyte-associated protein 4 (CTLA-4) inhibitor] in intermediate- or poor-risk advanced kidney cancer (Motzer et al., 2018). In prostate cancer, many studies reported that checkpoint inhibitors, such as nivolumab, pembrolizumab, enzalutamide, and avelumab, have no significant effect when used alone (Bolat & Haydaroğlu, 2019).

In testicular cancer, several studies (case reports, case series, and phase I–II clinical studies) reported a promising efficacy of checkpoint inhibitors, alone or in combined therapy, in testicular germ cells (Chovanec et al., 2019).

26.3.1.2 Anti-cytotoxic T lymphocyte-associated protein 4 antibodies

CTLA-4 is a molecule expressed on the surface of activated T cells, which bind B7.1 and B7.2, expressed by B-lymphocytes, DCs, and macrophages. CTLA-4 negatively regulates the immune response, and consequently, its inhibition, using anti-CTLA-4 antibodies, may increase the regulation of the immune response in bladder cancer. These antibodies could be used in the treatment of bladder cancer (Farina et al., 2017).

Small et al. reported for the first time PSA modulation and efficacy of ipilimumab in prostate cancer (Small et al., 2007). Also, a clinical study has shown the efficacy of ipilimumab on survival in patients with docetaxel-resistant prostate cancer and bone metastasis (Kwon et al., 2014), while another demonstrated the efficacy of tremelimumab, another anti-CTLA-4 agent, in patients with prostate cancer with PSA recurrence (McNeel et al., 2012).

26.3.2 Bacillus Calmette–Guerin

In 1974 bacillus Calmette–Guerin (BCG) was used for the first time against cancer in an animal model (Farina et al., 2017). In 1976 it was successfully used in bladder cancer (Morales et al., 1976), and in 1980 Lamm et al. reported that BCG therapy following transurethral resection of bladder tumors (TURBT) reduces the chance of relapse (Lamm et al., 1980). Currently, for nonmuscle invasive BC (NMIBC), high-grade papillary tumors, in situ cancer, and invasive plaque-proprious tumors, the standard treatment is TURBT, followed by intravesical treatment with BCG or chemotherapy (Zhang et al., 2020).

The effect of BCG on cancer cells could be a direct cytotoxicity or by secretion of toxic compounds such as TNF. The immune cells involved in this effect include CD4 + , CD8 + , NK cells, macrophages, granulocytes, and DCs (Zhang et al., 2020). Three groups of patients can be distinguished: BCG resistant, BCG relapsing, and BCG intolerant. Thus understanding the immunobiological mechanism of action of BCG is necessary to improve efficacy and reduce intolerance to this therapy.

26.3.3 Monoclonal antibodies

Enfortumab vedotin (PADCEV) is an ADC (monoclonal antibody associated to a drug). It binds to Nectin-4 protein on the surface of bladder cancer cells and allows the drug to enter in cells and kill them. It is used in people with advanced bladder cancer already treated with cisplatin and immunotherapy (PD-1/PD-L1 inhibitor) (Chang et al., 2021).

26.3.4 Combined Therapies

Combined therapies, that is, association of two or more methods of treatment, are one of the strategies used to treat cancer. In the case of NIMBC, combined therapies are mostly used, and they show more effectiveness with reduction of relapse and the risk of regression. In bladder cancer, the combination of Mitomycin C and BCG is widely used. For patients who are not eligible, cisplatin, pembrolizumab, or atezolizumab (checkpoint inhibitors) are recommended instead of cisplatin in the combination therapies cisplatin + gemcitabine and methotrexate + vinblastine + Adriamycin + cisplatin (Wołącewicz et al., 2020).

Also, it has been reported that combined therapy could have an important interest in patients with prostate cancer. Examples of these combinations include: vaccines + checkpoint inhibitors (Gulley et al., 2017), immunotherapy + enzalutamide (androgen inhibitor) (Beer et al., 2014), immunotherapy + abiraterone (Small et al., 2015), and immunotherapy + poly (ADP-ribose) polymérase inhibition (Karzai et al., 2017).

26.3.5 Other therapies

IL-12: Delivered along with chitosan, intravesical IL-12 stimulates the immune system against cancer cells as reported by animal studies (Wołącewicz et al., 2020). IL-12 acts by stimulating macrophages leading to release of interferon γ, which activates CD3 + , CD8 + , and CD4 + T cells and tumor-infiltrating lymphocytes. Additionally, it decreases the number of regulatory T cells and MDSCs (Wołącewicz et al., 2020).

COX-2 inhibitors: It has been shown that celecoxib, a cyclooxygenase-2 (COX-2) inhibitor, has an important chemo-preventive effect on various cancers, including bladder cancer. It acts by inhibiting proliferation, migration, invasion, and epithelial-to-mesenchymal transition. This effect becomes more important when celecoxib is associated with molecules that mimic microRNA-145 (Liu et al., 2019).

mammalian target of rapamycin (mTOR) kinase inhibitors: Everolimus and sirolimus are drugs used as immunosuppressive. They act by inhibiting mTOR kinase, responsible for the regulation of pathways involved in growth, cell proliferation, and angiogenesis. In vitro and in vivo studies reported the efficacy of everolimus in bladder cancer alone or combined with cisplatin. Furthermore, a phase II study revealed antitumor activity of the same drug in patients with metastatic urothelial carcinoma (Milowsky et al., 2013).

Vaccine therapy: Therapeutic vaccines are becoming increasingly used in urogenital cancers. This class is presented in another section of this chapter.

26.3.6 Perspectives

Several novel approaches are under study for their possible use in some urogenital cancers. They are enumerated as follows.

Epidermal growth factor receptor (EGFR)-inhibitor: Erlotinib, an EGFR inhibitor, and cetuximab, an anti-EGFR monoclonal antibody, have been shown to inhibit tumor cell proliferation in vitro (Aragon-Ching & Trump, 2017).

HER-2 inhibitors: a study on a DC-based vaccine suggested that HER-2 inhibitors could be used as a treatment for patients with HER2 + urothelial bladder cancer (Peethambaram et al., 2009).

Indirect activation of the immune system by costimulatory molecules: OX40 is a molecule expressed on the surface of CD4 + and CD8 + T cells. It may increase antitumor immunity by activation of these cells and recognition of a specific antigen (Curti et al., 2013).

Stem cells: It has been reported that stem cells might be a promising therapeutic tool to use against bladder cancer. However, molecular subtyping of carcinoma types is necessary in this case (Aghaalikhani et al., 2019).

Tumor-infiltrating lymphocytes (TIL): Poch et al. reported that the use of TIL, which secrete interféron-gamma in response to bladder cancer, is a promising method in the therapy against this type of tumor (Poch et al., 2018).

Chimeric PD-1 receptor (chPD-1): These molecules were made to avoid limited cytolytic activity and secretion in the tumor microenvironment due to PD-1 activation. Antitumor activity of chPD-1 T cells was reported in bladder cancer cell lines among others (Parriott et al., 2020).

Personalized therapy: Finally, combined and personalized therapies are becoming increasingly recommended since there is the matter of diversity and uniqueness of the patients to treat.

26.3.7 Alternative therapies

Roos et al. reported that, in bladder cancer cell cultures, curcumin inhibits cell growth and proliferation (Roos et al., 2019). Also, Sulforaphane, a natural compound produced by cruciferous vegetables such as Brussels sprouts and cabbages, has an important antitumor activity in vitro and in vivo. It acts by inhibiting histone deacetylases (HDACs) (Juengel et al., 2018), involved in the epigenetic regulation of gene expression. In fact, about 90% of cancers have been associated with epigenetic modifications (Aggarwal et al., 2009). Studies have reported that broccoli and cabbage consumption reduces bladder cancer risk (Mastuo et al., 2020).

26.4 Prostate and bladder cancers biomarkers

Biomarkers are defined by two functional categories, namely, prognostic and predictive. The former is measured objectively and can be correlated with an outcome for the patient (Slovin, 2016), and the latter plays a vital role in identifying which patients may be more likely to respond to a cancer therapy (Slovin, 2016).

For the purpose of sampling, urine is used as the clinical specimen of choice for many proteomic studies on bladder and prostate, added to the development of biomarkers for genitourinary cancers using tissue, blood, and cyst fluid (Chen et al., 2019). Molecular profiling using fluid and tissue is becoming more feasible with recent developments in next-generation sequencing technologies (Kojima et al., 2017). Currently, these profiling methods are beginning to be used for early detection, prediction of prognosis, and drug sensitivity (Kojima et al., 2017).

The tumor–immune cells interaction has been demonstrated by the analysis of immune infiltrates that may help in identifying patients who may be potential candidates for specific immune therapies. There has been approval of several checkpoint inhibitors for bladder cancer, many of which show correlation of response with immunohistochemical staining of PD-L1 or PD1. However, the success of these agents has been limited given the minimal expression of these biomarkers in prostate cancer (Slovin, 2017).

Another checkpoint molecule that is gaining wide interest is the V-domain immunoglobulin containing suppressor of T-cell activation, which has inhibitory effects both as a ligand on antigen presenting cells (APCs) and as a receptor on T cells. While its expression is increased in the tumor microenvironment, it participates in the inhibiting signals to reduce T-cell responses (Slovin, 2017).

Nuclear matrix proteins (NMPs): Several kinds of NMPs are overexpressed in urothelial tumors and released into the urine following apoptosis of tumor cells; NMP22 is more prevalent in malignant urothelial cells than in their normal counterpart (Kojima et al., 2017).

MicroRNAs (miRNAs): They are a group of short, noncoding RNAs that play an important role in gene silencing, acting on the posttranscriptional level. Up- or downregulation of miRNAs may influence bladder cancer tumorigenesis by acting as oncogenes or tumor-suppressor genes (Kojima et al., 2017). Of 15 miRNAs thought to be the most promising diagnostic and prognostic bladder cancer biomarkers, 11 were upregulated and 4 were downregulated (Kojima et al., 2017).

Furthermore, several researchers explored the miRNA expression from prostate cancer patients associating the tissue-restricted or circulating miRNAs expression with the occurrence of tumoral cells and the prognosis; the expression of 6sixmiRNAs is associated with induction of cell differentiation and tumor angiogenesis. On the other hand, the expression of 14 miRNAs is associated with the inhibition of cell proliferation and metastasis formation associated in the development of prostate cancer (Galvão-Lima et al., 2021).

DNA methylation: DNA methylation in cells obtained from urine is investigated to identify specific patterns associated with bladder cancer. For example, it commonly occurs in CpG-rich promoter regions, which contribute to gene inactivation. Because CpG hypermethylation does not occur in normal cells, methylation can be a good early diagnostic biomarker for bladder cancer (Kojima et al., 2017).

BCG, used for vaccination against tuberculosis, is also used in immunotherapy for bladder cancer treatment (Song et al., 2019). Increased TILs and CD4 + /CD8 + ratio on BCG induction have been linked to good therapeutic response, and pre-BCG treatment tumor-infiltrating macrophages are associated with poor treatment response (Song et al., 2019). Changes in DCs, NK cells, and urine leukocytes on BCG induction have also been suggested as potential predictors of BCG therapeutic response (Song et al., 2019). The induction of a TH1 immune response after BCG instillation, particularly from a TH2 baseline, is strongly associated with a good response (Song et al., 2019).

As genomic alterations in tumor tissues, FGFR3 mutations are common in low-grade and low-stage NMIBC (Kojima et al., 2017). A large prospective study reported a significantly higher risk of developing intravesical recurrence in patients having FGFR3-mutant tumors (Kojima et al., 2017). On the other hand, a significant association between FGFR3 mutation and recurrence-free survival was not found in two other studies (Kojima et al., 2017). Therefore a combination of FGFR3 and other genes is more promising to discriminate high-risk NMIBC patients (such as examining the FGFR3 mutation combined with a PIK3CA alteration) (Kojima et al., 2017).

Circulating tumor cells (CTCs): They have been suggested to play a critical role in the occurrence and progression of prostate cancer. A number of studies have shown that CTCs are necessary in the processes of tumor progression, including tumorigenesis, invasion, metastasis, and colonization. Moreover, CTCs can serve as potential prognostic targets in prostate cancer owing to their roles in regulating many processes associated with cancer metastasis (Yang et al., 2021).

Androgen receptor (AR): Androgens are involved in the normal development of the prostate gland, but also in prostate carcinogenesis. AR contributes to the control of the balance between cell proliferation and differentiation. Treatment of prostate cancer includes androgen signaling inhibition, either through androgen deprivation or AR activity block. Therefore analyzing AR status may be used as a good biomarker to improve the treatment of prostate cancer (Conteduca et al., 2021).

To conclude, these panels of biomarker targets look promising, and they need to be tested in a larger scale. The development of predictive molecular biomarkers is anticipated to improve genitourinary cancers' clinical management.

26.5 Renal cell carcinoma biomarkers

26.5.1 Pathologic and molecular subtypes of renal cell carcinoma

Clear cell RCC (ccRCC) accounts for over 75% of kidney cancer, while the other 25% can be classified as non−clear cell renal cell carcinoma (nccRCC) (Moch et al., 2016). These subtypes include papillary renal cell carcinoma (pRCC) (20%) and chromophobe renal cell carcinoma (chRCC) (5%), which are the most frequent nccRCC subtypes. On the other hand, hereditary leiomyomatosis and renal cell associated carcinoma, collecting duct carcinoma, renal medullary carcinoma, MiT family translocation carcinoma, succinate dehydrogenase-deficient RCC, mucinous tubular and spindle cell carcinoma, tubulocystic RCC, acquired cystic disease-associated RCC, clear cell papillary RCC, and RCC unclassified represent less common subtypes (Moch et al., 2016).

In the molecular side, similar genomic changes have been found in The Cancer Genome Atlas (TCGA) analysis of a ccRCC, showing recurrent alterations in the PI(3)K/AKT pathway and several epigenetic changes in DNA methylation (Brannon et al., 2010). Molecular stratification of ccRCC revealed two different subtypes: clear cell type A (ccA) and B (ccB), with ccA patients having a markedly better prognosis (Brooks et al., 2014; Cancer Genome Atlas Research Network et al., 2016). A second TCGA study aimed the papillary RCC (pRCC) and found that type 1 and type 2 pRCC are distinctly different diseases based on molecular features and that type 2 pRCC is a heterogeneous disease with at least three different subgroups (Davis et al., 2014). A third TCGA project focused on the chromophobe RCC (ChRCC) and found gene expression changes related to mitochondrial function and recurrent structural breakpoints within telomerase reverse transcriptase promoter region (Escudier et al., 2019). Likewise, a multilevel molecular characterization of the three TCGA RCC databases revealed nine major genomic RCC subtypes, each one distinct in terms of altered pathways and patient survival (Chen et al., 2016). Overlapping and subtype-specific genomic changes were observed, and good correlation with histologic subtypes was noticed. These molecular classes show substantial molecular diversity represented within each major histologic type, but importantly, actionable alterations also included PI3K and immune checkpoint pathways (Chen et al., 2016).

26.5.1.1 *Kidney cancer biomarkers*

26.5.1.1.1 Single-nucleotide polymorphisms

Many studies on genome have reported that the risk of an individual developing renal cell carcinoma may be increased by the single-nucleotide polymorphisms (SNPs) (Purdue et al., 2011) that include germline variation and somatic mutations within tumors, which may also help to explain observed differences in response and toxicity to anticancer agents.

In a study of 397 patients treated with pazopanib, 27 polymorphisms amongst 13 genes were evaluated. Two IL8 polymorphisms, linked to increased gene expression, were associated with a significantly shorter median PFS (27 weeks) than those carrying the wild-type genotype (48 weeks) ($P = 0.01$) (Xu et al., 2011). It is worth noting that IL-8 has recently been identified as a potential driver of resistance to tyrosine kinase inhibitors (Huang et al., 2010), making the results of biological relevance.

Another study aimed at the examining both response ($n = 89$) and toxicity ($n = 95$) to sunitinib in patients with ccRCC. A total of 16 polymorphisms were examined in nine genes. Using multivariable analysis, two VEGFR3 missense polymorphisms were associated with reduced PFS, and a high-metabolizing variant of CYP3A5*1 was associated with increased toxicity (Garcia-Donas et al., 2011).

26.5.1.2 *MicroRNA*

The alteration of the expression in the microRNA has been reported in a number of studies:

- *In the serum*

A composition of four mRNAs (miR-27, -28, -185, let-7f-2) was overexpressed in RCC specimens ($p < 0.05$) compared to healthy kidney (Gottardo et al., 2007).

Another study reported that 43 miRNAs were differently expressed in conventional RCC and in healthy kidney tissues. Indeed, 37 miRNAs were significantly underexpressed and the other six were overexpressed. The most important downregulation were observed in miRNA-141 and miRNA-200c (Nakada et al., 2008).

In another study, it was found that, miRNA-210 serum expression levels were significantly higher in patients with ccRCC than in healthy controls ($p = 0.001$) (Iwamoto et al., 2014).

The serum levels of miRNA-210 and miRNA-378 were analyzed in a study by Fedorko et al. in 2015. The analysis revealed that this combination of the serum level of these two miRNAs enabled the identification of patient with RCC (significant overexpression) with 80% sensitivity and 78% specificity if ($p < 0.0001$) (Fedorko et al., 2015).

- *In the urine*

Von Brandenstein et al., (2012), found that upregulated miRNA-15a can be measured in urine from patients with ccRCC, but it is barely detectable in cases of benign renal tumors (such as oncocytoma) and inflammation of the upper and lower urinary tracts.

Another study aimed at evaluating the expression of miRNA-15a in the urine of 67 adult patients with solid renal tumors before and after surgery (22 ccRCCs, 16 pRCCs, 14 chRCCs, 8 oncocytomas, 5 angiomyolipomas, and 2 papillary adenomas) compared to 15 healthy controls using polymerase chain reaction. It was found that miRNA-15a expression was significantly upregulated in RCC patients in comparison to benign tumors and healthy renal parenchyma ($p < 0.01$) (Mytsyk et al., 2017).

26.5.1.3 The change in the DNA

The loss of chromosome 3p (70%–80%) and gain of chromosome 5q (50%–60%) account for the most notable genetic abnormalities in relation with ccRCCS (Mytsyk et al., 2017). Loss-of-function mutations in the remaining VHL allele are thought to represent an early event in ccRCC development but are not sufficient alone to drive tumor growth.

Another major tumor suppressor gene (TSG) implicated in ccRCC is the SW1/SNF chromatin remodeling complex gene polybromo1 (PBRM1), with truncating mutations found in 41% of the 227 cases tested (Varela et al., 2011).

Mutations are also found in BRCA related protein-1 (BAP1), with inactivation of BAP1 protein in 15% of ccRCCs. Interestingly, mutations in PBRM1 and BAP1 were largely observed to occur exclusively, suggesting that simultaneous loss may be disadvantageous to the tumor (Peña-Llopis et al., 2012).

26.5.1.4 DNA methylation

Cancer cells often demonstrate TSG inactivation as a result of aberrant promoter hypermethylation (Jones & Baylin, 2002).

Indeed, the VHL TSG is inactivated via methylation in approximately 10%–30% of sporadic ccRCC cases (Young et al., 2009; Nickerson et al., 2008; Dulaimi et al., 2004). Methylation studies, including recent genome-wide based approaches, have identified numerous candidate TSGs inactivated by hypermethylation in ccRCC, which, in many cases, occur at high frequency within the studied sample sets (Ricketts et al., 2012; Morris et al., 2011).

For example, The Ras association domain family 1 gene, which codes for a protein ensuring the functions of a negative regulator of the cell cycle, is methylated in approximately 45% of cases (Dulaimi et al., 2004). Secreted frizzled related protein, which antagonizes Wnt signaling, is methylated in 34%–68% of ccRCC tumors (Dahl et al., 2007; Morris et al., 2010).

26.6 Recent trends in antitumor vaccines

It is obvious that the development of an antitumor vaccine must follow specific conditions and rules. Conventionally, a vaccine essentially consists in presenting antigens to the immune cells in order to encourage them to produce antibodies against the pathogens. However, in the case of tumors, the situation is different. It is worth noting that most of the antitumor vaccine types are curative, excluding the vaccines against cervical cancer, for example, viral-based preventive vaccines against the causal agent of the disease. On the other hand, tumors are part of the body, and thus they are part of the self and have the molecules of the major histocompatibility complex of class I (MHC 1). This allows them to escape the control of the immune system.

Compared to other cells, it is known that red blood cells do not carry MHC I, but they do have minor markers called agglutinogens. Monocytes, B lymphocytes, and DCs additionally have MHC class II. Since the identification of certain tumor antigens such as melanoma associated antigen A (MAGE-A1), it has been possible to carry out clinical trials based on these antigens. Unfortunately, the levels of clinical response and gain in survival after use of these vaccines have been disappointing. They vary between an exceptional level of four months of survival after use of the Provenge vaccine DCs loaded with prostate tumor antigens in phase III and the negative results of the vaccine with MAGE-A3 (melanoma-associated antigen-A3) (Depil et al., 2018).

These first disappointing results led to the adoption of a new paradigm, which consists in developing antitumor vaccination on the basis of mutated tumor-specific neo-antigens [mutation-associated neo-antigens, (MANA)], which will subsequently lead to the development of personalized antitumor vaccination (Leclerc, 2007; Fu et al., 2020). This is because tumor cells express mutated proteins that are not present in normal body cells. These proteins are called neo-antigens.

Furthermore, the degradation of these proteins results in peptides of various sizes, among which emerge tumor-specific neo-epitopes having a high affinity for the MHC and the T cell receptor (TCR). The presentation of these epitopes by the MHC on the surface of tumor cells allows recognition by the T lymphocytes via the TCR, and this leads to the proliferation and to a strong cytotoxicity of the CD8 + T lymphocytes (Leclerc, 2007; Fu et al., 2020). The development of vaccines from these epitopes depends on the ability to detect mutations and the results of cleavage of the mutated proteins that give rise to neo-antigens.

This development uses bioinformatics and modulation techniques associated with various techniques and protocols, namely, mass spectrometry (Ruffini et al., 2002), RNA sequencing, complementary DNA, protein–protein interactions, verifying the absence of interaction with self-proteins (binding tests) (Davis et al., 2014), immunogenicity tests, in vitro validation of in silico tests (Depil et al., 2018; Leclerc, 2007; Ruffini et al., 2002). At the same time, understanding the major role played by DCs in inducing immune responses has made these cells a key element in vaccine development. Targeting the antigen to DCs therefore represents a very important objective in vaccinology (Leclerc, 2007). All of these techniques help to carry out reverse vaccinology and allow important advances in the field of onco-vaccines.

DCs are obtained by in vitro derivation from monocytes. monocyte-derived DCs (MoDCs) are thus obtained (Fu et al., 2020), which sometimes have a functional limitation and are replaced by the use of exosomes derived from DCs for their resistance to suppression by tumors. However, the latter ones have also shown the weakness of their clinical effects because they do not produce a specific reaction to antigens such as T lymphocytes (Fu et al., 2020). Consequently, the production of antitumor vaccines has been directed toward the use of circulating CDs instead of the activated CDs in vitro, and particularly also the plasmacytoid CD, which make it possible to obtain lasting CD 8T cell immunity (Leclerc, 2007; Ruffini et al., 2002).

The results of the trials and uses of these vaccines are encouraging although mixed. Indeed, some major questions still need to be resolved. These include the choice of peptides to use, the number of these peptides, the role of CD4 and CD8, the level of application, the form and route of administration of the vaccines, and the possible risks of the development of the vaccine resistance. The lattermost point raises the importance of the fact that there is a great diversity of neo-antigens from tumor to tumor and therefore from patient to patient with the existence of subclonal epitopes. This diversity is double-edged; it is useful for ensuring better response, but on the other hand, it requires customization. However, it must be remembered that advanced tumors, stages for which many vaccine trials are carried out, set up immuno-suppression, which leads to systemic resistance to immunotherapy (Leclerc, 2007).

Regarding the place of this type of vaccine in cancer therapy, it is generally found that they are being tested as adjuvants and as neo-adjuvants with anti PD-1/PD-L1, with chemotherapy and surgery. Regarding urogenital cancers, trials have been conducted in patients with stage III/IV ovarian cancer following standard treatment of surgery and chemotherapy and phase I/II trial comparing autologous DC vaccine pulsed either with personalized peptides and translates a novel concept of NeoAg vaccine delivery from laboratory to the clinic, and implements a new personalized and agnostic epitope discovery pipeline, which relies on advanced bio-computational methodologies, exome and RNA sequencing, mass spectrometry-based immune-peptidomics, and validation of the potential epitopes through functional cell-based assays (Racle et al., 2019).

There are also other clinical trials in front-line kidney cancer patients with ipilimumab. While currently the main interest is in epitopes mutated from the single-nucleotide variant (SNV) to produce vaccines, other neo-antigens are conceivable for this use. These are peptides with splicing abnormalities or with insertion deletion (indel) mutations for which the possibility of having a large number of neo-antigens with high affinity for MHC compared to SNVs is expected. On the other hand, the expected benefit of these neo-antigen-based vaccines is their use as adjuvant and for the long-term control of residual disease by generating a memory immune response (Sarivalasis et al., 2019; Zahm et al., 2017). Consequently, for DC-based vaccination to gain a comprehensible and effective role in the therapeutic landscape of cancer, research should be focused on well-designed trials in the adjuvant setting, combinational strategies, and patient selection (Van Willigen et al., 2018; Gilboa, 2007).

References

Aggarwal, B. B., Vijayalekshmi, R. V., & Sung, B. (2009). Targeting inflammatory pathways for prevention and therapy of cancer: Short-term friend, long-term foe [Internet]. *Clinical Cancer Research*, *15*(2), 425–430, [cited 2021 Apr 8]. Available from https://pubmed.ncbi.nlm.nih.gov/19147746/.

Aghaalikhani, N., Rashtchizadeh, N., Shadpour, P., Allameh, A., & Mahmoodi, M. (2019). Cancer stem cells as a therapeutic target in bladder cancer. *Journal of Cellular Physiology*, *234*, 3197–3206.

Aragon-Ching, J. B., & Trump, D. L. (2017). Targeted therapies in the treatment of urothelial cancers. *Urologic Oncology: Seminars and Original Investigations*, *35*(7), 465–472.

Atkins, M. B., Lotze, M. T., Dutcher, J. P., Fisher, R. I., Weiss, G., Margolin, K., et al. (1999). High-dose recombinant interleukin 2 therapy for patients with metastatic melanoma: Analysis of 270 patients treated between 1985 and 1993. *Journal of Clinical Oncology*, *17*, 2105–2116, [cited 2021 Apr 8]. Available from https://pubmed.ncbi.nlm.nih.gov/10561265/.

Balkwill, F., & Mantovani, A. (2001). Inflammation and cancer: Back to Virchow? [Internet]. *Lancet*, *357*(9255), 539–545, [cited 2021 Apr 8]. Available from https://pubmed.ncbi.nlm.nih.gov/11229684/.

Beer, T. M., Armstrong, A. J., Rathkopf, D. E., Loriot, Y., Sternberg, C. N., Higano, C. S., et al. (2014). Enzalutamide in metastatic prostate cancer before chemotherapy [Internet]. *New England Journal of Medicine*, *371*, 424–433, [cited 2021 Apr 8]. Available from https://www.ncbi.nlm.nih.gov/pmc/articles/PMC4418931/.

Bladder, C., Be, C., Early, F., Signs, B. C., Stages, B. C., To, Q., et al. (2020). Bladder cancer early detection, diagnosis, and staging can bladder cancer be found early ? [Internet]. *American Cancer Society*, 1–24. Available from https://www.cancer.org/cancer/kidney-cancer/detection-diagnosis-staging/staging.html.

Bolat, D., & Haydaroğlu, A. (2019). Immunotherapy in prostate cancer. *Üroonkoloji Bülteni*, *18*, 67–72.

Bou-Dargham, M. J., Sha, L., Sang, Q. X. A., Sang, Q. X. A., & Zhang, J. (2020). Immune landscape of human prostate cancer: Immune evasion mechanisms and biomarkers for personalized immunotherapy. *BMC Cancer*, *20*, 1–10.

Brannon, A. R., Reddy, A., Seiler, M., Arreola, A., Moore, D. T., Pruthi, R. S., et al. (2010). Molecular stratification of clear cell renal cell carcinoma by consensus clustering reveals distinct subtypes and survival patterns [Internet]. *Genes and Cancer*, *1*, 152–163, [cited 2021 Jun 24]. Available from https://pubmed.ncbi.nlm.nih.gov/20871783/.

Brooks, S. A., Brannon, A. R., Parker, J. S., Fisher, J. C., Sen, O., Kattan, M. W., et al. (2014). ClearCode34: A prognostic risk predictor for localized clear cell renal cell carcinoma [Internet]. *European Urology*, *66*, 77–84, [cited 2021 Jun 24]. Available from https://pubmed.ncbi.nlm.nih.gov/24613583/.

Cancer Genome Atlas Research NetworkMarston Linehan, W., Spellman, P. T., Ricketts, C. J., Creighton, C. J., Fei, S. S., & Davis, C. (2016). Comprehensive molecular characterization of papillary renal-cell carcinoma [Internet]. *New England Journal of Medicine*, *374*, 135–145, [cited 2021 Jun 24]. Available from https://pubmed.ncbi.nlm.nih.gov/26536169/.

Chang, E., Weinstock, C., Zhang, L., Charlab, R., Dorff, S. E., Gong, Y., et al. (2021). FDA approval summary: Enfortumab vedotin for locally advanced or metastatic urothelial carcinoma [Internet]. *Clinical Cancer Research*, *27*(4), 922–927, [cited 2021 Apr 8]. Available from https://pubmed.ncbi.nlm.nih.gov/32962979/.

Chen, F., Zhang, Y., Şenbabaoğlu, Y., Ciriello, G., Yang, L., Reznik, E., et al. (2016). Multilevel genomics-based taxonomy of renal cell carcinoma [Internet]. *Cell Reports*, *14*, 2476–2489, [cited 2021 Jun 24]. Available from https://pubmed.ncbi.nlm.nih.gov/26947078/.

Chen, M. F., Lin, P. Y., Wu, C. F., Chen, W. C., & Wu, C. Te (2013). IL-6 expression regulates tumorigenicity and correlates with prognosis in bladder cancer [Internet]. *PLoS One*, *8*, e61901, [cited 2021 Apr 8]. Available from https://pubmed.ncbi.nlm.nih.gov/23637926/.

Chen, Y. T., Tsai, C. H., Chen, C. L., Yu, J. S., & Chang, Y. H. (2019). Development of biomarkers of genitourinary cancer using mass spectrometry-based clinical proteomics [Interenet]. *Journal of Food and Drug Analysis*, *27*, 387–403. Available from https://doi.org/10.1016/j.jfda.2018.09.005.

Chovanec, M., Mardiak, J., & Mego, M. (2019). Immune mechanisms and possible immune therapy in testicular germ cell tumours [Internet]. *Andrology*, *7*(4), 479–486, [cited 2021 Apr 8]. Available from https://pubmed.ncbi.nlm.nih.gov/31169364/.

Conteduca, V., Mosca, A., Brighi, N., de Giorgi, U., & Rescigno, P. (2021). New prognostic biomarkers in metastatic castration-resistant prostate cancer [Internet]. *Cells*, *10*(1), 193, [cited 2021 Mar 29]. Available from https://pubmed.ncbi.nlm.nih.gov/33478015/.

Curti, B. D., Kovacsovics-Bankowski, M., Morris, N., Walker, E., Chisholm, L., Floyd, K., et al. (2013). OX40 is a potent immune-stimulating target in late-stage cancer patients. *Cancer Research*, *73*, 7189–7198.

Dahl, E., Wiesmann, F., Woenckhaus, M., Stoehr, R., Wild, P. J., Veeck, J., et al. (2007). Frequent loss of SFRP1 expression in multiple human solid tumours: Association with aberrant promoter methylation in renal cell carcinoma [Internet]. *Oncogene*, *26*, 5680–5691, [cited 2021 Jun 27]. Available from https://pubmed.ncbi.nlm.nih.gov/17353908/.

Davis, C. F., Ricketts, C. J., Wang, M., Yang, L., Cherniack, A. D., Shen, H., et al. (2014). The somatic genomic landscape of chromophobe renal cell carcinoma [Internet]. *Cancer Cell*, *26*, 319–330, [cited 2021 Jun 24]. Available from https://pubmed.ncbi.nlm.nih.gov/25155756/.

Depil, S., Bonaventura, P., Alcazer, V., & Tonon, L. (2018). Nouvelles approches vaccinales en cancérologie [Internet]. *Bulletin du Cancer*, *105*, S113–S120, [cited 2021 Apr 8]. Available from https://pubmed.ncbi.nlm.nih.gov/30595192/.

Dulaimi, E., De Caceres, I. I., Uzzo, R. G., Al-Saleem, T., Greenberg, R. E., Polascik, T. J., et al. (2004). Promoter hypermethylation profile of kidney cancer [Internet]. *Clinical Cancer*

Research, *10*, 3972–3979, [cited 2021 Jun 24]. Available from https://pubmed.ncbi.nlm.nih.gov/15217927/.

Dunn, G. P., Bruce, A. T., Ikeda, H., Old, L. J., & Schreiber, R. D. (2002). Cancer immunoediting: From immunosurveillance to tumor escape [Internet]. *Nature Immunology*, *3*(11), 991–998, [cited 2021 Apr 8]. Available from https://pubmed.ncbi.nlm.nih.gov/12407406/.

Escudier, B., Porta, C., Schmidinger, M., Rioux-Leclercq, N., Bex, A., Khoo, V., et al. (2019). Renal cell carcinoma: ESMO clinical practice guidelines for diagnosis, treatment and follow-up [Internet]. *Annals of Oncology*, *30*, 706–720, [cited 2021 Jun 24]. Available from https://pubmed.ncbi.nlm.nih.gov/30788497/.

Farina, M. S., Lundgren, K. T., & Bellmunt, J. (2017). Immunotherapy in urothelial cancer: Recent results and future perspectives [Internet]. *Drugs*, *77*(10), 1077–1089, [cited 2021 Apr 8]. Available from https://pubmed.ncbi.nlm.nih.gov/28493171/.

Fedorko, M., Stanik, M., Iliev, R., Redova-Lojova, M., Machackova, T., Svoboda, M., et al. (2015). Combination of MiR-378 and MiR-210 serum levels enables sensitive detection of renal cell carcinoma [Internet]. *International Journal of Molecular Sciences*, *16*, 23382–23389, [cited 2021 Jun 24]. Available from https://www.ncbi.nlm.nih.gov/pmc/articles/PMC4632704/.

Fridman, W. H., Pagès, F., Saut̀s-Fridman, C., & Galon, J. (2012). The immune contexture in human tumours: Impact on clinical outcome [Internet]. *Nature Reviews. Cancer*, *12*(4), 298–306, [cited 2021 Apr 8]. Available from https://www.nature.com/articles/nrc3245.

Fu, C., Zhou, L., Mi, Q.-S., & Jiang, A. (2020). DC-based vaccines for cancer immunotherapy [Internet]. *Vaccines*, *8*, 706, [cited 2021 Apr 8].

Galvão-Lima, L. J., Morais, A. H. F., Valentim, R. A. M., & Barreto, E. J. S. S. (2021). miRNAs as biomarkers for early cancer detection and their application in the development of new diagnostic tools [Internet]. *Biomedical. Engineering Online*, *20*(1), 21, [cited 2021 Mar 29].

Garcia-Donas, J., Esteban, E., Leandro-García, L. J., Castellano, D. E., del Alba, A. G., Climent, M. A., et al. (2011). Single nucleotide polymorphism associations with response and toxic effects in patients with advanced renal-cell carcinoma treated with first-line sunitinib: A multicentre, observational, prospective study [Internet]. *The Lancet. Oncology*, *12*, 1143–1150, [cited 2021 Jun 24].

Gilboa, E. (2007). DC-based cancer vaccines [Internet]. *Journal of Clinical Investigation*, *117* (5), 1195–1203, [cited 2021 Apr 8].

Gottardo, F., Liu, C. G., Ferracin, M., Calin, G. A., Fassan, M., Bassi, P., et al. (2007). MicroRNA profiling in kidney and bladder cancers. *Urologic Oncology: Seminars and Original Investigations*, *25*, 387–392, [cited 2021 Jun 24].

Gulley, J. L., Madan, R. A., Pachynski, R., Mulders, P., Sheikh, N. A., Trager, J., et al. (2017). Role of antigen spread and distinctive characteristics of immunotherapy in cancer treatment. *Journal of the National Cancer Institute*, *109*, 1–9.

Huang, D., Ding, Y., Zhou, M., Rini, B. I., Petillo, D., Qian, C. N., et al. (2010). Interleukin-8 mediates resistance to antiangiogenic agent sunitinib in renal cell carcinoma [Internet]. *Cancer Research*, *70*, 1063–1071, [cited 2021 Jun 24].

Inman, B. A., Sebo, T. J., Frigola, X., Dong, H., Bergstralh, E. J., Frank, I., et al. (2007). PD-L1 (B7-H1) expression by urothelial carcinoma of the bladder and BCG-induced granulomata: Associations with localized stage progression [Internet]. *Cancer*, *109*, 1499–1505, [cited 2021 Apr 8].

Iwamoto, H., Kanda, Y., Sejima, T., Osaki, M., Okada, F., & Takenaka, A. (2014). Serum miR-210 as a potential biomarker of early clear cell renal cell carcinoma [Internet]. *International Journal of Oncology*, *44*, 53–58, [cited 2021 Jun 24].

Jagodinsky, J. C., Harari, P. M., & Morris, Z. S. (2020). The promise of combining radiation therapy with immunotherapy [Interent]. *International Journal of Radiation Oncology – Biology – Physics*, *108*, 6–16, [cited 2021 Apr 8].

Jones, P. A., & Baylin, S. B. (2002). The fundamental role of epigenetic events in cancer [Internet]. *Nature Reviews. Genetics*, *3*(6), 415–428, [cited 2021 Jun 24].

Juengel, E., Erb, H. H. H., Haferkamp, A., Rutz, J., Chun, F. K. H., & Blaheta, R. A. (2018). Relevance of the natural HDAC inhibitor sulforaphane as a chemopreventive agent in urologic tumors [Internet]. *Cancer Letters*, *435*, 121–126, [cited 2021 Apr 8].

Karzai, F., Madan, R. A., Owens, H., Hankin, A., Couvillon, A., Cordes, L. M., et al. (2017). Combination of PDL-1 and PARP inhibition in an unselected population with metastatic castrate-resistant prostate cancer (mCRPC). *Journal of Clinical Oncology*, *35*, 5026.

Kojima, T., Kawai, K., Miyazaki, J., & Nishiyama, H. (2017). Biomarkers for precision medicine in bladder cancer. *International Journal of Clinical Oncology*, *22*, 207–213.

Kwon, E. D., Drake, C. G., Scher, H. I., Fizazi, K., Bossi, A., Alfons, J. M., et al. (2014). Ipilimumab versus placebo after radiotherapy in patients with metastatic castration-resistant prostate cancer that had progressed after docetaxel chemotherapy (CA184-043): A multicentre, randomised, double-blind, phase 3 trial. *The Lancet Oncology*, *15*, 700–712.

Lamm, D. L., Thor, D. E., Harris, S. C., Reyna, J. A., Stogdill, V. D., & Radwin, H. M. (1980). Bacillus Calmette-Guerin immunotherapy of superficial bladder cancer [Internet]. *The Journal of Urology*, *124*, 38–42, [cited 2021 Apr 8].

Leclerc, C. (2007). L'apport des nouvelles technologies en vaccinologie [Internet]. *médecine/sciences*, *23*, 386–390, [cited 2021 Apr 8].

Liu, X., Wu, Y., Zhou, Z., Huang, M., Deng, W., Wang, Y., et al. (2019). Celecoxib inhibits the epithelial-to-mesenchymal transition in bladder cancer via the miRNA-145/TGFBR2/Smad3 axis. *International Journal of Molecular Medicine*, *44*, 683–693.

Lopez-Beltran, A., Cimadamore, A., Blanca, A., Massari, F., Vau, N., Scarpelli, M., et al. (2021). Immune checkpoint inhibitors for the treatment of bladder cancer. *Cancers (Basel)*, *13*, 131.

Mastuo, T., Miyata, Y., Yuno, T., Mukae, Y., Otsubo, A., Mitsunari, K., et al. (2020). Molecular mechanisms of the anti-cancer effects of isothiocyanates from cruciferous vegetables in bladder cancer. *Molecules.*, *25*, 575.

McNeel, D. G., Smith, H. A., Eickhoff, J. C., Lang, J. M., Staab, M. J., Wilding, G., et al. (2012). Phase I trial of tremelimumab in combination with short-term androgen deprivation in patients with PSA-recurrent prostate cancer [Internet]. *Cancer Immunology, Immunotherapy*, *61*, 1137–1147, [cited 2021 Apr 8].

Milowsky, M. I., Iyer, G., Regazzi, A. M., Al-Ahmadie, H., Gerst, S. R., Ostrovnaya, I., et al. (2013). Phase II study of everolimus in metastatic urothelial cancer [Internet]. *BJU International*, *112*, 462–470, [cited 2021 Apr 8].

Moch, H., Cubilla, A. L., Humphrey, P. A., Reuter, V. E., & Ulbright, T. M. (2016). The 2016 WHO classification of tumours of the urinary system and male genital organs—part A: Renal, penile, and testicular tumours [Internet]. *European Urology*, *70*, 93–105, [cited 2021 Jun 24].

Morales, A., Eidinger, D., & Bruce, A. W. (1976). Intracavitary Bacillus Calmette Guerin in the treatment of superficial bladder tumors [Internet]. *The Journal of Urology*, *116*, 180–182, [cited 2021 Apr 8].

Morris, M. R., Ricketts, C., Gentle, D., Abdulrahman, M., Clarke, N., Brown, M., et al. (2010). Identification of candidate tumour suppressor genes frequently methylated in renal cell carcinoma [Internet]. *Oncogene*, *29*, 2104–2117, [cited 2021 Jun 27].

Morris, M. R., Ricketts, C. J., Gentle, D., McRonald, F., Carli, N., Khalili, H., et al. (2011). Genome-wide methylation analysis identifies epigenetically inactivated candidate tumour suppressor genes in renal cell carcinoma [Internet]. *Oncogene, 30*, 1390–1401, [cited 2021 Jun 27].

Motzer, R. J., Tannir, N. M., McDermott, D. F., Arén Frontera, O., Melichar, B., Choueiri, T. K., et al. (2018). Nivolumab plus ipilimumab versus sunitinib in advanced renal-cell carcinoma [Internet]. *New England Journal of Medicine, 378*, 1277–1290, [cited 2021 Apr 8].

Murphy, K. A., James, B. R., Guan, Y., Torry, D. S., Wilber, A., & Griffith, T. S. (2015). Exploiting natural anti-tumor immunity for metastatic renal cell carcinoma [Internet]. *Human Vaccines & Immunotherapeutics, 11*, 1612–1620, [cited 2021 Apr 8].

Mytsyk, Y., Dosenko, V., Borys, Y., Ilchyshyn, O., Chernova, N., Mytsyk, O., et al. (2017). The possibility of application of detected in urine MicroRNA-15a for diagnostics of renal cell carcinoma. *Experimental and Clinical Physiology and Biochemistry, 2017*, 49–53.

Nakada, C., Matsuura, K., Tsukamoto, Y., Tanigawa, M., Yoshimoto, T., Narimatsu, T., et al. (2008). Genome-wide microRNA expression profiling in renal cell carcinoma: Significant down-regulation of miR-141 and miR-200c [Internet]. *The Journal of Pathology, 216*, 418–427, [cited 2021 Jun 24].

Nakanishi, J., Wada, Y., Matsumoto, K., Azuma, M., Kikuchi, K., & Ueda, S. (2007). Overexpression of B7-H1 (PD-L1) significantly associates with tumor grade and postoperative prognosis in human urothelial cancers [Internet]. *Cancer Immunology, Immunotherapy, 56*, 1173–1182, [cited 2021 Apr 8].

Nickerson, M. L., Jaeger, E., Shi, Y., Durocher, J. A., Mahurkar, S., Zaridze, D., et al. (2008). Improved identification of von Hippel-Lindau gene alterations in clear cell renal tumors [Internet]. *Clinical Cancer Research, 14*, 4726–4734, [cited 2021 Jun 24].

Parriott, G., Deal, K., Crean, S., Richardson, E., Nylen, E., & Barber, A. (2020). T-cells expressing a chimeric-PD1-Dap10-CD3zeta receptor reduce tumour burden in multiple murine syngeneic models of solid cancer [Internet]. *Immunology, 160*, 280–294, [cited 2021 Apr 8].

Peethambaram, P. P., Melisko, M. E., Rinn, K. J., Alberts, S. R., Provost, N. M., Jones, L. A., et al. (2009). A phase I trial of immunotherapy with lapuleucel-T (APC8024) in patients with refractory metastatic tumors that express HER-2/neu [Internet]. *Clinical Cancer Research, 15*, 5937–5944, [cited 2021 Apr 8].

Peña-Llopis, S., Vega-Rubín-De-Celis, S., Liao, A., Leng, N., Pavía-Jiménez, A., Wang, S., et al. (2012). BAP1 loss defines a new class of renal cell carcinoma [Internet]. *Nature Genetics, 44*, 751–759, [cited 2021 Jun 24].

Pierantoni, F., Maruzzo, M., Gardi, M., Bezzon, E., Gardiman, M. P., Porreca, A., et al. (2019). Immunotherapy and urothelial carcinoma: An overview and future prospectives [Internet]. *Critical Reviews in Oncology/Hematology, 143*, 46–55, [cited 2021 Apr 8].

Poch, M., Hall, M., Joerger, A., Kodumudi, K., Beatty, M., Innamarato, P. P., et al. (2018). Expansion of tumor infiltrating lymphocytes (TIL) from bladder cancer [Internet]. *Oncoimmunology, 7*, e1476816, [cited 2021 Apr 8].

Purdue, M. P., Johansson, M., Zelenika, D., Toro, J. R., Scelo, G., Moore, L. E., et al. (2011). Genome-wide association study of renal cell carcinoma identifies two susceptibility loci on 2p21 and 11q13.3 [Internet]. *Nature Genetics, 43*, 60–65, [cited 2021 Jun 24].

Racle, J., Michaux, J., Rockinger, G. A., Arnaud, M., Bobisse, S., Chong, C., et al. (2019). Robust prediction of HLA class II epitopes by deep motif deconvolution of immunopeptidomes [Internet]. *Nature Biotechnology, 37*, 1283–1286, [cited 2021 Apr 8].

Ricketts, C. J., Morris, M. R., Gentle, D., Brown, M., Wake, N., Woodward, E. R., et al. (2012). Genome-wide CpG island methylation analysis implicates novel genes in the pathogenesis of renal cell carcinoma [Internet]. *Epigenetics, 7*, 278–290, [cited 2021 Jun 24].

Roos, F., Binder, K., Rutz, J., Maxeiner, S., Bernd, A., Kippenberger, S., et al. (2019). The anti-tumor effect of curcumin in urothelial cancer cells is enhanced by light exposure in vitro. *Evidence-Based Complementary Alternative Medicine*, *2019*, 8.

Ruffini, P. A., Neelapu, S. S., Kwak, L. W., & Biragyn, A. (2002). Idiotypic vaccination for B-cell malignancies as a model for therapeutic cancer vaccines: From prototype protein to second generation vaccines [Internet]. *Haematologica*, *87*(9), 989–1001, [cited 2021 Apr 8].

Samstein, R. M., Lee, C. H., Shoushtari, A. N., Hellmann, M. D., Shen, R., Janjigian, Y. Y., et al. (2019). Tumor mutational load predicts survival after immunotherapy across multiple cancer types [Internet]. *Nature Genetics*, *51*(2), 202–206, [cited 2021 Apr 8].

Sarivalasis, A., Boudousquié, C., Balint, K., Stevenson, B. J., Gannon, P. O., Iancu, E. M., et al. (2019). A Phase I/II trial comparing autologous dendritic cell vaccine pulsed either with personalized peptides (PEP-DC) or with tumor lysate (OC-DC) in patients with advanced high-grade ovarian serous carcinoma [Internet]. *Journal of Translational Medicine*, *17*, 391, [cited 2021 Apr 8].

Slovin, S. F. (2016). Biomarkers for immunotherapy in genitourinary malignancies [Internet]. *Urologic Oncology: Seminars and Original Investigations*, *34*, 205–213. Available from https://doi.org/10.1016/j.urolonc.2015.02.007.

Slovin, S. F. (2017). The need for immune biomarkers for treatment prognosis and response in genitourinary malignancies. *Biomarkers in Medicine*, *11*, 1149–1159.

Small, E. J., Lance, R. S., Gardner, T. A., Karsh, L. I., Fong, L., McCoy, C., et al. (2015). A randomized phase II trial of sipuleucel-T with concurrent versus sequential abiraterone acetate plus prednisone in metastatic castration-resistant prostate cancer [Internet]. *Clinical Cancer Research*, *21*, 3862–3869, [cited 2021 Apr 8].

Small, E. J., Tchekmedyian, N. S., Rini, B. I., Fong, L., Lowy, I., & Allison, J. P. (2007). A pilot trial of CTLA-4 blockade with human anti-CTLA-4 in patients with hormone-refractory prostate cancer [Internet]. *Clinical Cancer Research*, *13*, 1810–1815, [cited 2021 Apr 8].

Solinas, G., Germano, G., Mantovani, A., & Allavena, P. (2009). Tumor-associated macrophages (TAM) as major players of the cancer-related inflammation [Internet]. *Journal of Leukocyte Biology*, *86*, 1065–1073, [cited 2021 Apr 8]. Available from http://doi.wiley.com/10.1189/jlb.0609385.

Song, D., Powles, T., Shi, L., Zhang, L., Ingersoll, M. A., & Lu, Y. (2019). Bladder cancer, a unique model to understand cancer immunity and develop immunotherapy approaches. *The Journal of Pathology*, *249*, 151–165.

Suttmann, H., Riemensberger, J., Bentien, G., Schmaltz, D., Stöckle, M., Jocham, D., et al. (2006). Neutrophil granulocytes are required for effective Bacillus Calmette-Guérin immunotherapy of bladder cancer and orchestrate local immune responses [Interenet]. *Cancer Research*, *66*, 8250–8257, [cited 2021 Apr 8]. Available from https://pubmed.ncbi.nlm.nih.gov/16912205/.

Van Der Horst, G., Bos, L., & Van Der Pluijm, G. (2012). Epithelial plasticity, cancer stem cells, and the tumor-supportive stroma in bladder carcinoma [Internet]. *Molecular Cancer Research*, *10*(8), 995–1009, [cited 2021 Apr 8].

Van Parijs, L., & Abbas, A. K. (1998). Homeostasis and self-tolerance in the immune system: Turning lymphocytes off [Internet]. *Science*, *280*, 243–248, [cited 2021 Apr 8].

Van Willigen, W. W., Bloemendal, M., Gerritsen, W. R., Schreibelt, G., De Vries, I. J. M., & Bol, K. F. (2018). Dendritic cell cancer therapy: Vaccinating the right patient at the right time [Internet]. *Frontiers in Immunology*, *9*, 2265, [cited 2021 Apr 8].

Varela, I., Tarpey, P., Raine, K., Huang, D., Ong, C. K., Stephens, P., et al. (2011). Exome sequencing identifies frequent mutation of the SWI/SNF Complex Gene PBRM1 in renal carcinoma [Internet]. *The Journal of Urology*, *186*(3), 1150, [cited 2021 Jun 24].

Von Brandenstein, M., Pandarakalam, J. J., Kroon, L., Loeser, H., Herden, J., Braun, G., et al. (2012). MicroRNA 15a, inversely correlated to PKCα, is a potential marker to differentiate between benign and malignant renal tumors in biopsy and urine samples [Internet]. *The American Journal of Pathology*, *180*, 1787–1797, [cited 2021 Jun 24].

Wołącewicz, M., Hrynkiewicz, R., Grywalska, E., Suchojad, T., Leksowski, T., Roliński, J., et al. (2020). Immunotherapy in bladder cancer: Current methods and future perspectives. *Cancers (Basel)*, *12*, 1–17.

Xu, C. F., Bing, N. X., Ball, H. A., Rajagopalan, D., Sternberg, C. N., Hutson, T. E., et al. (2011). Pazopanib efficacy in renal cell carcinoma: Evidence for predictive genetic markers in angiogenesis-related and exposure-related genes [Internet]. *Journal of Clinical Oncology*, *29*, 2557–2564, [cited 2021 Jun 24].

Yang, M., Zhang, X., Guo, L., Liu, X., Wu, J., & Zhu, H. (2021). Research progress for the clinical application of circulating tumor cells in prostate cancer diagnosis and treatment [Internet]. *Biomed Research International*, *2021*, 6230826, [cited 2021 Mar 29].

Young, A. C., Craven, R. A., Cohen, D., Taylor, C., Booth, C., Harnden, P., et al. (2009). Analysis of VHL gene alterations and their relationship to clinical parameters in sporadic conventional renal cell carcinoma [Internet]. *Clinical Cancer Research*, *15*, 7582–7592, [cited 2021 Jun 24].

Zahm, C. D., Colluru, V. T., & McNeel, D. G. (2017). Vaccination with high-affinity epitopes impairs antitumor efficacy by increasing PD-1 expression on CD8 + T cells [Internet]. *Cancer Immunology Research*, *5*, 630–641, [cited 2021 Apr 8].

Zhang, C., Berndt-Paetz, M., & Neuhaus, J. (2020). Identification of key biomarkers in bladder cancer: Evidence from a bioinformatics analysis [Internet]. *Diagnostics*, *10*, 66, [cited 2021 Apr 8].

Zhu, Z., Shen, Z., & Xu, C. (2012). Inflammatory pathways as promising targets to increase chemotherapy response in bladder cancer [Internet]. *Mediators of Inflammation*, *2012*, 528690, [cited 2021 Apr 8].

Chapter 27

The global genomic allelic heterogeneity of the HOXB 13 variants of prostate cancer and gene therapy application for different genealogical lineages of the Y-chromosome haplogroups and haplotypes of STR microsatellites

Ihsane Ali Mahasneh[1], Berjas Abumsimir[2,3], Moulay Mustapha Ennaji[4] and Yassine Kasmi[3]

[1]*Faculty of Science, Department of Applied Biology-Biotechnology Program, University of Sharjah, Sharjah, United Arab Emirates,* [2]*Pharmacological and Diagnostic Research Centre (PDRC), Department of Medical Laboratory Sciences, Faculty of Allied Medical Sciences, Al-Ahliyya Amman University (AAU), Amman, Jordan,* [3]*Team of Virology, Oncology, and Biotechnologies, Laboratory of Virology, Oncology, Biosciences, Environment and New Energies (LVO-BEEN), Faculty of Sciences and Techniques Mohammedia, University Hassan II of Casablanca, Casablanca, Morocco,* [4]*Group Leader Research team of Virology, Oncology, and Biotechnologies, Head of Laboratory of Virology, Oncology, Biosciences, Environment and New Energies (LVO-BEEN), Faculty of Sciences and Techniques Mohammedia, University Hassan II of Casablanca, Casablanca, Morocco*

27.1 Introduction

According to the World Health Organization (WHO) statistics, prostate cancer (PCa) is the second most prevalent cancer in males and the sixth cause of cancer-related deaths (https://www.who.int.). These statistics have prompted the scientific question that whether this high global rate of prevalence and incidence of the ancestral-based PCa mutations can be predicted and followed by the gene flow of males Y-haplogroups between different continents or through

Immunological Implications and Molecular Diagnostics of Genitourinary Cancer.
DOI: https://doi.org/10.1016/B978-0-323-85496-2.00011-7

migration tracking among the different populations. Therefore there is an urgent need for global genealogical profiling of the Y-chromosome haplogroups as associated with the epidemiology of PCa allelic heterogeneity as the obtained data will be a vital and valuable tool to enhance the diagnosis, therapy, and thus the overall management of the familial cancer disease in the region.

With regard to the future challenges and needs of PCa, it has been pointed out by several authors (see inside) that PCa has the highest heritability of any major cancer, and several genetic susceptibility loci have been identified, primarily in men of European and Asian descent. Therefore there is a pressing need to identify African-specific alleles and thereby elucidate the etiology of PCa in Afro-American and Afro-Caribbean men, who have the highest PCa mortality rates in the world.

Generally, a wide variety of strategies of gene therapy have been developed and found their way into the market commercially, including suicide, antiangiogenic, radioisotopic, and pro-apoptotic gene therapies. From practices' point of view, administration and delivery vectors can be constructed easily using various protocols of genetic engineering and cassette expression in which viral or nonviral vectors can yield impressive local gene expression and therapeutic effects.

About two decades ago, Harrington et al. (2001) concluded and reported that various therapeutic genes have proved activity against PCa in vitro and in vivo using nonviral (plasmid DNA, DNA-coated gold particles, liposomes, and polymer DNA complexes) and viral (adenovirus, retrovirus, adeno-associated virus, herpes virus, and poxvirus) vectors. They categorized therapeutic strategies as corrective, cytoreductive, and immunomodulatory gene therapy for the purpose of data analysis and comparison.

Jou et al. (2021) recently reported that the corrective gene therapy to restore normal patterns of tumor suppressor gene (p53, Rb, p21, and p16) expression or negate the effect of mutated tumor-promoting oncogenes (RAS, myc, erbB2, and bcl-2) have efficacy in animal models, but this approach suffers from the fact that each cancer cell must be targeted.

In conclusion, the genealogical profiling of PCa epidemiology and allelic heterogeneity is a vital and valuable tool to enhance the diagnosis, therapy, and thus the overall management of the familial cancer disease in the region. The practices discussed in this chapter will have the clinical potential of applications on PCa profiling among different population ancestry, which could be computed, inferred, and predicted by using its association with different genealogical lineages of the Y-chromosome haplogroups.

27.2 Background and hypothesis on the prostate cancer allelic heterogeneity associated with the genealogical lineages of populations

Recently, there has been worldwide growing interest in the heterogeneity of PCa variants between different populations and ethnic groups, as allelic heterogeneity on the PCa mutations has been reported to be associated with the ancestry of the population (Abumsimir et al., 2019; Brechka et al., 2017; Mahasneh, 2018; Mahasneh et al., 2021; William et al., 2021). For instance, the screening studies in different parts of Europe have shown that a high risk of PCa is directly associated with the European inheritance of a known germline mutation of HOXB13 in men of European ancestry (Laitinen et al., 2013; Xu et al., 2013, Karlsson et al., 2014; Kote-Jarai et al., 2015; Nyberg et al., 2019; Storebjerg et al., 2016). Furthermore, the genetic complexity of the families with three or more affected first- or second-degree relatives meet criteria for hereditary PCa. Evidently, a large genetic screening of cancer-prone families for the HOXB13 G84E germline mutation is now encompassed by National Comprehensive Cancer Network (NCCN) guidelines. For instance, William et al. (2021) studied the G84E germline mutation of HOXB13 predisposes to PCa and is clinically tested for familial cancer care. They investigated the HOXB locus to define a potentially broader contribution to PCa heritability and thus sought HOXB locus germline variants altering PCa risk in three European-ancestry case-control study populations (combined 7812 cases and 5047 controls). Another global pan-population study has been reported by Taitt (2018) to compare PCa data from various demographic regions to contextualize how disproportionate the incidence and mortality rates are among men from the African diaspora versus men of European, Hispanic, and Asian descent, as well as to highlight the need for more robust screening and treatment guidelines in developing countries.

PCa is the second most prevalent cancer in males and the sixth cause of cancer-related deaths since it was first reported and before the outset of the prevalence of the HOXB13-G84E mutation. Furthermore, the germline HOXB13-G84E mutation has consistently been associated with PCa risk among European pedigree (Maia et al., 2015; Pinhasi, 2012; Shang et al., 2013). More recently, in a wide-range population study that included results from the UK Biobank showed that the G84E mutation was found in 1545 (0.34%) subjects out of 460,224 participants of European pedigree (Wei et al., 2020)

Maia et al. (2015) provided further evidence to substantiate this assertion and showed that the G84E mutation was not found among PCa males of both African and Asian descent. For several years, our research outcomes on the Y-chromosome haplogroups of Arab genealogical lineages as determined by mutations of the short tandem repeats (STRs) of the nonrecombined region of the Y-chromosome showed that the epidemiology of cancers correlates with the genealogy and ethnicity of the population clusters (Mahasneh, 2018; Majasneh et al., 2018; Mahasneh and Zurigat, 2019). This has prompted the scientific question on whether the incidence of such ancestral-based mutation of PCa can be predicted by the gene flow in male haplogroups' genealogical lineages between different continents or through migration tracking among the different populations.

Currently, the research outcomes, using the latest technology such as next-generation sequencing and biochip microarray, have shown conclusively that the epidemiology of cancers is correlated to the genealogy and ethnicity of the population clusters around the world. Therefore the genealogical profiling of the PCa epidemiology and allelic heterogeneity will be a vital and valuable tool to enhance the diagnosis, therapy, and thus the overall management of the familial cancer disease in the region.

27.3 The landscape of the HOXB 13 gene cluster on chromosome 17

Chromosome 17 with a size of 81 Mb, poses about 3% of the total human genome and contains 1300–1400 genes, which play a crucial role in the development of body organs and maintaining numerous physiological activities. It also plays a major role in many other respects as it is implicated in a wide range of human genetic diseases including PCa causative gene cluster HOXB13 (Abumsimir et al., 2019, Mahasneh et al., 2021), early-onset breast cancer (BRCA1), neurofibromatosis (NF1), and the DNA damage response (TP53 encoding the p53 protein) (Zody et al., 2006). Chromosome 17 is highly rich in protein-coding genes, having the second-highest gene density in the genome. It is also enriched with segmental duplications, ranking third in density among the autosomes and the complexity rearrangements including duplication structure resulting in DNA rearrangements that are known to cause several well-studied microdeletion disorders and hereditary diseases (Bailey JA et al., 2002). The HOX13B G84E mutation, previously shown to be frequent among the European men with PCa, recently revealed to be absent among PCa Moroccan men (Abumsimir et al., 2019, Mahasneh et al., 2021).

The genomic landscape of chromosome 17 as constructed earlier (Brechka et al., 2017) (Fig. 27.1) shows the location of the HOXB13 gene (17q21.32) with genomic size 3988 base pair (bp) and the stretch of the HOXB13 gene (chr17:48,724,763–48,728,750) as available on the public domain of the Gene Cards (http://www.genecards.org) and NCBI (http://www.ncbi.nlm.nih.gov). This HOXB13 among other genes at the 5′ end of the 17q21–22 HOXB cluster consists of two exons and three known functional domains (accession number NC_000017/11 and ProtID Q92826). The HOXB13 transcript is 3987 bp long, and exons 1 and 2 are positioned at 157–757 bp and 1707–1960 bp, respectively.

27.4 The landscape of the Short tandem repeat microsatellite on the nonrecombined region of the Y-chromosome

The structure diagram of the Y-chromosome and the landscape of the STR microsatellites is shown in Fig. 27.1. The genome size of the Y-chromosome is the smallest in terms of the functional genes as composed of 59 Mbp, which is larger in size than the smallest chromosome 21 (spanning 48 Mbp) and composed of about 2%–3% of the total haploid genome (Zody et al.,

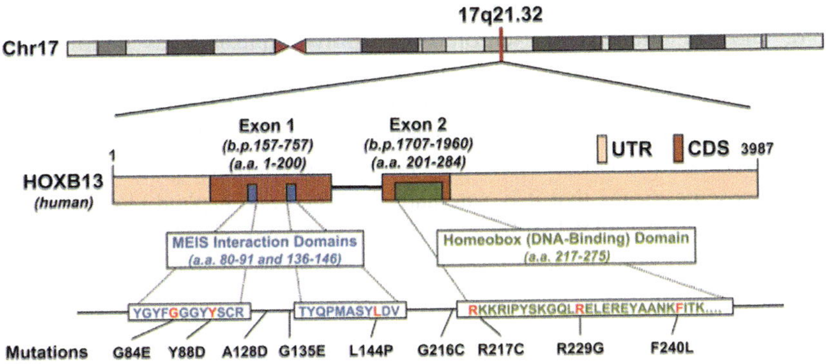

FIGURE 27.1 The genomic landscape of chromosome 17 shows the location of the HOXB13 gene 17q21.32. *Based on Brechka et al, 2017 Brechka, H., Bhanvadia, R. R., VanOpstall, C., Vander Griend, D. J. (2017). HOXB13 mutations and binding partners in prostate development and cancer: Function, clinical significance, and future directions.* Genes & Diseases, 4*(2), 75–87. https://doi.org/10.1016/j.gendis.2017.01.003.*

2006). Cytogenic banding studies of both Yp and Yq allowed for the identification of the three sites of the Y-chromosome known as pseudoautosomal (PAR1 and PAR2), euchromatic, and heterochromatic regions. The Y-chromosome contains the maleness development SRY gene, which triggers male development and is passed only from father to son; it carries an estimated 100–200 genes, with between 45 and 73 of this protein-coding. Male meiosis recombination takes place only in the pseudoautosomal regions at the tips of both arms of Y and X chromosomes (PAR1, with 2.6 Mb, and PAR 2, with 0.32 Mb). Along ~95% of its length, the Y-chromosome is male-specific and effectively haploid, since it is exempt from meiotic recombination. Therefore this Y-chromosome segment where X–Y crossing over is absent has been designated as the nonrecombining region of the Y-chromosome or NRY. Because of the high nonhomologous recombination occurring within this Y-chromosome, a specific region, a more appropriate name of a male-specific region or MSY is nowadays used to designate it.

27.4.1 Characteristics of the short tandem repeat microsatellites of Y-chromosome and its application in human ancestry and genealogical linages

In humans, the Y-chromosome spans 58 million BPs and represents approximately 0.38% of the total DNA in a human cell. The human Y-chromosome contains 86 genes (Pontes et al., 2004), and many of the genes on the Y-chromosome are involved in male sex determination and development (Brinkmann et al., 1998). The bulk of the Y-chromosome, which does not recombine is known as the nonrecombining region of the Y-chromosome or

NRY. This part of the human Y-chromosome is paternally inherited and haploid, and the interest in Y-chromosome polymorphisms has continuously increased (Pontes et al., 2004). The STRs are categorized in terms of the length of the repeated units described before (Butler, 2007); these are dinucleotide (CA), trinucleotide (TAT), tetranucleotide (TTTA), pentanucleotide (TAAAA), hexanucleotide (AGAGAT). The sex-determining function of the Y-chromosome means that it is paternally inherited and haploid (Jobling et al., 1997), and thus the STR loci have a uniform and dense distribution throughout the genome and exhibit a high level of relatively stable polymorphism (Agrawal & Khan, 2005).

27.4.2 Application of the Y-short tandem repeats in human ancestry and different genealogical lineages

The majority of Y-STRs are located within its nonrecombining region and are passed without recombination (Schoske et al., 2003). STR polymorphisms are abundant in the human genome and can be easily genotyped and scored (Zhivotovsky et al., 2004). The microsatellite (STRs) consist of variable numbers of tandem repeat units ranging from 1 to 6 bp in length and mutate via a particular mutation mechanism, which favors very small (usually one repeat unit) changes in array length (Schlecht et al., 2008), which can be readily amplified with PCR. The STR markers are dispersed throughout the genome and occur on average every 10,000 nucleotides (Schoske et al., 2003).

Applications of Y-STRs are becoming increasingly important because of their male specificity and the informativeness of the haplotypes they define (Fig. 27.1). Enough markers are available to provide useful discriminating power in individual identification work, and the geographical differentiation of Y-haplotypes (Parkin et al., 2006). Y-chromosomes are passed down from father to son unaltered except by the gradual accumulation of mutations. In principle, it is possible to reconstruct the histories of paternal lineages by comparing modern Y-chromosomes (Jobling et al., 1997). The STRs of the Y-chromosome have proved to be a very powerful tool in tracing the movements of males in human population history (Mukherjee et al., 2001). Application of the Y-STR polymorphism has become widespread in the forensic application, individual identification (Agrawal & Khan, 2005), evolutionary studies, and more recently in human association between the five most prevalent cancers including PCa and the genealogical lineages of ancestry. The analysis of the human Y-chromosome is also useful in solving evolutionary and anthropological problems, owing to its haploid nature and paternal inheritance. Therefore Y-STRs have key roles in the fields of forensic genetics, anthropological genetics, and genealogy because of their ability to discriminate between male lineages and provide information about the relationships between them (Lim et al., 2007). The Y-STR markers are available to provide useful discriminating power in the geographical differentiation of Y-haplotypes, which means that the information about the population of origin of the donor of a given Y-chromosome can often be deduced (Parkin et al., 2008). The Y-STR polymorphisms have become a powerful tool for human identification chromosome mapping and linkage analysis (Brinkmann et al., 1998). The Y-STR loci are also extremely useful in population genetics for the purpose of comparing closely related populations and constructing phylogenetic trees.

27.4.3 Global studies on short tandem repeat of different genealogical lineages of ancestry

Eleven Y-chromosome STR loci have been typed in the three main United Kingdom population groups (Caucasians, Afro-Caribbean, and South Asians), and clear differences for most loci were observed between the population group sampled; only a small proportion of haplotypes occur more than once (Ballared et al., 2005). In a small number of instances, haplotypes were shared between individuals in different population groups of 678 different haplotypes observed, and two were shared between South Asians and Caucasians, one between South Asians and Afro-Caribbean, and seven between Caucasians and Afro-Caribbean (Ballared et al., 2005).

A study of the 17 Y filer loci across 389 father–son sample pairs with approximately 100 each from US Caucasians, African Americans, Hispanics, and Asians found 24 differences between father and son. Thirteen resulted in the gain of a repeat in the son, while 11 resulted in the loss of a repeat (Butler et al., 2007). All were single repeat mutations except a two repeat loss at the GATA-H4 locus (allele 11 → 9). In addition, the researchers observed two sample pairs that exhibited two mutations across the 17 Y-STRs examined. An African American father–son pair had mutations at DYS458 (allele 18 → 19) and DYS635 (allele 23 → 22), and an Asian father–son pair had mutations at DYS439 (allele 13 → 12) and GATA-H4 (allele 12 → 11) (Butler et al., 2007). European populations with the exception of the loci DYS19 and DYS389II; The most frequent DYS19 allele was 16, while at the DYS389II the most frequent were alleles 30 and 31. The most frequent Y-chromosome haplotype (16–13–13–31–24–11–11–13) was found in 33 individuals (7.22%). One hundred and seventy-four haplotypes (38.07%) were observed in single copies.

In Northern Poland, 28 different haplotypes were observed, 12 of which were seen only once, and the haplotype diversity was found to be 0.805. The distribution of haplotypes of the studied loci is specific to the population of Northern Poland and distinguishes it from compared West-European populations.

In the northern region of Portugal, 101 unique haplotypes were found, and the haplotypic diversity was 0.998 ± 0.001, whereas the phylogenetic analysis showed that Portugal population can be included in the European Y-chromosome lineages distinct from the Asian ones (Pontes et al., 2004).

In the Arabian population in Africa, 51 samples for males were analyzed for 17 Y STR loci (Said, 2008). Fifty-one different haplotypes were observed, which were distributed as 16 haplotypes among Libyan, 11 haplotypes among Moroccans, 5 haplotypes among Egyptians, 4 hyplotypes among Algerian, 4 hyplotypes among Sudani, 4 haplotypes among Mauritanian, 4 hyplotypes among Tunisian, and 3 hyplotypes among Somali. There were significant differences at $p \leq 0.05$ level between the mean STR of different countries. This indicates that the mutation rate among the Arabian countries' population in Africa is less as it is clear from the narrow range of the SD value for each marker. Within the same Arabian population, but in Asia, 103 unrelated male samples were analyzed for 17 Y STR loci. From 10 countries (Saudi Arabia, Qatar, Oman, U.A.E, Bahrain, Yemen, Iraq, Kuwait, Syria, and Lebanon), 103 different hyplotypes were observed, which were distributed among Saudi Arabia (23), Yemen (14), Kuwait (14), Bahrain (13), Iraq (12), Oman (8), UAE (8), Syria (5), Qatar (4), and Lebanon (2). Higher homogeneity was observed in Oman (97%), Qatar (65%), Kuwait (58%), Saudi Arabia (52%), Bahrain (50%), and lower homogeneity was noted in UAE (49%), Lebanon (44%), Iraq (43%), Yemen (39%), Syria (33%). The (Minimal Haplotypes) MinHt is composed of seven STRs, which were observed in the Arabian Gulf countries, namely, Syria and Lebanon (Rajab, 2008).

In a study conducted in the Central Anatolia Region, Turkey, 11Y-STRs loci (DYS19, DYS385a-b, DYS389I, DYS389II, DYS390, DYS391, DYS392, DYS393, DYS438, and DYS439) were determined in a sample of 113 unrelated males from Anatolia (Fakir et al., 2004), and 106 different hyplotypes were found. The results demonstrated that these loci (DYS19, DYS393) will be useful for human identification in paternity and forensic tests in the Anatolia region (Fakir et al., 2004). In another study in Bangladesh (Dobashi et al., 2004), 11 Y-chromosome STR loci (DYS19, DYS385a-b, DYS389I, DYS389II, DYS390, DYS391, DYS392, DYS393, DYS438, and DYS439) were determined from 72 unrelated males. In this study, 71 haplotypes were demonstrated, out of which 70 were unique and one was found in two individuals. Also, 10 loci with Japanese, Chinese, and 8 loci compared with Koreans and Filipinos. The majority of the frequency distributions in Bangladesh were significantly different from those of four Asian populations (Dobashi et al., 2004). Another study examined the diversity of nine Y-chromosome STR in nine aboriginal tribes of Taiwanese (Hsieh et al., 2003). The STR loci were DYS19, DYS389I, DYS389II, DYS390, DYS391, DYS392, DYS393, DYS385, and DYS388. The populations studied included Ami, Atayal, Bunun, Paiwan, Puyuma, Rukai, Saisiat, Tsou, and Tao tribes. A total of 113 haplotypes for all nine Y-chromosome STR loci were found in 173 unrelated healthy males. The diversity of the nine Y-STR loci was more variable in the Chinese Han population than in the nine aboriginal tribes (Hsieh et al., 2003).

In Costa Rica, 100 unrelated male individuals were analyzed (Villalta et al., 2008) for 12 Y-chromosome STRs. In this study, a total of 86 different hyplotypes were identified, of which 76 were unique, and the most frequent hyplotype was found in four individuals, high hyplotype diversity was found (99.6%), being DYS385, representing two loci, the most diverse marker, and DYS393 presented the lowest gene diversity value (Villalta et al., 2008).

The hyplotypes of seven Y-chromosome STR loci (DYS19, DYS389I, DYS389II, DYS390, DYS391, DYS392, and DYS393) were determined in a study of 634 healthy Brazilian males, including 412 adult individuals and 222 father–son pairs (Soares et al., 2008). The 412 adults were unrelated, and among them, a total of 264 different seven-loci hyplotypes were identified, 210 of which were unique.

27.5 Global allelic heterogeneity of the HOXB 13 variants of prostate cancer among different genealogical lineages of populations

One of the largest and conclusive studies carried out on the heterogeneity of the PCa single-nucleotide polymorphism (SNP) variants is that reported by Shang at al. (2013), who demonstrated clearly and conclusively the presence of unique HOXB13 G84E mutation in men of European lineage across different geographic regions who had PCa during their attempt to test and extend the previous study reported by Bailey et al. (2002), who identified the rare and recurrent mutation (G84E) in homeobox B13 (HOXB13) (rs138213197) as prevailing among the European genealogical lineages of ancestry. Shang et al. (2013) conducted a large scanning of over 200 genes in the 17q21–22 region by sequencing germline DNA from 94 unrelated patients with familial PCa. Ewing et al. (2012) identified a rare but recurrent mutation (G84E) in homeobox B13 (HOXB13) (rs138213197), a homeobox transcription factor gene that is important in prostate development. In an attempt to confirm and expand the findings by Ewing et al., we completed a metaanalysis of HOXB13 G84E mutation in men of European lineage across different geographic regions who had PCa.

In another unique and recent study, we have shown conclusively the presence of G84E allelic heterogeneity of the European PCa SNP mutation of HOX13B-G84E associated with the European R-haplogroup of Y-chromosome and the absence of gene flow into Moroccan patients (Mahasneh et al., 2021). Also, we have identified for the first time five mutations, and their frequencies are shown in Table 27.1.

rs1197613952 (12%), rs1597934612 (4%), rs1597933874 (4%), rs1597933837 (4%) and rs867793282 (4%).

The European HOXB13-G84E (rs138213197) PCa mutation was not detected among Moroccan patients. The Y-chromosome genealogical haplotypes of the Western European (R1b1b2-M2G9) and the Eastern European

TABLE 27.1 Profiling of the most common HOXB13 nonsense mutations detected in Moroccan prostate cancer patients showing the SNP allelic heterogeneity in comparison with the European HOXB13 G84E (rs138213197) mutation.

Mutation location	CDS change	dbSNP number	Amino acid/ protein change	Frequency (%) n = 50
Chr17:48728333	c.261C>A		p. Tyr87Ter	(12)
Chr17:48728330	c.264C>A		p. Tyr88Ter	(4)
Chr17:48728053	c.541C>T		p. Gln181Ter	(4)
Chr17:48728042	c.552C>A		p. Cys184Ter	(4)
Chr17:48728010	c.585G>A		p. Trp195Ter	(4)

Source: Mahasneh, I A, Ennaji, M. M., Abumsimir, B., Kasmi, Y. (2021). Presence of G84E allelic heterogeneity of the European prostate cancer SNP mutation of HOX13B-G84E associated with the European R-Haplogroup of Y-chromosome and absence of gene flow into moroccans patients. Journal of Biosciences and Medicines, 09(05), 50–61. https://doi.org/10.4236/jbm.2021.95006.

(R191a-M-17) were not observed in Moroccan PCa patients. The patients had their own haplotypes E1b1 and J with a frequency of 55% and 35%, respectively. In this reciprocal comparative study that we have made; there are an absence of any gene flow of the European HOXB13 G84E into Moroccan genetic pool, and that is due to the absence of the gene flow of European-lineage haplogroups (R1a1a-M17 and R1b1b2-M269) into the Moroccan gene pool (Table 27.2) (Figs. 27.2, 27.5 and 27.6).

27.6 Practices on the genetic diagnosis of the haplotypes of microsatellite short tandem repeats and the haplogroups of genealogical lineages of the Y-chromosome

The microsatellite analysis of STRs of Y-chromosome can be conducted for any genealogical haplogroups and haplotypes of Y-chromosome using the STR DNA analysis.

27.6.1 Human genomic DNA extraction and purification

Human genomic DNA can be isolated from either blood or saliva samples following the manufacture protocol of Wizard Genomic DNA Purification Kit (Cat No. A1125, Promega). As described in the manufacturer's protocol, DNA was amplified using the AmpFlster Y filer PCR amplification Kit using the Gene Amp-PCR System 9700 Thermo Cycler (Applied Biosystem). Subsequently, PCR products were analyzed by capillary electrophoresis on an ABI 310 Genetic Analyzer using 310 Data Collection Software Version 3.1.

TABLE 27.2 Frequency (%) of the European prostate cancer mutations HOXB13 G84E and the European-lineages haplogroups (R1b1b2-M269 and R1a1a-M17) of the among prostate cancer Moroccan males as in comparison with other reported studies.

No	Population	HOXB13G84E (%)	R1a1a-M17(%)	R1b1b2-M269 (%)	(%)	(%)	References
1	Morocco	0.0	0.0	0.0	55	35	The present study
2	Morocco	NA*	4.4	0.0	54.0	19.6	Bekada et al. (2013)
3	British	1.5	9.38	88.6	3.0	4.0	Helgason (2000); Kote-Jarai et al. (2015); Wilson (2001); Chen et al. (2013)
4	Belgium	3.85	4.0	63.04	2.0	5.0	Rosser (2000); Chen et al. (2013)
5	Dutch	2.51	3.7	70.4	2.9	5.1	Semino (2000)
6	French		0.0	52.2	8.7	4.3	Semino (2000)
7	German	0.49	16	50	6.2	4.0	Semino (2000); Chen et al. (2013)
8	Italian			62.0	13.0	24.6	Rootsi (2004)
9	Portuguese		2.0	62.0	11.0	-	Rosser (2000)
10			2.0	65.0	9.0	2.1	Zalloua et al. (2008)
11		3.4	18	22.9	1.0	1.0	Chen et al. (2013)

**The HOXB13G84E was not found among Moroccan PCa pateints.*

Source: Mahasneh, I A, Ennaji, M. M., Abumsimir, B., Kasmi, Y. (2021). Presence of G84E allelic heterogeneity of the European prostate cancer SNP mutation of HOX13B-G84E associated with the European R-Haplogroup of Y-chromosome and absence of gene flow into moroccans patients. *Journal of Biosciences and Medicines, 09*(05), 50–61. https://doi.org/10.4236/jbm.2021.95006.

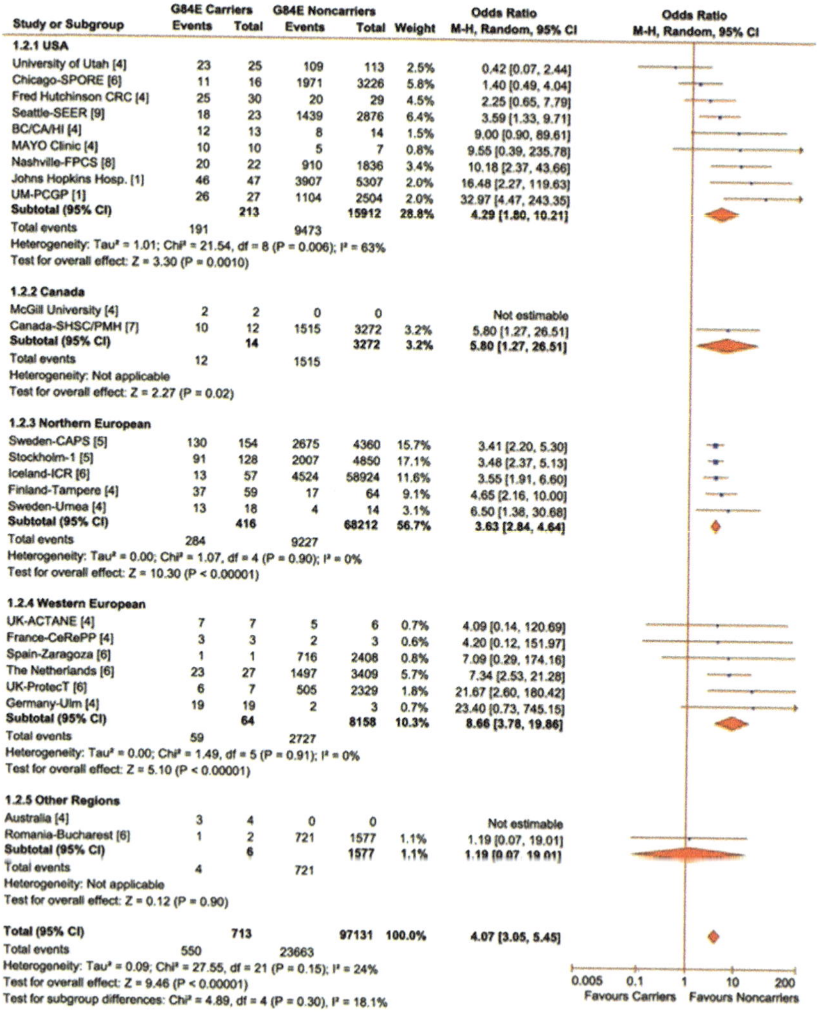

FIGURE 27.2 Forest plots for overall analysis (and region-based subgroup analysis) of prostate cancer risk in homeobox B13 gene (HOXB13) G84E carriers under the random effects model. *CI*, Confidence interval; *M-H*, Mantel–Haenszel method. *With acknowledgments: Shang, Z., Zhu, S., Zhang, H., Li, L., Niu, Y. (2013). Germline homeobox B13 (HOXB13) G84E mutation and prostate cancer risk in European descendants: A meta-analysis of 24 213 cases and 73 631 controls.* European Urology, 64*(1), 173–176. https://doi.org/10.1016/j.eururo.2013.03.007.*

Data were then analyzed using the Gene Mapper ID Software version 4. Alleles can be then determined according to the recommendations of the DNA Commission of the International Society for Forensic Genetics. Finally, the haplogroups of each haplotype were deduced using the Athey's Haplogroups Predictor version 3.16. The final data then can be used in the Analysis of

Molecular Variance (AMOVA) software as provided in the public database of the Y-Haplotype Reference Database (YHRD) (http://www.yhrd.org).

27.6.2 Protocol optimization details for short tandem repeats analysis are as follows

The DNA can be extracted either from either blood (EDTA anticoagulant vacutainers) or saliva samples, according to the protocol as described by the manufacture using the wizard genomic DNA kit part ® 050(PROMEGA, USA) in which the following practical steps were specified:

1. Take 300 μl of blood a sterile 1.5 ml centrifuge tube and add 900 μl of cell lyses solution.
2. Gently rock the tube of the mixture of the cell lyses solution by inversion the tube 5–6 times mix.
3. The mixture then incubated for 10 minutes at the room temperature (inverting 2–3 times; once during the incubation) to lyses the red blood cells. After that centrifuge at 13000 × g is done for 1 minute at the room temperature.
4. Discard the supernatant as much as possible without disturbing the visible white pellet.
5. Vortex vigorously until the white blood cells were suspended (10–15 seconds).
6. Add 300 μl Nuclei lyses solution to the tube containing suspended calls. The solution is pipetted 5–6 times to lyses the white blood cell.
7. Add 100 μl protein precipitation solution to the nuclear lyses and vortexe vigorously for 10–20 seconds.
8. Centrifugation to be followed at 13000 × g for 3 minutes at the room temperature.
9. Transfer the supernatant to 1.5 ml Centrifuge tube containing 300 μl Isopropanol.
10. Gently, the solution must be mixed by inversion until the white thread-like strand of DNA form visible mass.
11. Centrifugation at 13000 × g must be followed for 1 minute at the room temperature.
12. The supernatant must be decanted and 500 μl of 70% ethanol was added to the DNA. Then the tube must be gently inverted several times to wash the DNA pellet and the sides of the microcentrifuge tube. After that mixture must be centrifuged as in step 11.
13. Carefully, aspirate the ethanol using either a drawn Pasteur pipette or sequencing pipette tip inverting the tube on clean absorbent paper and air-dry the pellet for 10–15 minutes.
14. Add 100 μl Rehydration solution to the tube and incubation at 65°C for 1 hour.15. Finally, store the DNA at 2–8°C.

27.6.3 Quality control and DNA purity

The purity of DNA of the samples was detected using the Smart Spec Plus Spectrophotometer (BioRad, USA), on the abs 260/280 nm or any other spectrophotometer available with such range of wavelength.

27.6.4 Protocol optimization for DNA amplification polymerase chain reaction

Amplification of DNA was optimized for each sample, and the silver 96-well amp polymerase chain reaction (PCR) system with 9700 thermal cycles was used with the AmpFlSTR Y FILER amplification kit, composing 17 loci. The AmpFlSTR Y filer PCR Amplification Kit is an STR multiplex assay that amplifies 17 Y-STR loci in a single PCR reaction.

27.6.5 Genotyping of the short tandem repeat alleles on genetic analyzer and data analysis

Genetic profile for each amplification loci was diagnosed as shown in Figs. (27.3–27.5) using different machines of the Genetic Analyzer models such as ABI310 or ABI3500 (Applied Biosystems, USA) or any other equivalent to version, containing special software compatibilities such as data collection software V 3.0, Genemapper ID 3.2, Genescan 3.7.1 and Genotyper 3.7.

The AMOVA method was applied to measure the genetic distance (øst) between population samples and reference samples from YHRD. The analysis of variance (ANOVA) test was conducted, and Fst between each population was calculated. By using the YHRD site built in analyzing tool, (Fig. 27.3) the apportionment of within/among population variance between pairs of populations was calculated (http://www.yhrd.org).

Allele frequencies were calculated for each locus by simple gene counting, and then haplotype frequencies were computed for haplotype frequency calculation. Haplotype diversity was also calculated by any in-house-built program or by an online diversity calculator Fig. 27.4.

27.6.5.1 World Health Organization online data on the global prevalence of prostate cancer

The prevalence of PCa in different genealogical lineages of different geographic areas was used for comparison purposes for population (http://www.who.int). WHO online-software data was used to conduct statistical analysis (http://www.who.int). The sets of the analysis were selected as clusters of several genetically interrelated populations and compared worldwide Fig. 27.5.

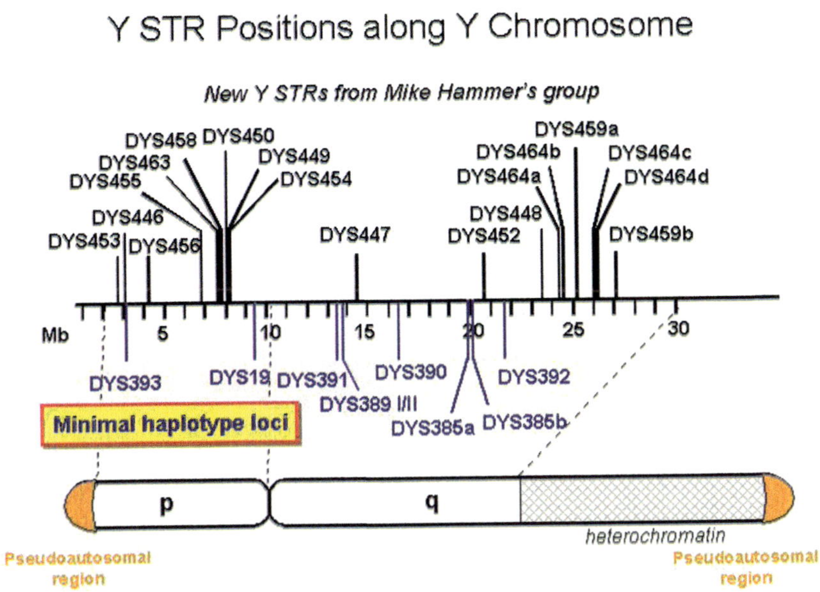

FIGURE 27.3 The landscape of the Y-short tandem repeat along Y-chromosome. *With acknowledgment: Butler (2007).*

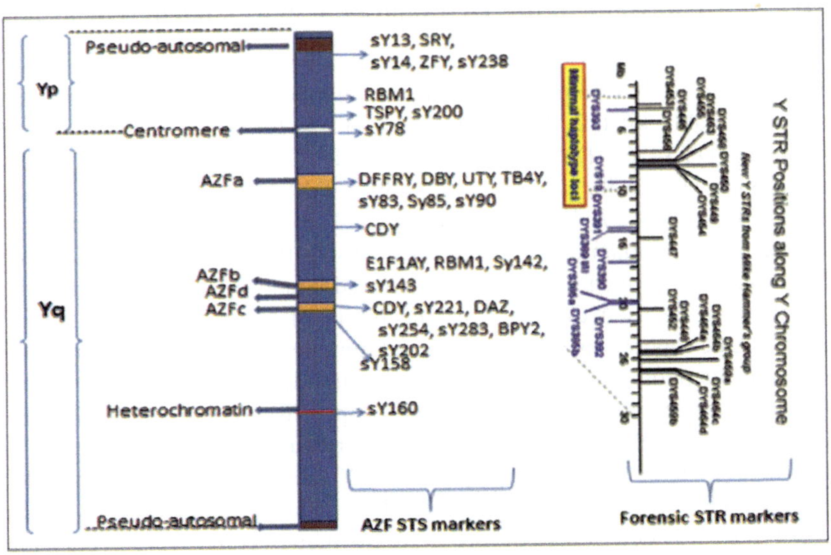

FIGURE 27.4 The diagnostic STS and short tandem repeat markers for the Y-chromosome.

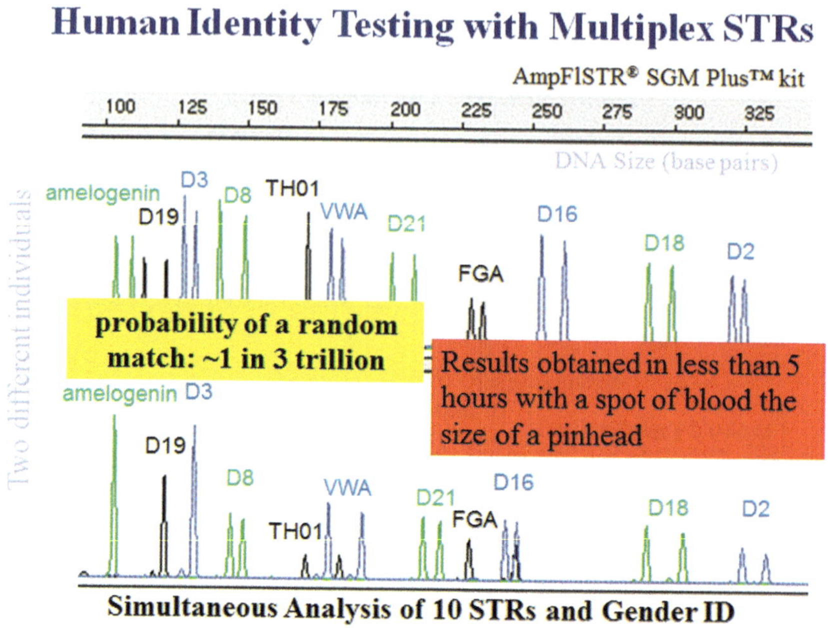

FIGURE 27.5 Human identity testing with multiplex short tandem repeats: simultaneous analysis of 10 short tandem repeats and gender ID using the Amp-FlSTR SGM Plus kit.

27.7 Practices on the genetic diagnosis of prostate cancer

27.7.1 Genotyping of the Y-chromosome short tandem repeats and haplogroup lineage prediction

The extracted DNA helped determine any number of STRs in the commercially available kit (12, 17, 36, 67, and 111 STRs) of the respective loci such as DYS456, DYS389i, DYS390, DYS389ii, DYS458, DYS19, DYS385a, DYS385b, DYS393, DYS391, DYS439, DYS635, DYS392, TAGA H4, DYS437, DYS438, and DYS448. DNA can then be purified according to the manufacturer's protocols using the Wizard Genomic DNA Isolation-Kit (Promega, USA). The BioRad Smart-Spec-Plus spectrophotometer can be used to determine the purity of DNA for quality control check. Electrophoreses was carried out on the HORIZON 58 apparatus required for photographing the Ethidium bromide-stained gel. Gene amplification was conducted on the Gene-Amp-PCR System 9700 Thermo-Cycler (Applied BioSystem) (using any other equivalent PCR commercially available systems) and the Amp FlSTR Y filer PCR Amplification Kit (AmpFlSTRR Y filer) containing the allelic ladder. Next, the STRs allelic genotyping was determined according to the manufacturer's protocols using any of the available machines of Genetic Analyzer such as the ABI

Prism310, ABI Prism3101, or ABI Prism3500 Genetic Analyzer (Applied BioSystems) as equipped with the Gene Scan-500 Internal Lane Size Standard (LIZ-500), Data Collection Software Version 3.1, and Gene Mapper ID Software Version 4. The allelic data were created using the Genetic Analyzer, collected by the Data Collection Software Version 3.1, and analyzed by Gene Mapper-ID software Version 4 (Gene Scan analysis software and Genotyper software). Alleles were determined according to the recommendations of the DNA Commission of the International Society for Forensic Genetics. The Y-chromosome haplogroups of the genealogical lineages were determined using the Athey's Haplogroups Predictor Version 3.16 (Abumsimir et al., 2020; Brechka et al., 2017; Pinhasi, 2012; Mahasneh and Zurigat, 2019; Bailey et al., 2002; Parkin et al., 2006; Ballard et al., 2005; Shang et al., 2013; Helgason, 2000; Kote-Jarai et al., 2015; Wilson, 2001; Chen et al., 2013; Rosser, 2000; Semino, 2000; Butler, 2007).

Prostate biopsies were derived from patients who were treated with PCa for DNA extraction and processing for genotyping using standard techniques by following the protocols specified in the manufacturing kit. DNA samples were obtained from PCa tissues, where $\leq$ 25 mg of minced tissue was placed into a sterile microcentrifuge tube, and DNA was separated from tissue samples using pure link Invitrogen Genomic DNA Mini-Kit, Thermo Fisher USA, according to the manufacturer's protocol. DNA was quantified using the NanoDrop spectrophotometer. Samples with a DNA concentration of 20–50 ng/μL or above were selected to perform the PCR. The Specific HOXB13 gene accession, (NM_006361.5) exon 1 and exon 2 were targeted by PCR using specific primers described elsewhere (Akbari et al., 2012). PCR reaction composed of 15 μL total volume and containing genomic DNA (8 ng), 2 × Taq PCR master mix kit Qiagen USA, 10 μmol forward and reverse primers. PCR products were then purified before genotyping of the HOXB13 G84E (rs138213197) SNP using forward and reverse primers as customized by the manufacturer on then ABPrism Genetic Analyzer 3130, and the BigDye X Terminato Purification Kit (Applied Biosystems, Foster City, CA). The resulting mutations were compared with Refseq reference (NM_006361.5), and all the observed novel mutations were submitted to ClinVar-NCBI Database and registered as clinical relevance variants with the given respective condition accession numbers Fig. 27.6.

27.7.2 Data deposition and availability in the international gene/banks

We recommend that all authors register STRs of different SNP mutations of PCa in the YHRD (http://www.yhrd.org) and the NCBI (http://www.ncbi.nlm.nih.gov).

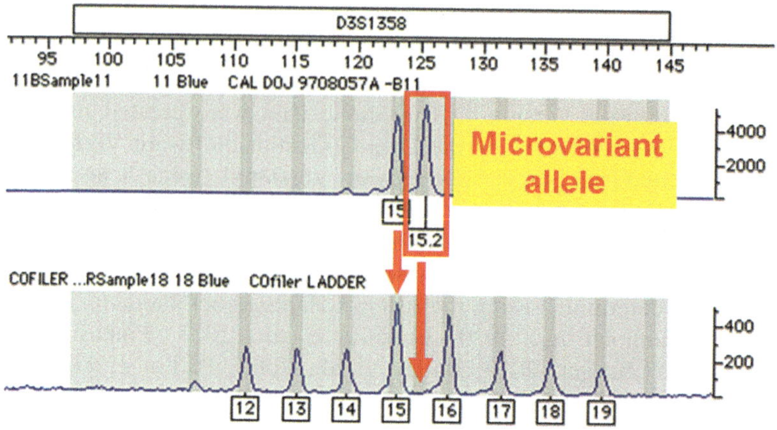

- **STR genotyping is performed by comparison of sample data to allelic ladders**

FIGURE 27.6 Short tandem repeat genotyping is performed by comparison of sample data to allelic ladders.

27.8 Gene therapy applications and future challenges against prostate cancer in different ethnicities of Y-chromosome

Currently, there has been a worldwide growing interest in gene therapy as the most sustainable therapeutic approach for cancers as well as genetic diseases (Mahasneh, 2018; Mahasneh et al., 2021). The research outcomes, using the latest technology such as next-generation sequencing and biochip microarray have shown conclusively that the epidemiology of cancers is correlated to the genealogy and ethnicity of the population's clusters around the world. Therefore the genealogical profiling of cancers will be a vital and valuable tool to enhance the diagnosis, therapy, and thus the overall management of the familial cancer disease in the region. An example of the PCa ancestry allelic heterogeneity has been shown between the European and Moroccan populations (Mahasneh et al., 2021) as they have reported the presence of G84E allelic heterogeneity of the European PCa SNP mutation of HOX13B-G84E associated with the European R-Haplogroup of Y-Chromosome and absence of gene flow into Moroccan patients.

A second example is that the prevailing rate of congenital genetic diseases and disorders are being directed by the genealogical landscape all over the Arabs countries. In fact, the vast majority of their internal marriages occur within the first-cousin relationship, which remarkably increases the prevalence of autosomal recessive disorders in particular.

Recent sequencing studies have shown that the nucleotide repeat expansions (NRTEs) disorders (such as CAG, CCG, CGG, CAACAG) comprise a heterogeneous group of diseases that result from the expansion of specific repetitive DNA microsatellite sequences, as the pathogenic expansions can occur in coding or noncoding regions of genes, known as "junk-DNA," where the main cause for such diseases includes: transcriptional regulation, mRNA splicing, and metabolism, RNA binding protein distribution, signal transduction, and cellular homeostatic pathways (Maia et al., 2015).

The genetic complexity of PCa is not far from the genetic complexity, and pathogenesis of the repeated expansion mutations have unexpectedly caused at least 22 inherited neurological diseases including some of the most common inherited diseases, such as Huntington's disease (HD) and myotonic dystrophy, neuraxis, the X-linked disorders fragile X syndrome of mental retardation (FMR1), X-linked spinal, and bulbar muscular atrophy SBMA, as caused by expansion of the (CAG/polyglutamine tracts) (Pinhas 2012, Shang et al., 2013). Furthermore, microsatellites' instability has been reported to cause colorectal cancer, and that STRs represent the hypermutable region in the human genome that are linked to human diseases such as chronic prostatitis/chronic pelvic pain syndrome (Maia et al., 2015).

References

Abumsimir, B., Mrabti, M., Laraqui, A., Ameur, A., Koraishi, S. I., Mzibrie, M., Benchekroun, M. N., Bessi, H., Tiabi, I., Almahasneh, I., & Ennaji, M. M. (2020). Most frequent mutational events of home box 13 gene in prostatic adenocarcinoma and correlation with tumor characteristics. *Meta Gene*, 23. Available from https://doi.org/10.1016/j.mgene.2019.100637.

Agrawal, S., & Khan, F. (2005). Reconstructing recent human phylogenies with forensic STR loci: A statistical approach. *BMC Genetics*, 6. Available from https://doi.org/10.1186/1471-2156-6-47.

Ali Almahasneh, I., Abumsimir, B., & Mustapha Ennaji, M. (2018). DNA sequencing and genotyping profile of the microsatellites of Y-STRs of the Beer-Alsabaa bedouins of Jordan as part of the Arabian genome project since 1995. *International Journal of Molecular Biology*. Available from https://doi.org/10.15406/ijmboa.2018.03.00067.

Bailey, J. A., Gu, Z., Clark, R. A., Reinert, K., Samonte, R. V., Schwartz, S., Adams, M. D., Myers, E. W., Li, P. W., & Eichler, E. E. (2002). Recent segmental duplications in the human genome. *Science*, *297*(5583), 1003–1007. Available from https://doi.org/10.1126/science.1072047.

Balaresque, P., Parkin, E. J., Roewer, L., Carvalho-Silva, D. R., Mitchell, R. J., van Oorschot, R. A. H., Henke, J., Stoneking, M., Nasidze, I., Wetton, J., de Knijff, P., Tyler-Smith, C., & Jobling, M. A. (2009). Genomic complexity of the Y-STR DYS19: Inversions, deletions and founder lineages carrying duplications. *International Journal of Legal Medicine*, *123*(1), 15–23. Available from https://doi.org/10.1007/s00414-008-0253-3.

Ballard, D. J., Phillips, C., Thacker, C. R., Robson, C., Revoir, A. P., & Syndercombe Court, D. (2005). Y chromosome STR haplotypes in three UK populations. *Forensic Science International*, *152*(2–3), 289–305. Available from https://doi.org/10.1016/j.forsciint.2004.10.006.

Barać, L., Peričić, M., Klarić, I. M., Janićijević, B., Parik, J., Rootsi, S., & Rudan, P. (2003). Y chromosome STRs in Croatians. *Forensic Science International*, *138*(1–3), 127–133. Available from https://doi.org/10.1016/j.forsciint.2003.09.004.

Brechka, H., Bhanvadia, R. R., VanOpstall, C., & Vander Griend, D. J. (2017). HOXB13 mutations and binding partners in prostate development and cancer: Function, clinical significance, and future directions. *Genes & Diseases*, *4*(2), 75–87. Available from https://doi.org/10.1016/j.gendis.2017.01.003.

Brinkmann, B., Klintschar, M., Neuhuber, F., Hühne, J., & Rolf, B. (1998). Mutation rate in human microsatellites: Influence of the structure and length of the tandem repeat. *American Journal of Human Genetics*, *62*(6), 1408–1415. Available from https://doi.org/10.1086/301869.

Butler, J. M., Hill, C. R., Decker, A. E., Kline, M. C., Reid, T. M., Vallone, P. M. (2007). New autosomal and Y-chromosome STR loci: Characterization and potential uses, biochemical science division, national institute of standards and technology. In: *Proceedings of the 18th International Symposium on Human Identification.*

Chen, Z., Greenwood, C., Isaacs, W. B., Foulkes, W. D., Sun, J., Zheng, S. L., Condreay, L. D., & Xu, J. (2013). The G84E mutation of HOXB13 is associated with increased risk for prostate cancer: Results from the REDUCE trial. *Carcinogenesis*, *34*(6), 1260–1264. Available from https://doi.org/10.1093/carcin/bgt055.

Dupont, W. D., Breyer, J. P., Johnson, S. H., Plummer, W. D., & Smith, J. R. (2021). Prostate cancer risk variants of the HOXB genetic locus. *Scientific Reports*, *11*(1). Available from https://doi.org/10.1038/s41598-021-89399-7.

Ewing, C. M., Ray, A. M., Lange, E. M., Zuhlke, K. A., Robbins, C. M., Tembe, W. D., Wiley, K. E., Isaacs, S. D., Johng, D., Wang, Y., Bizon, C., Yan, G., Gielzak, M., Partin, A. W., Shanmugam, V., Izatt, T., Sinari, S., Craig, D. W., Zheng, S. L., & Cooney, K. A. (2012). Germline mutations in HOXB13 and prostate-cancer risk. *New England Journal of Medicine*, *366*(2), 141–149. Available from https://doi.org/10.1056/NEJMoa1110000.

Fakir, A. H., Celebioglu, A., Yardimci, E., & Haplotypes, Y.-S. (2004). *Central Anatolia Region of Turkey*, *144*, 59–64.

Harrington, K. J., Spitzweg, C., Bateman, A. R., Morris, J. C., & Vile, R. G. (2001). Gene therapy for prostate cancer: Current status and future prospects. *Journal of Urology*, *166*(4), 1220–1233. Available from https://doi.org/10.1016/s0022-5347(05)65742-4.

Helgason, A., Sigurðardottir, S., Nicholson, J., Sykes, B., Hill, E. W., Bradley, D. G., Bosnes, V., Gulcher, J. R., Ward, R., & Stefánsson, K. (2000). Estimating Scandinavian and gaelic ancestry in the male settlers of Iceland. *American Journal of Human Genetics*, *67*(3), 697–717. Available from https://doi.org/10.1086/303046.

Hsieh, H. M., Shen, R. K., Yuen, T. Y., Tsai, L. C., Huang, N. E., Shih, R. T. P., Chang, J. C., Ko, Y. C., Linacre, A., & Lee, J. C. (2003). Screening of Y-chromosome STR Loci in Taiwanese populations. *Forensic Science Journal*, *2*, 69–76.

Jezierski, G., & Pawlowski, R. (2001). Y chromosome related anomalies detected with Y chromosome STR systems. *Z Zagadnien Nauk Sadowych*, *47*, 340–344.

Jobling, M. A., Pandya, A., & Tyler-Smith, C. (1997). The Y chromosome in forensic analysis and paternity testing. *International Journal of Legal Medicine*, *110*(3), 118–124. Available from https://doi.org/10.1007/s004140050050.

Jou, J., Harrington, K. J., Zocca, M. B., Ehrnrooth, E., & Cohen, E. E. W. (2021). The changing landscape of therapeutic cancer vaccines-novel platforms and neoantigen identification. *Clinical Cancer Research*, *27*(3), 689–703. Available from https://doi.org/10.1158/1078-0432.CCR-20-0245.

Karlsson, R., Aly, M., Clements, M., Zheng, L., Adolfsson, J., Xu, J., Grönberg, H., & Wiklund, F. (2014). A population-based assessment of germline HOXB13 G84E mutation and prostate cancer risk. *European Urology*, *65*(1), 169–176. Available from https://doi.org/10.1016/j.eururo.2012.07.027.

Kayser, M., & Sajantila, A. (2001). Mutations at Y-STR loci: Implications for paternity testing and forensic analysis. *Forensic Science International*, *118*(2–3), 116–121. Available from https://doi.org/10.1016/S0379-0738(00)00480-1.

Kote-Jarai, Z., Mikropoulos, C., Leongamornlert, D. A., Dadaev, T., Tymrakiewicz, M., Saunders, E. J., Jones, M., Jugurnauth-Little, S., Govindasami, K., Guy, M., Hamdy, F. C., Donovan, J. L., Neal, D. E., Lane, J. A., Dearnaley, D., Wilkinson, R. A., Sawyer, E. J., Morgan, A., Antoniou, A. C., & Eeles, R. A. (2015). Prevalence of the HOXB13 G84E germline mutation in British men and correlation with prostate cancer risk, tumour characteristics and clinical outcomes. *Annals of Oncology*, *26*(4), 756–761. Available from https://doi.org/10.1093/annonc/mdv004.

Laitinen, V. H., Wahlfors, T., Saaristo, L., Rantapero, T., Pelttari, L. M., Kilpivaara, O., Laasanen, S.-L., Kallioniemi, A., Nevanlinna, H., Aaltonen, L., Vessella, R. L., Auvinen, A., Visakorpi, T., Tammela, T. L. J., & Schleutker, J. (2013). HOXB13 G84E mutation in Finland: Population-based analysis of prostate, breast, and colorectal cancer risk. *Cancer Epidemiology Biomarkers & Prevention*, *22*(3), 452–460. Available from https://doi.org/10.1158/1055-9965.EPI-12-1000-T.

Lim, S. K., Xue, Y., Parkin, E. J., & Tyler-Smith, C. (2007). Variation of 52 new Y-STR loci in the Y chromosome consortium worldwide panel of 76 diverse individuals. *International Journal of Legal Medicine*, *121*(2), 124–127. Available from https://doi.org/10.1007/s00414-006-0124-8.

Mahasneh, I. (2018). Genetic profiling of the 5-top cancers among Arabian populations in relation to their genealogical landscape: Towards establishment of gene therapy platform in the region. *International Journal of Molecular Biology: Open Access*, *3*(2), 52–54.

Mahasneh, I. A., & Zuriegat, Q. H. (2019). Genetic profiling of the short tandem repeats (STRs) of Y-chromosome of populations of south Jordan. *Journal of Forensic Medicine*, *4*(1), 1–16.

Mahasneh, I. A., Ennaji, M. M., Abumsimir, B., & Kasmi, Y. (2021). Presence of G84E allelic heterogeneity of the European prostate cancer SNP mutation of HOX13B-G84E associated with the European R-Haplogroup of Y-chromosome and absence of gene flow into moroccans patients. *Journal of Biosciences and Medicines*, *09*(05), 50–61. Available from https://doi.org/10.4236/jbm.2021.95006.

Maia, S., Cardoso, M., Pinto, P., Pinheiro, M., Santos, C., Peixoto, A., Bento, M. J., Oliveira, J., Henrique, R., Jerónimo, C., Teixeira, M. R., & Prokunina-Olsson, L. (2015). Identification of two novel HOXB13 germline mutations in Portuguese prostate cancer patients. *PLoS One*, *10*(7), e0132728. Available from https://doi.org/10.1371/journal.pone.0132728.

Mukherjee, N., Nebel, A., Oppenheim, A., & Majumder, P. P. (2001). High-resolution analysis of Y-chromosomal polymorphisms reveals signatures of population movements from Central Asia and West Asia into India. *Journal of Genetics*, *80*(3), 125–135. Available from https://doi.org/10.1007/BF02717908.

N.d. https://doi.org/10.1086/303046. PMC 1287529. PMID 10931763.

Nyberg, T., Govindasami, K., Leslie, G., Dadaev, T., Bancroft, E., Ni Raghallaigh, H., Brook, M. N., Hussain, N., Keating, D., Lee, A., McMahon, R., Morgan, A., Mullen, A., Osborne, A., Rageevakumar, R., Kote-Jarai, Z., Eeles, R., & Antoniou, A. C. (2019). Homeobox B13 G84E mutation and prostate cancer risk. *European Urology*, *75*(5), 834–845. Available from https://doi.org/10.1016/j.eururo.2018.11.015.

Parkin, E. J., Kraayenbrink, T., Opgenort, J. R. M. L., van Driem, G. L., Tuladhar, N. M., de Knijff, P., & Jobling, M. A. (2007). Diversity of 26-locus Y-STR haplotypes in a Nepalese population sample: Isolation and drift in the Himalayas. *Forensic Science International*, *166*(2–3), 176–181. Available from https://doi.org/10.1016/j.forsciint.2006.05.007.

Pinhasi, R., Thomas, M. G., Hofreiter, M., Currat, M., & Burger, J. (2012). The genetic history of Europeans. *Trends in Genetics*, *28*(10), 496–505. Available from https://doi.org/10.1016/j.tig.2012.06.006.

Pontes, M. L., Peña, J. A., Alfonso Sanchez, M. A., Abrantes, D., Lima, G., Pereira, M. J., Fernández-Fernández, I., Castro, A., Pinheiro, M. F., & Martínez de Páncorbo, M. (2004). Y chromosome STRs in the north of Portugal. *International Congress Series, 1261*(C), 350–352. Available from https://doi.org/10.1016/s0531-5131(03)01839-9.

Rajab, B. A. M. (2008). STRs analysis of Y-chromosome among the Arabian Gulf countries. *Syria and Lebanon*, 18–40.

Rębała, K., Kapińska, E., & Szczerkowska, Z. (2003). Analysis of polymorphism of three human Y-chromosome STR loci: DYS390, DYS392 and DYS393 in the population of northern Poland. *Journal of Applied Genetics*, *44*(2), 219–223.

Rebbeck, T. R. (2017). Prostate cancer genetics: Variation by race, ethnicity, and geography. *Seminars in Radiation Oncology*, *27*(1), 3–10. Available from https://doi.org/10.1016/j.semradonc.2016.08.002.

Redd, A. J., Agellon, A. B., Kearney, V. A., Contreras, V. A., Karafet, T., Park, H., De Knijff, P., Butler, J. M., & Hammer, M. F. (2002). Forensic value of 14 novel STRs on the human Y chromosome. *Forensic Science International*, *130*(2–3), 97–111. Available from https://doi.org/10.1016/S0379-0738(02)00347-X.

Rootsi, S. (2004). Human Y-chromosomal variation in European populations. PhD diss.

Rosser, Z. H., Zerjal, T., Hurles, M. E., Adojaan, M., Alavantic, D., Amorim, A., Amos, W., Armenteros, M., Arroyo, E., Barbujani, G., Beckman, G., Beckman, L., Bertranpetit, J., Bosch, E., Bradley, D. G., Brede, G., Cooper, G., Côrte-Real, H. B. S. M., de Knijff, P., & Jobling, M. A. (2000). Y-chromosomal diversity in Europe is clinal and influenced primarily by geography, rather than by language. *American Journal of Human Genetics*, *67*(6), 1526–1543. Available from https://doi.org/10.1086/316890.

Said, M. A. (2008). *STRs analysis of Y-Chromosome among Arabian population in Africa* (pp. 19–26).

Schoske, R., Vallone, P. M., Ruitberg, C. M., & Butler, J. M. (2003). Multiplex PCR design strategy used for the simultaneous amplification of 10 y chromosome short tandem repeat (STR) loci. *Analytical and Bioanalytical Chemistry*, *375*(3), 333–343. Available from https://doi.org/10.1007/s00216-002-1683-2.

Semino, O., Passarino, G., Oefner, P. J., Lin, A. A., Arbuzova, S., Beckman, L. E., De Benedictis, G., Francalacci, P., Kouvatsi, A., Limborska, S., Marcikiae, M., Mika, A., Mika, B., Primorac, D., Santachiara-Benerecetti, A. S., Cavalli-Sforza, L. L., & Underhill, P. A. (2000). The genetic legacy of paleolithic Homo sapiens sapiens in extant Europeans: A Y chromosome perspective. *Science*, *290*(5494), 1155–1159. Available from https://doi.org/10.1126/science.290.5494.1155.

Shang, Z., Zhu, S., Zhang, H., Li, L., & Niu, Y. (2013). Germline homeobox B13 (HOXB13) G84E mutation and prostate cancer risk in European descendants: A meta-analysis of 24 213 cases and 73 631 controls. *European Urology*, *64*(1), 173–176. Available from https://doi.org/10.1016/j.eururo.2013.03.007.

Spanish population data and forensic usefulness of a novel Y-STR set. (n.d.). *International Journal of Legal Medicine*, *117*, 306–311.

Storebjerg, T. M., Høyer, S., Kirkegaard, P., Bro, F., Ørntoft, T. F., Borre, M., & Sørensen, K. D. (2016). Prevalence of the HOXB13 G84E mutation in Danish men undergoing radical prostatectomy and its correlations with prostate cancer risk and aggressiveness. *BJU International*, *118*(4), 646–653. Available from https://doi.org/10.1111/bju.13416.

Taitt, H. E. (2018). Global trends and prostate cancer: A review of incidence, detection, and mortality as influenced by race, ethnicity, and geographic location. *American Journal of Men's Health*, *12*(6), 1807–1823. Available from https://doi.org/10.1177/1557988318798279.

Villalta, M., Rodriguez, A., González, L., Arce, V., Arrieta, G., Morales, A., Gusmão, L., & Espinoza, M. (2008). Haplotype data for 12 Y-chromosome STR loci from Costa Rica. *Forensic Science International: Genetics Supplement Series, 1*(1), 252–254. Available from https://doi.org/10.1016/j.fsigss.2007.10.101.

Wei, J., Shi, Z., Na, R., Wang, C.-H., Resurreccion, W. K., Zheng, S. L., Hulick, P. J., Cooney, K. A., Helfand, B. T., Isaacs, W. B., & Xu, J. (2020). Germline HOXB13 G84E mutation carriers and risk to twenty common types of cancer: Results from the UK Biobank. *British Journal of Cancer, 123*(9), 1356–1359. Available from https://doi.org/10.1038/s41416-020-01036-8.

Wilson, J. F., Weiss, D. A., Richards, M., Thomas, M. G., Bradman, N., & Goldstein, D. B. (2001). Genetic evidence for different male and female roles during cultural transitions in the British Isles. *Proceedings of the National Academy of Sciences of the United States of America, 98*(9), 5078–5083. Available from https://doi.org/10.1073/pnas.071036898.

Zalloua, P. A., Platt, D. E., El Sibai, M., Khalife, J., Makhoul, N., Haber, M., Xue, Y., Izaabel, H., Bosch, E., Adams, S. M., Arroyo, E., López-Parra, A. M., Aler, M., Picornell, A., Ramon, M., Jobling, M. A., Comas, D., Bertranpetit, J., Wells, R. S., & Tyler-Smith, C. (2008). Identifying genetic traces of historical expansions: Phoenician footprints in the Mediterranean. *The American Journal of Human Genetics, 83*(5), 633–642. Available from https://doi.org/10.1016/j.ajhg.2008.10.012.

Zarrabeitia, M. T. (2003). Spanish population data and forensic usefulness of a novel Y-STR set (DYS437, DYS438, DYS439, DYS460, DYS461, GATA A10, GATA C4, GATA H4). *International Journal of Legal Medicine, 117*(5), 306–311.

Zody, M. C., Garber, M., Adams, D. J., Sharpe, T., Harrow, J., Lupski, J. R., Nicholson, C., Searle, S. M., Wilming, L., Young, S. K., Abouelleil, A., Allen, N. R., Bi, W., Bloom, T., Borowsky, M. L., Bugalter, B. E., Butler, J., Chang, J. L., Chen, C. K., & Nusbaum, C. (2006). DNA sequence of human chromosome 17 and analysis of rearrangement in the human lineage. *Nature, 440*(7087), 1045–1049. Available from https://doi.org/10.1038/nature04689.

Chapter 28

Impact of vitamin D status on breast cancer prognosis

Hasna Azmi[1], Najwa Hassou[1] and Moulay Mustapha Ennaji[2]
[1]Team of Virology, Oncology, and Biotechnologies, Laboratory of Virology, Oncology, Biosciences, Environment and New Energies (LVO-BEEN), Faculty of Sciences and Techniques Mohammedia, University Hassan II of Casablanca, Casablanca, Morocco, [2]Group Leader Research team of Virology, Oncology, and Biotechnologies, Head of Laboratory of Virology, Oncology, Biosciences, Environment and New Energies (LVO-BEEN), Faculty of Sciences and Techniques Mohammedia, University Hassan II of Casablanca, Casablanca, Morocco

28.1 Introduction

Breast cancer is the most common cancer with over 2.2 million cases reported worldwide in 2020. One in 12 women develops breast cancer in their lifetime. It is the first cause of cancer death in women. Almost 685,000 women died of breast cancer in 2020 (World Health Organization, 2021). Certain parameters are incriminated in the genesis of breast cancer, and vitamin D status is one of them. Vitamin D has been reported to have extra-bony effects.

Epidemiological studies have indicated a negative correlation between the risk of developing breast cancer and serum vitamin D (Bauer et al., 2013; Wang et al., 2013). Biological studies have reported that pharmacological levels of calcitriol inhibit cancer cell proliferation, particularly in tissue culture models (Feldman et al., 2014; Narvaez et al., 2014). Metastatic disease is the main cause of treatment failure and worse prognosis in breast cancer patients.

The determination of the correlation cause between therapeutic failures and vitamin D deficiency may contribute to enhance the care of breast cancer patients by enabling the development of novel therapeutic strategies.

In this sense, we propose to study the status impact of vitamin D on breast cancer prognosis.

28.2 Vitamin D

28.2.1 Intakes of vitamin D

Vitamin D is a lipophilic vitamin provided by the diet ensuring 10%–20% of the needs. Skin synthesis is the main source of UVB radiation in the deep

Immunological Implications and Molecular Diagnostics of Genitourinary Cancer.
DOI: https://doi.org/10.1016/B978-0-323-85496-2.00024-5

Vitamin D
Recommended Daily Intake and Food Sources

	Infants, Children, and Adolescents
Vitamin D (IU/d)	400 Infants, children, and adolescents who do not obtain 400 IU/day vitamin D through diet should take a 400 IU/day vitamin D supplement, according to recent recommendations issued by the American Academy of Pediatrics.

Some food sources:	
Cod liver oil, 1 tbsp = 1360 IU	Margarine, fortified, 1 tbsp = 60 IU
Salmon, cooked, 3.5 oz = 360 IU	Egg, 1 whole (vitamin D in yolk) = 20 IU
Tuna, canned in oil, 3 oz = 200 IU	Liver (beef), cooked, 3.5 oz = 15 IU
Milk, fortified, nonfat, reduced fat, and whole, 1 cup = 98 IU	

Wagner CL, et al. *Pediatrics*. 2008;122:1142-1152. Dietary Supplement Fact Sheet: Vitamin D. Office of Dietary Supplements, National Institutes of Health. Available at: http://ods.od.nih.gov/factsheets/vitamind.asp. Accessed on: August 14, 2009.

FIGURE 28.1 Vitamin D recommended daily intake and food sources (Wagner & Greer, 2008). *From Wagner, C.L., & Greer, F.R. (2008). American academy of pediatrics section on breastfeeding; American academy of pediatrics committee on nutrition. Prevention of rickets and vitamin D deficiency in infants, children, and adolescents.* Pediatrics, 122*(5), 1142–1152.*

layers of the epidermis (Garabédian, 2008). Vitamin D2 (ergocalciferol) is of vegetable origin (fungi), and vitamin D3 (cholecalciferol) is of animal origin (fatty fish, liver, eggs, and dairy products) (Lansiaux et al., 2018) (Fig. 28.1). The endogenous synthesis of vitamin D by sun exposure means that vitamin D status can fluctuate with seasons (Tonnel, 2016) and according to latitudes, sex (lower concentration in women), age, body mass index, dress habits, eating habits, physical activity, time spent outside the home, smoking, phototype, and pollution level (Bouvard et al., 2010). It is noted that daily sun exposure for 30 min of approximately 30% of the body between the months of June and October provides only 10,000 UI of vitamin D, which is not sufficient to cover a patient's annual needs (Balvers et al., 2015).

28.2.2 Vitamin D metabolism

Absorption of dietary vitamin D takes place in the proximal part of the small intestine in the presence of CD36, NPC1L1, and SR-B1 cholesterol carriers (Reboul et al., 2011). After absorption, plasmatic transport of dietary vitamin D depends on its incorporation into the chylomicrons that transport vitamin

D to the liver. Vitamins D2 and D3 have identical metabolism and depend on the same enzymes (Haddad et al., 1993). Vitamin D from endogenous synthesis is transported by vitamin D–binding protein (VDBP). It is a 2-globulin synthesized by the liver, which binds not only vitamin D but also its metabolites (25-hydroxyvitaminD and 1,25 dihydroxy vitamin D).

Their binding to VDBP prolongs their plasma half-life and stabilizes their plasma concentrations (Safadi et al., 1999). Once transported in the bloodstream, either by chylomicrons or by VDBP, vitamin D is taken up in the liver, where it is hydroxylated on carbon 25 to form 25-hydroxyvitamin D 25 (OH) D having a long half- life of three to four weeks. This first hydroxylation involves different enzymes from the cytochrome P450 family, namely, CYP2R1, CYP27A1, CYP3A4, and CYP2J2 (Schuster, 2011).

25 (OH) circulates in the blood after this first hydroxylation, linked to VDBP. Arrived at the renal level, the 25 (OH) D-VDBP complex undergoes endocytosis in the renal proximal tubule cells after glomerular filtration (Nykjaer et al., 1999).

Once in the cell, VDBP is degraded, and 25 (OH) D is partly re-excreted in the bloodstream. The other part undergoes hydroxylation at position 1 at the renal level, synthesizing 1,25-dihydroxyvitamin D (1,25 (OH) 2D), called calcitriol, the active form of vitamin D (Dusso et al., 2005). The half-life of 1,25 (OH) 2D is very short (approximately 4 h), and its concentration is very low compared to 25 (OH) D (Girgis et al., 2013). This form of vitamin D is active and is able to enter the target cell and bind to its specific VDR receptor. The vitamin D / VDR couple is translocated to the nucleus, where it will activate or inactivate gene expression.

1,25 (OH) D can also be generated extra-renally in the epidermis, aortic endothelium, growth cartilage, osteoblasts, brain, immune system cells, and the feto-placental unit (Rizk-Rabin et al., 1994) (Fig. 28.2).

28.2.3 Target cells

VDR is present on the surface of different cells: bone tissue, intestine, kidney, cartilage, thyroid, parathyroid, brain, pituitary, adrenal, testis, ovary, prostate, breast, pancreas, immune cells, muscles, cardiac tissue, lungs, digestive tract, and skin. This explains the different vitamin D effects, bone, and extra-bone either by a direct mechanism or by the 1,25(OH)2D produced by the kidney and acting via the general circulation on the target tissue or by the 1,25(OH) 2D produced locally and acting on the cells (Garabédian, 2008).

Long regarded as a useful hormone in the regulation of phosphocalcic metabolism and bone mineralization, it turns out more and more that vitamin D is incriminated in cancer pathology.

Our interest will focus on the relationship between vitamin D and the most common cancer in women, namely, breast cancer.

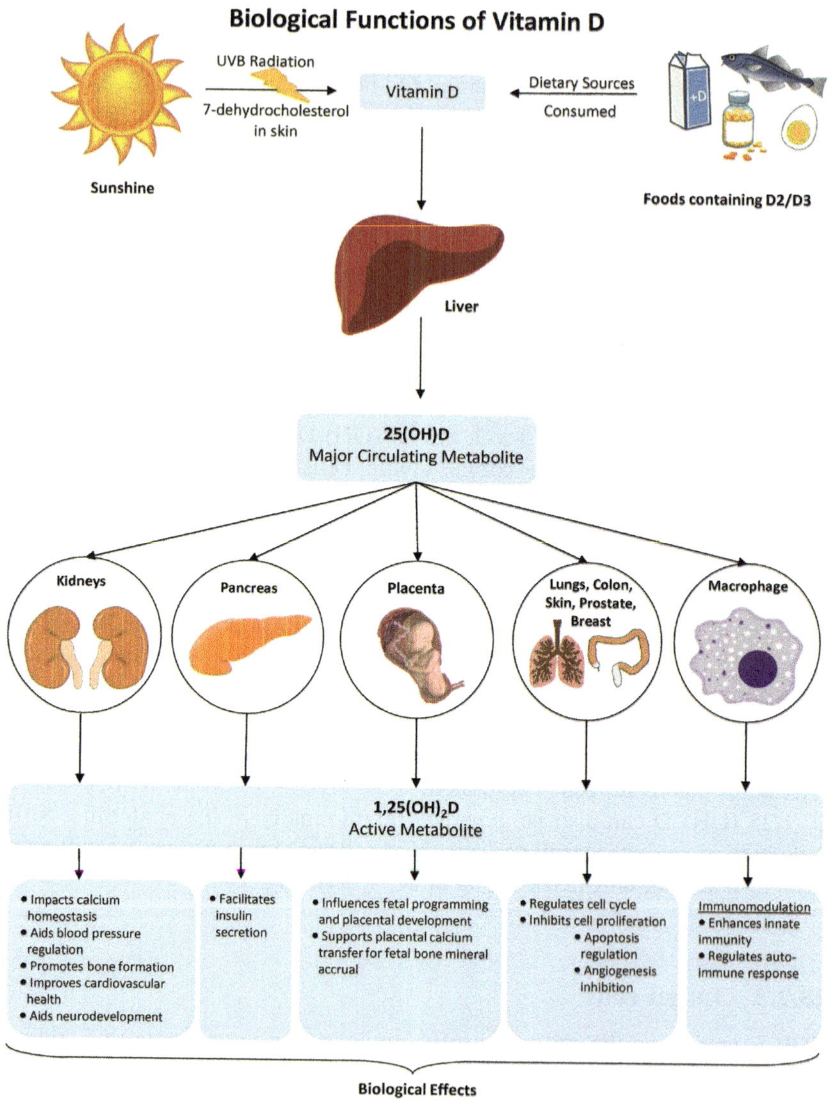

FIGURE 28.2 Sources, synthesis, and biological functions of vitamin D.

28.3 Vitamin D and breast cancer relationship

28.3.1 Vitamin D pathophysiology and link to cancer

Vitamin D acts on cell differentiation and proliferation: it inhibits the proliferation of tumor cells by blocking them in G1 phase, by activating the synthesis of p21 and p27 proteins. It modulates the production of proto-oncogenes and promotes apoptosis of certain cancer cells by blocking the production of the Bcl-2 protein (Bouillon et al., 2006). Vitamin D is also likely to promote differentiation of these tumor cells and reduce angiogenesis (Ooi et al., 2010).

More than 80% of breast tumors have VDR; previous studies have reported a protective effect of vitamin D against tumor growth (Colston et al., 1989; Pendas-Franco et al., 2007). In addition, VDR polymorphism has been linked to different survivorship in patients with breast cancer and may influence tumor progression (Lundin et al., 1999).

Knight et al. studied another mechanism that accounts for blood levels of progesterone and estradiol. They observed that a 10 nmol/L increase of 25 (OH)D3 caused progesterone to decrease proportionately by a factor of 10% and estradiol by a factor of 3.

A high rate of 25(OH)D could decrease progesterone and oestradiolemia in women between 18 and 22 years old, explaining the decrease in breast cancer risk (Knight et al., 2010).

28.3.2 Sun exposure and breast cancer relationship

Vitamin D is mainly synthesized at the skin level after sun exposure to UVB. Various studies have sought to demonstrate the link between lack of sun exposure and increased risk of breast cancer. John et al. showed that the decrease in breast cancer risk is greater in US regions with the highest solar exposures (John et al., 1999).

According to the E3N cohort study, women who live in the French regions most exposed to UV rays have a lower incidence of breast cancer. It also demonstrates that women in the south of France have a lower risk of breast cancer than women in the north (Engel et al., 2011).

In addition, a 2008 study of 107 countries identified a higher breast cancer incidence for countries with latitudes far from the equator (Mohr et al., 2008). Knight et al. reported that exposure to vitamin D during breast development would protect against breast cancer. Significant solar exposure between the ages of 10 and 19 years was linked to a reduced risk of breast cancer (Knight et al., 2007).

28.3.3 Link between vitamin D-rich diet and breast cancer

Rossi et al. and Lee et al. reported a reduced risk of breast cancer in women who consumed more vitamin D (Lee et al., 2011; Rossi et al., 2009). Mc Cullough et al. found this association only for estrogen receptor-positive breast tumors (Mc Cullough et al., 2005).

Two studies confirmed this link only in nonmenopausal patients (Abbas et al., 2007; Kawase et al., 2010).

28.3.4 Vitamin D supplementation and breast cancer relationship

The Women's Health Initiative trial that randomized postmenopausal women into a 400 IU vitamin D supplemented group and a 1000 mg calcium daily placebo group did not show a decrease in breast cancer risk after supplementation (Chlebowski et al., 2008). Randomized trial Randomised Evaluation of Calcium or Vitamin D (RECORD) found no decrease in cancer incidence (breast, colorectal, lung, prostate, and other) in patients supplemented with 800 IU/d of vitamin D compared to the placebo group (Avenell et al., 2012).

In contrast, Lappe et al. showed a reduction in the incidence of cancers (breast, colon, lung, blood, and uterus) in calcium-supplemented patients with a dose of 1000 IU/d vitamin D in comparison to the placebo group (Anderson et al., 2010).

28.3.5 Link between total vitamin D intake and breast cancer

Shin et al. reported that total vitamin D intakes greater than 500 IU/d were associated with a lower risk of breast cancer in postmenopausal women than intakes less than or equal to 150 IU/d (Shin et al., 2002). For total intakes exceeding 800 IU/d, Robien et al. showed a reduction in breast cancer risk (Robien et al., 2007).

According to Chen et al.'s metaanalysis, there is an inverse correlation between vitamin D intake and the risk of breast cancer (Chen et al., 2010). However, Gissel et al., 2008 did not find this association.

28.3.6 Link between serum 25(OH)D and breast cancer

Janowsky et al. conducted a control study and reported no significant association between the 25(OH)D concentration and the occurrence of breast cancer (Janowsky et al., 1999).

Other case-control researches reported a decrease in breast cancer risk with elevated serum levels of 25(OH)D (Abbas et al., 2008; Abbas et al., 2009; Lowe et al., 2005). Chung et al.'s metaanalysis showed that the risk of breast cancer does not decrease with the increase in blood levels of 25(OH)D (Chung et al., 2011).

28.4 Vitamin D and breast cancer prognosis

28.4.1 Vitamin D and local breast cancer recurrence

The study by Jacobs et al. did not demonstrate a relationship between the blood level of 25(OH)D and the risk of breast cancer repetition (Jacobs et al., 2011). In Kim et al.'s research, vitamin D deficiency appears as an independent prognostic indicator of breast cancer recurrence (Kim et al., 2011).

For Vrieling et al., low levels of vitamin D are closely linked to a high risk of recurrence (Vrieling et al., 2011).

28.4.2 Vitamin D and metastatic spread of breast cancer

Various studies have investigated the impact of vitamin D signaling on breast cancer metastases. Flanagan et al. found that VDR agonists not only reduced tumor growth but suppressed metastatic spread as well (Flanagan et al., 2003). In an in vitro study of mice with breast tumors, VDR suppression was linked to more extensive metastases in the liver and lungs, B-catenin-induced effect (Johnson et al., 2015). Ooi et al. demonstrated that metastatic osteolytic lesions appear earlier and are significantly higher in mice with vitamin D deficiency than in mice with normal vitamin D levels (Ooi et al., 2010). Zhang et al. studied human breast cancer tumor cells and mouse breast tumor cells with metastases and demonstrated that VDR expression was negatively correlated with metastases. Additionally, they reported that overexpression of VDR in tumor cells reduced metastatic growth by inhibiting the release of tumor necrosis factor by tumor-associated macrophages (Zhang et al., 2014).

28.4.3 Breast cancer survival and vitamin D

Goodwin et al. pointed to increased mortality in patients with vitamin D deficiency (Goodwin et al., 2009). Vrieling et al. indicated that lower concentrations of 25(OH)D are linearly linked to a higher risk of death (Vrieling et al., 2011).

A large prospective study conducted in Northern California (USA) called the Pathways cohort on 1666 women with breast cancer had a better prognosis when the serum rate of 25(OH)D was high. Women with high levels of 25(OH)D had better overall survival, and premenopausal women had better breast cancer-specific, relapse-free, and invasive disease-free survival.

Inversely proportional relationship between vitamin D and tumor stage and grade has been identified. Among premenopausal women, vitamin D levels were the lowest in women with triple-negative breast cancer, an aggressive subtype of the disease. Premenopausal women with high rates of 25(OH)D developed less triple-negative breast cancer compared to those with lower rates, thereby confirming the significance of vitamin D status in breast cancer survivors (JoEllen, 2018; Yao et al., 2017).

28.4.4 Prognosis of vitamin D and breast cancer by hormonal status (menopausal and nonmenopausal)

28.4.4.1 Postmenopausal women

Vrieling et al.'s study of 2177 postmenopausal breast cancer patients reported that low concentrations of circulating 25(OH)D were associated with a high risk of overall mortality, breast cancer-specific mortality, breast cancer mortality (Vrieling et al., 2014).

For overall mortality, four studies (Goodwin et al., 2009; Haste et al., 2012; Jacobs et al., 2011; Villasenor et al., 2013) observed an increased risk with lower 25(OH)D concentrations. Low rates in 25(OH)D were reported as being linked to a significantly high risk of recidivism at a distance (Goodwin et al., 2009).

Another study identified a significant association with disease-free survival (Kim et al., 2011).

28.4.4.2 Women in premenopause

In premenopausal women, the relation between vitamin D and breast cancer prognosis may be linked to the joint link between vitamin D and insulin-like growth factors. IGF-I is a mitogenic, antiapoptotic peptide that can enhance proliferation of the epithelial cells of the breast by increasing the risk of neoplastic conversion (Christopoulos et al., 2015). The active metabolite of vitamin D blocks the mitogenic effects of IGF-I, leading to a reduced cell proliferation and an increase in apoptosis (Ameri et al., 2013). As IGF decreases physiologically with aging (Gomez, 2006), the interaction between IGF pathways and vitamin D is stronger in premenopausal women, resulting in a better prognosis of breast cancer when vitamin D concentrations are high (Chlebowski, 2011).

28.4.5 Vitamin D and breast cancer prognosis by tumor hormone receptor status

A few researchers have reported that the protective effect of vitamin D on breast cancer is independent of the status of tumor hormone receptors (Abbas et al., 2008; Grew et al., 2009). A study conducted on the health of nurses reported that high concentrations of vitamin D positively influenced the prognosis of tumors with negative hormone receptors but not those with positive hormone receptors (Bertone-Johnson et al., 2005). The Iowa Women's Health study revealed a stronger protective effect of vitamin D supplements in women with negative rather than positive breast cancer hormone receptors (Robien et al., 2007).

These studies are important because triple-negative breast cancer has no effective chemotherapy, and vitamin D may improve the prognosis.

28.5 Conclusion

Vitamin D deficiency is becoming more common worldwide, and its extrabony effects are becoming more and more evident. Currently, the bibliography of vitamin D and breast cancer is very rich. New data have been reported in terms of risk factor and prognosis. It turns out that vitamin D status influences breast cancer prognosis. Unfortunately, current recommendations seem insufficient for breast cancer patients. Randomized clinical studies must clarify the best method to quickly correct vitamin D deficiency and the optimal rate that prevents recurrence.

References

Abbas, S., Linseinsen, J., & Chang-Claude, J. (2007). Dietary vitamin D and calcium intake and premenopausal breast cancer risk in a German case-control study. *Nutrition and Cancer, 59* (1), 54–61.

Abbas, S., Linselsen, J., Slanger, T., Kropp, S., Mutschelknauss, E. J., Flesch-Janys, D., et al. (2008). Serum 25-hydroxyvitamin D and risk of post-menopausal breast cancer-results of a large case-control study. *Carcinogenesis, 29*(1), 93–99.

Abbas, S., Chang-Claude, J., & Linselsen, J. (2009). Plasma 25-hydroxyvitamin D and premenopausal breast cancer risk in a German case-control study. *International Journal of Cancer. Journal International du Cancer, 124*(1), 250–255.

Ameri, P., et al. (2013). Interactions between vitamin D and IGF-I: From physiology to clinical practice. *Clinical Endocrinology (Oxf), 79*, 457–463.

Anderson, L. N., Cotterchio, M., Vieth, R., & Knight, J. A. (2010). Vitamin D and calcium intakes and breast cancer risk in pre-and postmenopausal women. *The American Journal of Clinical Nutrition, 91*(6), 1699–1707.

Avenell, A., Mac Lennan, G. S., Jenkinson, D. J., Mc Pherson, G. C., Mc Donald, A. M., Pant, P. R., et al. (2012). Long-term follow-up for mortality and cancer in a randomized placebo-controlled trial of vitamin D3 and /or calcium (RECORD trial). *The Journal of Clinical Endocrinology and Metabolism, 97*(2), 614–622.

Balvers, M. G., Browwer-Brolsma, E., Enderburg, S., et al. (2015). Recommended intakes of vitamin D to optimize health, associated circulating 25-hydroxyvitamin D concentrations and dosing regimens to treat deficiency: Workshop report and overview of current literature. *Journal of Nutritional Science, 4*, e231–e238.

Bauer, S. R., Hankinson, S. E., Bertone-Johnson, E. R., & Ding, E. L. (2013). Plasma vitamin D levels, menopause and risk of breast cancer: Dose-response meta-analysis of prospective studies. *Medicine, 92*(3), 123–131.

Bertone-Johnson, E. R., Chen, W. Y., Holick, M. F., et al. (2005). Plasma 25-hydroxyvitaminD and 1,25-dihydroxyvitaminD and risk of breast cancer. *Cancer Epidemiology Biomarkers and Prevention, 14*(8), 1991–1997.

Bouillon, R., Eelen, G., Verlinden, L., et al. (2006). Vitamin D and cancer. *The Journal of Steroid Biochemistry and Molecular Biology, 102*, 156–162.

Bouvard, B., Annveiller, C., Sallé, A., Beauchet, O., Chappard, D., Audran, M., & Legrand, E. (2010). Les effets extra-osseux de la vitamine D: Faits, questions et controverses. *Revue du Rhumatisme, 775*, A18–A25, Joint Bone Spine, 78 (2010) A18-A25.

Chen, P., Hu, P., Xie, D., Qin, Y., Wang, F., & Wang, H. (2010). *Meta*-analysis of vitamin D, calcium and the prevention of breast cancer. *Breast Cancer Research and Treatment, 121*(2), 469–477.

Chlebowski, R. T., Johnson, K. C., Kooperberg, C., Pettinger, M., Waetawski-Wende, J., Rohan, T., et al. (2008). Calcium plus vitamin D supplementation and the risk of breast cancer. *Journal of the National Cancer Institute, 100*(22), 1581–1591.

Chlebowski, R. T. (2011). Vitamin D and breast cancer: Interpreting current evidence. *Breast Cancer Research: BCR, 3*, 217.

Christopoulos, P.F., Msaouel, P., Koutsilieris, M. (2015). The role of the insulin-like growth foctor-1 system in breast cancer, *Molecular cancer, 15*(14), 43.

Chung, M., Lee, J., Terasawa, T., Lau, J., & Trikalinos, T. A. (2011). Vitamin D with or without calcium supplementation for prevention of cancer and fractures: An updated meta-analysis for the US preventive services task force. *Annals of Internal Medicine, 155*(12), 827–838.

Colston, K. W., Berger, U., & Coombes, R. C. (1989). Possible role for vitamin D in controlling breast cancer cell proliferation. *Lancet, 1*(8631), 188–191.

Dusso, A. S., Brown, A. J., & Slatopolsky, E. (2005). Vitamin D. *American Journal of Physiology. Renal Physiology, 289*(1), F8–F28.

Engel, P., Fagherazzi, G., Mesrine, S., Boutron-Ruault, M.-C., & Clavel-Chapelon, F. (2011). Joint effects of dietary vitamin D and sun exposure on breast cancer risk:results from the French E3N cohort. *Cancer Epidemiology, Biomarkers & Prevention: A Publication of the American Association for Cancer Research, Cosponsored by the American Society of Preventive Oncology, 20*(1), 187–198.

Feldman, D., Krishnan, A. V., Swami, S., Giovannucci, E., & Feldman, B. J. (2014). The role of vitamin D in reducing cancer risk and progression. *Nature Reviews. Cancer, 14*(5), 342–357.

Flanagan, L., Packman, K., Juba, B., O'Neill, S., Tenniswood, M., & Welsh, J. (2003). Efficacy of vitamin D compounds to modulate estrogen receptor negative breast cancer growth and invasion. *The Journal of Steroid Biochemistry and Molecular Biology, 84*, 181–192.

Garabedian, M. (2008). *La vitamine D. Traité des maladies métaboliques osseuses de l'adulte* (pp. 89–105). Paris: Médecine Sciences Flammarion.

Girgis, C. M., Clifton-Bligh, R. J., Hamrick, M. W., Holick, M. F., & Gunton, J. E. (2013). The roles of vitamin D in skeletal muscle: Form, function, and metabolism. *Endocrine Reviews, 34*(1), 33–83.

Gissel, T., Rejnmark, L., Mosekilde, L., & Vestergaard, P. (2008). Intake of vitamin D and risk of breast cancer-a meta-analysis. *The Journal of Steroid Biochemistry and Molecular Biology, 111*(3–5), 195–199.

Gomez, M. (2006). The role of insulin-like growth factor I components in the regulation of vitamin D. *Current Pharmaceutical Biotechnology, 7*, 125–132.

Goodwin, P. J., Ennis, M., Pritchard, K. I., Koo, J., & Hood, N. (2009). Prognostic effects of 25-hydroxyvitamin D levels in early breast cancer. *Journal of Clinical Oncology: Official Journal of the American Society of Clinical Oncology, 27*(23), 3757–3763.

Grew, K. D., Gammon, M. D., Steck, S. E., et al. (2009). Association between plasma 25-hydroxyvitamin 1 and breast cancer risk. *Cancer Prevention Research, 2*, 598–604.

Haddad, J. G., Matsuoka, L. Y., Hollis, B. W., Hu, Y. Z., & Wortsman, J. (1993). Human plasma transport of vitamin D after its endogenous synthesis. *The Journal of Clinical Investigation, 91*(6), 2552–2555.

Haste, S., Lambrechts., Verstuyi, A., et al. (2012). Vitamin 1 status at breast cancer diagnosis: Correlation coith tumor characteristics, disease outcome, and geuetic determinants of vitamin D insufficiency. *Careinogenesis, 33*, 1319–1326.

Jacobs, E. T., Thomson, C. A., Flatt, S. W., Al-Delainy, W. K., Hibler, E. A., Jones, L. A., et al. (2011). Vitamin D and breast cancer recurrence in the women's healthy eating and living (WHEL) study. *The American Journal of Clinical Nutrition, 93*(1), 108–117.

Janowsky, E. C., Lester, G. E., Weinberg, C. R., Millikan, R. C., Schildkrant, J. M., Garrett, P. A., et al. (1999). Association between low levels of 1,25-dihydroxyvitamin D and breast cancer risk. *Public Health Nutrition, 2*(3), 283–291.

JoEllen, W. (2018). Vitamin D and breast cancer: Past and present. *The Journal of Steroid Biochemistry and Molecular Biology*, Mars; 177-15-20.

John, E. M., Schwartz, G. G., Dreon, D. M., & Koo, J. (1999). Vitamin D and breast cancer risk: The NHANES I.Epidemiologic follow-up study,1971–1975 to 1992. National health and nutrition examination survey. *Cancer Epidemiology, Biomarkers & Prevention: A Publication of the American Association for Cancer Research, Cosponsored by the American Society of Preventive Oncology*, *8*(5), 399–406.

Johnson, A. L., Zinser, G. M., & Waltz, S. E. (2015). Vitamin D3-dependent VDR signaling delays ron-mediated breast tumorigenesis through suppression of beta-catenin activity. *Oncotarget*, *6*, 16304–16320.

Kawase, T., Matsuo, K., Suzuki, T., Hirose, K., Hosono, S., Watanabe, M., et al. (2010). Association between vitamin D and calcium intake and breast cancer risk according to menopausal status and receptor status in Japan. *Cancer Science*, *101*(5), 1234–1240.

Kim, H. J., Lee, Y. M., Ko, B. S., Lee, J. W., Yu, J. H., Son, B. H., et al. (2011). Vitamin D deficiency is correlated with poor outcomes in patients with luminal-type breast cancer. *Annals of Surgical Oncology*, *18*(7), 1830–1836.

Knight, J. A., Lesosky, M., Barnett, H., Rabond, J. M., & Vieth, R. (2007). Vitamin D and reduced risk of breast cancer: A population -based case-control study. *Cancer Epidemiology, Biomarkers & Prevention: A Publication of the American Association for Cancer Research, Cosponsored by the American Society of Preventive Oncology*, *16*(3), 422–429.

Knight, J. A., Wong, J., Blackmore, K. M., Raboud, J. M., & Vieth, R. (2010). Vitamin D association with estradiol and progesterone in young women. *Cancer Causes & Control: CCC*, *21*(3), 479–483.

Lansiaux, E., Pebaij, P. P., Picard, J. L., & Forget, J. (2018). Vitamin D: Classic and novel actions. *Annals of Nutrition & Metabolism*, *72*(2), 87–95.

Lee, M. S., Huang, Y. C., Wahlqvist, M. L., Wu, T. Y., Chou, Y. C., Wu, M. H., et al. (2011). Vitamin D decreases risk of breast cancer in premenopausal women of normal weight in subtropical Taiwan. *Journal of Epidemiology/Japan Epidemiological Association*, *21*(2), 87–94.

Lowe, L. C., Guy, M., Mansi, J. L., Peckitt, C., Bliss, J., Wilson, R. G., et al. (2005). Plasma 25-hydroxyvitamin D concentrations, vitamin D receptor genotype and breast cancer risk in a UK Caucasian population. *European Journal of Cancer*, *41*(8), 1164–1169.

Lundin, A. C., Soderkvist, P., Eriksson, B., Bergman-Jungestrom, M., & Wingran, S. (1999). Association of breast cancer progression with a vitamin D receptor gene polymorphism. South-east Sweden breast cancer group. *Cancer Research*, *59*(10), 2332–2334.

Mc Cullough, M. L., Rodriguez, C., Diver, W. R., Feigelson, H. S., Stevens, V. L., Thun, M. J., et al. (2005). Dairy, calcium, and vitamin D intake and postmenopausal breast cancer risk in the cancer prevention study II nutrition Cohort. *Cancer Epidemiology, Biomarkers & Prevention: A Publication of the American Association for Cancer Research, Cosponsored by the American Society of Preventive Oncology*, *14*(12), 2898–2904.

Mohr, S. B., Garland, C. F., Gorham, E. D., Grant, W. B., & Garland, F. C. (2008). Relationship between low ultraviolet B irradiance and higher breast cancer risk in 107 countries. *The Breast Journal*, *14*(3), 255–260.

Narvaez, C. J., Matthews, D., Laporta, E., Simmons, K. M., Beaudin, S., & Welsh, J. (2014). The impact of vitamin D in breast cancer: Genomics, pathways, metabolism. *Frontiers in Physiology*, *5*, 213.

Nykjaer, A., Dragun, D., Walther, D., Vorim, H., Jacobsen, C., Herz, J., et al. (1999). An endocytic pathway essential for renal uptake and activation of the steroid 25(OH) vitamin D3. *Cell*, *96*(4), 507–515.

Ooi, L. L., Zhou, H., Kalak, R., et al. (2010). Vitamin D deficiency promotes human breast cancer growth in a murine model of bone metastasis. *Cancer Research*, *70*, 1835–1844.

Pendas-Franco, N., Gonzalez-Sancho, J. M., Suarez, Y., Aguilera, O., Steinmeyer, A., Gamallo, C., et al. (2007). Vitamin D regulates the phenotype of human breast cancer cells. *Differentiation; Research in Biological Diversity*, *75*(3), 193–207.

Reboul, E., Goncalves, A., Comera, C., Bott, R., Nowicki, M., Landrier, J. F., et al. (2011). Vitamin D intestinal absorption is not a simple passive diffusion:evidences for involvement of cholesterol transporters. *Molecular Nutrition & Food Research*, *55*(5), 691–702.

Rizk-Rabin, M., Zineb, R., Zhor, B., et al. (1994). Synthesis of and response to 1,25 dihydroxycholecalciferol by subpopulations of murine epidermal keratinocytes: Existence of a paracrine system for 1,25 dihydrocholecalciferol. *Journal of Cellular Physiology*, *159*, 131–141.

Robien, K., Cutler, G. J., & Lazovich, D. (2007). Vitamin D intake and breast cancer risk in postmenopausal women: The lowa women's health study. *Cancer Causes & Control: CCC*, *18*(7), 775–782.

Rossi, M., Mc Laughlin, J. K., Lagion, P., Bosetti, C., Talamini, R., Lipworth, L., et al. (2009). Vitamin D intake and breast cancer risk: A case -control study in Italy. *Annals of Oncology: Official Journal of the European Society for Medical Oncology / ESMO*, *20*(2), 374–378.

Safadi, F. F., Thornton, P., Magiera, H., Hollis, B. W., Gentile, M., Haddad, J. G., et al. (1999). Osteopathy and resistance to vitamin D toxicity in mice null for vitamin D binding protein. *The Journal of Clinical Investigation*, *103*(2), 239–251.

Schuster, I. (2011). Cytochromes P450 are essential players in the vitamin D signaling system. *Biochimica et Biophysica Acta*, *1814*(1), 186–199.

Shin, M.-H., Holmes, M. D., Hankinson, S. E., Wu, K., Colditz, G. A., & Willet, W. C. (2002). Intake of dairy products, calcium, and vitamin D and risk of breast cancer. *Journal of the National Cancer Institute*, *94*(17), 1301–1311.

Tonnel, A. B. (2016). Lumière, vitamin D et allergie. *Revue française d'allergologie*, *56*, 196–198.

Villasenor, A., Ballard-Barbash, R., Ambs, A., et al. (2013). Associations of scrum 25-hydroxyvitamin D with overall and breast cancer-specific mortality in a multiethnic cohort of breast cancer survivors. *Cancer Causes & Control: CCC*, *24*, 759–767.

Vrieling, A., Hein, R., Abbas, S., Schneeweiss, A., Flesch-Janys, D., & Chang-Claude, J. (2011). Serum 25-hydroxyvitamin D and post-menopausal breast cancer survival: A prospective patient cohort study. *Breast Cancer Research: BCR*, *13*(4), R74.

Vrieling, A., Scibold, P., Johnson, T. S., Heinz, J., Obi, N., Kaaks, R., Flesch-Janys, D., & Chang-Claude, J. (2014). Circulating 25-hydroxyvitamin D and postmenopausal breast cancer survival: Influence of tumor characteristics and lifestyle factors? *International Journal of Cancer*, *134*(12), 2972–2983.

Wagner, C. L., & Greer, F. R. (2008). American academy of pediatrics section on breastfeeding; American academy of pediatrics committee on nutrition. Prevention of rickets and vitamin D deficiency in infants, children, and adolescents. *Pediatrics*, *122*(5), 1142–1152. Available from https://doi.org/10.1542/peds.2008-1862. Erratum in: Pediatrics. 2009 Jan;123(1):197. PMID: 18977996.

Wang, D., Velez de-la-Paz, O. I., Zhai, J. X., & Liu, D. W. (2013). Serum 25-hydroxyvitamin D and breast cancer risk: A meta-analysis of prospective studies. *Tumour Biology: The Journal of the International Society for Oncodevelopmental Biology and Medicine*, *34*(6), 3509–3517.

Yao, S., Kwan, M. L., Ergas, I. J., Roh, J. M., Cheng, T. D., et al. (2017). Association of serum level of vitamin D at diagnosis with breast cancer survival: A case–cohort analysis in the pathways study. *JAMA Oncology*, *3*, 351–357.

World Health Organization. (2021). *Cancer du sein*. Breast Cancer. Retrieved July 22, 2021 from https://www.who.int/fr/news-room/fact-sheets/detail/breast-cancer.

Zhang, Y., Guo, Q., Zhang, Z., Bai, N., Liu, Z., et al. (2014). VDR status arbitrates the prometastatic effects of tumor-associated macrophages. *Molecular Cancer Research*, *12*, 1181–1191.

Index

Note: Page numbers followed by "*f*" and "*t*" refer to figures and tables, respectively.

C

D

G

I

J

K

N

O

R

S

9780323854962